REPRINTS

The New England Journal of Medicine

Clinical Studies

AIDS: Epidemiological and Clinical Studies

Library of Congress Cataloging-in-Publication Data

AIDS: epidemiological and clinical studies.

(Clinical studies)
Reprints, the New England journal of medicine.

Reprints of articles from various issues of the *New England Journal of Medicine*, 1981–1987.
Includes index.
1. AIDS (Disease). 2. AIDS (Disease) — Epidemiology.
I. Massachusetts Medical Society. II. New England Journal of Medicine.
III. Series: Clinical studies (Waltham, Mass.) [DNLM: 1. Acquired Immunodeficiency Syndrome — collected works. WD 309 A28762]
RC607.A26A34575 1987 614.5′993 87-18480

ISBN 0-910133-19-0

Printed in the United States of America
5 4 3 2 1

This book was set in Baskerville No. 2 type and produced by the in-house Composition department of the Massachusetts Medical Society.

Clinical Studies

AIDS: Epidemiological and Clinical Studies

Epidemiology and Public Health Issues

Diagnosis and Early Identification of AIDS

AIDS Transmission via Transfusion and Dialysis

Heterosexual Transmission, Intravenous Drug Use, and Other Transmission Concerns

General Public Health Issues Related to AIDS

Clinical Studies

Immune Deficiency Manifestations and Classifications

Epstein–Barr Virus, Cytomegalovirus, and Herpes Virus Related to AIDS

Transmission of AIDS and the Blood-Brain Barrier

Experimental Treatment and General Follow-up

INTRODUCTION

The first few cases of the disorder that later came to be called AIDS were briefly recorded in the June 5, 1981, issue of the Centers for Disease Control's *Morbidity and Mortality Weekly Report* and then described in more detail in the *New England Journal of Medicine* on December 10, 1981.

Today, six years later, AIDS is a household word, the subject of intense medical investigation and growing public debate. It claims not only the largest share of space in the general medical journals (like *NEJM*), but prominent and almost daily coverage in the popular media.

The extraordinary rapidity and force with which this new disorder has seized our attention is without parallel in medical annals. It reflects, in part, the frightening, still largely unmitigated lethality of AIDS and the size of its ever-widening circle of victims. But AIDS is also a major scientific challenge, with far-reaching biological implications. Investigators are drawn not simply by the urgency of the clinical problem but by the expectation that the ultimate deciphering of the AIDS riddle will provide important new insights into basic phenomena in virology and immunology.

The complex of social issues created by the AIDS epidemic is also unprecedented. Here is a slowly progressive but usually deadly disease, caused by a new and unusual virus that has already infected an estimated 1.5 to 2 million Americans and continues to spread. We do not yet know how many of those infected will ultimately develop the disease and die. The virus was at first rapidly disseminated among intravenous drug abusers and male homosexuals through social and sexual behavior generally considered deviant. Then it was transmitted to many recipients of transfused blood and blood products. Now it seems to be spreading slowly among prostitutes and heterosexual partners of infected persons. To what extent it will ultimately penetrate the so-called "low-risk" population by these means (and by accidental blood-to-blood transmission) remains to be seen. In any case, there are few precedents to help our society deal with such a threat. Difficult questions of public health policy and private behavior, of politics, economics, and ethics, must be faced — so it was inevitable that AIDS would become one of the dominant and most divisive public issues of our time.

From the very beginning the *NEJM* has received, reviewed, and published a large share of the original, important new medical developments on AIDS. In its pages over the past six years can be traced the steady evolution of our clinical understanding of the disease. We have also published a number of discussions of the public health and ethical issues. The story is still unfolding, but it seemed to the editors that readers might be interested in having at hand a convenient collection of the most notable of the articles we have published to date.

Reading these articles in sequence affords a unique perspective on a modern plague that is testing our society as never before. What will future historians say about the intelligence and resolution with which we attacked the medical riddle, and how will they judge our wisdom and compassion in dealing with the political and moral dilemma of AIDS?

Arnold S. Relman, M.D.
Editor, *New England Journal of Medicine*

Epidemiology and Public Health Issues

Diagnosis and Early Identification of AIDS

ORIGINAL ARTICLE

PNEUMOCYSTIS CARINII PNEUMONIA AND MUCOSAL CANDIDIASIS IN PREVIOUSLY HEALTHY HOMOSEXUAL MEN

Evidence of a New Acquired Cellular Immunodeficiency

MICHAEL S. GOTTLIEB, M.D., ROBERT SCHROFF, PH.D., HOWARD M. SCHANKER, M.D., JOEL D. WEISMAN, D.O., PENG THIM FAN, M.D., ROBERT A. WOLF, M.D., AND ANDREW SAXON, M.D.

Abstract Four previously healthy homosexual men contracted *Pneumocystis carinii* pneumonia, extensive mucosal candidiasis, and multiple viral infections. In three of the patients these infections followed prolonged fevers of unknown origin. In all four cytomegalovirus was recovered from secretions. Kaposi's sarcoma developed in one patient eight months after he presented with esophageal candidiasis. All patients were anergic and lymphopenic; they had no lymphocyte proliferative responses to soluble antigens, and their responses to phytohemagglutinin were markedly reduced. Monoclonal-antibody analysis of peripheral-blood T-cell subpopulations revealed virtual elimination of the Leu-3+ helper/inducer subset, an increased percentage of the Leu-2+ suppressor/cytotoxic subset, and an increased percentage of cells bearing the thymocyte-associated antigen T10. The inversion of the T helper to suppressor/cytotoxic ratio suggested that cytomegalovirus infection was an important factor in the pathogenesis of the immunodeficient state. A high level of exposure of male homosexuals to cytomegalovirus-infected secretions may account for the occurrence of this immune deficiency.

ACQUIRED T-cell defects are well known to occur in adults with untreated Hodgkin's disease, sarcoidosis, and viral infections.[1,2] These noniatrogenic T-cell deficiencies are marked by cutaneous anergy and diminished proliferative responses to mitogens and antigens in vitro. Opportunistic infections rarely occur in the absence of immunosuppressive therapy. We recently treated several young, previously healthy, homosexual men for multiple episodes of *Pneumocystis carinii* pneumonia, extensive mucosal candidiasis, and severe viral infections.[3] The clinical manifestations and studies of cellular immune function in these patients indicated a similar severe acquired T-cell defect. Several lines of evidence suggested that cytomegalovirus infection was a major factor in the pathogenesis of the immunocompromised state. This syndrome represents a potentially transmissible immune deficiency.

METHODS

Antibody Assays

Antibodies to cytomegalovirus, adenovirus, and herpes simplex were determined by complement fixation. Antibody to cytomegalovirus was measured in Patient 2 by the anticomplement immunofluorescence method. Hepatitis B surface antigen and antibodies to hepatitis B surface and core antigens were determined by radioimmunoassay. Antibodies to Epstein–Barr virus were measured in the laboratory of Dr. Werner Henle.

Lymphocyte Separation and Identification

Peripheral blood was collected in heparin, and lymphocytes were separated on a Ficoll–Hypaque gradient as previously described.[4] T lymphocytes were identified by their ability to form spontaneous rosettes with sheep erythrocytes (E rosettes).[5] B lymphocytes were identified by staining immunoglobulin-bearing cells with a fluorescein-conjugated polyvalent goat antihuman immunoglobulin antiserum.[6,7]

Stimulation of Lymphocytes by Phytohemagglutinin and Antigens

Blastogenic stimulation of peripheral-blood lymphocytes by phytohemagglutinin (Burroughs–Wellcome) was tested as previously described.[5] The lymphocyte response to candida antigen (Hollister–Stier Laboratories, Spokane, Wash.) and streptokinase-streptodornase (Varidase, Lederle Laboratories) was assayed by mixing antigens with 2×10^5 Ficoll–Hypaque-purified peripheral-blood lymphocytes in 0.2 ml of RPMI 1640 supplemented with L-glutamine, streptomycin, penicillin, and 10 percent heat-inactivated human AB serum in round-bottom microtiter plates. The candida antigen was used at a final concentration of 1:20, and the Varidase antigen at 20 units of streptokinase and 5 units of streptodornase per 0.2 ml. The cells were cultured for six days and pulsed with [^{3}H]thymidine for 16 hours. The phytohemagglutinin and antigens were titrated to obtain maximum stimulation.

Viral Identification

Viral cultures were performed in human-embryonic-lung fibroblasts (WI38), human-foreskin fibroblasts (Flow 7000), and primary cultures of African-green-monkey-kidney cells. The cultures were maintained at 36°C for five weeks. All isolates were presumptively identified by characteristic cytopathic effect and subsequently confirmed by neutralization[8] or immunofluorescence staining[9] with specific antiserums.

Monoclonal Antibodies

Leu-1, Leu-2, and Leu-3 antibodies were generously provided by Becton-Dickinson (Mountain View, Calif.). Leu-1 recognizes the same surface antigen that monoclonal antibodies OKT-1 and T101 recognize; this antigen is present on mature circulating T cells.[10-12] Leu-2 recognizes the same surface antigen as OKT-8; this antigen is reportedly present on T cells that mediate cytotoxic and immunosuppressive events.[11,13,14] Leu-3a recognizes the same surface antigen as OKT-4, and this antigen is found on T cells showing helper and inducer activity.[13-15] Previous studies in our laboratory have indicated that Leu-2 and OKT-8 define very similar or identical T-cell subsets. Likewise, Leu-3 and OKT-4 recognize equivalent subpopulations. T10 is present on 95 percent of thymocytes and on less than 5 percent of peripheral-blood T cells.[16] All monoclonal antibodies were stored at 4°C before their use. Purified mouse myeloma

From the Division of Clinical Immunology/Allergy, the Department of Medicine, and the Department of Microbiology/Immunology, UCLA School of Medicine; and the Rheumatology Section, Wadsworth Medical Center, Los Angeles.

Supported in part by grants (AI-16694, AI-15332, and CA-12800) from the National Institutes of Health. Dr. Saxon is the recipient of an Allergic Diseases Academic Award (AI-00326) from the National Institute of Allergy and Infectious Diseases, and Dr. Schroff is supported by a grant (CA-09120) from the National Institutes of Health and by The Concern Foundation of Los Angeles.

protein of the IgG2a class (RPC 5, Bionetics, Kensington, Md.) served as a negative control for immunofluorescence assays.

Direct Immunofluorescence Assays

Cells were washed twice before analysis; 0.5×10^6 cells were used for each assay. After incubation for 45 minutes at 4°C in 100 μl of medium with 2 percent heat-inactivated neonatal-calf serum and 5 μl of monoclonal-antibody solution, cells were washed twice by centrifugation and resuspended in 100 μl of medium containing 3 μg of fluorescein-conjugated goat antimouse IgG (TAGO, Burlingame, Calif.). After another 45-minute incubation at 4°C, the cells were washed twice in medium containing 0.2 percent sodium azide and resuspended in one drop of 30 percent glycerol in phosphate-buffered saline (0.1 M phosphate, pH 7.4) plus 0.2 percent sodium azide. The cells were examined on a fluorescence microscope equipped with epi-illumination. A minimum of 200 cells were examined for surface immunofluorescence.

Patients

Tests of cellular immune function were conducted in the Clinical Research Laboratory of the UCLA School of Medicine.

Patient 1

A 33-year-old homosexual man was transferred to the UCLA Medical Center on March 16, 1981, for evaluation of recurrent fever and mucocutaneous candidiasis. He had been well until October 1980, when he was admitted to another hospital because of fever and cervical lymphadenopathy. The white-cell count was 6600, with 65 percent neutrophils, 6 percent band forms, 23 percent lymphocytes, and 6 percent monocytes. Atypical lymphocytes were absent. Test results for latex fixation, antinuclear antibody, venereal disease reaction level (VDRL), Monospot, toxoplasmosis titer, and febrile agglutinins were negative. The antibody profile to Epstein–Barr virus indicated remote infection. The serum contained antibodies to hepatitis B surface and core antigens, but hepatitis B surface antigenemia was absent. The serum aspartate aminotransferase was 388 IU per liter (3.12 $\mu mol \cdot sec^{-1}$ per liter).

The patient received prednisone for two weeks, during which the fever resolved. In December 1980 fever (temperatures to 39°C) recurred, and a two-month course of daily prednisone was administered. Severe oral and perianal candidiasis developed, and the drug dose was rapidly tapered and discontinued. Because of continued fever (39 to 40°C), the patient was transferred to UCLA. Findings included generalized alopecia, moist superficial gluteal erosions, oral thrush, and fungating lesions of the distal index fingers. Rash and lymphadenopathy were absent. Tests of liver enzymes, chest x-ray films, and an upper-gastrointestinal-tract series gave normal results. Cytomegalovirus was recovered from the urine, but not from the blood buffy coat. Herpes simplex and *Candida albicans* were cultured from the pharynx, perianal area, and both fingertip lesions. Serum levels of IgG and IgM were normal, but IgA was elevated to 961 mg per deciliter (normal, 121 to 563 mg per deciliter). Circulating immune complexes, determined by the polyethylene glycol method, were 730 μg per milliliter (normal, <310 μg per milliliter). The patient was anergic to a battery of five recall antigens, including candida.

Ketoconazole (200 mg twice daily) produced marked improvement of the gluteal and fingertip lesions; however, daily episodes of fever continued. After a five-day course of intravenous acyclovir (9-[2-hydroxyethoxymethyl] guanine) (250 mg per square meter of body-surface area, give three times daily) herpes simplex was no longer recovered from the previously infected sites; however, cytomegalovirus was still cultured from the urine. The patient was discharged but was readmitted one month later with a three-day history of dyspnea, dry cough, and fever. The fingers and perianal lesions were nearly healed. A chest film showed diffuse interstitial infiltrates. Silver stains of bronchial brushings contained numerous *P. carinii* organisms, and smears and cultures for bacteria, acid-fast bacilli, and fungi were negative. Herpes simplex was recovered from bronchial washings. The percentages of both T and B lymphocytes in the peripheral blood were depressed (Table 1). Despite intravenous trimethoprim–sulfamethoxazole (TMP–SMZ), the x-ray findings and arterial oxygenation worsened. A 10-day course of acyclovir (500 mg per square meter, three times daily) was administered. Bronchial brushings and a biopsy specimen obtained on April 24, 1981, were negative for *P. carinii,* acid-fast bacilli, fungi, and *Legionella pneumophila.* Cytomegalovirus was cultured from both specimens. Because of clinical deterioration, TMP–SMZ was stopped and pentamidine was given. An open-lung biopsy performed on May 1 revealed *P. carinii* and morphologic evidence of CMV infection. The patient died two days later. Autopsy findings included extensive *P. carinii* and culture-proved cytomegalovirus pneumonia, with histologic evidence of cytomegalovirus retinitis.

Patient 2

A 30-year-old homosexual man was referred to UCLA Medical Center in March 1981 with a four-month history of daily fever and malaise. He had been hospitalized elsewhere in February 1981, at which time generalized lymphadenopathy without hepatosplenomegaly was present. The white-cell count was 4200, with 77 percent neutrophils, 10 percent lymphocytes, 8 percent monocytes, and 5 percent eosinophils. Atypical lymphocytes were absent. The sedimentation rate was 126 mm per hour. The level of IgG was 2647 mg per deciliter; IgM, 448 mg per deciliter; and IgA, 721 mg per deciliter (the normal upper limits are 1700, 400, and 280 mg, respectively). Circulating immune complexes were elevated to 1530 μg per milliliter. Delayed skin tests to five recall antigens were negative. The serum aspartate aminotransferase was 113 IU per liter (0.91 $\mu mol \cdot sec^{-1}$ per liter). A liver biopsy showed mild focal nonspecific hepatitis. Inclusion bodies were absent. The level of antibody to cytomegalovirus, determined by the anticomplement immunofluorescence method, rose from <1:16 to >1:128. Cytomegalovirus was cultured from samples of urine and buffy coat. Antibody evidence of past infection with Epstein–Barr and hepatitis B viruses was detected.

On April 21, 1981, the patient was admitted to UCLA Medical Center, after four days of nonproductive cough, dyspnea, rising

Table 1. Levels of Lymphocyte Surface Markers in Patients with Cellular Immunodeficiency.

Marker	Patient 1		Patient 2		Patient 3		Patient 4	Normal Range
	Sample 1 (3/18/81)	Sample 2 (4/16/81)	Sample 1 (4/21/81)	Sample 2 (5/4/81)	Sample 1 (1/30/81)	Sample 2 (4/22/81)	Sample 1 (6/5/81)	
White-cell count (cells/mm³)	3800	4800	3200	2200	2300	1600	4400	4800–10,800
Peripheral lymphocyte count (cells/mm³)*	342	480	320	484	690	480	132	1440–3040
E-rosette formation								
Percentage	62	39	65	44	67	45	44	59–74
Absolute number (cells/mm³)	212	187	208	232	462	216	62	849–2249
Surface immunoglobulin-bearing cells								
Percentage	3	2	†	10	9	14	10	5–10
Absolute number (cells/mm³)	10	10	†	48	62	67	13	72–304

*Calculated by multiplying the total leukocyte count by the percentage of lymphocytes in the differential count.

†Quantity was insufficient to perform test.

fever, and chills. He reported the recent onset of rectal and oral thrush. He appeared acutely ill, with a temperature of 39°C. The arterial partial pressure of oxygen during breathing of ambient air was 44 mm Hg, and a chest film showed a diffuse interstitial pattern. Silver staining of bronchial brushings revealed numerous *P. carinii* organisms. A 14-day course of intravenous TMP-SMZ led to resolution of the pneumonia. The white-cell count declined to 1900, with 10 percent lymphocytes; the platelet count was 80,000. A bone-marrow aspirate and a biopsy specimen were normocellular, with slightly increased numbers of plasma cells. A urine culture grew adenovirus. On June 24, 1981, funduscopic examination revealed multiple discrete white retinal opacities that were consistent with the occurrence of microinfarction of the nerve-fiber layer of the retina. There was no history of visual disturbance. On serial follow-up examinations the lesions had not progressed. The patient was readmitted on August 15, 1981 with gradually increasing dyspnea, cough, and interstitial infiltrates. Bronchial brushings were negative for *P. carinii;* however, numerous pneumocysts were found on open-lung biopsy. Cytomegalovirus was cultured from the tissue specimen. The patient's condition deteriorated despite five days of pentamidine therapy. The fever and pulmonary infiltrates cleared only after a four-week course of high-dose TMP-SMZ, and low-dose prophylaxis was instituted after recovery.

Patient 3

A 30-year-old, previously healthy, homosexual man was admitted to the UCLA Medical Center with a one-month history of pain on swallowing, oral thrush, leukopenia, and a weight loss of 12 kg. Endoscopy performed after admission revealed distal esophageal erosions and two gastric ulcers. A biopsy specimen of the esophageal mucosa contained intranuclear inclusions but no yeast forms. Virus was not recovered from the initial biopsy sample. The white-cell count was 2300, with 34 percent neutrophils, 19 percent band forms, 30 percent lymphocytes, and 16 percent monocytes. Atypical lymphocytes were present.

Bone-marrow aspiration and biopsy revealed a slight reduction in the ratio of myeloid to erythroid cells. Serum IgG and IgM were normal, but IgA was elevated to 1061 mg per deciliter (normal, 121 to 563). Circulating immune complexes were elevated at 785 μg per milliliter.

Treatment with amphotericin B reduced the odynophagia. The patient was discharged on February 17, 1981, but was readmitted five days later with fever (temperatures reaching 40°C), dyspnea, and dry cough. The arterial partial pressure of oxygen (room air) was 57 mm Hg, and a chest film showed bilateral interstitial infiltrates. Silver stain of a transbronchial biopsy specimen revealed abundant *P. carinii.* Viral inclusion bodies were absent on tissue sections. An adenovirus was recovered from the bronchial washings and from the stool on two occasions. Treatment with intravenous TMP-SMZ led to prompt resolution of the pneumonia. The percentage of peripheral E-rosette-forming cells was then markedly decreased (Table 1). The patient was discharged on March 11, 1981, but was readmitted on April 22 because he had severe difficulty in swallowing. Endoscopy revealed confluent plaques of candida and erosions. Additional doses of amphotericin B were administered, producing improvement clinically and endoscopically. Cytomegalovirus was cultured from an esophageal-biopsy specimen. Ophthalmologic examination on May 20 revealed multiple discrete retinal opacities that were asymptomatic. At follow-up examination on May 26 the lesions had increased in size and number. Atypical candidal chorioretinal lesions could not be excluded, and additional amphotericin B (1500 mg) was administered, with little effect on the lesions. On subsequent evaluations, these lesions were thought to represent microinfarctions of the nerve-fiber layer of the retina.

On June 20, dyspnea developed and bilateral lower-lobe interstitial infiltrates were seen on the chest film. A transbronchial biopsy specimen was positive for pneumocystis, which responded to treatment with pentamidine. Cytomegalovirus was cultured from the urine and the biopsy specimen, but not from buffy coat. After recovery, TMP-SMZ prophylaxis was instituted. The patient was readmitted on September 15, 1981, because of progressive cachexia. A violaceous plaque (3 cm in diameter) with a central nodule, which had not been present on previous examinations, was noted on the left wall of the chest; three similar lesions were located in the esophagus. Biopsies revealed Kaposi's sarcoma.

Patient 4

A 29-year-old homosexual man was referred to UCLA Medical Center on June 5, 1981, with an eight-month history of high fever, lymphadenopathy, fatigue, and a weight loss of 11 kg. He had been hospitalized elsewhere on four occasions in 1981 for diagnostic studies, which were inconclusive. In November 1980 the white-cell count had been 2900, with 73 percent neutrophils, 10 percent band forms, 7 percent lymphocytes, 9 percent monocytes, and 1 percent eosinophils. The level of antibody to cytomegalovirus on complement fixation had risen from 1:64 in November 1980 to 1:256 in February 1981. Two biopsies of lymph nodes showed reactive changes, and biopsy of normal-appearing skin revealed a nonspecific perivascular infiltrate. A whole-body computerized tomogram, an abdominal angiogram, and a lymphangiogram for evaluation of possible neoplasia and vasculitis were negative.

On admission the patient reported a two-month history of dysphagia and a two-week history of exertional dyspnea and a morning cough with clear sputum. He appeared cachectic and was febrile (39.5°C). Oral thrush was present. The white-cell count was 4400, with 88 percent neutrophils, 6 percent band forms, 3 percent monocytes, and 3 percent lymphocytes. Serum levels of IgG and IgM were normal; IgA was elevated to 536 mg per deciliter (normal upper limit, 366). Circulating immune complexes were elevated to 1570 μg per deciliter. The patient was anergic to a battery of five recall antigens. Cytomegalovirus was recovered from the urine. Complement-fixing antibodies to cytomegalovirus, herpes simplex, and adenovirus were not detected. Antibody evidence of past infection with Epstein–Barr and hepatitis B viruses was present. Endoscopy of the upper gastrointestinal tract revealed white plaques in the lower esophagus, and cultures of biopsy specimens grew *C. albicans.* Amphotericin B was given, for a total dose of 300 mg. In view of the uniform occurrence of *P. carinii* pneumonia in the previous three patients, bronchoscopy was performed despite an essentially negative chest film. Numerous pneumocystis organisms were found on bronchial brushings. Treatment with TMP-SMZ was begun and continued for prophylaxis after hospital discharge. On complete ophthalmologic examination the patient was noted to have multiple discrete white retinal opacities, consistent with microinfarction at the level of the nerve-fiber layer ("cotton-wool spots"). He had no visual symptoms.

After discharge the patient remained chronically ill. He was readmitted two months later for recurrence of fever and severe mucosal candidiasis, which responded to amphotericin B.

Results

Marked lymphopenia was present in all four patients (Table 1). At the first evaluation Patients 1, 2,

Table 2. Stimulation of Mononuclear Cells by Antigens and Phytohemagglutinin in Normal Subjects and Patients.

Group	Stimulator			
	Medium Alone	Phytohemagglutinin	Candida Antigen	Streptokinase-Streptodornase
	counts per minute			
Normal subjects (n = 32 [mean ±SD])	1,312 ±565	155,983 ±53,652	74,500 ±38,759	87,408 ±24,365
Patients				
1 (3/18/81)	522	27,000	1,594	1,264
2 (4/21/81)	777	81,186	1,930	1,852
3 (5/8/81)	820	5,000	938	*
4 (6/5/81)	666	6,142	*	*

*Not determined.

and 3 had normal percentages of E-rosette-forming cells. In Patients 1 and 2 E-rosette-forming cells were subsequently markedly depressed at the time of *P. carinii* pneumonia. The depressed percentage of T cells in Patient 3 (Sample 2) and Patient 4 had no obvious clinical correlates. The percentage of B lymphocytes was normal except in Patient 1. The four patients had a diminished proliferative response to phytohemagglutinin (Table 2). In those tested, the response to candida and streptokinase-streptodornase was virtually absent. Cells bearing the surface antigen recognized by monoclonal antibodies OKT4 and Leu-3 make the maximal proliferative response to phytohemagglutinin and nearly all the proliferative response to soluble antigens.[15] Thus the results of the mitogen and antigen stimulation studies suggested that these patients had a deficiency of the Leu-3/OKT4 helper/inducer subset. We therefore analyzed peripheral-blood mononuclear cells from these patients with monoclonal antibodies to T-cell subsets on indirect immunofluorescence.

Table 3 shows that peripheral lymphocytes from all four patients contained reduced percentages and total numbers of T cells (Leu-1). Helper/inducer Leu-3+ cells were virtually absent. The percentage of Leu-2+ cytotoxic/suppressor T cells was uniformly increased although the absolute numbers (per cubic millimeter) were below normal. The ratio of Leu-3+/Leu-2+ cells was markedly depressed in all patients, relative to the normal control ratio of 1.6. The percentage of cells bearing T10 was increased in all four patients.

Discussion

These patients presented a distinct and unusual clinical syndrome. All were exclusively homosexual and had been in excellent health before late 1980. Their medical histories did not suggest preexisting immunodeficiency. All were anergic and had infections in which cell-mediated immunity plays the major part in host defense. *P. carinii* pneumonia, extensive mucosal candida infections, and chronic viral shedding were uniformly present. Cytomegalovirus was recovered from secretions in all four patients. A significant rise in specific antibody (Patients 2 and 4) indicated recent infection or reactivation. The presentation in Patient 3 differed in that protracted fever did not precede the development of esophageal candidiasis and pneumocystis pneumonia. The initial illness in Patients 1, 2, and 4 resembled primary cytomegalovirus-induced mononucleosis in previously healthy adults.[17,18] However, the persistence of fever for more than three months and the occurrence of leukopenia, lymphopenia, and opportunistic infection are not features of the cytomegalovirus-mononucleosis syndrome in the normal host. These patients' clinical courses resemble those of primary cytomegalovirus infections in some renal-transplant recipients in whom iatrogenic immunosuppression undoubtedly enhances the severity of infection.[19,20] Although the prednisone administered early in the course of infection in Patient 1 may have impaired the host response to cytomegalovirus, systemic viral infection persisted despite discontinuation of corticosteroids three months before his death. The chronic viral infections in Patients 2, 3, and 4 were clearly unrelated to the administration of immunosuppressive agents. The retinal lesions (cotton-wool spots) observed in Patients 2, 3, and 4 did not appear to represent ocular infection, since they frequently resolved spontaneously. These lesions are seen in patients with systemic lupus erythematosus, uncontrolled hypertension, or diabetes mellitus. They are described in association with florid cytomegalovirus-retinitis but not as an isolated finding in systemic cytomegalovirus infections. These lesions represent microinfarctions and could be related to the circulating immune complexes documented in these patients. Analysis of the immune complexes for antigenic content is in progress. The explanation for the elevated IgA levels in these patients remains unclear.

The fact that this illness was first observed in homosexual men is probably not due to coincidence. It suggests that a sexually transmitted infectious agent or exposure to a common environment has a critical role in the pathogenesis of the immunodeficient state. Sexually transmitted infections, including cytomegalovirus, are highly prevalent in the male homosexual community.[21-23] In a recent study, 94 percent of exclusively homosexual men had serologic evidence of cytomegalovirus infection, as compared with 54 percent of heterosexual men attending the same venereal-disease clinic.[24] The shedding of virus for prolonged periods in many secretions, including semen, facilitates sexual transmission.[25] The four patients described in this report did not know each other. In-depth interviews did not reveal common contacts or knowledge of sexual partners who had been ill. There were no differences among the patients with respect to history of sexually transmitted disease. Patient 3 was highly sexually active and frequented homosexual bars and bathhouses. Patient 2 had lived with one partner for seven years, and Patients 2 and 4 had several regular partners. All patients had serologic evi-

Table 3. Characterization of T-Lymphocyte Subsets.

Group	Lymphocyte Subset				Leu 3/ Leu 2 Ratio
	Leu 1	Leu 2	Leu 3	T10	
	percent lymphocytes reactive with monoclonal antibodies				
Patients					
1	45	57	0	59	0
2	47	52	0	59	0
3	49	57	10	79	0.18
4	67	47	2	81	0.04
Mean ±SD	52* ±10.1	53.3* ±4.7	3.0† ±4.76	69.5† ±12.1	0.05 ±0.08*
Normal subjects (n = 16 [mean ±SD])	71.0 ±10.0	28.0 ± 8.0	46.0 ±12.0	15.0 ±6.6	1.6 ±0.74

*Significantly different from value in normal subjects ($P<0.003$).

†Significantly different from value in normal subjects ($P<0.0001$).

dence of hepatitis B infection in the distant past; however, none had chronic liver disease or hepatitis B antigenemia. There was no history of exposure to a common prescribed or illicit drug.

An increased predisposition to other opportunistic infections has been suspected in immunocompromised hosts who have had cytomegalovirus infection. Coincident pneumocystis pneumonia and cytomegalic inclusion disease was recognized in premature or otherwise debilitated European infants who died in the 1930s and 1940s with what was then termed "interstitial plasma cell pneumonia."[26] After renal and cardiac transplantation, primary cytomegalovirus infection has been associated with greater mortality and an increased incidence of pulmonary super-infection, including *P. carinii*.[27-29] In normal mice, infection with murine cytomegalovirus produces marked immunosuppression and increased mortality from doses of bacteria or candida that are usually not lethal.[30]

In normal subjects cytomegalovirus-induced mononucleosis is associated with in vitro alterations of cellular immune function, which include depressed lymphocyte proliferation and interferon production in response to mitogens and herpesvirus antigens.[31,32] Depression of T-cell numbers and of proliferative responses to the degree observed in our patients (Table 2) has not been reported to occur in cytomegalovirus-induced syndromes in normal persons.

Our patients had a marked imbalance of peripheral-blood T-cell subsets, as defined with monoclonal antibodies. The most striking abnormalities were nearly total elimination of Leu-3+ helper/inducer cells and an abnormally increased percentage of Leu-2+ suppressor/cytotoxic cells. Thus, the normal ratio of T helper cells to T suppressor/cytotoxic cells was markedly inverted. The absolute numbers of cells in both subsets were decreased. A very similar reversal of the normal ratio of helper T cells to suppressor/cytotoxic T cells has recently been reported as a uniform occurrence in uncomplicated cytomegalovirus-induced infectious mononucleosis.[33] Although this abnormality was most pronounced during the acute phase of the illness, it persisted in some patients for at least 10 months. The virtual absence of the Leu-3+ subset was undoubtedly the major contributing factor to the severe immune deficiency observed in our patients. The mechanism of this differential effect on the Leu-3+ subset is still unclear, since cytomegalovirus has not been shown to infect subpopulations of lymphocytes directly.[34] Increased immune suppression due to a relative excess of cells with the suppressor phenotype could compound the deficiency. In addition, suppressor monocytes, which have been demonstrated in the peripheral blood of normal persons with cytomegalovirus mononucleosis,[31] could have contributed to the immune deficiency in our patients. The percentage of cells with the thymocyte-associated surface antigen T10 was markedly elevated in all our patients. High percentages of peripheral-blood lymphocytes bearing T10 have been reported in Epstein–Barr virus-induced mononucleosis and in toxoplasmosis.[35,36] We suspect that the increase in T10+ cells in our patients was due to the documented cytomegalovirus infection, since there was no evidence of toxoplasmosis or reactivation of Epstein–Barr virus.

Patient 3 had Kaposi's sarcoma eight months after he had presented with mucosal candida and pneumocystis pneumonia. A recent report described a large number of cases of Kaposi's sarcoma in young homosexual men, four of whom also had pneumocystis pneumonia.[37] In older adults, this neoplasm is associated with serologic evidence of chronic cytomegalovirus infection.[38,39] We recently studied the peripheral-blood T cells of two young homosexual men who presented with exclusively lymphadenopathic Kaposi's sarcoma with no evidence of infection. The pattern was similar to that observed in the four patients described above, with respect to inversion of the Leu-3+/Leu-2+ ratio (0.46 and 0.6). This finding further suggests a relation between the immunodeficiency syndrome and the recent appearance of Kaposi's sarcoma in the homosexual population. Complete evaluation of our other three patients, including endoscopy of the upper and lower gastrointestinal tracts, disclosed no evidence of Kaposi's sarcoma; however, they remain under observation because of the possibility that it will develop.

The reason for the appearance of these two unusual illnesses in male homosexuals remains unclear. It is known that after infection with cytomegalovirus, very high titers of the virus may be shed in the semen of asymptomatic subjects for more than a year.[25] In a recent study cytomegalovirus viruria was detected in 14 percent of homosexual men 18 to 29 years old.[24] Since urine samples were cultured only once, the true incidence may be even higher. It is therefore likely that sexually active, young homosexual men are frequently reinfected through exposure to semen and urine of sexual partners. Such reinfection with large inoculums of virus before recovery from the cellular immune dysfunction induced by previous cytomegalovirus infection could conceivably lead to overwhelming chronic infection and immunodeficiency or Kaposi's sarcoma. In mice, induction of cytomegalovirus infection by large inoculums of virus leads to destruction of lymphoid elements and profound depression of immune responses.[40,41] The possibility also exists that these syndromes are related to a particular strain of cytomegalovirus transmitted initially within the male homosexual population. We acknowledge the possibility that cytomegalovirus infection was a result rather than a cause of the T-cell defect, and that some other exposure to an undetected microorganism, drug, or toxin made these patients susceptible to infection with opportunistic organisms, including cytomegalovirus. However, at this time cytomegalovirus is highly suspect, in view of its prevalence among male homosexuals and its previously documented potential for immunosuppression.

To date there has been no indication of spontaneous

recovery of celluar immunocompetence in our surviving patients. All have continued to have a severe wasting syndrome despite intensive supportive measures. Pneumocystis pneumonia recurred in two of the three patients who did not receive TMP-SMZ prophylaxis. We therefore believe that long-term TMP-SMZ prophylaxis should be initiated in such patients after the first episode of pneumocystis. At present it is unclear whether antiviral and antifungal agents, intensive nutritional support, or immunostimulators will prove useful in the management of this syndrome.

Note added in proof: Since submission of this manuscript we have documented this syndrome in an additional four homosexual patients and in two exclusively heterosexual men. Cytomegalovirus was cultured from the semen of one of the heterosexual cases. The latter cases are under intensive study for environmental exposures in common with homosexual patients. To date, we have not encountered female patients with this syndrome.

We are indebted to Dr. William J. Martin (Clinical Microbiology Laboratory, UCLA Center for the Health Sciences) and Violet Fiacco and Dr. Marjorie Miller (Clinical Virology Section) for their efforts; to the UCLA medical house staff for their assistance in caring for these patients; to Diane Smith and Loretta Chai for excellent technical assistance; to Drs. Eugene Rogolsky, Michael Roth, and Jay Sugerman for referring patients; to Drs. Gary Holland and Thomas Petit for performing the ophthalmologic examinations; to Dr. Lowell S. Young for reviewing the manuscript; and to the Medical Immunology Laboratory (Dr. John Fahey, Director) for performing tests of cellular immune function.

References

1. Dent PB. Immunodepression by oncogenic viruses. Prog Med Virol 1972; 14:1-35.
2. Woodruff JF, Woodruff JJ. The effect of viral infections on the function of the immune system. In: Notkins AL, ed. Viral immunology and immunopathology. New York: Academic Press, 1975:393-418.
3. Gottlieb MS, Schanker H, Fan P, et al. Pneumocystis pneumonia — Los Angeles. MMWR 1981; 30:250-2.
4. Böyum A. Isolation of mononuclear cells and granulocytes from human blood. Scand J Clin Lab Invest [Suppl] 1968; 97:77-89.
5. Portaro JK, Glick GI, Zighelboim J. Population immunology and immune cell parameters. Clin Immunol Immunopathol 1978; 11:339-45.
6. Frøland SS, Natvig JB. Surface-bound immunoglobulin on lymphocytes from normal and immunodeficient humans. Scand J Immunol 1972; 1:1-12.
7. Winchester RJ, Fu SM. Lymphocyte surface membrane immunoglobulin. Scand J Immunol [Suppl] 1976; 5:77-82.
8. Lennette EH, Schmidt NJ, eds. Diagnostic procedures for: viral, rickettsial and chlamydial infections. 5th ed. Washington, D.C.: American Public Health Association, 1979:241-7, 327-36.
9. Stagno S, Pass RF, Reynolds DW, Moore MA, Nahmias AJ, Alford CA. Comparative study of diagnostic procedures for congenital cytomegalovirus infection. Pediatrics 1980; 65:251-7.
10. Engleman EG, Levy R. Studies of a human T lymphocyte antigen recognized by a monoclonal antibody. Clin Res 1980; 28:502A. abstract.
11. Reinherz EL, Kung PC, Goldstein G, Schlossman SF. A monoclonal antibody with selective reactivity with functionally mature human thymocytes and all peripheral human T cells. J Immunol 1979; 123:1312-7.
12. Royston I, Majda JA, Baird SM, Meserve BL, Griffiths JC. Human T cell antigens defined by monoclonal antibodies: the 65,000-dalton antigen of T cells (T65) is also found on chronic lymphocytic leukemia cells bearing surface immunoglobulin. J Immunol 1980; 125:725-31.
13. Ledbetter JA, Evans RI, Lipinski M, Cunningham-Rundles C, Good RA, Herzenberg LA. Evolutionary conservation of surface molecules that distinguish T lymphocyte helper/inducer and cytotoxic/suppressor subpopulations in mouse and man. J Exp Med 1981; 153:310-23.
14. Evans RL, Wall DW, Platsoucas CD, et al. Thymus-dependent membrane antigens in man: inhibition of cell-mediated lympholysis by monoclonal antibodies to T_{H2} antigen. Proc Natl Acad Sci USA 1981; 78:544-8.
15. Reinherz EL, Kung PC, Goldstein G, Schlossman SF. Separation of functional subsets of human T cells by a monoclonal antibody. Proc Natl Acad Sci USA 1979; 76:4061-5.
16. Reinherz EL, Schlossman SF. The differentiation and function of human T lymphocytes. Cell 1980; 19:821-7.
17. Klemola E, Kääriäinen L. Cytomegalovirus as a possible cause of a disease resembling infectious mononucleosis. Br Med J 1965; 2:1099-102.
18. Klemola E, von Essen R, Wager O, Haltia K, Koivuniemi A, Salmi I. Cytomegalovirus mononucleosis in previously healthy individuals: five new cases and follow-up of 13 previously published cases. Ann Intern Med 1969; 71:11-9.
19. Ho M, Suwansirikul S, Dowling JN, Youngblood LA, Armstrong JA. The transplanted kidney as a source of cytomegalovirus infection. N Engl J Med 1975; 293:1109-12.
20. Spencer ES. Clinical aspects of cytomegalovirus infection in kidney-graft recipients. Scand J Infect Dis 1974; 6:315-23.
21. Drusin LM, Magagna J, Yano K, Ley AB. An epidemiologic study of sexually transmitted diseases on a university campus. Am J Epidemiol 1974; 100:8-19.
22. Fluker JL. A 10-year study of homosexually transmitted infection. Br J Vener Dis 1976; 52:155-60.
23. Venereal aspects of gastroenterology. West J Med 1979; 130:236-46.
24. Drew WL, Mintz L, Miner RC, Sands M, Ketterer B. Prevalence of cytomegalovirus infection in homosexual men. J Infect Dis 1981; 143:188-92.
25. Lang DJ, Kummer JF, Hartley DP. Cytomegalovirus in semen: persistence and demonstration in extracellular fluids. N Engl J Med 1974; 291:121-3.
26. Gajdusek DC. *Pneumocystis carinii* — etiologic agent of interstitial plasma cell pneumonia of premature and young infants. Pediatrics 1957; 19:543-65.
27. Rubin RH, Cosimi AB, Tolkoff-Rubin NE, Russell PS, Hirsch MS. Infectious disease syndromes attributable to cytomegalovirus and their significance among renal transplant recipients. Transplantation 1977; 24:458-64.
28. Lopez C, Simmons RL, Park BH, Najarian JS, Good RA. Cell-mediated and humoral immune responses of renal transplant patients with cytomegalovirus infections. Clin Exp Immunol 1974; 16:565-73.
29. Rand KH, Pollard RB, Merigan TC. Increased pulmonary superinfections in cardiac-transplant patients undergoing primary cytomegalovirus infection. N Engl J Med 1978; 298:951-3.
30. Hamilton JR, Overall JC Jr, Glasgow LA. Synergistic effect on mortality in mice with murine cytomegalovirus and *Pseudomonas aeruginosa, Staphylococcus aureus,* or *Candida albicans* infection. Infect Immun 1976; 14:982-9.
31. Rinaldo CR Jr, Carney WP, Richter BS, Black PH, Hirsch MS. Mechanisms of immunosuppression in cytomegaloviral mononucleosis. J Infect Dis 1980; 141:488-95.
32. Levin MJ, Rinaldo CR Jr, Leary PL, Zaia JA, Hirsch MS. Immune response to herpesvirus antigens in adults with acute cytomegalovirus mononucleosis. J Infect Dis 1979; 140:851-7.
33. Carney WP, Rubin RH, Hoffman RA, Hansen WP, Healey K, Hirsch MS. Analysis of T lymphocyte subsets in cytomegalovirus mononucleosis. J Immunol 1981; 126:2114-6.
34. Rinaldo CR Jr, Richter BJ, Black PH, Callery R, Chess L, Hirsch MS. Replication of herpes simplex virus and cytomegalovirus in human leukocytes. J Immunol 1978; 120:120-30.
35. De Waele M, Thielemans C, Van Camp BKG. Characterization of immunoregulatory T cells in EBV-induced infectious mononucleosis by monoclonal antibodies. N Engl J Med 1981; 304:460-2.
36. *Idem.* Immunoregulatory T cells in mononucleosis and toxoplasmosis. N Engl J Med 1981; 305:228.
37. Kaposi's sarcoma and *Pneumocystis* pneumonia among homosexual men — New York City and California. MMWR 1981; 30:305.
38. Giraldo G, Beth E, Kourilsky FM, et al. Antibody patterns to herpesvirus in Kaposi's sarcoma: serological association of European Kaposi's sarcoma with cytomegalovirus. Int J Cancer 1975; 15:839-48.
39. Giraldo G, Beth E, Henle W, et al. Antibody patterns to herpesvirus in Kaposi's sarcoma. II. Serological association of American Kaposi's sarcoma with cytomegalovirus. Int J Cancer 1978; 22:126-31.
40. Howard RJ, Narjarian JS. Cytomegalovirus-induced immune suppression. I. Humoral immunity. Clin Exp Immunol 1974; 18:109-18.
41. Howard RJ, Miller J, Najarian JS. Cytomegalovirus-induced immune suppression. II. Cell-mediated immunity. Clin Exp Immunol 1974; 18:119-26.

ORIGINAL ARTICLE

AN OUTBREAK OF COMMUNITY-ACQUIRED *PNEUMOCYSTIS CARINII* PNEUMONIA

Initial Manifestation of Cellular Immune Dysfunction

Henry Masur, M.D., Mary Ann Michelis, M.D., Jeffrey B. Greene, M.D., Ida Onorato, M.D., Robert A. Vande Stouwe, M.D., Ph.D., Robert S. Holzman, M.D., Gary Wormser, M.D., Lee Brettmen, M.D., Michael Lange, M.D., Henry W. Murray, M.D., and Susanna Cunningham-Rundles, Ph.D.

Abstract Eleven cases of community-acquired *Pneumocystis carinii* pneumonia occurred between 1979 and 1981 and prompted clinical and immunologic evaluation of the patients. Young men who were drug abusers (seven patients), homosexuals (six), or both (two) presented with pneumonia. Immunologic testing revealed that absolute lymphocyte counts, T-cell counts, and lymphocyte proliferation were depressed, and that humoral immunity was intact. Of the 11 patients, one was found to have Kaposi's sarcoma, and another had angioimmunoblastic lymphadenopathy. Eight patients died. In the remaining three, no diagnosis of an immunosuppressive disease was established, despite persistence of immune defects. These causes of pneumocystosis suggest the importance of cell-mediated immune function in the defense against *P. carinii*. The occurrence of this infection among drug abusers and homosexuals indicates that these groups may be at high risk for this infection.

PNEUMOCYSTIS CARINII is a ubiquitous organism that infects human beings by a respiratory route. The organism appears to be relatively avirulent, since it rarely if ever causes disease in immunologically competent persons.[1,2] In North America, almost all cases have occurred in patients who have had diagnoses of primary congenital immunodeficiencies or who have received immunosuppressive chemotherapy for malignant neoplastic disease or organ transplantation.[1,2]

Despite the rarity of *P. carinii* pneumonia in previously healthy persons, we recently recognized 11 cases of this disease in young men with no previous history to suggest immunologic dysfunction. All 11 men were drug abusers or homosexuals or both. Each was found to have similar immunologic defects indicative of abnormal cell-mediated immunity. The clinical, epidemiologic, and immunologic features of this population are the subject of this report.

Methods

Selection of Patients

Between July 1979 and April 1981, infectious-disease consultants in the New York metropolitan area became aware of several cases of *P. carinii* pneumonia in adults with no history suggestive of immunologic incompetence. Consultants from several medical institutions, who regularly meet at an intercity infectious-disease conference, were queried about similar cases. Thirteen patients were reported from nine hospitals: 11 patients at seven hospitals were made available for this study. A diagnosis of *P. carinii* pneumonia was accepted only if abundant *P. carinii* organisms (identified by methenamine silver or Gram–Weigert stain) were present in areas of lung tissue, if an inflammatory cellular or exudative response was present, and if no other coexistent organisms were demonstrated by pathological examination, by cultivation (for bacteria, fungi, and mycobacteria), or by serology. Serologic studies for infectious agents were performed as indicated by the clinical situation. Nine patients were evaluated by complement-fixation testing for titers of cytomegalovirus antibody more than two weeks after lung biopsy. Viral cultivations were not attempted. The pathological features of any available nonpulmonary tissue were also reviewed in order to assess the presence or absence of underlying systemic disease.

Selection of Controls

The control group for in vitro mononuclear-cell studies consisted of healthy hospital personnel (matched for age, but not for sex or race) who were not known to be drug addicts or homosexuals and who were not taking medications. Subjects were excluded if they had had an acute illness during the week before testing. Historical control values were used for other studies.

Immunologic Testing

Ten of the 11 patients had all immunologic testing performed at the same laboratories of the New York Hospital, Rockefeller University, and Memorial Sloan–Kettering Cancer Center. Patient 8 was studied only at Downstate Medical Center and the Brooklyn Veterans Administration Medical Center. At the time of testing, nine patients had received no immunosuppressive chemotherapy; a single patient had received a two-day course of prednisone (60 mg per day) 10 days before his first test, and another had received a nine-day course of prednisone that ended 11 days before his first test. Five patients who survived their initial hospitalization (Patients 1, 2, 6, 7, and 10) were tested on at least two occasions, the last of which occurred one month or more after discharge from the hospital, when they appeared to be well. Two patients (Patients 3 and 4) who survived the initial hospitalization but died subsequently had their only testing performed at least two months after the resolution of their pneumocystosis. Among four patients who did not survive the initial hospitalization, one was studied on two occasions separated by more than two weeks (Patient 5) and three were studied only once during the acute illness (Patients 8, 9 and 11).

Mononuclear cells were separated from heparinized venous blood by centrifugation on a Ficoll–Hypaque cushion. T cells were counted by rosette formation with sheep erythrocytes after incubation at 4°C for one hour. B cells were enumerated by detection of cells bearing surface immunoglobulins, with a polyvalent rabbit $f(ab)_2$-fragment antiserum to human immunoglobulin. The number of monocytes was determined as the percentage of mononuclear cells ingesting latex particles. The viability of cells, as determined by exclusion of trypan blue dye, always exceeded 90 percent of the total. Enumeration of these different mononuclear-cell populations,

From the departments of Medicine, The New York Hospital–Cornell, Rockefeller University, New York University, Queens Hospital Center Affiliation Long Island Jewish–Hillside Medical Center, St. Luke's–Roosevelt Hospital Center, Bronx Veterans Administration Medical Center, Brooklyn Veterans Administration Medical Center, and Memorial Sloan–Kettering Cancer Center, New York.

Drs. Masur and Murray are recipients of the Teacher-Scientist Award from the Andrew W. Mellon Foundation. Dr. Michelis is a recipient of the Arthritis Foundation Fellowship.

Table 1. Clinical Features of 11 Men with *Pneumocystis carinii* Pneumonia.*

Clinical Feature	Patient No.				
	1	2	3	4	5
Age (yr)	27	37	39	40	34
Race/ethnic group	Black	White	Black	Black	White
Occupation	Hospital guard	Drug dealer	Hospital clerk	Mover	Teacher
Sexual preference	Homosexual	Heterosexual	Heterosexual	Heterosexual	Homosexual
Drugs abused	None	Heroin	Alcohol	Heroin	None
Onset of PCP (mo/yr)	4/79	4/80	2/80	6/80	11/80
Duration of symptoms	2 mo	5 mo	5 mo	1 mo	3 days
Date of lung biopsy (mo/yr)	6/79	9/80	7/80	7/80	11/80
Outcome of PCP	Survived	Survived	Survived	Survived	Survived
Other infections					
Before PCP	Oral candidiasis	None	Epididymitis	None	Oral candidiasis
After PCP	Candidia esophagitis, amebiasis, PCP	*Mycobacterium avium*	Klebsiella sepsis	None	Cryptococcosis, CMV, polybacterial sepsis, PCP
Follow-up (mo after biopsy)	6	10	8	8	3
Current status	Dead	Dead	Dead	Alive	Dead
Clinical and pathological findings	Autopsy: candida esophagitis, PCP	LAP: mycobacterium avium	Marrow biopsy, CTT of abdomen lymph-node biopsy: AILD	CTT of abdumen, LSS, LAP, marrow biopsy: NAD	Autopsy: Kaposi's sarcoma, CMA, PCP, cryptococcosis

as previously described,[3] was kindly performed by Dr. B. Koziner. Monocyte antitoxoplasmic activity was assessed as previously described.[4] T-cell function was measured in vivo by delayed cutaneous reactivity after intradermal administration of at least four of the following antigens: candida, mumps, tetanus-toxoid, trichophyton, tuberculin, and streptokinase-streptodornase. Lymphocyte transformation was measured by incorporation of [^{14}C]thymidine in response to stimulation with mitogens, antigens, and allogeneic cells, as previously described.[5,6] The mitogens used and the final concentrations were as follows: phytohemagglutinin at 175-3 μg per milliliter, concanavalin A at 114-3 μg per milliliter, and pokeweed mitogen at 142-3 μg per milliliter. Antigens used included the following microbial activators, prepared as previously described[7] and used in multiple dilutions of their respective stock solutions: ultracentrifuged and sonicated extract of *Candida albicans* Type A at 1 g per milliliter (wet weight), pools of treated extracts of common *Escherichia coli* and common *Staphylococcus aureus,* each resuspended at 10^9 cells per milliliter, and purified protein derivative of tuberculin at a range of final concentrations of 0.5 to 4.5 μg per milliliter. Allogeneic cells pooled from donors who were of at least six different HLA types were also used as stimulators, added (in concentrations ranging from 3000 to 50,000 cells per milliliter) to 50,000 responder cells from patients or controls. Results of lymphocyte-proliferation studies are expressed as the net counts per minute: those in a stimulated culture minus those in the unstimulated culture.

For statistical evaluation, lymphoproliferative responses were analyzed with the median counts per minute of the maximal response elicited to a range of concentrations of each cell activator. P values as given in the text were determined by the paired t-test, comparing each patient's response with his simultaneously tested control's response.[8]

The preformed-antibody response was determined by measurement of isohemagglutinin titers to antigens of the ABO blood group. Most of the patients were tested for the ability to make a specific antibody response by determination of antibody levels after administration of diphtheria–tetanus vaccine with a hemagglutination assay (kindly performed by the Centers for Disease Control, Atlanta) or after administration of pneumococcal polysaccharide vaccine with a radioimmunoassay (kindly performed by Dr. Gerald Schiffman) or with both procedures.

Standard techniques were used for measurement of serum immunoglobulins, absolute lymphocyte number, serum complement, resting-cell nitroblue tetrazolium testing, and myeloperoxidase staining. Latex fixation for rheumatoid factor and indirect immunofluorescence for antinuclear antibody were also performed.

Results

Patient Population

The clinical features of these 11 patients are summarized in Table 1. The 11 patients were all men 27 to 40 years old. Four were black, five were white, and two were Hispanic. Each patient was a drug user (seven patients), a homosexual (six), or both (two). Abused substances at the time of illness included heroin (four patients), methadone (one), alcohol (one), and alcohol plus cocaine (one). All patients were residents of New York City who had no social or occupational contacts with one another. The time of lung biopsy was randomly distributed (as calculated by Poisson distribution) over a 21-month period for the group as a whole, although four homosexual men presented to one hospital between February and April 1981. None of the patients had a history of unusual, severe, or recurrent infections in themselves or their families. Four patients had had oral candidiasis several weeks before the onset of *P. carinii* pneumonia, and one had had localized herpes zoster eight months before his pulmonary disease.

Clinical Illness

Four patients (Patients 3, 5, 6, and 8) had had nonrespiratory symptoms for three to 19 months before presenting with a pulmonary syndrome. These symptoms included fever, anorexia, and weight loss in each patient and voluminous diarrhea in Patient 5. All pa-

Table 1. (Continued.)

Patient No.					
6	7	8	9	10	11
31	27	34	31	35	27
Black	White	Hispanic	Hispanic	White	White
Carpenter	Waiter	Clerk	None	Horticulturist	None
Heterosexual	Homosexual	Heterosexual	Homosexual	Homosexual	Homosexual
Alcohol, cocaine	None	Methadone	Heroin	None	Heroin
11/80	9/80	7/80	2/81	4/81	1/81
7 days	5 mo	6 mo	2 mo	21 days	2 mo
11/80	2/81	12/80	4/81	4/81	3/81
Survived	Survived	Died	Died	Survived	Died
Herpes zoster	Oral candidiasis	None	None	Oral candidiasis	None
None	PCP, CMV	Candida and aspergillus esophagitis, gram-negative bacillary pneumonia	Gram-negative bacillary pneumonia, CMV, herpes esophagitis, PCP	Oral candidiasis	Gram-negative bacillary pneumonia
10	7	1	1	5	1
Alive	Dead	Dead	Dead	Alive	Dead
Marrow biopsy, CTT of chest: NAD	Autopsy: PCP, CMV	LSS, marrow biopsy, CTT of abdomen, IVP, LAG, gallium scan: NAD	Autopsy: CMV, herpes esophagitis, PCP	Marrow biopsy, LSS, CTT of abdomen: NAD	None

*PCP denotes *Pneumocystis carinii* pneumonia, CTT computed transaxial tomography, LAG lymphangiogram, LSS liver-spleen scan, LAP laparotomy, IVP intravenous pyelogram, AILD angioimmunoblastic lymphadenopathy, CMV cytomegalovirus, and NAD no apparent disease.

tients eventually had a respiratory illness characterized by nonproductive cough. Seven of the patients also had marked dyspnea. One patient had pleuritic chest pain, and one had rigors. The pulmonary syndrome had persisted for two to eight months before lung biopsy in eight patients and for three to seven days in three. Ten of the 11 patients had a history of fever before admission.

Initial physical examination revealed that 10 of these patients had fever (temperatures above 38.0°C) and that all had either diffuse fine rales or rhonchi. Two patients who were found to have neoplastic disorders were the only ones with remarkable extrapulmonary findings. Patient 5, who had malabsorption, was markedly cachectic on admission; Patient 3 had both generalized lymphadenopathy and epididymitis.

Routine Laboratory Evaluation

Seven patients had mild anemia (hematocrit, 31 to 39 percent), but all had normal granulocyte and platelet counts on admission. Lymphopenia was detected in all patients except one (Patient 4). Leukopenia (1060 to 3000 white cells per cubic millimeter) subsequently developed in five patients (Patients 1, 4, 5, 7, and 10) after therapy with trimethoprim–sulfamethoxazole. Patient 5's chemistry profile was consistent with marked malabsorption, as evidenced by hypoalbuminemia (2.3 g per deciliter) and reduced folate and vitamin B_{12} stores. The other patients' chemistry profiles were remarkable only for mild elevations in transaminases (less than twice normal) in three patients, mild hypoalbuminemia (3.0 to 3.3 g per deciliter) in three, and hypocalcemia (4.2 mg per deciliter [1.0 mmol per liter]) in one. Measurements of arterial blood gases while patients were breathing room air showed that the partial pressure of oxygen at admission ranged from 33 to 91 mm Hg. Chest radiographs at admission showed a diffuse interstitial or reticulonodular pattern in 10 cases, three of which were initially asymmetrical. Patient 6 presented with a 3-by-3-cm right-lower-lobe nodule, which progressed to a diffuse reticulonodular pattern after lung biopsy.

Diagnosis of *P. carinii* Pneumonia

Ten patients were initially treated with a broad-spectrum antibacterial regimen without resolution of their pulmonary illness. Patient 6 underwent a lung biopsy before the institution of antimicrobial therapy. The diagnosis of *P. carinii* pneumonia was established by transbronchial biopsy in five patients and by open-lung biopsy in six. In 10 patients there was a patchy distribution of mononuclear-cell infiltration with eosinophilic intra-alveolar exudate. Patient 6, who presented with a nodular lesion, had areas of necrosis, infarction, and atypical granulomas surrounding abundant *P. carinii* organisms.

Treatment and Outcome

All 11 patients were initially treated for pneumocystosis with oral or intravenous trimethoprim–sulfamethoxazole. Five patients responded promptly, whereas five responded poorly and were treated with pentamidine instead of the trimethoprim–sulfamethoxazole or in addition to it. Patient 6, who initially presented with a nodular lesion, had diffuse infiltrates, which resolved spontaneously before trimethoprim–sulfamethoxazole was instituted.

All patients had extensive serologic, radiologic, and histologic evaluations for the presence of immunosuppressive diseases. Patient 3 had angioimmunoblastic lymphadenopathy documented by lymph-node and bone-marrow biopsy. In Patient 5, a cutaneous lesion was noted during hospitalization; this lesion was demonstrated by biopsy to be Kaposi's sarcoma. Both patients survived their pneumocystosis but died of other infectious processes eight months and three months later, respectively.

Three patients died early in the course of their disease: Patient 9 of autopsy-proved progressive pneumocystosis and Patients 8 and 11 after acquiring nosocomial gram-negative pneumonia. Five others died after more prolonged illnesses. Patient 1 apparently responded promptly to therapy, with clearance of infiltrates and improvement in blood gases, but he continued to have debilitating fever for six months. The only diseases identified during this period were esophageal candidiasis and intestinal amebiasis. The patient died suddenly at home; at autopsy he was found to have extensive pneumocystis pneumonia but no evidence of an immunosuppressive disease. Patient 2 died 10 months after lung biopsy because of a progressive febrile disease (disseminated *Mycobacterium avium* infection), but no underlying disease was found at laparotomy. Fatal klebsiella sepsis developed in Patient 3, and an autopsy was not performed. Patient 5 died of an overwhelming cryptococcal infection that developed after his initial presentation. At autopsy, pneumocystis and cytomegalovirus were also present in the lungs. Patient 7 died seven months after lung biopsy because of another episode of *P. carinii* pneumonia; autopsy did not reveal an underlying disease.

The three survivors have been well and free of severe infectious diseases since discharge. One has had persistent oral candidiasis. These three patients include one homosexual and two drug abusers. They have been followed for five to 10 months.

Immunologic Evaluation

None of the patients had cutaneous reactivity to any of the antigens tested. This anergy was present during the acute illness, and it persisted in the patients who were tested for delayed hypersensitivity more than two weeks after the *P. carinii* pneumonia had clinically resolved (Patients 1 to 4 and 6 to 8). Patients 1, 2, 3, 4, 6, 7, and 10 underwent lymphocyte-transformation studies after the clinical resolution of the pneumocystosis. Patients 5, 8, 9, and 11 were studied during their acute illness, as described above.

As seen in Figure 1, the patients had lower proliferative responses to various mitogens, antigens, and allogeneic cells than did a simultaneously tested age-matched control group. These responses represent the maximal lymphocyte proliferation that could be elicited with a range of concentrations of stimulating substances and cells. Since only pooled normal human serum was used to supplement the lymphocyte-culture mediums, it is not possible that serum suppressor factors had a role in these abnormally low responses. An impaired cellular immune response in the patients, as compared with the controls, was observed in in vitro studies of lymphocytes cultured with nonspecific inducers of T-lymphocyte activation: phytohemagglutinin ($P<0.0001$), concanavalin A ($P<0.0001$), and the T-cell-dependent inducer of mitosis in B lymphocytes, pokeweed mitogen ($P<0.0001$) (Fig. 1*A*). Lymphocyte responses to the microbial activators *C. albicans* ($P<0.0001$), *Staph. aureus* ($P<0.003$), *Esch. coli* ($P<0.004$), and purified protein derivative of tuberculin ($P<0.025$) were also depressed, as seen in Figure 1*B*. Alloreactivity (Fig. 1*C*) was similarly depressed in these patients ($P<0.0001$), as indicated by their low response to pooled lymphocytes as compared with that of the controls. With the exception of Patients 5, 8, 9, and 11, these tests of lymphocyte proliferation were performed when the patients were not acutely ill. In addition, repeated evaluation in Patients 1, 2, 5, 6, 7, and 10 more than one month after the first evaluation confirmed the same type of abnormally depressed responses.

In Table 2, the responses of patients with *P. carinii* pneumonia to phytohemagglutinin are compared with the total lymphocyte count, the percentage of sheep-erythrocyte-rosetting lymphocytes, and the percentage of mononuclear phagocytic cells. These data illustrate that the depressed phytohemagglutinin re-

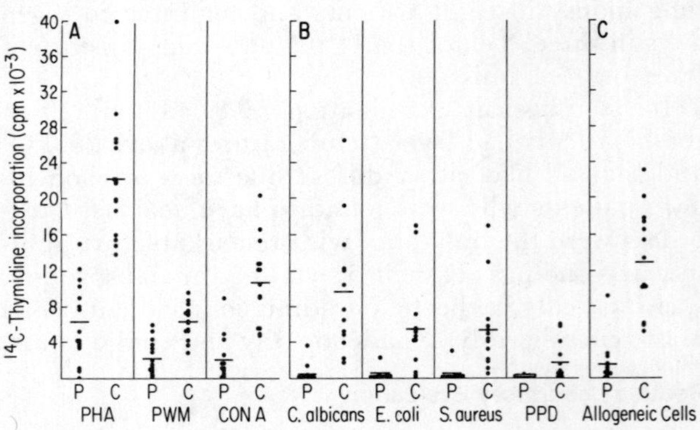

Figure 1. Maximal Proliferation of Lymphocytes from Patients with *Pneumocystis carinii* Pneumonia and from Healthy Controls in Response to Several Mitogens (A), Antigens (B), and Pooled Allogeneic Cells (C).

Five patients were studied once, and six were studied twice. Lymphocytes (5×10^4) were cultured in triplicate with multiple dilutions for each cell activator tested. Each culture was pulse-labeled with 0.04 μCi of ^{14}C-thymidine at time points predetermined from normal control studies to represent the time of maximum proliferative activity for the particular cell activator used. Cells were harvested 16 to 18 hours later onto glass-fiber filter paper and counted in a scintillation counter. Data are given as net counts per minute (cpm). Bars indicate the arithmetic mean in each group for each activator tested. PHA denotes phytohemagglutinin, PWM pokeweed mitogen, CON A concanavalin A, PPD purified protein derivative of tuberculin, P patients, and C controls.

Table 2. Comparison of Maximal Response to Phytohemagglutinin with Lymphocyte Count, Percentage of T-Cell Rosettes, and Percentage of Mononuclear Phagocytic Cells in Patients with *Pneumocystis carinii* Pneumonia.

Patient No.	Time of Test After Diagnosis	Total Lymphocyte Count*	Sheep-Erythrocyte Rosettes†	Mononuclear Phagocytic Cells‡	Patient's Phytohemagglutinin Response§	Control's Phytohemagglutinin Response§
	mo	*cells/mm³*	%		$cpm \times 10^{-3}$	
1	1	225	44	29	9,025	15,415
1	2½	1444	67	13	14,988	21,772
2	1	220	63	21	11,113	15,975
2	4	576	19	ND	10,396	14,768
3	3½	825	55	27	4,220	19,698
4	4	2065	73	3	8,013	13,810
5	½	540	24	25	3,504	21,975
5	1½	480	12	6	100	26,330
6	2	972	71	20	5,235	29,500
6	5	1002	40	33	4,252	19,838
7	1	630	67	12	1,198	18,635
7	3	480	46	ND	908	26,678
8	2	588	22	ND	12,229	39,784
9	<1	735	10	0	3,987	22,150
10	<1	665	75	4	7,780	22,150
10	2	983	71	7	3,920	25,738
11	<1	82	11	0	ND	—

*Normal range, 1500 to 4000 cells per cubic millimeter.
†Normal mean range ±SD, 72±11.
‡Normal mean range ±SD, 17±8. ND denotes not determined.
§Value represents [^{14}C]thymidine incorporation.

sponses in the patients with pneumocystis infection were associated with low lymphocyte counts, ranging from 82 to 1444 cells per cubic millimeter in all but Patient 4, whose lymphocyte count of 2065 was normal. Nine of the 11 patients had a diminished sheep-erythrocyte-rosetting population on one or more determinations. It is important to note that the degree of impairment of an individual patient's phytohemagglutinin response did not directly relate to the level of reduction of sheep-erythrocyte-rosetting lymphocytes or to the number of mononuclear phagocytic cells. The impaired phytohemagglutinin responses in these patients are consistent with a defect in T cells, T-cell subsets, monocytes, or a combination of these cells.

The evaluation of antibody-mediated immunity in these patients is presented in Table 3. Quantitation of serum immunoglobulins revealed normal or elevated levels of some of the immunoglobulin classes in nine patients. Two patients had slight decreases in their IgG or IgM levels. No monoclonal proteins were detected by serum immunoelectrophoresis. Isohemagglutinins to antigens of the ABO blood group were present in normal titers. Protective levels of tetanus antitoxin were found in Patients 2 to 7 and 9 to 11; protective levels of diphtheria antitoxin were found in Patients 2 to 5, 7, 9, and 10. Patients 1 to 4, who were immunized with pneumococcal vaccine, acquired a substantial level of antibody to at least 11 serotypes two weeks after immunization. More important, six of the 10 patients had titers of anti-pneumocystis antibody ⩾1:16. B-cell quantitation, determined as the number of surface-immunoglobulin-positive cells,

Table 3. Evaluation of Antibody-Mediated Immunity in Patients with *Pneumocystis carinii* Pneumonia.*

Variable (Normal Range)	Patient No. 1	2	3	4	5	6	7	8	9	10	11
Serum immunoglobulins											
IgG (616–1647 mg/100 ml)	817	1150	2400	1560	600	1700	560	1390	1590	1360	1300
IgA (59–371 mg/100 ml)	93	370	320	780	200	260	195	710	410	640	220
IgM (57–343 mg/100 ml)	115	170	160	310	100	478	40	380	362	360	146
IgE (<41.0 μg/ml)	15	5.5	83	82	ND	ND	109	0	44	833	20
Isohemagglutinins (titer >1:4 after 1 yr of age)											
Anti-A	1:32	—	1:32	—	0†	ND	—	ND	1:32	1:128	1:8
Anti-B	—	1:64	—	1:64	0†	ND	1:32	—	1:32	1:64	1:4
Specific antibody response											
Tetanus (⩾0.01 antitoxin units/ml)	ND	⩾0.35	0.09	⩾0.35	0.04	⩾0.35	⩾0.35	ND	⩾2.8	0.18	1.4
Diphtheria (⩾0.01 antitoxin units/ml)	ND	⩾6.0	0.05	⩾6.0	0.02	⩽0.01	0.38	ND	0.05	0.09	⩽0.01
Pneumococcal polysaccharides (substantial antibody rise in 12 serotypes tested)	Present	Present	Present	Present	ND	ND	ND	ND	ND	ND	ND
Pneumocystis	1:16	1:64	1:16	1:16	1:16	Negative	Negative	ND	Negative	1:32	Negative
B-cell quantitation											
Ig-bearing lymphocytes (150–960 cells/mm³)	217	196	388	620	418	156	214	ND	ND	147	73

*ND denotes not done.
†Blood type AB.

showed normal B-lymphocyte counts in seven patients. Plasma cells were detected by marrow examination in eight patients (Patients 1 and 3 to 9).

The phagocytic cells of these patients were assessed by the neutrophil count, nitroblue tetrazolium testing of unstimulated neutrophils and monocytes, and tests of the monocytes' ability to phagocytose and kill *Toxoplasma gondii;* these cells were found to be normal in all patients. Total hemolytic complement, C3 and C4, or both were also measured, and the levels were not depressed. Rheumatoid factor and antinuclear antibodies were absent in all patients.

Discussion

P. carinii pneumonia is usually a disease of persons with previously recognized immunosuppressive disorders. In adults, pneumocystosis is usually associated with hematologic neoplasia or organ transplantation, although the widespread use of immunosuppressive chemotherapy (especially corticosteroids) has facilitated its occurrence in patients with a wide range of malignant neoplastic and inflammatory diseases.[1,2] In children, pneumocystosis has also been associated with primary congenital immunodeficiency syndromes and protein-calorie malnutrition.[1,2,9,10]

Pneumocystosis has only rarely been recognized as the initial manifestation of an immunologic abnormality. Five infants have had pneumocystosis during the first year of life, and each was found to have a congenital hypogammaglobulinemia.[11-14] Infants and young children with severe protein-calorie malnutrition but no history of severe or recurrent infection have also had *P. carinii* pneumonia either during nursery epidemics in Eastern Europe or, more recently, as isolated cases among Asian refugees.[1,2,15] In a recent preliminary report, five homosexual men had *P. carinii* pneumonia with evidence of cytomegalovirus infection, and three of these patients had cellular immune dysfunction.[16] Six of our 11 patients were homosexuals, but only two of the five homosexuals tested had serologic evidence of cytomegalovirus.

The 11 patients in this series all had profound defects in the cell-mediated immune response. All patients were anergic, had T-lymphocyte depletion, and had markedly depressed lymphoproliferative responses to mitogens, antigens, and allogeneic cells. The reduction in the response of these patients' lymphocytes to phytohemagglutinin could not be correlated with the percentage of sheep-erythrocyte rosettes or with the percentage of latex-ingesting cells, suggesting that the impaired phytohemagglutinin response was more probably related to T-cell or monocyte dysfunction than to the cell number. Repeat testing in some of these patients, months after the acute *P. carinii* pneumonia, demonstrated persistence of immunologic abnormalities. In addition, five of these patients had oral candidiasis or herpes zoster before the *P. carinii* pneumonia, at least three had histopathologic evidence of concurrent cytomegalovirus infection, and five had mycobacterial, protozoan, or invasive fungal disease after their initial presentation with pneumocystosis. Infection with these opportunistic agents in vivo clearly supports the in vitro evidence of defective cellular immunity.

In contrast to cellular immunity, humoral immunity, phagocytosis, and complement levels all appeared intact in the persons tested.

Evaluation of the relative importance of cell-mediated and humoral immunity in adults with *P. carinii* pneumonia has previously been difficult, because both are usually suppressed by the complex interaction of effects of the underlying immunosuppressive disease, chemotherapy, or protein-calorie malnutrition.[1,2,8] In children with primary congenital immunodeficiencies, pure B-cell defects have clearly been associated with pneumocystis disease.[1,2,10] However, patients with combined T-cell and B-cell deficiencies seem more predisposed to pneumocystosis than patients with pure B-cell dysfunction.[9] There has been only one reported case of a pure T-cell defect associated with pneumocystosis.[17]

Our study supports the importance of cell-mediated immune function in host defenses against pneumocystis infection. This concurs with studies that have shown in vitro that the human-lymphocyte-antibody response to pneumocystis antigen is dependent on the presence of both T lymphocytes and adherent cells.[18] These observations supplement previous studies that have shown that the degradation of pneumocystis trophozoites by murine cells is dependent on specific anti-pneumocystis serum for opsonization and on intact mononuclear phagocytes for killing.[19]

In two of the 11 patients, the observed immune dysfunction could have been associated with malignant neoplastic disorders: angioimmunoblastic lymphadenopathy and Kaposi's sarcoma. The cause of the immune abnormalities in the remaining nine patients has not been established. Perhaps, given sufficient time, all would have had a recognizable disease that caused their immunosuppression. A common environmental substance that might have been a factor in the immunosuppression in this group of young men could not be identified. They did not live near each other or use similar medications; their close associates were not clinically affected. Narcotic abuse has been reported to cause in vitro immune defects similar to those described here,[20,21] yet it has not previously been associated with pneumocystosis. Certain viral diseases common in the homosexual community, such as cytomegalovirus, can depress the immune response; yet, these viral processes have not previously been associated with opportunistic superinfection in this population.[23,24] Moreover, in patients with evidence of cytomegalovirus infection, it is unclear whether the viral process was the precipitating cause of the immune depression or the result of reactivation subsequent to the initial immunosuppressive process. We are not aware of previous data suggesting that immunosuppression has been frequent among homosexuals. The results of this study and of other preliminary reports suggest that immunologic evaluation of homosexuals and drug abusers should be reassessed in conjunction with epidemiologic investigations of factors that could subject subpopulations to unusual risks for neoplastic disease or opportunistic infections.[16,22]

Serologic data and limited autopsy studies have suggested that pneumocystis is a ubiquitous organism to which many people are exposed early in life.[25,26] Studies in animals have demonstrated that murine transmission can occur through a respiratory route.[27] Nursery epidemics in economically disadvantaged regions and clusters of cases of pneumocystis pneumonia among oncology patients at three separate hospitals have suggested that person-to-person spread does occur, probably by a respiratory route, and that normal, healthy persons can serve as vectors.[1,28,29] Healthy medical personnel and family contacts of patients have not been documented to have *P. carinii* pneumonia, despite close contact with sporadic cases or hospital epidemics, although Watanabe et al. described an intriguing cluster of respiratory illnesses in two healthy family members of a patient who died of pneumocystosis.[30] In fact, diffuse *P. carinii* pneumonia has never been convincingly demonstrated to occur in an immunologically normal adult. Three adults and two children have been reported to have *P. carinii* pneumonia and to have had no immunosuppressive disease discovered at autopsy.[30-34] However, these patients had only limited immunologic studies performed. Subsequently, one seven-month-old child survived *P. carinii* pneumonia and was found by Rao et al. to have several normal markers of cell-mediated and humoral immunity.[35]

At present, there is insufficient evidence to determine whether the *P. carinii* pneumonia in these patients was due to pneumocystis infection that was latent and then reactivated or to infection that was recently acquired. Since homosexuals are suddenly contracting a variety of opportunistic fungal, viral, and mycobacterial infections, it seems unlikely that this outbreak has been due exclusively to a new virulent or resistant strain of pneumocystis. This outbreak was more probably related to the immunologic consequences of some unknown process. The high mortality rate also seems more likely to have been due to the immunologic lesion than to virulence or resistance of the specific organism or to peculiarities of clinical management.

This outbreak of community-acquired *P. carinii* pneumonia among young male homosexuals and drug abusers raises questions about increased exposure to pneumocystis as well as about the prevalence and origin of abnormal cellular immune responses in these populations. An awareness of the association should prompt further study of the epidemiology of pneumocystis infection and an aggressive diagnostic approach to diffuse pneumonias that occur in these groups of patients.

References

1. Burke BA, Good RA. *Pneumocystis carinii* infection. Medicine (Baltimore) 1973; 52:23-51.
2. Hughes WT. *Pneumocystis carinii* pneumonia. N Engl J Med 1977; 297:1381-3.
3. Koziner B, Filippa SA, Mertelsmann R, et al. Characterization of malignant lymphomas in leukemic phase by multiple differentiation markers of mononuclear cells: correlation with clinical features and conventional morphology. Am J Med 1977; 63:556-67.
4. Wilson CB, Tsai V, Remington JS. Failure to trigger the oxidative metabolic burst by normal macrophages: possible mechanism for survival of intracellular pathogens. J Exp Med 1980; 151:328-46.
5. Cunningham-Rundles S, Cunningham-Rundles C, Siegal FP, et al. Defective cellular immune response *in vitro* in common variable immunodeficiency. J Clin Immunol 1981; 1:65-72.
6. Bryan CF, Cunningham-Rundles S, Ashikari H, et al. Immunologic status of peripherla blood and regional lymph node lymphocytes in breast cancer patients. In: Schleslinger D, ed. Microbiology 1981. Washington, D.C.: American Society for Microbiology 1981:308-10.
7. Cunningham-Rundles S, Hansen JA, Dupont B. Lymphocyte transformation *in vitro* in response to mitogens and antigens. In: Bach F, Good RA, eds. Clinical immunobiology. Vol. 3. New York: Academic Press, 1976:151-94.
8. Snedecor GW, Cochran WG. Statistical methods. 6th ed. Ames, Iowa: Iowa State University Press, 1967:94.
9. Walzer PD, Perl DP, Krogstad DJ, Rawson PG, Schultz MG. *Pneumocystis carinii* pneumonia in the United States: epidemiologic, diagnostic, and clinical features. Ann Intern Med 1974; 80:83-93.
10. Hughes WT, Price RA, Sisko F, et al. Protein-calorie malnutrition: a host determinant for *Pneumocystis carinii* infection. Am J Dis Child 1974; 128:44-52.
11. Gentry LO, Remington JS. Pneumocystis carinii pneumonia in siblings. J Pediatr 1970; 76:769-72.
12. Jose DG, Gatti RA, Good RA. Eosinophilia with *Pneumocystis carinii* pneumonia and immune deficiency syndromes. J Pediatr 1971; 79:748-54.
13. Whisnant JK, Buckley RJ. Successful pyrimethamine-sulfadiazine therapy of pneumocystis pneumonia in infants with X-linked immunodeficiency with hyper IgM. Natl Cancer Inst Monogr 1976; 43:211-7.
14. Saulsbury FT, Bernstein MT, Winkelstein JA. *Pneumocystis carinii* pneumonia as the presenting infection in congenital hypogammaglobulinemia. J Pediatr 1979; 95:559-61.
15. Giebink GS, Sholler L, Keenan TP, Franciosi RA, Quie PG. *Pneumocystis carinii* pneumonia in two Vietnamese refugee infants. Pediatrics 1976; 58:115-8.
16. Pneumocystis pneumonia — Los Angeles. Morbid Mortal Weekly Rep 1981; 30:250-2.
17. DiGeorge AM. Congenital absence of the thymus and its immunologic consequences: concurrence with congenital hypoparathyroidism. Birth Defects 1968; 4:116-23.
18. Herrod HG, Valenski WR, Woods DR, Pifer LL. The *in vitro* response of human lymphocytes to *Pneumocystis carinii* antigen. J Immunol 1981; 126:59-61.
19. Masur H, Jones TC. The interaction in vitro of *Pneumocystis carinii* with macrophages and L-cells. J Exp Med 1978; 147:157-70.
20. McDonough RJ, Madden JJ, Falek A, et al. Alteration of T and null lymphocyte frequencies in the peripheral blood of human opiate addicts: *in vivo* evidence for opiate receptor sites on T lymphocytes. J Immunol 1980; 125:2539-43.
21. Brown SM, Stimmel B, Taub RN, Kochwa S, Rosenfield RE. Immunological dysfunction in heroin addicts. Arch Intern Med 1974; 134:1001-6.
22. Follow-up on Kaposi's sarcoma and pneumocystis pneumonia. MMWR 1981; 30:409-10.
23. Reinherz EL, O'Brien C, Rosenthal P, Schlessman SF. The cellular basis for viral-induced immunodeficiency: analysis by monoclonal antibodies. J Immunol 1980; 125:1269-74.
24. Ho M. The lymphocyte in infections with Epstein–Barr virus and cytomegalovirus. J Infect Dis 1981; 143:857-62.
25. Pifer LL, Hughes WT, Stagno S, Woods D. *Pneumocystis carinii* infection: evidence for high prevalence in normal and immunosuppressed children. Pediatrics 1978; 61:35-41.
26. Meuwissen JHE, Tauber I, Leeuweuberg ADEM, Beckers PJA, Sieben M. Parasitologic and serologic observations of infection with *pneumocystis* in humans. J Infect Dis 1977; 136:43-9.
27. Walzer PD, Schnelle V, Armstrong D, Rosen PP. Nude mouse: a new experimental model for *Pneumocystis carinii* infection. Science 1977; 197:177-9.
28. Singer C, Armstrong D, Rosen PP, Schottenfeld D. *Pneumocystis carinii* pneumonia: A cluster of eleven cases. Ann Intern Med 1975; 82:772-7.
29. Ruebush TK II, Weinstein RA, Baehner RL, et al. An outbreak of pneumocystis pneumonia in children with acute lymphocytic leukemia. Am J Dis Child 1978; 132:143-8.

30. Watanabe J, Chinchinian H, Weitz C, McIlvanie SK. *Pneumocystis carinii* pneumonia in a family. JAMA 1965; 193:685-6.
31. Reye RDK, ten Seldam REJ. Pneumocystis pneumonia. J Pathol Bacteriol 1956; 72:451-8.
32. Anderson CD, Barrie HJ. Fatal pneumocystis pneumonia in an adult: report of a case. Am J Clin Pathol 1960; 34:365-70.
33. Hennigar GR, Vinijchaikul K, Roque AL, Lyons HA. *Pneumocystis carinii* pneumonia in an adult: report of a case. Am J Clin Pathol 1961; 35:353-64.
34. Huneycutt HC, Anderson WR, Hendry WS. *Pneumocystis carinii* pneumonia: case studies with electron microscopy. Am J Clin Pathol 1964; 41:411-8.
35. Rao M, Steiner P, Victoria MS, et al. *Pneumocystis carinii* pneumonia: occurrence in a healthy American infant. JAMA 1977; 238:2301.

SPECIAL REPORT

EPIDEMIOLOGIC ASPECTS OF THE CURRENT OUTBREAK OF KAPOSI'S SARCOMA AND OPPORTUNISTIC INFECTIONS*

SINCE June 1981, the Centers for Disease Control (CDC) has learned of an increased occurrence of Kaposi's sarcoma, *Pneumocystis carinii* pneumonia, and other serious opportunistic infections concentrated among homosexual men in the United States. After receiving the initial reports,[1,2] the CDC formed a task force to undertake surveillance for these disorders and conduct epidemiologic and laboratory investigations. This report describes these surveillance activities and summarizes current knowledge of the epidemiologic aspects of this outbreak.

Surveillance and Reporting Methods

Case-report forms were completed for biopsy-proved cases of Kaposi's sarcoma in persons under 60 years of age without underlying immunosuppressive disease or therapy. Reports were also completed on all life-threatening or fatal opportunistic infections documented by biopsy or culture from patients with no known underlying illness or history of immunosuppressive therapy. The cases summarized below fit this case definition and were reported to the CDC between June 1 and November 10, 1981. For each case reported, an epidemiologist interviewed the attending physician by telephone and recorded both demographic data (age, race, marital status, sexual preference, and residence) and clinical information (e.g., illnesses, dates and methods of diagnoses, presence and dates of onset of signs and symptoms, history of predisposing conditions, and outcome of therapy).

To examine the incidence of Kaposi's sarcoma before 1980, we contacted epidemiologists associated with selected tumor registries in New York, California, and Georgia. Information was obtained from the National Cancer Institute Surveillance Epidemiology and End Results registries in the San Francisco Bay and Atlanta areas through 1979. Additional data were provided by the New York State Tumor Registry, the New York University Coordinated Cancer Registry, and the University of California Tumor Registry.

Task-force epidemiologists or officers of the CDC's Epidemic Intelligence Service actively surveyed physicians in 18 major metropolitan areas in the United States by letter and telephone to inquire about Kaposi's sarcoma in persons under 60 years of age or opportunistic infections in patients without a known predisposing factor since January 1979. At a minimum, heads of infectious disease, dermatology, oncology, and pathology departments from all major hospitals in these communities were contacted. In several of the metropolitan areas, physicians who served large numbers of homosexual men were known by the staff of clinics for sexually transmitted diseases or by other health-care personnel. When we obtained the names of these physicians, we attempted to contact them as well. In early August 1981, a formal request was made to all state health departments to notify the CDC of illnesses suspected of fitting the case definition. Several of these agencies have begun active surveillance.

Since November 1967, the CDC has been the sole United States supplier of pentamidine isethionate for the therapy of *P. carinii* pneumonia. Although trimethoprim–sulfamethoxazole has replaced pentamidine as the initial therapeutic agent, many patients still require pentamidine therapy. Routinely collected data on the patients' underlying conditions were reviewed from January 1, 1976, to November 10, 1981.

Results

There were 159 documented cases of Kaposi's sarcoma, *P. carinii* pneumonia, and other serious opportunistic infections reported to the CDC between June 1 and November 10, 1981 (Table 1). Sixteen additional cases have been excluded because of possible predisposing illnesses or systemic immunosuppressive therapy. The majority of the cases were detected through follow-up of reports to the CDC and requests for pentamidine or through active surveillance in New York City and California. Active surveillance in 15 metropolitan areas outside New York and California revealed no cases fitting the case definition that had not been reported previously. Searches of available tumor registries in New York, California, and Georgia indicated that Kaposi's sarcoma was an uncommonly reported cancer in these areas, rarely occurring in persons under the age of 50. No increased incidence of Kaposi's sarcoma was noted through 1979. From January 1, 1976, through June 1980 there was one questionable request to the CDC for pentamidine isethionate to treat an adult without an underlying disorder. From July through December 1980, there were nine such requests, all of which are included in this report. At this writing in 1981, 42 requests for pentamidine have been filled for men without underlying disorders. This represents 37 percent of all the requests for pentamidine for the treatment of adults in the United States in 1981 (42 of 114 requests).

The high mortality rate among the patients with *P. carinii* pneumonia accurately reflects the severity of their illness as well as the general debilitation of many of these men. Among 76 men with *P. carinii* pneumo-

Table 1. Outcome of Cases of Kaposi's Sarcoma, *Pneumocystis carinii* Pneumonia, and Other Serious Opportunistic Infections Reported to the Centers for Disease Control from June 1 to November 10, 1981.

Disease	No. Alive	No. Dead	Total No.	% Dead
Kaposi's sarcoma	62	1	73	15.1
P. carinii pneumonia	24	37	61	60.7
Both	8	7	15	46.7
Other infections	4	6	10	60.0
Total	98	61	159	38.4

*Report of the Centers for Disease Control Task Force on Kaposi's Sarcoma and Opportunistic Infections:

The members of the Task Force include David M. Auerbach, M.D., John V. Bennett, M.D., Philip S. Brachman, M.D., Glyn C. Caldwell, M.D., Salvatore J. Crispi, James W. Curran, M.D. (Coordinator), William W. Darrow, Ph.D., Henry Falk, M.D., David S. Gordon, M.D., Mary E. Guinan, M.D., Harry W. Haverkos, M.D., Clark W. Heath, Jr., M.D., Roy T. Ing, M.D., Harold W. Jaffe, M.D., Bonnie Mallory Jones, Dennis D. Juranek, D.V.M., Alexander Kelter, M.D., J. Michael Lane, M.D., Dale N. Lawrence, M.D., Richard Ludlow, Cornelia R. McGrath, James M. Monroe, David M. Morens, M.D., John P. Orkwis, Martha F. Rogers, M.D., Wilmon R. Rushing, Richard W. Sattin, M.D., Mary Ellen Shapiro, Thomas J. Spira, M.D., John A. Stewart, M.D., Pauline A. Thomas, M.D., and Hilda Westmoreland.

nia, 30 (39.5 percent) died of the initial infection. Of 46 survivors, 13 subsequently died, including four of the eight who had recurrent *P. carinii* pneumonia. The remainder of the subsequent deaths were attributed to Kaposi's sarcoma or to other opportunistic infections. Forty-three of 76 initial episodes of *P. carinii* pneumonia and all eight recurrent episodes required therapy with pentamidine. Among the 15 patients with both Kaposi's sarcoma and *P. carinii* pneumonia, Kaposi's sarcoma was diagnosed first in six, *P. carinii* pneumonia was diagnosed first in six, and the diagnoses were made during the same month in the remaining three. In some patients, the diagnosis of *P. carinii* pneumonia preceded that of Kaposi's sarcoma by six months or longer.

The 10 patients with other serious opportunistic infections included four with progressive or disseminated herpes simplex virus infections, three with toxoplasmosis of the central nervous system, one with cryptococcal meningitis, and two with disseminated

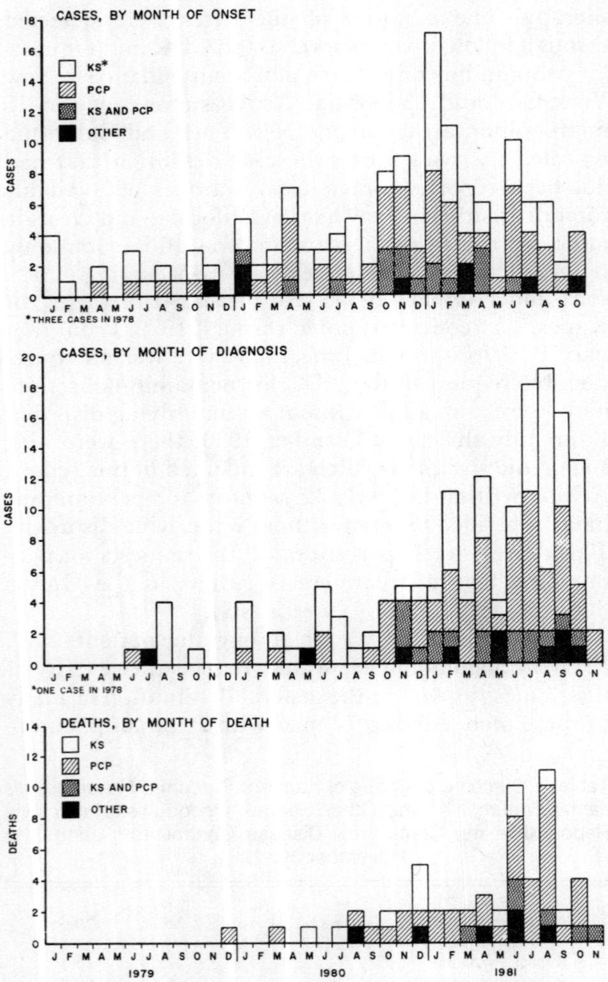

Figure 1. Incidence of Kaposi's Sarcoma (KS), *Pneumocystic carinii* Pneumonia (PCP), and Other Opportunistic Infections in the United States, 1979–1981.

Table 2. Signs or Symptoms Reported in Patients with Kaposi's Sarcoma, *P. carinii* Pneumonia, or Both.

Sign or Symptom	% with Sign or Symptom		
	Kaposi's Sarcoma (N = 73)	*P. carinii* Pneumonia (N = 61)	Both (N = 15)
Skin or mucosal lesions	80.8	8.2	86.7
Lymphadenopathy	43.8	23.0	40.0
Fever	23.3	93.4	86.7
Weight loss	19.2	70.5	53.3
Diarrhea	17.8	34.4	40.0
Dyspnea	5.5	88.5	100.0
Oral thrush	6.8	41.0	26.7

cytomegalovirus infection. Over 40 percent of the remaining 149 patients with Kaposi's sarcoma, *P. carinii* pneumonia, or both were reported to have other serious opportunistic infections, including 10 of 73 patients with Kaposi's sarcoma alone, 42 of 61 with *P. carinii* pneumonia alone, and 12 of 15 with both Kaposi's sarcoma and *P. carinii* pneumonia. Patients with *P. carinii* pneumonia alone were significantly more likely to be reported as having opportunistic infections than were those with Kaposi's sarcoma alone ($P<0.00001$ by Fisher's exact test). These infections include 24 clinically important cytomegalovirus infections confirmed by virus isolation or biopsy, six progressive or disseminated herpes simplex virus infections, five cryptococcal meningitis infections, 12 invasive gastrointestinal candida infections, seven disseminated mycobacterial infections (two with *Mycobacterium tuberculosis* and five with other species), and 10 other infections. These data are incomplete; they reflect only the coexisting infections that were well documented and were reported to the CDC.

Data generated by CDC surveillance indicate a secular increase in the number of reported cases by month of onset, month of confirmed diagnosis, and month of death (Fig. 1). The patients with both Kaposi's sarcoma and *P. carinii* pneumonia are represented in the diagnosis curve according to their first diagnosed illness. A considerable delay occurred between the initial onset of symptoms and diagnosis in both the Kaposi's sarcoma and *P. carinii* pneumonia groups. For Kaposi's sarcoma, the time from the onset of symptoms to diagnosis ranged from one to 30 months (median, 5.5); for *P. carinii* pneumonia, the range was one to 18 months (median, 3.5). Fifty-three percent of the patients (84 of 159) had the onset of their illness after January 1981, whereas 88 percent became ill after January 1980. Seventy-five percent of the cases (119 of 159) were diagnosed during 1981, and 74 percent of the deaths (45 of 61) occurred during 1981. The decline in the onset curve probably reflects the average three to six-month delay from the onset of symptoms to diagnosis. Late declines in the diagnosis and death curves may represent delay in reports to the CDC.

Table 2 shows selected signs or symptoms in patients with Kaposi's sarcoma, *P. carinii* pneumonia, or both. The frequency of lymphadenopathy, fever, and weight loss in the group with Kaposi's sarcoma attests to the often generalized nature of the disease. In each group, many patients were reported to have had a prodromal illness lasting for weeks to months and characterized by weight loss, lymphadenopathy, fever, and diarrhea. This prodrome was more consistently present and severe in patients with *P. carinii* pneumonia.

All but one of the 159 reported cases occurred in men. Ninety-two percent of these men (136 of 148) were reported to be homosexual or bisexual when sexual preference was known (Table 3). Patients' ages ranged from 15 to 57 years, with a median of 35. Eighty-two percent of the men were in the 25 to 44-year-old group. Seventy percent of the men were white (not Hispanic), 16 percent Hispanic, and 14 percent black. There were no significant differences in age or race between the disease categories.

Although cases were reported from 15 states, the District of Columbia, and two foreign countries, over three fourths of the patients were living in New York City, San Francisco, or Los Angeles at the time of diagnosis (Table 4). Since over half the cases were reported from the New York City metropolitan area, we compared the residence of patients whose onset of symptoms was early with that of patients whose symptoms began later in the epidemic. There was no significant difference in residence in metropolitan New York City between patients whose symptoms began before January 1, 1980 (17 of 24, 70.8 percent), and those whose symptoms began after that date (70 of 135, 51.9 percent) ($P>0.10$).

Discussion

The current outbreak of Kaposi's sarcoma, *P. carinii* pneumonia, and other opportunistic infections is highly unusual. Kaposi's sarcoma is a rare, malignant neoplasm, predominantly affecting elderly men and seldom causing death.[3] Although precise rates are unavailable, the annual incidence in the United States has been estimated to be 0.021 to 0.061 per 100,000 population.[4,5] In one large series, Safai et al. reported a 3:1 male-to-female ratio and a mean age of 63 years among patients with Kaposi's sarcoma.[6] Precise incidence estimates specific for sexual preference are not available, because the number of homosexual men living in cities where Kaposi's sarcoma has occurred is unknown. Nonetheless, the highly localized occurrence of 88 cases among men under 60 suggests at least a 100-fold increase in age-specific risk among homosexual men in the cities reporting cases, as compared with previous estimates of incidence. Although *P. carinii* causes several hundred cases of severe pneumonia in the United States annually, these cases were previously found almost exclusively in patients whose immunity was severely compromised by underlying disease, immunosuppressive therapy, or both.[7,8] After reviewing requests for pentamidine in the period from 1967 to 1970, when pentamidine was the only recommended treatment for *P. carinii* pneumonia, Walzer et al. discovered only one case of confirmed *P. carinii* pneumonia in a patient without a known underlying condition.[7] Our recent review of requests for pentamidine confirms the rarity with which this disease has been previously diagnosed among adults without underlying conditions.

Table 3. Sexual Preference of Men with Kaposi's Sarcoma, *P. carinii* Pneumonia, or Other Serious Opportunistic Infections Reported to the CDC.

Disease	Homosexual or Bisexual	Heterosexual	Unknown	Total
		no. of patients		
Kaposi's sarcoma	66	2	5	73
P. carinii pneumonia	49	9	3	61
Both	15	—	—	15
Other infections	6	1	2	9
Total	136	12	10	158

Table 4. Metropolitan Area of Residence at the Time of Diagnosis in Patients with Kaposi's Sarcoma, *P. carinii* Pneumonia, or Other Serious Opportunistic Infections.

Disease	New York City	San Francisco	Los Angeles	Other	Total
			no. of patients		
Kaposi's sarcoma	40	12	4	17	73
P. carinii pneumonia	34	5	10	12	61
Both	7	2	2	4	15
Other infections	6	0	1	3	10
Total	87	19	17	36	159

The simultaneous occurrence of Kaposi's sarcoma and *P. carinii* pneumonia among homosexual men of the same age and racial groups who live in the same geographic areas strongly suggests the occurrence of a single epidemic of underlying immunosuppression in these men. As noted previously, *P. carinii* pneumonia is typically a disease of immunocompromised patients. The incidence of Kaposi's sarcoma is greatly increased among recipients of renal allografts[9-12] and others receiving immunosuppressive therapy.[13-15] The natural history of the currently reported cases of Kaposi's sarcoma among these homosexual men is similar to that among transplant recipients, in that it more frequently involves the visceral organs and has a poor prognosis.[12,15a] When Kaposi's sarcoma occurs in allograft recipients, the tumor often spontaneously regresses with cessation or reduction of immunosuppressive therapy.[10,12]

The high mortality rate among young men with these disorders indicates a serious public-health problem. The magnitude of the current epidemic understated by the data presented on biopsy-confirmed cases of Kaposi's sarcoma and *P. carinii* pneumonia. Young men presenting with interstitial pneumonia without an underyling disorder may not have received a definite diagnosis or specific therapy for *P. carinii* pneumonia; others may have received empirical therapy with trimethoprim–sulfamethoxazole. The rather benign, inconspicuous appearance of many of the skin and mucous-membrane lesions of Kaposi's sarcoma in these men suggests that this disease may also be underdiagnosed.

If immunosuppression is the underlying cause of these conditions, then Kaposi's sarcoma and *P. carinii* pneumonia may represent the "tip of the iceberg" including other conditions that are less readily recognized or have longer latency periods. While investigating this outbreak, we have received numerous physicians' reports on young homosexual men with nonfatal opportunistic infections, unexplained prolonged lymphadenopathy, or lymphoreticular neoplasias. Although sporadic case reports of lymphoreticular neoplasms are difficult to interpret, these reports are a cause for concern, since Safai et al. have noted that Kaposi's sarcoma is frequently associated with other primary tumors.[6] In their series, 37 percent of the patients with Kaposi's sarcoma had other primary cancers; specifically, the authors noted a 20-fold increase in lymphoreticular neoplasms. Clinicians caring for homosexual men should be alert for signs and symptoms of other infections and neoplasms associated with immunodepression, in addition to Kaposi's sarcoma and *P. carinii* pneumonia.

Although it is possible that the concentration of reported Kaposi's sarcoma, *P. carinii* pneumonia, and other opportunistic infections among homosexual men living in New York and California represents a reporting artifact, we consider this possibility unlikely. Most of the reported cases were from tertiary-care facilities — the same type of facility included in our survey of 18 cities. If the geographic clustering of cases is in fact real, it suggests that risk factors for these diseases are not randomly distributed in the homosexual community.

Giraldo et al. first suggested an association between Kaposi's sarcoma and cytomegalovirus infection when they isolated cytomegalovirus from one of eight tissue-culture cell lines from patients with Kaposi's sarcoma.[16] They subsequently demonstrated a serologic association of Kaposi's sarcoma with cytomegalovirus in American and European patients, but not in African patients.[17,18] Finally, they found that three of eight tumor-biopsy samples were positive for cytomegalovirus DNA by DNA-DNA reassociation kinetics.[19] Cytomegalovirus is often associated with *P. carinii* pneumonia in immunosuppressed hosts, especially among renal-transplant recipients.[20] Furthermore, cytomegalovirus induces transient abnormalities in cellular immune function in otherwise healthy persons.[21] Since serologic evidence of cytomegalovirus infection and active shedding of cytomegalovirus in the urine have been shown to be more common among homosexual men than among heterosexual men of the same age,[22] further investigation of cytomegalovirus in the cases reported here is important. On the other hand, cytomegalovirus infection is very common in the United States and has not been shown to have such devastating effects on other populations. Since reactivation of cytomegalovirus is common among immunocompromised hosts, the role of this virus will not be easily defined in this outbreak.

In a recently published study, Masur et al. described 11 cases of *P. carinii* pneumonia in immunocompromised men without underlying disorders or therapy.[23] Although six of these men were homosexual, five others were reported to be drug abusers (using heroin, methadone, alcohol, or cocaine). Opiate addiction has been associated with alterations in cellular immune status in vitro,[24,25] but it had not previously been associated with *P. carinii* pneumonia.

The interest in a causal role for inhalants containing amyl nitrite or isobutyl nitrite or both ("poppers," as they are commonly called) stems from the hypothesis that they are used as sexual stimulants or recreational drugs by some homosexual men. In a recent survey of 420 men attending clinics for sexually transmitted diseases in New York, San Francisco, and Atlanta, we found that 86.4 percent of homosexual and bisexual men (242 of 279), as compared with 14.9 percent of heterosexual men (21 of 141), reported the use of nitrite inhalants within five years. However, the frequency of nitrite use was closely correlated with the number of sexual partners reported during the previous month. This suggests that the use of nitrites may be associated with other hypothetical etiologic factors, such as sexually transmitted infections, antimicrobial agents for treatment or prevention of these infections, types of sexual behavior, attendance at places where partners are encountered, and perhaps the use of other drugs. Studies undertaken to determine what role (if any) nitrites may have as risk factors for Kaposi's sarcoma and *P. carinii* pneumonia and immunosuppression must carefully consider the confounding effects of these other variables.

In collaboration with investigators in New York, California, and Georgia, the CDC task force is completing a national case-control study to identify risk factors for Kaposi's sarcoma and *P. carinii* pneumonia among homosexual men. We are continuing surveillance for these disorders and conducting other clinical and laboratory investigations.

This sudden, highly focal occurrence of Kaposi's sarcoma and *P. carinii* pneumonia provides an opportunity to investigate the relations among life style, environment, host immune responses, and oncogenesis and suggests the potential for prevention of these diseases if risk factors can be identified.

Note added in proof: Between November 10, 1981, and January 13, 1982, 57 additional cases were reported, bringing the total to 216 (89 cases of Kaposi's sarcoma, 91 of *P. carinii* pneumonia, 18 of both, and 18 of other infections). At least 88 (40.8 percent) of these patients have died.

We are indebted to the physicians reporting cases and to Drs. Donald F. Austin, Erwin Braff, James W. Buehler, James Chin, J. Lyle Conrad, Selma Dritz, Diane M. Dwyer, Shirley L. Fannin, Yehudi M. Felman, Stephen M. Friedman, Robert A. Gunn, John P. Hanrahan, Robert J. Kingon, Michael D. Malison, Stanley I. Music, Mark A. Roberts, Alain J. Roisin, Richard B. Rothenberg, and R. Klein Sikes for their roles in active surveillance.

References

1. *Pneumocystis* pneumonia — Los Angeles. MMWR 1981; 30:250-2.
2. Kaposi's sarcoma and *Pneumocystis* pneumonia among homosexual men — New York City and California. MMWR 1981; 30:305-8.
3. Safai B, Good RA. Kaposi's sarcoma: a review and recent developments. CA 1981; 31:2-12.
4. Oettle AG. Geographical and racial differences in the frequency of Kaposi's sarcoma as evidence of environmental or genetic causes. Acta Unio Int Contra Cancrum 1962; 18:330-63.
5. Rothman S. Remarks on sex, age, and racial distribution of Kaposi's sarcoma and on possible pathogenetic factors. Acta Unio Int Contra Cancrum 1962; 18:326-9.
6. Safai B, Miké V, Giraldo G, Beth E, Good RA. Association of Kaposi's sarcoma with second primary malignancies: possible etiopathogenic implications. Cancer 1980; 45:1472-9.
7. Walzer PD, Perl DP, Krogstad DJ, Rawson PG, Schultz MG. *Pneumocystis carinii* pneumonia in the United States: epidemiologic, diagnostic, and clinical features. Ann Intern Med 1974; 80:83-93.
8. Hughes WT. *Pneumocystis carinii* pneumonia. N Engl J Med 1977; 297:1381-3.
9. Harwood AR, Osoba D, Hofstader SL, et al. Kaposi's sarcoma in recipients of renal transplants. Am J Med 1979; 67:759-65.
10. Stribling J, Weitzner S, Smith GV. Kaposi's sarcoma in renal allograft recipients. Cancer 1978; 42:442-6.
11. Myers BD, Kessler E, Levi J, Pick A, Rosenfeld JB. Kaposi sarcoma in kidney transplant recipients. Arch Intern Med 1974; 133:307-11.
12. Penn I. Kaposi's sarcoma in organ transplant recipients: report of 20 cases. Transplantation 1979; 27:8-11.
13. Grange RW, Jones EW. Kaposi's sarcoma and immunosuppressive therapy: an appraisal. Clin Exp Dermatol 1978; 3:135-46.
14. Klepp O, Dahl O, Stenwig JT. Association of Kaposi's sarcoma and prior immunosuppressive therapy: a 5-year material of Kaposi's sarcoma in Norway. Cancer 1978; 42:2626-30.
15. Hoshaw RA, Schwartz RA. Kaposi's sarcoma after immunosuppressive therapy with prednisone. Arch Dermatol 1980; 116:1280-2.

15a. Gottlieb GJ, Ragaz A, Vogel JV, et al. A preliminary communication on exclusively disseminated Kaposi's sarcoma in young homosexual men. Am J Dermatopathol 1981; 3:111-4.

16. Giraldo G, Beth E, Haguenau F. Herpes-type virus particles in tissue culture of Kaposi's sarcoma from different geographical regions. J Natl Cancer Inst 1972; 49:1509-13.
17. Giraldo G, Beth E, Kourilsky FM, et al. Antibody patterns to herpesviruses in Kaposi's sarcoma: serological association of European Kaposi's sarcoma with cytomegalovirus. Int J Cancer 1975; 15:839-48.
18. Giraldo G, Beth E, Henle W, et al. Antibody patterns to herpesvirus in Kaposi's sarcoma. II. Serologic association of American Kaposi's sarcoma with cytomegalovirus. Int J Cancer 1978; 22:126-31.
19. Giraldo G, Beth E, Huang ES. Kaposi's sarcoma and its relationship to cytomegalovirus (CMV). III. CMV DNA and CMV early antigens in Kaposi's sarcoma. Int J Cancer 1980; 26:23-9.
20. Ryning FW, Mills J. *Pneumocystis carinii, Toxoplasma gondii*, cytomegalovirus and the compromised host. West J Med 1979; 130:18-34.
21. Rinaldo CR Jr, Carney WP, Richter BS, Black PH, Hirsch MS. Mechanisms of immunosuppression in cytomegaloviral mononucleosis. J Infect Dis 1980; 141:488-95.
22. Drew WL, Mintz L, Miner RC, Sands M, Ketterer B. Prevalence of cytomegalovirus infection in homosexual men. J Infect Dis 1981; 143:188-92.
23. Masur H, Michelis M, Greene JB, et al. An outbreak of community-acquired *Pneumocystis carinii* pneumonia: initial manifestation of cellular immune dysfunction. N Engl J Med 1981; 305:1431-8.
24. McDonough RJ, Madden JJ, Falek A, et al. Alteration of T and null lymphocyte frequencies in the peripheral blood of human opiate addicts: *in vivo* evidence for opiate receptor sites on T lymphocytes. J Immunol 1980; 125:2539-43.
25. Brown SM, Stimmel B, Taub RN, Kochwa S, Rosenfield RE. Immunologic dysfunction in heroin addicts. Arch Intern Med 1974; 134:1001-6.

ORIGINAL ARTICLE

LYMPHADENOPATHY-ASSOCIATED VIRAL ANTIBODY IN AIDS

Immune Correlations and Definition of a Carrier State

JEFFREY LAURENCE, M.D., FRANÇOISE BRUN-VEZINET, M.D., STEVEN E. SCHUTZER, M.D., CHRISTINE ROUZIOUX, PH.D., DAVID KLATZMANN, M.D., FRANÇOISE BARRÉ-SINOUSSI, PH.D., JEAN-CLAUDE CHERMANN, PH.D., AND LUC MONTAGNIER, M.D.

Abstract We investigated whether serologic evidence of lymphadenopathy-associated virus (LAV), an exogenous human T-cell lymphotropic and cytopathic retrovirus, correlated with the acquisition and transmission of the acquired immunodeficiency syndrome (AIDS). Serum from 17 of 25 patients with AIDS contained circulating IgG anti-LAV antibody (all of 5 adults with cancer and 6 of 12 adults and 6 of 8 children with opportunistic infections, with or without Kaposi's sarcoma). All of eight homosexual men with generalized lymphadenopathy or the AIDS-related complex and five homosexual men with AIDS prodromes who subsequently had AIDS were also sero-positive. The anti-LAV antibody was not found in 99 of 100 healthy blood donors or in 23 patients with genetic immunodeficiencies, supporting the contention that LAV is unlikely to represent simply another opportunistic microorganism. An AIDS carrier state was indicated by the probable transfer of LAV from asymptomatic, immunologically competent mothers to their offspring. These data offer a basis for the hypotheses that LAV is a marker for AIDS, may be carried and transmitted in the absence of clinical findings or in vitro T-cell abnormalities, and is probably an etiologically important agent in AIDS and its prodromes.

LYMPHADENOPATHY-associated virus (LAV) is a newly identified exogenous human T-cell lymphotropic retrovirus, first isolated from nodal tissue of a homosexual man[1] and subsequently recovered from T cells of hemophiliacs and other patients with the acquired immunodeficiency syndrome (AIDS).[2,3] IgG antibodies to LAV core antigen have been detected in a large percentage of patients with unexplained generalized hyperplastic lymphadenopathy and risk factors for AIDS, as well as in a smaller fraction of patients with opportunistic infections or malignant disorders characteristic of clinical AIDS.[3] The preference of LAV for a subset of the helper/inducer (Leu-3a+ or OKT4+) T-lymphocyte subpopulation, its capacity to produce cytopathic changes in these cells,[4] and the serum immunoglobulin profiles of antibodies to LAV in persons with AIDS or at risk for AIDS make this virus an attractive etiologic candidate. In a preliminary survey employing a specific enzyme-linked immunosorbent assay for extracts of total LAV protein,[5] the incidence of LAV-specific IgG antibody among patients with AIDS and lymphadenopathy was shown to be increased over that recorded in previous studies.[6,7] In the following report the incidence of such seroreactivity is established as equivalent to the incidence of antibody to HTLV-III in AIDS.[8-10] HTLV-III is a new type of the human T-cell lymphotropic virus (HTLV), now considered to be identical to LAV by virtue of competitive radioimmunoassay of their core proteins, as well as by other criteria.[11]

A simple description of a new virus with increased prevalence in patients with AIDS does not, of course, negate the possibility that the virus is yet another opportunistic pathogen to which these persons are acutely susceptible. In the absence of an in vivo model, serial analysis of serum samples from subjects who are initially healthy and serologically negative for the agent in question, and who then become positive for AIDS or its prodromes, would be invaluable. Defining a carrier state for this agent would require the identification of seropositive asymptomatic persons who were linked with transmission of AIDS directly to persons without other risk factors for the disease. In this paper we summarize several such informative associations, correlated with T-cell–subset phenotype ratios and DNA synthesis in response to a T-cell–dependent mitogen.

From the Division of Hematology–Oncology, Department of Medicine, New York Hospital–Cornell Medical Center, and the Department of Immunology, Rockefeller University, New York; Laboratoire de Virologie, Hôpital Claude Bernard, Paris; Laboratoire d'Immunologie Nephrologique et de Transplantåtion, UER Pitié-Salpétrière, Paris; and Institut Pasteur, Départemente de Virologie, Paris.

Supported by grants from the New York affiliate of the American Heart Association, the New York Community Trust, the New York State AIDS Institute, and a grant (CA 35018-01) from the National Institutes of Health. Dr. Laurence is a Clinician-Scientist of the American Heart Association and an Academic Fellow of the William S. Paley Foundation.

METHODS

Subjects

Serum samples were obtained from 25 patients with clinically documented AIDS: 17 adults with either cancer (4 with Kaposi's sarcoma and 1 with poorly differentiated lymphocytic lymphoma of the B-cell phenotype in whom *Pneumocystis carinii* pneumonia developed six months after diagnosis of the lymphoma) or opportunistic infection (10 with *P. carinii* pneumonia, 1 with herpes simplex encephalitis, and 1 with *Cryptococcus neoformans* meningitis), with or without Kaposi's sarcoma; and 8 children 8 to 24 months old (7 with *P. carinii* pneumonia, and 1 with cytomegaloviral pneumonia). The mothers of five children were current intravenous-drug abusers, and the mothers of three children were former abusers on methadone-maintenance regimens.

Five patients with an AIDS prodrome, defined retrospectively upon the development of AIDS, were also studied. In these patients, AIDS developed within 2 to 11 months after the initial serum sample was collected. Other subjects studied were 8 homosexual men with generalized lymphadenopathy, 6 of whom fulfilled the recommended criteria for diagnosis of the AIDS-related complex[12]; 9 healthy persons with risk factors for AIDS; and 23 patients with congenital immunodeficiencies (5 with common variable immunodeficiency who had some humoral response to antigen, and 18 with IgA deficiency). Serum specimens from these subjects were collected from 1981 through early 1984, before the institution of intravenous gamma globulin therapy. Three of the five patients with common variable immunodeficiency had evidence of T-cell–associated immunosuppression, documented by depressed T4/T8 ratios and the ability of isolated T cells to inhibit polyclonal immunoglobulin production in vitro when added to a pokeweed-mitogen–driven assay system using normal peripheral-blood mononuclear cells, as previously described.[13] One hundred randomly selected blood donors from two Paris hospitals were also studied.

LAV Serology

LAV was propagated in phytohemagglutinin-stimulated OKT4+ cells obtained from healthy heterosexual donors or umbilical-cord blood. The virus was concentrated by 10 percent polyethylene glycol 6000 precipitation and banded to equilibrium in a 20 to 60 percent sucrose gradient. Viral antigens, disrupted in 0.5 percent sodium dodecyl sulfate at 37°C for 15 minutes, were used to coat 96-well Immulon plates. Serum samples diluted at 1:40 in phosphate-buffered saline were tested against the antigens as well as a control, crude cytoplasmic extract of uninfected lymphocytes from the same donors. Virus-specific fixed IgG was revealed by a peroxidase-conjugated goat antihuman IgG in an enzymatic reaction employing orthophenylene diamine as substrate. Correlation with a recently described radioimmunoprecipitation assay for LAV confirmed the validity of the results of the enzyme-linked immunosorbent assay and established the core protein of LAV as the main immunogen.[2]

Lymphocyte Phenotypes and Function

T-lymphocyte–membrane phenotypes were determined by indirect immunofluorescence using monospecific antibodies to helper/inducer (Leu-3a+ or OKT4+) and suppressor/cytotoxic (Leu-2a+ or OKT8+) T-cell subsets and a rhodamine-conjugated rabbit antimouse IgG, as previously detailed.[13] The response to a T-cell–dependent B-cell lectin — pokeweed mitogen — was assessed by incubating 3×10^5 peripheral-blood mononuclear cells for five days in flat-bottom microwells containing the mitogen at varying dilutions (1:100 to 1:400). Sixteen hours before culture termination, 1.0 μCi of [^{3}H]methylthymidine (specific activity, 1.9 Ci per millimole) was added. The contents of each well were harvested onto fiberglass filters, and cell-associated radioactivity was measured. The results are expressed as mean counts per minute (cpm) of triplicate wells containing the dilution of pokeweed mitogen providing the highest response. The normal range for healthy heterosexual controls is 20,000 to 100,000 cpm for adults and 30,000 to 150,000 cpm for children below the age of 36 months.

Results

Of the 25 patients with AIDS, 17 (68 percent) were seropositive for anti-LAV antibody (Table 1). A higher proportion of adults with cancer alone, as compared with those with opportunistic infections in the presence or absence of Kaposi's sarcoma, had a positive reaction in this assay (100 vs. 50 percent). Two of the eight seronegative patients with AIDS had Kaposi's sarcoma in addition to an opportunistic infection. All of the eight homosexual men with generalized lymphadenopathy or AIDS-related complex had anti-LAV antibody.

Serologic studies of LAV among the affected offspring of mothers who were clinically healthy but at risk for the development of AIDS was of particular value in defining an AIDS carrier state (Table 2). In Mother 1, a former intravenous-drug abuser, the phenotypic T_{helper}:$T_{suppressor}$ ratio (T_H:T_S) and blastogenic response to pokeweed mitogen were within normal limits. She has remained asymptomatic over 16 months of follow-up. Her daughter died of *P. carinii* pneumonia at the age of nine months after a prodromal phase of failure to thrive, fever, oral candidiasis, and hepatomegaly. Although the pokeweed mitogen–stimulation values for this child remained normal, the T_H:T_S ratio declined from 0.87 to 0.25 within two months. There was no evidence of acute infection with or prior exposure to several viral agents with potential etiologic links to AIDS, including adenovirus, cytomegalovirus, Epstein–Barr virus, and hepatitis B virus. An extensive immunologic investigation antemortem and a postmortem examination did not delineate a known immunodeficiency syndrome. The clinical and immunologic features of Mother 1 and Child 1 have been described in detail elsewhere.[14] Both mother and child were seropositive for LAV. The serologic and immunologic profiles of two other affected infants of mothers with a history of intravenous-drug abuse are also shown in Table 2. The fact that one infant with AIDS (Child 2) was born to a seropositive mother and yet had no detectable IgG antibody to LAV during a phase of marked T-cell lymphopenia and antemortem infection makes simple

Table 1. IgG Anti-LAV Antibody in Serum from Patients with AIDS, Patients at Risk of AIDS, and Controls.

Group	T_H:T_S Ratio	Prevalence of Antibody
	mean (range)	*% (no. positive/no. tested)*
AIDS		
Kaposi's sarcoma or B-cell lymphoma	0.34 (0.00–2.0)	68 (17/25)
Opportunistic infection (with or without Kaposi's sarcoma)	0.22 (0.03–0.26)	100 (5/5)
Adults	0.18 (0.02–0.72)	50 (6/12)
Children	0.63 (0.03–2.0)	75 (6/8)
Risk of AIDS		
Prodrome*	0.58 (0.27–1.0)	100 (5/5)
Lymphadenopathy	0.77 (0.15–1.13)	100 (8/8)
Controls†		
Health, with AIDS risk factors‡	1.20 (0.50–2.30)	0 (0/9)
Sexual contacts of AIDS patients	1.09 (0.59–1.78)	40 (2/5)
Healthy mothers of children with AIDS§	1.12; 0.36; 1.14	100 (3/3)
Healthy children with LAV-negative mothers, with AIDS risk factors§	Not determined	0 (0/2)
Common variable immunodeficiency	1.52 (1.20–2.0)	0 (0/5)
IgA deficiency	Not determined	0 (0/18)

*AIDS developed in all five subjects during 2 to 11 months of follow-up (Table 3).

†Other controls tested were 100 healthy blood donors, of whom 1 was positive for LAV.

‡The nine controls were six sexually active homosexual men and two men and one woman who were former intravenous-drug abusers.

§All mothers were currently or formerly intravenous-drug abusers.

Table 2. T-Cell Phenotype and Function in Children with AIDS and Their Mothers.

	T_H:T_S Ratio*	Lymphocyte Stimulation†		IgG Antibody to LAV
		medium	pokeweed mitogen	
		mean cpm		
Mother 1 — clinically healthy; intravenous-drug abuser	1.12	5,117	23,680	+
Child 1 — daughter; AIDS; death at age of 9 mo	0.25	2,378	66,888	+
Mother 2 — clinically healthy; intravenous-drug abuser	0.36	9,421	11,519	+
Child 2 — daughter; AIDS	0.77	2,918	6,663	–
Mother 3 — clinically healthy; intravenous-drug abuser	1.14	5,383	11,801	+
Child 3 — daughter; AIDS	0.86	21,599	72,839	–

*Normal value in infants and adults, 1.8±0.7.

†Normal value in adults, 20,000 to 100,000 cpm; in infants, 30,000 to 150,000 cpm.

transplacental carryover of anti-LAV antibody, rather than LAV infection, unlikely. The high level of DNA synthesis by lymphocytes from Child 3 in the absence of pokeweed mitogen may correspond to the elevated spontaneous B-cell activity of peripheral-blood mononuclear cells described in patients with AIDS.[15]

Serial antibody-reactivity patterns were determined in two subjects at risk for AIDS. One patient, a homosexual man with AIDS-related complex (a three-month history of generalized lymphadenopathy, low-grade fever, malaise, and depressed T_H:T_S ratio), was initially negative for antibody to LAV but became positive four months later. He has remained seropositive despite gradual resolution of the lymphadenopathy, constitutional symptoms, altered T_H:T_S ratio, and disappearance of initially high titers of SSF-AIDS, a soluble factor released by peripheral-blood mononuclear cells of certain patients with AIDS-related complex or AIDS that is capable of abrogating T-cell–dependent immune responses.[13,16] Another homosexual man with lymphadenopathy, malaise, and a low T_H:T_S ratio was initially positive for anti-LAV antibody but became seronegative upon the development of *P. carinii* pneumonia, Kaposi's sarcoma, and leukopenia with profound depression of the absolute number of OKT4+ peripheral lymphocytes.

The clinical and immunologic features of the patients with a true AIDS prodrome, defined retrospectively upon the development of clinical AIDS, are described in Table 3. All five of these patients were positive for IgG antibody to LAV.

Discussion

Three lines of evidence have been presented in support of an etiologic role for LAV in AIDS. The identification of IgG antibodies to LAV in a large proportion of patients with AIDS or its prodromes, both putative (i.e., the AIDS-related complex) and definitive (i.e., prodromes based on the histories of patients in whom clinical AIDS developed during the course of this study), extends recently reported serologic studies on anti-LAV antibody in AIDS. It also answers a previous objection[17] concerning the relatively low levels of positivity (38 percent) first reported in AIDS.[6] The description of a carrier state for LAV, with development of seropositivity and AIDS in infants born to clinically healthy, anti-LAV antibody–positive mothers, strengthens the pathogenic role of this virus. It also illuminates two recent case reports in which acquisition of anti-LAV antibody appeared to be linked to the transmission of AIDS in a mother–infant pair[18] and a blood-donor–recipient pair.[19]

The presence of antibody to LAV and the concurrent or subsequent recognition of clinical AIDS in a few patients with T_H:T_S ratios and mitogen-stimulation indexes in the normal range are consistent with the finding that only a small fraction of OKT4+ lymphocytes are susceptible to LAV infection.[3] The association also underscores the fact that phenotypic T-lymphocyte ratios and blastogenic responses to lectin are unreliable indicators of AIDS or its prodromes.

Our subject with clinical and in vitro immunologic evidence of AIDS-related complex, seroconversion to LAV positivity within three months of the onset of symptoms, and gradual resolution of clinical and laboratory abnormalities despite persistence of anti-LAV titers may serve as a model for one class of response to the AIDS-associated agent. It is hoped that this pattern will prove dominant among asymptomatic homosexual men with antibody to LAV[7] or HTLV-III.[10] Indeed, in one series the majority of homosexual men with decreased T_H:T_S ratios and depressed lymphocyte proliferation in response to T-cell mitogens, many of whom would be expected to have antibody to LAV on the basis of the present study and others, later had normalization of these values.[20] Clearly, however, the development of anti-LAV antibody is inadequate to

Table 3. Clinical, Serologic, and Immunologic Correlates of Prodromal AIDS.

Patient No.	Clinical Presentation*	T_H:T_S Ratio*	IgG Antibody to LAV	Months between Blood Sampling & Clinical AIDS
1	Lymphadenopathy, no constitutional symptoms	1.00	+	11
2	Epistaxis; immune thrombocytopenic purpura	0.50	+	11
3	Lymphadenopathy, fever, malaise	0.60	+	2
4	Lymphadenopathy, fever, oral candidiasis	0.53	+	5
5	Healthy	0.27	+	9

*Status on date that serum was obtained.

mitigate the effects of the carrier state for AIDS, and mother-to-infant transmission occurs in the presence of such immunoglobulin (Table 2). This is consistent with the finding that antibody to HTLV-I or HTLV-II[21] and HTLV-III (Gallo RC: personal communication) has minimal or no viral neutralizing capacity in vitro in the presence or absence of complement. Complement alone appears to be a natural defense mechanism against horizontal retroviral infection in animals and human beings[22]; the HTLV family and LAV may represent the only known retroviruses resistant to its action.

The relatively lower incidence of antibody to LAV in patients with AIDS as compared with those with the putative prodromes of AIDS need not be a deterrent to defining the etiologic role of the antibody. Although isohemagglutinin titers, serum immunoglobulin levels, and specific secondary antibody responses may be normal or increased in AIDS,[23] primary antibody responses to antigens such as keyhole-limpet hemocyanin[15] or pneumococcal polysaccharide[24] are markedly diminished, rendering serologic analysis of this population imperfect. Among patients with AIDS, the more pronounced depression of T_H:T_S ratios in the group with opportunistic infection, as compared with groups with other manifestations and prodromes of AIDS,[25] may also make serologic identification of the former group difficult. Direct isolation of a virus will not resolve this problem since only a small fraction (5 to 12 percent[3]) of OKT4+ lymphocytes are susceptible to LAV infection — a population that may be destroyed late in the disease, before the virus has been identified. In addition, patients with AIDS whose mitogen-stimulation responses and T_H:T_S ratios are in the normal range have been identified in this and in other studies, although these values tend to reverse as the syndrome progresses (as in Child 1 and women connected with drug abuse[26]). This reversal is probably related to the measurement of total OKT4+ populations, whereas the defect in AIDS appears to be limited to a portion of T cells within the T4/Leu-8+ subset.[27] Of interest in this regard is the ability of LAV to infect, by a co-cultivation protocol detailed elsewhere,[3] both T4/Leu-8+ and T4/Leu-8− T-lymphocyte subsets derived from normal donors (Chermann J-C: unpublished observations).

Finally, the disappearance of the anti-LAV antibody in one patient with AIDS may be important. Studies are in progress to determine whether a decrease in anti-LAV titer signals a poor prognosis in AIDS. However, antibody to a 110,000-dalton LAV glycoprotein has been found in all patients with AIDS, including the ten who lose detectable anti-LAV core antibody as the disease progresses (Chermann J-C: unpublished data).

The absence of LAV-reactive antibody in serum collected from healthy controls and patients with genetic immunodeficiency over a period contemporary with the AIDS epidemic in the United States, identification of an AIDS carrier state implicated in maternal–infant transmission, and serologic data in this and in other reports lend credence to the concept that LAV is at least a marker for AIDS, and strengthens the argument for a pathophysiologic association.

We are indebted to Drs. Anit Warren and Charlotte Cunningham-Rundles for supplying several patients' samples.

References

1. Barré-Sinoussi F, Chermann J-C, Rey F, et al. Isolation of a T-lymphotropic retrovirus from a patient at risk for acquired immune deficiency syndrome (AIDS). Science 1983; 220:868-71.
2. Vilmer E, Barré-Sinoussi F, Rouzioux C, et al. Isolation of new lymphotropic retrovirus from two siblings with hemophilia B, one with AIDS. Lancet 1984; 2:753-7.
3. Montagnier L, Chermann J-C, Barré-Sinoussi F, et al. A new human T-lymphotropic retrovirus: characterization and possible role in lymphadenopathy and acquired immune deficiency syndromes. In: Gallo RC, Essex M, Gross L, eds. Human T-cell leukemia/lymphoma viruses. Cold Spring Harbor, N.Y.: Cold Spring Harbor Press (in press).
4. Klatzmann D, Barré-Sinoussi F, Nugeyre MT, et al. Selective tropism of lymphadenopathy associated virus (LAV) for helper-inducer T lymphocytes. Science 1984; 225:59-62.
5. Kalyanaraman VS, Cabradilla CD, Getchell JP, et al. Antibodies to the core protein of lymphadenopathy-associated virus (LAV) in patients with AIDS. Science 1984; 225:321-3.
6. Brun-Vezinet F, Rouzioux C, Barré-Sinoussi F, et al. Detection of IgG-antibodies to lymphadenopathy-associated virus in patients with AIDS or lymphadenopathy syndrome. Lancet 1984; 1:1253-6.
7. Levy JA, Hoffman AD, Kramer SM, Landis JA, Shimabukuro JM, Oshiro LS. Isolation of lymphocytopathic retroviruses from San Francisco patients with AIDS. Science 1984; 225:840-2.
8. Schüpbach J, Popovic M, Gilden RV, Gonda MA, Sarngadharan MG, Gallo RC. Serological analysis of a subgroup of human T-lymphotropic retroviruses (HTLV-III) associated with AIDS. Science 1984; 224:503-5.
9. Sarngadharan MG, Popovic M, Bruch L, Schupbach J, Gallo RC. Antibodies reactive with human T-lymphotropic retroviruses (HTLV-III) in the serum of patients with AIDS. Science 1984; 224:506-8.
10. Safai B, Sarngadharan MG, Groopman JE, et al. Seroepidemiological studies of human T-lymphotropic retrovirus type III in acquired immunodeficiency syndrome. Lancet 1984; 1:1438-40.
11. Des Jarlis DC, Marmor M, Cohen H, et al. Antibodies to a retrovirus etiologically associated with acquired immunodeficiency syndrome (AIDS) in populations with increased incidences of the syndrome. MMWR 1984; 33:377-9.
12. Krause RM. Koch's postulates and the search for the AIDS agent. Rev Infect Dis 1984; 6:270-9.
13. Laurence J, Gottlieb AB, Kunkel HG. Soluble suppressor factors in patients with acquired immune deficiency syndrome and its prodromes: elaboration in vitro by T lymphocyte-adherent cell interactions. J Clin Invest 1983; 72:2072-81.
14. Schutzer SE. Immune deficiency in children and its association with the acquired immune deficiency syndrome. In: Friedman-Kien A, Laubenstein L, eds. AIDS: the epidemic of Kaposi's sarcoma and opportunistic infections. New York: Masson, 1984:305-15.
15. Lane HC, Masur H, Edgar LC, Whalen G, Rook AH, Fauci AS. Abnormalities of B-cell activation and immunoregulation in patients with the acquired immunodeficiency syndrome. N Engl J Med 1983; 309:453-8.
16. Laurence J, Mayer L. Immunoregulatory lymphokines of T hybridomas from AIDS patients: constitutive and inducible suppressor factors. Science 1984; 225:66-9.
17. The cause of AIDS? Lancet 1984; 2:1053-4.
18. Gilmer E, Fischer A, Griscelli C, et al. Possible transmission of a human lymphotropic retrovirus (LAV) from mother to infant with AIDS. Lancet 1984; 1:229-30.
19. Feorino PM, Kalyanaraman VS, Haverkos HW, et al. Lymphadenopathy associated virus infection of a blood donor-recipient pair with acquired immunodeficiency syndrome. Science 1984; 225:69-72.
20. Gerstoft J, Dickmeiss E, Bentsen K, et al. The prognosis of asymptomatic homosexual men with decreased T-helper to T-suppressor ratio. Scand J Immunol 1984; 19:275-80.
21. Hoshino H, Tanaka H, Miwa M, Okada H. Human T-cell leukaemia virus is not lysed by human serum. Nature 1984; 310:324-5.
22. Bartholomew RM, Esser AF, Müller-Eberhard HJ. Lysis of oncornaviruses by human serum: isolation of the viral complement (C1) receptor and identification as p15E. J Exp Med 1978; 147:844-53.
23. Masur H, Michelis MA, Greene JB, et al. An outbreak of community-acquired *Pneumocystis carinii* pneumonia: initial manifestation of cellular immune dysfunction. N Engl J Med 1981; 305:1431-8.

24. Ammann AJ, Schiffman G, Abrams D, Volberding P, Ziegler J, Conant M. B-cell immunodeficiency in acquired immune deficiency syndrome. JAMA 1984; 251:1447-9.
25. Fahey JL, Prince H, Weaver M, et al. Quantitative changes in T helper or T suppressor/cytotoxic lymphocyte subsets that distinguish acquired immune deficiency syndrome from other immune subset disorders. Am J Med 1984; 76:95-100.
26. Masur H, Michelis MA, Wormser GP, et al. Opportunistic infection in previously healthy women: initial manifestations of a community-acquired cellular immunodeficiency. Ann Intern Med 1982; 97:533-9.
27. Nicholson JKA, McDougal JS, Spira TJ, Cross GD, Jones BM, Reinherz EL. Immunoregulatory subsets of the T helper and T suppressor cell populations in homosexual men with chronic unexplained lymphadenopathy. J Clin Invest 1984; 73:191-201.

ORIGINAL ARTICLE

PREDICTORS OF THE ACQUIRED IMMUNODEFICIENCY SYNDROME DEVELOPING IN A COHORT OF SEROPOSITIVE HOMOSEXUAL MEN

B. Frank Polk, M.D., Robin Fox, M.S., Ron Brookmeyer, Ph.D., Sukon Kanchanaraksa, Ph.D., Richard Kaslow, M.D., Barbara Visscher, M.D., Dr.P.H., Charles Rinaldo, Ph.D., and John Phair, M.D.*

Abstract In a cohort of 1835 homosexual men who were seropositive for human immunodeficiency virus (HIV) on entry into a prospective study, the acquired immunodeficiency syndrome (AIDS) developed in 59 during a median follow-up of 15 months. We matched 5 seropositive controls to each case according to study center and date of enrollment and performed a case–control analysis to determine factors predictive of AIDS.

In a multivariate analysis, a decreased number of T helper lymphocytes, an increased number of T suppressor lymphocytes, a low level of antibody to HIV, a high titer of cytomegalovirus antibody, and a history of sex with someone in whom AIDS developed were independently associated with subsequent AIDS. Separate analyses of risk factors for Kaposi's sarcoma and opportunistic infections failed to support previously reported associations between the use of nitrites or an elevated cytomegalovirus-antibody titer and Kaposi's sarcoma.

These variables may be markers rather than determinants of disease progression. A vigorous antibody response to HIV infection may confer at least temporary protection against the progression of immunodeficiency to AIDS, or a low level of antibody to HIV may reflect a later stage of infection. The increased risk associated with a history of sex with someone in whom AIDS developed may indicate earlier infection in cases or infection with a more virulent strain of HIV. These results may be useful in counseling HIV-seropositive persons and in designing studies of clinical interventions.

RISK factors for infection with human immunodeficiency virus (HIV) have been identified and widely publicized.[1] However, the risk that the acquired immunodeficiency syndrome (AIDS) will develop in a given period following HIV infection has been estimated only in small, selected populations.[2-7] Estimates of the risk of AIDS among HIV-infected populations range from 6.4 percent in 61 months[2] to 34 percent in three years.[5] Methodologic reasons for the observed differences include selection criteria, duration of follow-up, analytic techniques, and unknown duration of infection among persons with prevalent HIV infection. Suggested determinants of risk include age,[2] the use of nitrite inhalants,[3] and the geographic location of the study[5]; the markers reported to be most strongly predictive of disease progression include the number of T helper lymphocytes,[7] antigen-stimulated lymphocyte proliferation,[4] and gamma-interferon generation.[4] However, differences in the design and analysis of these disparate, small studies make comparisons difficult. Neither determinants of risk nor markers of disease progression have been systematically explored in prospective studies. We tried to determine which factors were associated with or predictive of subsequent AIDS in a large cohort of homosexual men who were seropositive at the time of enrollment in a longitudinal follow-up study.

Methods

Population

The Multicenter AIDS Cohort Study enrolled 4955 homosexual and bisexual men from four cities during the period April 1984 through March 1985. Other than sexual orientation, the only eligibility criteria were that the subjects had to be more than 17 years old and give informed consent. The only exclusion criterion was a prior diagnosis of AIDS. Study participants were recruited through general publicity, announcements in the gay press, meetings and forums, and word-of-mouth communication in the gay community. Study centers were located in Baltimore (n = 1153), Chicago (n = 1102), Pittsburgh (n = 1063), and Los Angeles (n = 1637). The study was approved by institutional review boards in all the affiliated institutions. The confidentiality of the data was assured by certificates of confidentiality issued by the Secretary of Health and Human Services to each study center.

Study Design

Participants were seen every six months in their respective study centers. At each visit, they were interviewed and examined, and specimens were taken for laboratory studies. Data collection at base line and at each follow-up visit included demographic information, a directed physical examination, and a questionnaire administered by a trained interviewer. The questionnaire asked about past and recent medical history, medicinal and recreational drug use, any history of travel to high-prevalence areas, specific sexual practices, and any changes in these practices.

The overall one-year follow-up rate was 91 percent in Baltimore, 82 percent in Chicago, 83 percent in Los Angeles, and 80 percent in Pittsburgh. As of December 16, 1985, 59 incident cases of AIDS had been diagnosed, all in participants who were seropositive for HIV at base line. The median observation period for all partici-

*The following investigators participated in the study: *Baltimore* — The Johns Hopkins University School of Hygiene and Public Health: B. Frank Polk, M.D., M.Sc. (principal investigator); Robin Fox, M.S.; and Ron Brookmeyer, Ph.D.; University of Maryland Cancer Center: Richard Leavitt, M.D.; *Chicago* — Howard Brown Memorial Clinic–Northwestern University Medical School: John P. Phair, M.D. (principal investigator); Joan S. Chmiel, Ph.D.; and David G. Ostrow, M.D., Ph.D.; *Los Angeles* — University of California, Los Angeles, Schools of Public Health and Medicine: Roger Detels, M.D., M.S. (principal investigator); Barbara R. Visscher, M.D., Dr.P.H.; John L. Fahey, M.D., M.S.; Janis V. Giorgi, Ph.D.; and Jan Dudley, M.P.H.; *Pittsburgh* — University of Pittsburgh, Graduate School of Public Health and School of Medicine: Charles R. Rinaldo, Jr., Ph.D. (principal investigator); Monto Ho, M.D.; Lawrence A. Kingsley, Dr.P.H.; Ronald O. Valdiserri, M.D.; David W. Lyter, M.D.; and Alan Winkelstein, M.D.; *Bethesda* — National Institutes of Allergy and Infectious Diseases: Richard A. Kaslow, M.D., M.P.H.; Alfred J. Saah, M.D., M.P.H.; Mark J. Van Raden, M.A.; and Rachel E. Solomon, M.H.S.; National Cancer Institute: Andrew A. Monjan, Ph.D., M.P.H.; and A.R. Patel, Ph.D.

Supported by research contracts AI-32511, AI-32513, AI-32520, and AI-32535.

pants in the study through December 1985 was 15 months. All AIDS cases were verified by a pathology report, with the exception of one whose cause of death was listed on the death certificate as AIDS. One case had an unknown date of diagnosis and was not included in the time-dependent analyses.

Each case was matched with five seropositive controls according to study center and enrollment date (within three weeks). Controls were selected by means of a random-numbers table from among the eligible persons. An AIDS case could serve as a control for another AIDS case if his disease was diagnosed after that of the case for which he was selected as a control (this occurred in three instances).

Definition of Study Variables

Base-line information about the following selected variables was included in the analysis: age, race (white or nonwhite), body-mass index (weight/height^2), and the presence of lymphadenopathy at any two or more noncontiguous sites other than the inguinal region. Interview variables selected for analysis were the use of nitrites during sex within two years (yes/no); herpes zoster infection within six months (yes/no); ever having had sex with someone with AIDS or in whom AIDS later developed (yes/no); and having had anal-receptive sex within two years (with none, one/some, or most/all of their male partners). The AIDS-related complex variable was defined as the presence of two or more of the following: self-reported fatigue or diarrhea or fever higher than 37.8°C lasting two or more weeks within the preceding six months; self-reported unintentional weight loss of 4.5 kg or more within the preceding six months; and potassium hydroxide–confirmed oral thrush on physical examination.

Laboratory variables included the hemoglobin level; platelet count; monocyte count; presence of hepatitis B surface antigen; level of antibody to cytomegalovirus (International Diagnostic Technology, San Jose, Calif.); levels of IgA, IgG, and IgM (International Diagnostic Technology); and presence of anti-HIV antibody demonstrated by enzyme-linked immunosorbent assay (ELISA) (E.I. DuPont, Wilmington, Del.).[8] Total numbers of T cells (Leu-4), T helper/inducer cells (Leu-3), and T suppressor/cytotoxic cells (Leu-2) were determined by direct immunofluorescence with use of monoclonal antibodies (Becton Dickinson, Mountain View, Calif.) and two-color flow cytometry (Coulter Epics-C) on either whole-blood or Ficoll–Hypaque separated mononuclear cells.[9] Absolute numbers of T cells were calculated with use of the white-cell count and differential.

Statistical Analysis

Relative odds and significance levels were calculated by matched case–control methods.[10] Patients whose disease was diagnosed shortly after their base-line visit (0 to 9 months) were separated from those whose disease was diagnosed later (10 to 18 months). Such a time stratification may distinguish variables predictive of an early diagnosis of AIDS from those predictive of a later diagnosis.

A multivariate conditional logistic regression analysis was performed to determine which factors, when considered together, were the best predictors of subsequent AIDS within the follow-up period of 18 months. Interaction effects with the length of time after enrollment were also included in the logistic regression model. These time-interaction terms enabled us to identify variables for which the effect on the risk of AIDS varied with the length of time after enrollment.

Results

The median age of all participants at base line was 32 years. Ninety-five percent were white, 76 percent were employed full-time, and 87 percent had attended at least some college. The overall prevalence of antibody to HIV was 36 percent, with considerable variability among study centers (Baltimore, 31 percent; Chicago, 43 percent; Pittsburgh, 21 percent; and Los Angeles, 51 percent).

After a median follow-up of this cohort of approximately 15 months, AIDS had developed in 59 of the 1835 participants who were seropositive on entry. The approximate annual incidence rates were 2.6 percent in the 637 asymptomatic men, 3.2 percent in the 1094 with lymphadenopathy at their first visit, and 8.6 percent in the 104 with AIDS-related complex. The AIDS cases and the proportion of the seropositive men in whom AIDS developed were distributed according to center as follows: Baltimore, 13 (3.6 percent); Chicago, 9 (1.9 percent); Pittsburgh, 6 (2.7 percent); and Los Angeles, 31 (3.7 percent). Thirty-four of the cases presented with an opportunistic infection (24 with *Pneumocystis carinii* pneumonia, 4 with cryptococcal meningitis, 3 with cerebral toxoplasmosis, 2 with cryptosporidiosis, and 1 with esophageal candidiasis). Twenty-three presented with Kaposi's sarcoma alone, 1 had both Kaposi's sarcoma and pneumocystis pneumonia, and 1 (identified on his death certificate as having had AIDS) had no specific diagnosis.

The crude relative odds for the variables analyzed are shown in Table 1. Factors predicting AIDS that will develop at some distant time will probably be of greater interest and utility than factors predicting AIDS that will develop in the near future. Accordingly, as Table 1 shows, we have attempted to identify separately the predictors of AIDS that developed within nine months of enrollment (23 patients) and the predictors of AIDS that developed 10 to 18 months after enrollment (35 patients). The following 10 base-line variables were significantly associated with the development of AIDS in the analysis not stratified according to time: a history of sex with someone with AIDS or in whom AIDS later developed, the presence of AIDS-related complex, a reduced hemoglobin level, a reduced platelet count, a lowered monocyte count, a reduced number of T helper lymphocytes, elevated levels of serum IgA and IgM, a higher serum titer of cytomegalovirus antibody, and a lower serum "level" of HIV antibody. The following were not significantly associated with the development of AIDS in the analysis not stratified according to time: age, race, the number of partners in the previous two years, the frequency of anal-receptive intercourse in the previous two years, the use of nitrites ("poppers") during sex in the previous two years, a history of herpes zoster in the previous two years, the body-mass index, the presence of lymphadenopathy, the T suppressor lymphocyte count, the serum IgG level, and the presence of hepatitis B surface antigen.

When we stratified the univariate analysis according to the length of time since diagnosis, 10 base-line variables were associated with the "early onset" (within nine months of enrollment) of AIDS: a large number of partners in the two years before study enrollment; the presence of AIDS-related complex; a decreased hemoglobin level; reduced numbers of platelets, monocytes, and T helper lymphocytes; increased serum IgA, IgM, and cytomegalovirus antibody; and a reduced level of HIV antibody. Six variables were associated with the "late onset" (10 to 18 months after enrollment) of AIDS: a history of sex with someone with AIDS or in whom AIDS subsequently developed,

Table 1. Crude Relative Odds ($\widehat{RO}$) for AIDS at Any Time, within 9 Months of Enrollment, and 10 to 18 Months after Enrollment.*

Base-Line Variable	Overall (N = 59) $\widehat{RO}$	Overall P Value	≤9 Months (N = 23) $\widehat{RO}$	≤9 Months P Value	10–18 Months (N = 35) $\widehat{RO}$	10–18 Months P Value
Age (yr)						
≤30	1.00		1.00		1.00	
31–40	1.68	0.21	1.14	0.35	2.23	0.19
>40	1.90		1.49		1.94	
Race						
White	1.00		1.00		1.00	
Nonwhite	0.70	0.42	0.99	1.00	0.57	0.37
No. of partners in previous 2 yr						
≤20	1.00		1.00		1.00	
21–100	1.49	0.29	2.45	0.05	1.09	0.85
>100	1.81		4.54		0.82	
Anal-receptive intercourse in previous 2 yr						
None	1.00		1.00		1.00	
Some partners	0.70	0.45	0.62	0.28	1.03	0.98
Most partners	0.50		0.27		0.94	
Used nitrites during sex in previous 2 yr						
No	1.00		1.00		1.00	
Yes	0.69	0.31	0.58	0.30	1.00	1.00
Herpes zoster in previous 2 yr						
No	1.00				1.00	
Yes	3.33	0.16	None reported		3.33	0.16
Sex with someone in whom AIDS developed						
No	1.00		1.00		1.00	
Yes	2.74	<0.01	1.96	0.16	3.63	<0.01
Body-mass index†						
≤0.030	1.00		1.00		1.00	
0.031–0.035	0.76	0.55	0.79	0.65	0.66	0.62
>0.035	1.07		1.29		1.84	
Lymphadenopathy						
No	1.00		1.00		1.00	
Yes	1.18	0.62	1.11	0.85	1.43	0.41
AIDS-related complex						
No	1.00		1.00		1.00	
Yes	4.44	<0.01	6.39	<0.01	1.28	0.84
Hemoglobin (g/dl)						
≤13.5	1.00		1.00		1.00	
13.6–15.5	0.16	<0.01	0.06	<0.01	0.28	0.03
>15.5	0.14		0.09		0.17	
Platelets (per mm³)						
≤150,000	1.00		1.00		1.00	
151,000–300,000	0.74	<0.01‡	0.51	<0.01‡	0.90	<0.71‡
>300,000	0.58		0.26		2.00	
Monocytes (per mm³)						
≤100	1.00		1.00		1.00	
101–150	0.35	<0.01	0.35	<0.01	0.32	0.17
>150	0.26		0.10		0.49	
T helper lymphocytes (per mm³)						
≤300	1.00		1.00		1.00	
>300	0.06	<0.01	0.02	<0.01	0.10	<0.01
T suppressor lymphocytes (per mm³)						
≤600	1.00		1.00		1.00	
601–1000	1.10	0.37	0.55	0.47	2.01	0.05
>1000	1.65		0.59		3.69	
IgG (mg/dl)						
≤1730	1.00		1.00		1.00	
1731–2360	1.49	0.32	1.31	0.41	1.84	0.43
>2360	1.75		2.16		1.71	
IgA (mg/dl)						
≤220	1.00		1.00		1.00	
221–370	1.57	<0.01	1.54	<0.01	1.55	<0.01
>370	6.80		8.64		5.77	
IgM (mg/dl)						
≤130	1.00		1.00		1.00	
131–200	1.87	<0.01‡	2.60	0.03‡	1.80	0.02‡
>200	2.04		1.37		3.16	
CMV antibody (mg/dl)						
≤300	1.00		1.00		1.00	
>300	1.94	0.03	2.88	0.02	1.41	0.39
HIV antibody (OD)§						
<2.2	1.00		1.00		1.00	
2.2–3.0	0.40	<0.01	0.32	0.02	0.45	0.07
>3.0	0.14		0.11		0.18	
HBsAg						
No	1.00		1.00		1.00	
Yes	1.43	0.42	1.14	0.87	1.61	0.37

*The reference category for crude relative odds ($\widehat{RO}$) is RO = 1.00. CMV denotes cytomegalovirus, and HBsAg hepatitis B surface antigen.

†Body-mass index = weight in pounds/height in inches^2.

‡The P value is based on a test for linear trend; all other P values are based on statistical tests for differences among categories.

§HIV antibody was assayed with licensed DuPont ELISA kits; the results are reported in optical-density (OD) units.

a reduced hemoglobin level, a decreased number of T helper lymphocytes, an increased number of T suppressor lymphocytes, elevated serum IgA, and elevated serum IgM.

The analysis was repeated separately for cases presenting with Kaposi's sarcoma and for cases presenting with opportunistic infection (Table 2). The participant who presented with both was included with the cases of Kaposi's sarcoma. Variables associated with both types of presentation included a decreased hemoglobin level, a decreased number of T helper lymphocytes, and an increased serum IgA level. Variables associated only with AIDS presenting as an opportunistic infection were a history of herpes zoster in the two years preceding enrollment, a history of sex with someone in whom AIDS developed, the presence of AIDS-related complex, a reduced monocyte count, an elevated level of cytomegalovirus antibody, and a reduced level of HIV antibody. It is worthy of note that neither the use of nitrites during sexual activity in the previous two years nor an elevated titer of cytomegalovirus antibody was associated with Kaposi's sarcoma.

All the variables that were significant in the univariate analysis were used to develop a multiple logistic regression model. The final multivariate model is shown in Table 3. A few variables that were significant in one of the univariate analyses were not significant in the final model, suggesting a correlation between or among variables. Those that did not continue to be significant included the presence of AIDS-related complex, a decreased hemoglobin level, decreased numbers of monocytes and platelets, elevated serum IgA and IgM, a history of herpes zoster, and the number of partners in the previous two years. Significant independent predictors of AIDS included a reduced number of T helper lymphocytes, an increased number of T suppressor lymphocytes, a reduced amount of serum antibody to HIV, an elevated amount of serum antibody to cytomegalovirus, and a history of

Table 2. Crude Relative Odds ($\widehat{RO}$) for AIDS with Kaposi's Sarcoma and with Opportunistic Infection*

Base-Line Variable	Kaposi's Sarcoma (N = 24)		Opportunistic Infection (N = 34)	
	$\widehat{RO}$	P value	$\widehat{RO}$	P value
Age (10-yr increment)	1.05	0.20	1.03	0.17
Race				
White	1.00		1.00	
Nonwhite	0.92	0.90	0.59	0.35
No. of partners in previous 2 yr				
≤20	1.00		1.00	
21–100	1.58	0.57	1.36	0.70
>100	1.74		1.56	
Anal-receptive intercourse in previous 2 yr				
None	1.00		1.00	
Some partners	0.71	0.49	0.70	0.89
Most partners	0.39		0.66	
Used nitrites during sex in previous 2 yr				
No	1.00		1.00	
Yes	0.42	0.09	0.97	0.96
Herpes zoster in previous 2 yr				
No	None reported		1.00	
Yes			10.00	0.02
Sex with someone in whom AIDS developed				
No	1.00		1.00	
Yes	1.64	0.27	4.07	<0.01
Body-mass index†				
≤0.030	1.00		1.00	
0.031–0.035	0.97	0.86	0.73	0.27
>0.035	0.70		1.48	
Lymphadenopathy				
No	1.00		1.00	
Yes	0.52	0.22	1.72	0.22
AIDS-related complex				
No	1.00		1.00	
Yes	4.32	0.06	4.51	<0.01
Hemoglobin (g/dl)				
≤13.5	1.00		1.00	
13.6–15.5	0.11	<0.01	0.16	<0.01
>15.5	0.13		0.12	
Platelets (per mm³)				
≤150,000	1.00		1.00	
151,000–300,000	0.73	0.82	0.65	0.79
>300,000	1.02		0.79	
Monocytes (per mm³)				
≤100	1.00		1.00	
>100	0.41	0.12	0.20	<0.01
T helper lymphocytes (per mm³)				
≤300	1.00		1.00	
301–600	0.03	<0.01	0.15	<0.01
>600	0.01		0.03	
T suppressor lymphocytes (per mm³)				
≤600	1.00		1.00	
601–1000	1.49	0.68	0.76	0.30
>1000	1.83		1.52	
IgG (mg/dl)				
≤1730	1.00		1.00	
>1730	2.32	0.11	1.23	0.63
IgA (mg/dl)				
≤370	1.00		1.00	
>370	7.04	<0.01	5.07	<0.01
IgM (mg/dl)				
≤200	1.00		1.00	
>200	1.25	0.63	1.75	0.15
CMV antibody (mg/dl)				
≤300	1.00		1.00	
>300	1.09	0.86	2.91	<0.01
HIV antibody (OD)‡				
<2.2	1.00		1.00	
2.2–3.0	0.34	0.07	0.45	<0.01
>3.0	0.18		0.11	
HBsAg				
No	1.00		1.00	
Yes	2.34	0.18	1.04	0.95

*The reference category for crude relative odds ($\widehat{RO}$) is RO = 1.00. CMV denotes cytomegalovirus, and HBsAg hepatitis B surface antigen.

†Body-mass index = weight in pounds/height in inches².

‡HIV antibody was assayed with licensed DuPont ELISA kits; the results are reported in optical density (OD) units.

Table 3. Risk Factors for the Development of AIDS in a Cohort of Homosexual Men Seropositive for HIV.

	β*	P Value†
No. of T helper lymphocytes‡	−7.09	0.01
T helper lymphocytes × months since base line	0.36	0.03
No. of T suppressor lymphocytes‡	1.68	0.01
HIV antibody "level"§	−1.45	0.02
CMV antibody level¶	0.002	0.02
History of sex with someone with AIDS or in whom AIDS later developed‖	0.96	0.05

*Estimated regression coefficients in linear logistic regression model.
†Level of significance in the final multivariate logistic regression model.
‡Continuous, per 10 lymphocytes. §Continuous, per 0.1 OD (optical density unit).
¶Continuous, per 10 mg per deciliter. ‖No = 0, yes = 1.

sex with someone in whom AIDS developed. One interaction term is included: the number of T helper lymphocytes times the number of months since study enrollment. This term entered the model after the main effect of the number of T helper lymphocytes, suggesting the especially strong predictive power of a reduced number of T helper lymphocytes just before the diagnosis of AIDS is made.

Discussion

Our objective was to identify independent predictors of incident AIDS in a cohort of seropositive homosexual men and to distinguish markers of the progression to AIDS from determinants of that progression over a given observation period. In the final multiple logistic model, five independent variables and one interaction term were significant independent predictors of the development of AIDS: a reduced number of T helper lymphocytes; an interaction between T helper lymphocytes and the time since enrollment; an elevated number of T suppressor lymphocytes; a reduced level of HIV serum antibody; an elevated titer of cytomegalovirus antibody; and a history of sex with someone with AIDS or in whom AIDS later developed. In a study of only 59 cases, the finding of five independent, significantly associated variables is somewhat striking and suggests strong associations. Three of the final five variables are almost certainly markers of disease progression rather than determinants of disease — namely, an increased number of T suppressor lymphocytes, a decreased number of T helper lymphocytes, and an increased level of antibody to cytomegalovirus. These may simply indicate that a person infected with HIV has progressive immunodeficiency. As others have suggested, the number of T suppressor lymphocytes may be an early indicator,[11] whereas a decrease in the number of T helper lymphocytes is an especially strong indicator later in the course of HIV infection.[12] As cell-mediated immunity declines, reactivation and systemic infection with cytomegalovirus infection is common,[13] stimulating the production of specific antibody to cytomegalovirus. It is noteworthy that a number of variables that are well known to be associated with the risk of HIV infection (frequency of anal-receptive intercourse, number of sex partners) are not associated with the development of AIDS, once a person is infected.

A reduced level of serum antibody to HIV is also significantly predictive of the development of AIDS. The simplest (and perhaps most likely) explanation is that the level of antibody to HIV declines as the burden of infection with this virus is progressively reduced as a consequence of declining numbers of its target cells — T helper lymphocytes and monocytes.[14] Others have suggested that, as acquired immunodeficiency progresses, the quantity of virus present declines.[15] An alternative and somewhat more provocative explanation is that a vigorous humoral response to HIV infection may protect against the progression of immunodeficiency to AIDS, at least temporarily. Finally, the decline in antibody to HIV may be the result of B-lymphocyte dysfunction,[16] although the increased titer of antibody to cytomegalovirus argues against this explanation.

The significant association between a history of sex with someone in whom AIDS developed and the development of AIDS in the cases is noteworthy. This exposure variable may simply be a marker of infection of longer standing, since the cases who gave positive responses to this question had had the infection long enough for AIDS to develop in both themselves and at least one sex partner. Somewhat more intriguing is the possibility that some strains of HIV are more virulent than others. Comparative studies of base-line HIV isolates from cases and controls might be of considerable interest.

A few variables that were significantly associated with the subsequent development of AIDS in the univariate analysis did not continue to be significant in the final model. These included the presence of AIDS-related complex, a decreased hemoglobin level, a decreased monocyte count and platelet count, and elevated serum IgA and IgM levels. It is likely that the information contained in these variables is captured by the lymphocyte (T helpers and T suppressors) and antibody (cytomegalovirus and HIV) variables. If so, the former may be useful surrogates, since tests for them are more widely available and less expensive than studies of T-cell subsets and semiquantitative serologic studies. Furthermore, our failure to find a statistically significant association in some instances may be the result of the small number of AIDS cases, especially when they were divided into subsets.

A major limitation to case–control studies of subjects with prevalent HIV infection is the lack of information about the date of infection.[17] We do not know how long the participants who were seropositive at enrollment had been infected with HIV. All the variables we have identified as significant predictors of AIDS could be surrogates for the duration of infection. We attempted to account for this, in part, by matching according to study center, since epidemiologic data suggest that the epidemic of HIV infection began earlier in Los Angeles than in our other sites. However, this matching probably failed to control adequately for the confounding by the duration of infection. Only prospective studies of incident HIV infection will clarify this point.

We failed to confirm the association between the use of nitrites and the development of Kaposi's sarcoma that has been observed by some investigators.[18] It should be noted that we asked about nitrite use only within two years of entry into the study and that we did not attempt to quantify usage in this analysis. It is thus possible that we have missed or obscured a meaningful association; future analyses of quantitative data on nitrite use from our study should resolve this issue.

Future nested case–control studies within the Multicenter AIDS Cohort Study with larger numbers of cases will markedly improve our statistical power to identify additional significant predictors. Moreover, early predictors of AIDS that will develop later in the course of HIV infection are obviously of more interest than markers that appear just before diagnosis, especially since some of the former may be disease determinants or effect modifiers. Our current results may be useful in counseling seropositive persons and in designing clinical-intervention studies, and they should help to refine currently available disease classifications.[19-21] Variables predictive of AIDS in this population of homosexual men may not be predictive in other groups, such as intravenous drug users. Only comparable studies in disparate populations will clarify this point. We will confirm our observations with prospective analyses of cohorts of seropositive participants stratified according to predictors identified in this nested case–control analysis. Obviously, the future analysis of participants who were seronegative on entry into the study and then seroconverted should provide the most information bearing on the central question of our natural-history study: why AIDS develops in some persons infected with HIV and not in others, at least for a long time. The answer to this question is one of the major variables that will determine the ultimate magnitude of the epidemic of AIDS.

References

1. Curran JW, Morgan WM, Hardy AM, Jaffe HW, Darrow WW, Dowdle WR. The epidemiology of AIDS: current status and future prospects. Science 1985; 229:1352-7.
2. Jaffe HW, Darrow WW, Echenberg DF, et al. The acquired immunodeficiency syndrome in a cohort of homosexual men: a six-year follow-up study. Ann Intern Med 1985; 103:210-4.
3. Mathur-Wagh U, Mildvan D, Senie RT. Follow-up at 4½ years on homosexual men with generalized lymphadenopathy. N Engl J Med 1985; 313:1542-3.
4. Murray HW, Hillman JK, Rubin BY, et al. Patients at risk for AIDS-related opportunistic infections: clinical manifestations and impaired gamma interferon production. N Engl J Med 1985; 313:1504-10.
5. Goedert JJ, Biggar RJ, Weiss SH, et al. Three-year incidence of AIDS in five cohorts of HTLV-III–infected risk group members. Science 1986; 231:992-5.
6. Jaffe HW, Sarngadharan MG, DeVico AL, et al. Infection with HTLV-III/LAV and transfusion-associated acquired immunodeficiency syndrome: serologic evidence of an association. JAMA 1985; 254:770-3.
7. Stevens CE, Taylor PE, Zang EA, et al. Human T-cell lymphotropic virus type III infection in a cohort of homosexual men in New York City. JAMA 1986; 255:2167-72.
8. Sàrngadharan MG, Popovic M, Bruch L, Schüpbach J, Gallo RC. Antibodies reactive with human T-lymphotropic retrovirus (HTLV-III) in the serum of patients with AIDS. Science 1984; 224; 224:506-8.
9. Reinherz EL, King PC, Goldstein G, Schlossman SF. Further characterization of the human inducer T cell subset defined by monoclonal antibody. J Immunol 1979; 123:2894-6.
10. Breslow NE, Day NE. Statistical methods in cancer research. Vol. 1. The analysis of case-control studies. Lyon: International Agency for Research on Cancer, 1980. (IARC scientific publication no. 32.)
11. Schwartz K, Visscher BR, Detels R, Taylor J, Nishanian P, Fahey JL. Immunological changes in lymphadenopathy virus positive and negative symptomless male homosexuals: two years of observation. Lancet 1985; 2:831-2.
12. Goedert JJ, Biggar RJ, Melbye M, et al. Effect of T4 count and cofactors on incidence of AIDS in homosexual men infected with human immunodeficiency virus. JAMA (in press).
13. Ho M. Cytomegalovirus: biology and infection. New York: Plenum, 1982: 309.
14. Smith PD, Ohura K, Masur H, Lane HC, Fauci AS, Wahl SM. Monocyte function in the acquired immune deficiency syndrome: defective chemotaxis. J Clin Invest 1984; 74:2121-8.
15. Salahuddin SZ, Markham PD, Popovic M, et al. Isolation of infectious human T-cell leukemia/lymphotropic virus type III (HTLV-III) from patients with acquired immunodeficiency syndrome (AIDS) or AIDS-related complex (ARC) and from healthy carriers: a study of risk groups and tissue sources. Proc Natl Acad Sci USA 1985; 82:5530-4.
16. Lane HC, Depper JM, Greene WC, Whalen G, Waldmann TA, Fauci AS. Qualitative analysis of immune function in patients with the acquired immunodeficiency syndrome: evidence for a selective defect in soluble antigen recognition. N Engl J Med 1985; 313:79-84.
17. Brookmeyer R, Gail M, Polk BF. The prevalent cohort study and the acquired immunodeficiency syndrome. Am J Epidemiol (in press).
18. Haverkos HW, Pinsky PF, Drotman DP, Bregman DJ. Disease manifestations among homosexual men with acquired immunodeficiency syndrome (AIDS): a possible role of nitrites in Kaposi's sarcoma. Sex Transm Dis 1985; 12:203-8.
19. Haverkos HW, Gottlieb MS, Killen JY, Edelman R. Classification of HTLV-III/LAV-related diseases. J Infect Dis 1985; 152:1095.
20. Redfield RR, Wright DC, Tramont EC. The Walter Reed staging classification for HTLV-III/LAV infection. N Engl J Med 1986; 314:131-2.
21. CDC classification system for human T-lymphotropic virus type III/lymphadenopathy-associated virus infections. MMWR 1986; 35:334-9.

ORIGINAL ARTICLE

ACQUIRED IMMUNE DEFICIENCY IN HAITIANS

Opportunistic Infections in Previously Healthy Haitian Immigrants

Jeffrey Vieira, M.D., Elliot Frank, M.D., Thomas J. Spira, M.D., and Sheldon H. Landesman, M.D.

Abstract We describe acquired immune deficiency manifested by opportunistic infections in 10 previously healthy heterosexual Haitian men. The opportunistic pathogens included *Toxoplasma gondii* (in four patients), *Cryptococcus neoformans* (in one), *Pneumocystis carinii* (in four patients), and *Candida albicans* (in three). Six of the patients also had *Mycobacterium tuberculosis.* Immunologic studies of three patients showed a decrease in the numbers and activity of helper T cells, with normal or increased populations of suppressor T cells. Serologic markers for previous infections from hepatitis A, cytomegalovirus, and herpes simplex virus were detected in several patients. Six of the patients died despite specific antimicrobial therapy. The clinical and immunologic findings in these 10 Haitians are similar to those reported in drug addicts and homosexuals with the acquired immune-deficiency syndrome.

SINCE June 1981, over 700 cases of acquired immune-deficiency syndrome (AIDS) have been reported to the Centers for Disease Control.[1-5] The syndrome has been manifested clinically by Kaposi's sarcoma or opportunistic infections (or both) in previously healthy persons. Approximately 80 percent of the cases have involved homosexual or bisexual men; the remainder have occurred in heterosexual men and women, most of whom were drug addicts.

Coincident with the unprecedented epidemic in the homosexual community are reports of 34 cases among Haitian immigrants.[6] In this article we present the clinical and immunologic features of 10 Haitians with AIDS and opportunistic infections who were evaluated at Kings County Hospital–Downstate Medical Center between January 1981 and July 1982. This outbreak was unique in that it occurred within a single ethnic group of previously healthy men without histories of homosexuality or drug abuse.

Methods

Patients were seen at Kings County Hospital–Downstate Medical Center between January 1981 and July 1982. They were evaluated and followed during their hospitalization by one of us. All patients in this series met the criteria for AIDS as defined by the Centers for Disease Control — i.e., "a disease, at least moderately predictive of a defect in cell-mediated immunity, occurring in a person with no known cause for diminished resistance to that disease."[7]

Immunologic and serologic studies were performed through the courtesy of the Centers for Disease Control. Mononuclear cells were separated by Ficoll–Hypaque (LSM Solution, Litton Bionetics, Kensington, Md.) density-gradient centrifugation. T-lymphocyte subpopulations were quantitated by indirect immunofluorescence, using commercially available monoclonal antibodies (OKT3 for T cells, OKT4 for helper/inducer T cells, and OKT8 for suppressor/cytotoxic T cells) (Ortho Diagnostic Systems, Raritan, N.J.) and a fluorescein-conjugated antimouse immunoglobulin (Centers for Disease Control) on a fluorescence-activated cell sorter (FACS IV, Becton–Dickinson, Sunnyvale, Calif.).[8] B lymphocytes were quantitated by a peroxidase-staining method, using a peroxidase-conjugated antihuman immunoglobulin (Cappel Laboratories, West Chester, Pa.).[9]

Lymphocyte-transformation responses were quantitated by a micromethod, using the mitogens phytohemagglutinin (PHA-P, Difco Laboratories, Detroit), concanavalin A (Calbiochem–Behring, La Jolla, Calif.), and pokeweed mitogen (Gibco, Grand Island, N.Y.) and the antigens candida (Hollister–Stier Laboratories, Spokane, Wash.), tetanus (Massachusetts Public Health Biologic Laboratories, Boston), streptolysin O (Difco), herpes simplex virus (Centers for Disease Control), and cytomegalovirus (Centers for Disease Control). Mononuclear cells in RPMI 1640 medium supplemented with glutamine, penicillin, streptomycin, and 10 percent heat-inactivated AB+ serum, at a concentration of either 5×10^4 or 2.5×10^4 cells per well, were incubated with optimal concentrations of the mitogens or antigens for three days (phytohemagglutinin and concanavalin A) or for six days (pokeweed mitogen and antigens) in a total volume of 0.125 ml. Sixteen hours before termination of the incubation period, the cultures were pulsed with 0.25 μCi methyl [^{3}H]thymidine (specific activity, 6.7 μCi per millimole, New England Nuclear, Boston). Cultures were harvested on glass-fiber filter paper, using a multiple automated cell harvester (Titertek, Flow Laboratories, Rockville, Md.), and filter-paper disks were placed in scintillation fluid and counted in a Beckman liquid-scintillation counter. Cultures were set up in triplicate. Mitogen-stimulation responses were normalized by comparison with mononuclear cells, frozen down in bulk, from a single normal donor. These cells were used as a control each time a patient's cells were studied. The following formula was used to express the normalized mitogen response:

$$\frac{(\text{cpm}_{\text{stimulated}} - \text{cpm}_{\text{unstimulated}})\ \text{patient}}{(\text{cpm}_{\text{stimulated}} - \text{cpm}_{\text{unstimulated}})\ \text{control}} \times 100.$$

Antigen responses were expressed as stimulation ratios — i.e., $\text{cpm}_{\text{stimulated}}/\text{cpm}_{\text{unstimulated}}$. A stimulation ratio of 3 or more was considered normal.

Titers of antibodies to cytomegalovirus,[10] herpes simplex virus,[11] syphilis (rapid plasma reagin card test), toxoplasma,[12] and hepatitis A and B virus (hepatitis B surface antigen, antibody to hepatitis B surface antigen, and antibody to hepatitis A virus) (AUSRIA II, AUSAB, and HAVAB, Abbott Laboratories, North Chicago) were quantitated as previously described.

Biopsy specimens were prepared for viral culture by washing the tissue in a balanced salt solution. The tissues were ground and a 10 percent suspension in antibiotic-containing medium was inoculatd into diploid fibroblast, monkey kidney cells, and human heteroploid cells. Cytomegalovirus was identified by its ability to grow only in human diploid cells.

Results

The clinical data concerning the 10 patients are summarized in Table 1. All were heterosexual Haitian men, and all stated that they had not used parenteral or inhalational drugs. The mean age at the time of

From the Department of Medicine, Division of Infectious Diseases, State University of New York–Downstate Medical Center, Brooklyn, and the Centers for Disease Control, Division of Immunology, Atlanta.

Table 1. Opportunistic Infections in 10 Heterosexual Haitian Men.

Patient No.	Age	Time in U.S.	Pathogens	Treatment*	Outcome
1	29	2 yr	*T. gondii* (brain abscess)	Pyrimethamine/sulfa	Died
2	25	3 mo	Miliary *M. tuberculosis*, *T. gondii* (brain abscess)	INH/rifampin	Died
3	27	1½ yr	*M. tuberculosis* (adenitis), *C. albicans* (esophagitis), *P. carinii* (pneumonitis), Cytomegalovirus (retinitis)	INH/rifampin, Ketoconazole, TMP/SMX	Died
4	34	2 yr	*P. carinii* (pneumonitis)	TMP/SMX	Died
5	39	3 yr	*M. tuberculosis* (adenitis), *P. carinii* (pneumonitis)	INH/rifampin, TMP/SMX	Survived
6	29	2 yr	*M. tuberculosis* (adenitis), *P. carinii* (pneumonitis)	INH/rifampin, TMP/SMX	Died
7	36	8 yr	Disseminated *C. neoformans*	Amphotericin B/ 5-flucytosine	Died
8	28	2 yr	*T. gondii* (brain abscess), *C. albicans* (esophagitis)	Pyrimethamine/sulfa, Ketoconazole	Survived (sick)
9	24	4 yr	*M. tuberculosis* (liver, bone marrow), *C. albicans* (esophagitis)	INH/rifampin Ketoconazole	Survived
10	28	2 yr	*T. gondii* (brain abscess), *M. tuberculosis* (pneumonitis)	Pyrimethamine/sulfa, INH/rifampin	Survived (sick)

*INH denotes isoniazid and TMP/SMX trimethoprim/sulfamethoxazole.

diagnosis was 29.3 years, with a range of 24 to 39 years. The mean duration of residence in the United States before the illness was 2.7 years, with a range of 3 months to 8 years. Six of the ten patients died, and two of the survivors were ill at follow-up. None of the survivors have been followed for more than six months.

Six of the patients presented with nonspecific symptoms of fever and weight loss. Several had mild gastrointestinal symptoms, including nausea, vomiting, and diarrhea. Three patients had localized lymphadenopathy due to *Mycobacterium tuberculosis;* one had generalized lymphadenopathy due to *Cryptococcus neoformans*. All four patients who presented with intracerebral lesions due to *Toxoplasma gondii* had focal neurologic deficits with or without seizure activity. Six patients presented initially with infections from *M. tuberculosis*. In all six an opportunistic infection developed weeks to months after initiation of therapy with isoniazid and rifampin; all *M. tuberculosis* isolates were susceptible to the two drugs. All 10 patients were anergic to various combinations of skin-test antigens, including intermediate-strength purified protein derivative, candida, trichophyton, and mumps.

Table 2 summarizes the findings of the lymphocyte-subset analysis and proliferative studies of specimens from Patients 3, 5, and 10. These patients had been receiving therapy with isoniazid and rifampin for *M. tuberculosis* for six weeks, six months, and five months, respectively, before the onset of an opportunistic infection. The relative proportions of B and T lymphocytes were normal, although all three patients had lymphopenia. There was a marked decrease in the number of helper/inducer lymphocytes (OKT4+), whereas the relative number of suppressor/cytotoxic lymphocytes (OKT8+) was normal or increased. The ratios of helper to suppressor cells were decreased more than 10-fold as compared with normal heterosexual men.

Mitogen stimulation was impaired (the stimulation ratio was less than 3) in all three patients. Antigenic stimulation of blastogenesis revealed uniformly depressed incorporation of [^{3}H]thymidine when challenge was performed with candida, herpes simplex virus, tetanus-toxoid, cytomegalovirus, or streptolysin-O antigens. The [^{3}H]thymidine counts for unstimulated cells from the patients, in both the mitogen-stimulation and antigen-stimulation tests, were invariably low compared with those of the normal controls. This result may represent diminished spontaneous mitogenesis or premature death of the cells in culture.

Table 2. Lymphocyte-Subset Analysis and Functional Assays in Three Haitian Men with Opportunistic Infections.

	Patient 3	Patient 5	Patient 10	Control
Cell counts				
Leukocytes (cells/mm^3)	2200	4200	5800	4800–10,600
Lymphocytes (cells/mm^3)*	352	378	638	1200–3000
Surface immunoglobulin-bearing lymphocytes (%)†	5 (19)	15 (53)	4 (26)	6–21 (64–475)
OKT3+ (pan T) (%) †	49 (185)	36 (127)	82 (523)	53–81 (867–1897)
OKT4+ (T helper) (%)†	2 (8)	2 (7)	3 (19)	30–56 (468–1433)
OKT8+ (T suppressor) (%)†	50 (189)	28 (99)	71 (453)	15–32 (192–726)
OKT4+/OKT8+	0.04	0.07	0.04	1.2–2.5
Mitogen stimulation (%)‡				
Phytohemagglutinin	1	0	0	75–155
Concanavalin A	0	0	0	43–218
Pokeweed	1	0	0	37–187
Stimulation ratio§				
Candida	0.6	0.6	0.9	>3
Tetanus toxoid	0.9	0.6	1.4	>3
Streptolysin O	0.6	1.3	0.8	>3
Herpes simplex	0.7	0.5	2.0	>3
Cytomegalovirus	1.4	1.1	1.0	>3

*The total lymphocyte count was determined by multiplying the leukocyte count by the number of lymphocytes on the differential cell count.

†Numbers in parentheses represent absolute counts.

‡Calculation of the normalized mitogen response is described in the Methods section.

§Calculation of the stimulation ratio is described in the Methods section.

Table 3. Serologic Markers in 10 Haitian Men with Opportunistic Infections.*

Patient No.	Cytomegalovirus		Herpes Simplex		*Toxoplasma gondii*	RPR	HbsAg	Anti-HAV
	CF	IHA	CF	IHA (HSV-1)/ HSV-2)	IFA			
1	Not done		Not done		Not done	1:1	–	–
2	Not done		Not done		Not done	1:2	–	Not done
3	Not done		Not done		1:8	Not done	–	+
5	1:32	1:8192	1:32	1:16,384/ 1:16,384	1:32	1:1	–	+
7	1:16	1:2048	1:16	1:8192/ 1:1024	1:8	1:16	–	Not done
8	Not done		Not done		Not done	1:1	–	–
9	Not done		Not done		1:256	1:1	Not done	Not done
10	1:16	1:256	1:32	1:8192/ 1:128	1:512	1:16	–	+

*RPR denotes rapid plasma reagent card test, HbsAg hepatitis B surface antigen, anti-HAV antibody to hepatitis A virus, CF complement fixation test, IHA indirect hemagglutination test, HSV_1 and HSV_2 herpes simplex virus Types 1 and 2, and IFA indirect fluorescent-antibody test.

Serologic markers for previous infections with cytomegalovirus, herpes simplex virus, toxoplasmosis, or hepatitis-A virus were positive in several patients tested (Table 3).

Discussion

In these 10 Haitian men AIDS was manifested by a variety of opportunistic infections. The infections present were those against which cell-mediated immunity normally plays the major part in host defense — i.e., *M. tuberculosis, Pneumocystis carinii, T. gondii, C. neoformans,* and *Candida albicans* infections. Unlike other patients with AIDS,[1-5,13] our patients were neither homosexual nor addicted to drugs.

Six of the ten patients presented with tuberculosis. This disease is endemic among Haitian immigrants; its prevalence is 8 per 1000 population between 24 and 39 years of age.[14] The incidence of resistant isolates of *M. tuberculosis* among recent Haitian immigrants is about 30 percent[14]; however, we observed no resistance among the isolates from our patients. In all cases the syndrome was controlled with isoniazid and rifampin.

There was a marked reduction in the number of helper/inducer (OKT4+) T cells, with a normal or increased proportion of suppressor/cytotoxic (OKT8+) lymphocytes in the three patients whose lymphocytes were evaluated in detail. Helper/suppressor cell ratios were markedly decreased. In vitro lymphocyte stimulation with plant lectins and specific antigens showed an impaired lymphocyte proliferative capacity. Skin-test anergy was uniformly observed. These immunologic findings are characteristic of AIDS among drug addicts, homosexuals, and now Haitians.[13,15] Serologic studies in several patients showed high antibody titers to cytomegalovirus, herpes simplex virus, and *T. gondii*. None of the seven patients tested had hepatitis B surface antigen; however, other markers of hepatitis B infection were not routinely sought. Three of five patients tested had anti-hepatitis-A antibody.

The pathogenesis of the AIDS syndrome remains speculative. The epidemiologic features common to most of the cases in homosexuals and drug abusers, including multiple sexually transmitted infections and frequent use of prescription or recreational drugs, were generally absent in the Haitians. There is a high level of exposure of homosexual men to cytomegalovirus[2,16]; 94 percent of homosexuals have serologic evidence of prior cytomegalovirus infection.[16] Acute cytomegaloviral infections are known to result in a marked and occasionally prolonged depression of cell-mediated immunity with inversion of the normal ratio of helper to suppressor cells.[17,18] Like the homosexual patients with AIDS, only one of our patients had clinical evidence of an acute or reactivated infection with cytomegalovirus. Patient 3 had monocular blindness and hemorrhagic perivascular retinal lesions consistent with cytomegalovirus retinitis. Cytomegalovirus was subsequently isolated from his urine. Biopsy specimens from 6 of the 10 patients were submitted for viral culture and histologic examination for intranuclear viral inclusions. None contained cytomegalovirus on culture or histologic examination. Buffy-coat, urine, and semen samples were not routinely cultured for cytomegalovirus, however, and therefore we cannot exclude the possible contribution of this agent to immunosuppression in these patients. Cytomegaloviral antibody titers were measured in three patients and were elevated in all three.

Recreational drugs, such as marijuana, cocaine, and amyl or butyl nitrite are used commonly by homosexuals.[13] Some of these agents may have immunosuppressive effects in vivo.[19] Because of recurrent venereal infections, homosexuals are also likely to take repeated courses of antibiotics, including tetracyclines, metronidazole, and trimethoprim–sulfamethoxazole. These agents may be immunosuppressive at therapeutic doses,[20] although the clinical relevance of this observation is speculative. All the Haitians described in our series stated that they did not use illicit drugs and none were taking antibiotics before presenting to us. However, 5 of the 10 patients had received rifampin for the treatment of tuberculosis for weeks to months before the onset of an opportunistic superinfection. Rifampin is another agent that has been shown to have immunosuppressive effects in vitro and in vivo.[21,22]

The depression of the OKT4/OKT8 ratio observed in our patients is a sensitive and characteristic component of the immunologic alteration that occurs in patients with AIDS, particularly those with opportunistic infections. However, depressed OKT4/OKT8 ratios are not specific for AIDS, and many diseases, particularly viral infections, can induce an abnormal ratio. It is possible, but highly improbable, that tuberculosis or the therapy for tuberculosis (isoniazid or rifampin) induced the altered ratios, given the severity of the OKT4/OKT8 abnormality, its similarity to the OKT4/OKT8 abnormalities seen in other AIDS patients, the other accompanying immunologic alterations not usually seen with localized tuberculosis but commonly seen with AIDS, and the presence of other AIDS-associated opportunistic infections that are a consequence rather than a cause of the depressed immune status and abnormal OKT4/OKT8 ratios.

The recent report of 11 cases of Kaposi's sarcoma[23] and central-nervous-system toxoplasmosis in Port-au-Prince, Haiti (Curran J: personal comunication) suggests that the syndrome of acquired immunodeficiency among Haitians may not be limited to the United States. Unfortunately, our knowledge of the incidence of opportunistic infections in Haiti is inadequate to assess the extent of the problem. The geographic distribution of Haitian cases in the United States (22 from Dade County, Fla.; 10 from Brooklyn; and 1 each from New Jersey, California, and Georgia) suggests that AIDS is spread throughout the Haitian community in this country. The wide range of duration of residence before the onset of disease (three months to eight years) indicates that AIDS is not limited to Haitians who have recently immigrated.

It is possible, though unlikely, that the pathogenesis of AIDS among homosexuals is distinct from that among Haitians. Different infectious or environmental agents acting by way of a final common pathway may produce similar immunologic abnormalities. On the other hand, a single transmissible agent, such as a virus, may induce the basic immunologic defect, the ultimate expression of which depends on other variables, such as nutritional status, other infections or chronic illnesses, environmental agents, or genetic predisposition. If a viral agent were imported into the United States from Haiti by vacationing homosexuals, it might quickly spread within the homosexual community by means of frequent, often anonymous sexual encounters in bathhouses and elsewhere. Homosexual drug addicts, in turn, might introduce the agent via the parenteral route into the heterosexual addict population. To substantiate any hypothesis about the pathogenesis of AIDS with respect to Haitians, we will need to learn more about the Haitian life style in both the United States and Haiti. The assumption that heterosexual Haitians and homosexual Americans have little in common may prove erroneous when epidemiologic and anthropologic surveys are completed.

The occurrence of acquired immunodeficiency in patients who are neither homosexual nor addicted to drugs suggests that immunity is not conferred or guaranteed by virtue of a traditional life style. The possibility that the syndrome is due to a transmissible agent should dispel any sense of complacency that this is a homosexual or Haitian disease that does not have potentially serious public-health ramifications for everyone. The recent report of three cases of AIDS among hemophiliacs[24] underscores the public-health hazard of the syndrome and raises the possibility that products derived from blood may be contaminated with a transmissible agent responsible for the disease.

An interesting common epidemiologic feature linking the Haitians, homosexuals, intravenous-drug abusers, and hemophiliacs is a high incidence of hepatitis B viral markers. About 86 percent of Haitians reportedly have one or more serologic markers of hepatitis B infection (Johnson J: personal communication). There is no evidence to date suggesting that hepatitis viruses are themselves causally involved in AIDS. A reasonable but as yet unproved interpretation is that the transmissible agent causing AIDS has certain epidemiologic characteristics in common with hepatitis B virus — i.e., transmission by blood or body fluids and a prolonged incubation period or a carrier state (or both).

As a practical matter, the clinician caring for Haitians must be aware of the possibility of opportunistic infection. Aggressive evaluation is indicated if the diagnosis is not readily apparent or if empiric therapy fails to induce a favorable response promptly.

We are indebted to Bonnie M. Jones, Cornelia R. McGrath, Dr. Janet K. Nicholson, G. David Cross, and Marjorie R. Hubbard of the Centers for Disease Control, for technical assistance with immunologic testing; and to Drs. John A. Stewart, Paul M. Feorino, Kenneth Walls, Sandra A. Larsen, Donald P. Francis, Leo Kaufman, and Steven McDougal of the Centers for Disease Control, for serologic testing of specimens.

References

1. Gottlieb MS, Schanker HM, Fan PT, et al. *Pneumocystis* pneumonia — Los Angeles. MMWR 1981; 30:250-2.
2. Gottlieb MS, Schroff R, Schanker HM, et al. *Pneumocystis carinii* pneumonia and mucosal candidiasis in previously healthy homosexual men: evidence of a new acquired cellular immunodeficiency. N Engl J Med 1981; 305:1425-31.
3. Masur H, Michelis MA, Greene JB, et al. An outbreak of community-acquired *Pneumocystis carinii* pneumonia: initial manifestation of cellular immune dysfunction. N Engl J Med 1981; 305:1431-8.
4. Siegal FP, Lopez C, Hammer GS, et al. Severe acquired immunodeficiency in male homosexuals, manifested by chronic perianal ulcerative herpes simplex lesions. N Engl J Med 1981; 305:1439-44.
5. Update on Kaposi's sarcoma and opportunistic infections in previously healthy persons — United States. MMWR 1982; 31:294, 300-1.
6. Opportunistic infections and Kaposi's sarcoma among Haitians in the United States. MMWR 1982; 31:353-4, 360-1.
7. Update on acquired immune deficiency syndrome (AIDS) — United States. MMWR 1982; 31:507-8, 513-4.
8. Hoffman RA, Kung PC, Hansen WP, Goldstein G. Simple and rapid measurement of human T lymphocytes and their subclasses in peripheral blood. Proc Natl Acad Sci USA 1980; 77:4914-7.
9. Chan WC, Check IJ, Heffner LT, Gordon D, Whitsett C, Brynes RK. Prolymphocytic leukemia of helper cell phenotype: report of a case and review of the scientific literature. Am J Clin Pathol 1982; 77:643-7.
10. Waner JL, Weller TH, Stewart JA. Cytomegalovirus. In: Rose NR, Friedman H, eds. Manual of clinical immunology. Washington, D.C.: American Society of Microbiology, 1976:423-7.
11. Stewart JA, Herrmann KL. Herpes simplex virus. In: Rose NR, Friedman H, eds. Manual of clinical microbiology. Washington, D.C.: American Society of Microbiology, 1976:416-20.
12. Walls KW, Barnhart ER. Titration of human serum antibodies to *Toxoplasma gondii* with a simple fluorometric assay. J Clin Microbiol 1978; 7:234-5.
13. Friedman-Kien AE, Laubenstein LJ, Rubinstein P, et al. Disseminated Kaposi's sarcoma in homosexual men. Ann Intern Med 1982; 96:693-700.

14. Pitchenik AE, Russell BW, Cleary T, Pejovic I, Cole C, Snider DE Jr. The prevalence of tuberculosis and drug resistance among Haitians. N Engl J Med 1982; 307:162-5.
15. Mildvan D, Mathur U, Enlow RW, et al. Opportunistic infections and immune deficiency in homosexual men. Ann Intern Med 1982; 96: 700-4.
16. Drew WL, Mintz L, Miner RC, Sands M, Ketterer B. Prevalence of cytomegalovirus infection in homosexual men. J Infect Dis 1981; 143: 188-92.
17. Reinherz EL, O'Brien C, Rosenthal P, Schlossman SF. The cellular basis of viral-induced immunodeficiency: analysis by monoclonal antibodies. J Immunol 1980; 125:1269-74.
18. Rinaldo CR Jr, Carney WP, Richter BS, Black PH, Hirsch MS. Mechanisms of immunosuppression in cytomegaloviral mononucleosis. J Infect Dis 1980; 141:488-95.
19. Goedert JJ, Neuland GY, Wallen WC, et al. Amyl nitrite may alter T lymphocytes in homosexual men. Lancet 1982; 1:412-6.
20. Finch R. Immunomodulating effects of antimicrobial agents. J Antimicrob Agents Chemother 1980; 6:691-3.
21. Serrou B. Rifampicin and immunosuppression. Lancet 1974; 2:172.
22. Serrou B, Solassol C, Joyeux H, Pujol H, Romieu C. Immunosuppressive effect of rifampicin. Transplantation 1972; 14:654-5.
23. Liataud B, Laroche J, Duvivier J, Pean-Guichard C. Le sarcome de Kaposi (maladie de Kaposi) est-il frequent en Haiti? Presented at the 18th Congres des Medecins francophones de l'hemisphere americain, Port au Prince, Haiti, April 12-16, 1982.
24. *Pneumocystis carinii* pneumonia among persons with hemophilia A. MMWR 1982; 31:365-7.

ORIGINAL ARTICLE

CHARACTERISTICS OF THE ACQUIRED IMMUNODEFICIENCY SYNDROME (AIDS) IN HAITI

JEAN W. PAPE, M.D., BERNARD LIAUTAUD, M.D., FRANCK THOMAS, M.D., JEAN-ROBERT MATHURIN, M.D., MARIE-MYRTHA A. ST. AMAND, M.D., MADELEINE BONCY, VERGNIAUD PEAN, M.D., MOLIERE PAMPHILE, M.D., A. CLAUDE LAROCHE, M.D., AND WARREN D. JOHNSON, JR., M.D.

Abstract To identify the characteristics of the acquired immunodeficiency syndrome (AIDS) as it occurs in Haiti, we studied 61 previously healthy Haitians who had diagnoses of either Kaposi's sarcoma (15), opportunistic infections (45), or both (1) established in Haiti between June 1979 and October 1982. The first cases of Kaposi's sarcoma and opportunistic infections in Haiti were recognized in 1978-1979, a period that coincides with the earliest reports of AIDS in the United States. We do not believe that AIDS existed in Haiti before this period. The types of opportunistic infections and the clinical course in Haitians with Kaposi's sarcoma and opportunistic infections were similar in most aspects to those in patients with AIDS in the United States. The median age of Haitians with Kaposi's sarcoma and opportunistic infections was 32 years, and 85 percent were men. The interval between diagnosis and death was six months in 80 percent of the patients. Diarrhea was the most common reason for seeking medical attention in patients with opportunistic infections. Lymphopenia and skin-test anergy were observed in 86 and 100 percent of patients, respectively. Potential risk factors (bisexual activity or blood transfusions) were identified in 17 percent of male and 22 percent of female patients. Demographic information suggests that patients belonged to all socioeconomic strata of Haitian society.

OPPORTUNISTIC infections and Kaposi's sarcoma have been described in homosexuals, illicit drug users, Haitian immigrants, and patients with hemophilia in the United States.[1-8] During the period June 1981 to March 1983, over 1200 cases of opportunistic infections or Kaposi's sarcoma associated with the acquired immunodeficiency syndrome (AIDS) have been reported to the Centers for Disease Control.[9]

This report describes 61 patients in Haiti with either opportunistic infections or Kaposi's sarcoma and discusses the spectrum of infectious diseases, the clinical course, laboratory studies, and demographic data.

METHODS

The 61 patients were seen in Port-au-Prince, Haiti, between June 1979 and October 1982 by five of us who are Haitian clinicians (J.W.P., an internist and infectious-diseases specialist; B.L., a dermatologist; F.T., a surgeon and endoscopist; J.-R.M., an internist and cardiologist; and M.-M.A.S., an internist and gastroenterologist). The other Haitian authors of this paper include two pathologists (V.P. and A.C.L.), an epidemiologist (M.P.) and a medical technologist (M.B.). The Haitian Study Group on Kaposi's Sarcoma and Opportunistic Infection (GHESKIO) was formed in May 1982. This action was prompted by our independent experiences in establishing these diagnoses in previously healthy Haitians.

Fifty-one patients (44 with opportunistic infections and 7 with Kaposi's sarcoma) were initially seen as outpatients; 30 of these were referred by other physicians, and 21 were referred through other channels. Only one patient had previously been treated by a member of the Haitian Study Group. Nine additional patients (one with opportunistic infections and eight with Kaposi's sarcoma) were seen at the State University Hospital in Port-au-Prince. No active case finding was employed.

The diagnosis of Kaposi's sarcoma was established by biopsy or autopsy in 15 of 16 patients and was confirmed by American and French pathologists. The 46 cases of opportunistic infection involved 31 patients who met the strict Centers for Disease Control criteria for AIDS and 15 patients with probable AIDS.[5] The 31 patients with confirmed AIDS had histologic and parasitologic diagnoses of *Pneumocystis carinii* pneumonia (four patients), central nervous system toxoplasmosis (two patients), anogenital herpes infection (five patients), disseminated cytomegalovirus infection (six patients), and cryptosporidiosis (three patients). These diagnoses were confirmed by either Dr. Janet Mouradian (New York Hospital–Cornell Medical Center, New York) or Drs. George Hensley and Lee Moskowitz (Jackson Memorial Hospital, Miami). Esophageal candidiasis was diagnosed by esophagoscopy, with positive smears and cultures obtained in 24 living patients. Two patients were diagnosed at autopsy. A diagnosis of tuberculosis was made in 11 of the 31 confirmed AIDS cases on the basis of culture (three patients), biopsy or autopsy (six patients), or a finding of acid-fast bacilli in sputum smears (two patients). The species of the mycobacterial cultures were not identified because the method for doing so is not available in Haiti. A clinical diagnosis of *P. carinii* pneumonia was made in two additional patients with severe dyspnea and chest x-ray films revealing diffuse interstitial pneumonia compatible with *P. carinii* pneumonia. No patients were considered to have confirmed AIDS solely on the basis of a clinical diagnosis of *P. carinii* pneumonia or tuberculosis. The five patients with herpes infection had extensive anogenital ulcerations of at least six months' duration. Culture of the lesion in one patient (Patient 26) was positive for herpes simplex Type 2.

Fifteen patients were considered to have probable AIDS on the basis of a clinical diagnosis of esophageal candidiasis (culture-documented thrush and severe dysphagia). Two of these patients had compatible esophagrams. All these patients were anergic to skin testing with purified protein derivative and candida and mumps antigens, and 13 of 15 were lymphopenic (<1500 mm^3). None had received antimicrobial or immunosuppressive drugs during the two months preceding the onset of their symptoms. Six of these patients were also thought to have *P. carinii* pneumonia on the basis of findings of severe dyspnea and x-ray films revealing diffuse interstitial pneumonia. Four patients with either pulmonary infiltrates or cavities and sputum smears containing acid-fast bacilli were thought to have tuberculosis.

Demographic data were obtained through a questionnaire administered to 21 patients (5 with Kaposi's sarcoma and 16 with opportunistic infections) who were seen after August 1982 by the Haitian Study Group clinician treating the patient. The approach to questions of a personal nature (concerning sex or drug abuse) was not standardized. Demographic data on the remaining 40 patients were obtained from physicians' records.

Thirty-nine healthy subjects (37 men and 2 women) served as controls for delayed-type skin hypersensitivity testing with purified

From the Haitian Study Group on Kaposi's Sarcoma and Opportunistic Infection, Port-au-Prince, Haiti, and the Division of International Medicine, Department of Medicine, Cornell University Medical College, New York.

Table 1. Infections in 46 Haitians with Confirmed or Probable Diagnoses of AIDS.*

Patient No.	Age/Sex	Date of Diagnosis	CE	ASP	CRY	PCP	TOXO	CRYPT	TB	HI	CMV
1†	15/F	2/80	3‡								
2	54/F	3/80	1						5		
3	29/M	6/80	1								
4†	25/M	7/80	3								
5	30/F	9/80	5		5						
6	36/M	3/81	1			3			2		
7†	25/M	7/81	3								
8†	38/M	9/81	3			3			2		
9†	27/M	9/81	3			3			2		
10	35/M	9/81	1								
11	33/M	10/81	1						2	5	
12	30/M	11/81	1								
13†	45/M	12/81	3			3					
14	32/M	12/81	1	4					5		5
15†	29/M	1/82	3						2		
16†	24/M	1/82	3			3			2		
17	62/F	1/82							5		5
18	32/M	2/82	1			5					5
19	34/M	2/82	1						5		
20	44/F	3/82	1								
21	30/M	4/82	3			5			5		5
22	40/M	4/82	1						4		
23	37/M	4/82	1								
24	62/M	4/82	1								
25	26/M	5/82	1								
26	28/M	6/82	3							4	
27	39/M	7/82	1				5				
28†	25/M	8/82	3								
29	24/M	8/82	1			3					
30	39/M	8/82	5			5				5	5
31	65/M	9/82	1						4		
32†	40/M	9/82	3			3					
33†	29/M	9/82	3								
34†	37/M	9/82	3								
35†	29/M	9/82	3								
36	64/M	9/82	1		5				6		
37	30/M	9/82	1						4		
38	27/M	9/82					5				5
39†	35/F	9/82	3								
40	57/M	10/82	1						5		
41†	33/M	10/82	3			3					
42	29/M	10/82	1								
43	29/M	10/82	1								
44	34/M	10/82						6		5	
45	47/M	10/82	1					6		5	
46	28/M	10/82	1			5					

*CE denotes candida esophagitis, ASP aspergillosis, CRY cryptococcosis, PCP *Pneumocystis carinii* pneumonia, TOXO central nervous system toxoplasmosis, CRYPT cryptosporidiosis, TB tuberculosis, HI anogenital herpes infection, and CMV disseminated cytomegalovirus infection.

†Patient with probable AIDS.

‡The methods used to establish the diagnoses were esophagoscopy with smear and culture (1), sputum microscopy (2), clinical methods (3), culture (4), biopsy or autopsy (5), and stool microscopy (6).

protein derivative (5 tuberculin units) and candida and mumps antigens. These controls were patients' friends and physicians' employees. They were from 20 to 40 years old and approximated the socioeconomic status of the patient population.

Results

Opportunistic Infections

The clinical data in the 46 patients with opportunistic infections are summarized in Table 1. There were 40 male and 6 female patients with an age range of 15 to 65 years. The median ages of patients with confirmed and probable opportunistic infections were 34 and 29 years, respectively. Diagnoses were established in five patients during 1980 and in nine patients during 1981. Twelve patients were identified as having opportunistic infections during the first six months of 1982, and 20 patients were seen during the next four months. An additional 20 patients with opportunistic infections were seen from November 1982 through March 1983 but are not included in this report.

The diagnoses in the 31 confirmed cases included candida esophagitis, 26 cases; aspergillosis, 1; disseminated cryptococcosis, 2; *P. carinii* pneumonia, 6; central nervous system toxoplasmosis, 2; cryptosporidiosis, 3; tuberculosis, 11; anogenital herpes infection, 5; and disseminated cytomegalovirus infection, 6. A total of 62 infections were diagnosed in these 31 patients. The 11 patients with tuberculosis had either pulmonary tuberculosis (6 patients), miliary tuberculosis (3 patients), or tuberculous lymphadenitis (2 patients). Tuberculosis preceded other infections in most patients. Autopsies performed in 11 patients with opportunistic infections (Patients 14, 17, 18, 21, 27, 30, 36, 38, 40, 43, and 46 in Table 1) did not reveal any evidence of malignant disease. Patient 45, with candida esophagitis, cryptosporidiosis, and anogenital herpes infection, was found at autopsy to have had previously unrecognized Kaposi's sarcoma of the small intestine and skin. The 15 patients with probable AIDS all had candida esophagitis; additional diagnoses of *P. carinii* pneumonia and tuberculosis were made in six and four patients, respectively. Only 3 of the 46 patients with opportunistic infections were alive as of this writing. The interval between the diagnosis of opportunistic infection and death was less than six months in 76 percent of patients, and none survived for more than 24 months.

The physical findings observed in the patients with opportunistic infections differed according to their diseases. Clinical data on lymph-node examinations of 25 patients indicated that there was generalized enlargement in 2 patients, cervical lymphadenopathy in 8 patients, and no enlargement in 15 patients. Pruritic maculopapular or nodular lesions involving the extremities and occasionally the face were observed in 61 percent of patients with opportunistic infections. This finding usually occurred late in the clinical illness. Biopsies in three patients revealed perivascular infiltration of the skin and subcutaneous tissue with mononuclear cells (one patient) and eosinophils (two patients).

Weight loss and diarrhea were presenting signs in 100 percent and 91 percent of patients with opportunistic infections, respectively. A mean weight loss of 12 kg was documented in 27 patients. Diarrhea occurred during the course of the illness in all patients with opportunistic infections. The mean duration of diarrhea before the diagnosis of opportunistic infections was 6.6 months, with an average of 6.9 stools daily.

The stools were watery in 92 percent of patients, with blood observed in 8 percent. Stool examinations for ova and parasites and stool cultures were performed in three quarters and one half of the patients with opportunistic infections, respectively. Enteric pathogens were detected in 11 patients and included the following: *Shigella boydii*, 1 patient; *S. sonnei*, 2; salmonella species, 2; *Giardia lamblia*, 6; cryptosporidium, 3; *Entamoeba histolytica*, 3; *Ascaris lumbricoides*, 1; and *Trichuris trichiura*, 1. Stool acid-fast staining was performed in only three patients, and in all three, stools were positive for cryptosporidia for at least two months. Bloody diarrhea was more common in patients with either shigellosis or amebiasis, but otherwise there was no apparent correlation between the duration, severity, and character of diarrhea and the presence or absence of enteric pathogens. At autopsy, the small and large intestines of 10 patients appeared grossly normal, but histologic examination revealed diffuse infiltration of the lamina propria by mononuclear cells and plasma cells. Two of us who are Haitian pathologists (V.P. and A.C.L.) have observed similar findings in patients with severe chronic diarrhea and weight loss but have not associated them with a specific pathogen. Viral inclusions compatible with cytomegalovirus were seen in the colon and rectum of four patients in whom autopsies were performed.

Fever and dysphagia were present at the time of the initial visit in 89 and 72 percent of patients with opportunistic infections, respectively. Fever had been present for less than three months in 34 percent of patients, for three to six months in 29 percent, and for longer than six months in 37 percent of patients. Dysphagia had been present for less than three months in 67 percent of patients, for three to six months in 24 percent, and for longer than six months in only 9 percent.

Laboratory and clinical findings in the 46 patients with opportunistic infections included anemia, with hemoglobin of less than 10 g per deciliter in all 38 patients tested; lymphopenia, with absolute counts of less than 1500 mm^3 in 38 of 44 patients; elevated levels of alkaline phosphatase in 12 of 18 patients; elevated levels of serum aspartate and alanine aminotransferase in 11 of 30 patients; hypoalbuminemia and hyperglobulinemia in 25 of 26 patients; and abnormal chest films in 20 of 43 patients. Delayed-type skin hypersensitivity reactions to purified protein derivative (5 tuberculin units) and to candida and mumps antigens were negative in all 34 patients tested. Similar testing in 39 healthy control subjects revealed positive reactions to purified protein derivative in 100 percent of the subjects and reactions to mumps and candida antigens in 95 percent. In addition, positive reactions to purified protein derivative were obtained in each of 25 ambulatory male patients (mean age, 23 years) with active pulmonary tuberculosis or lymphadenitis who did not represent suspected cases of AIDS (Georges MRL: personal communication).

Kaposi's Sarcoma

The 16 patients with Kaposi's sarcoma included 13 men and 3 women, with an age range of 21 to 68 years (median, 31). The years of diagnosis and number of patients seen annually were as follows: 1979, two; 1980, two; 1981, seven; and 1982 (through October), five. One additional patient with Kaposi's sarcoma was seen between November 1982 and March 1983 but is not included in this report. The first patient with Kaposi's sarcoma in this series was a 28-year-old woman from the northwestern region of Haiti who was hospitalized in Port-au-Prince in June 1979 after six months of severe edema of the lower extremities. Multiple nodular and papular lesions were present over the face, trunk, and extremities. Biopsy revealed the presence of Kaposi's sarcoma. The patient did not respond to antineoplastic therapy and died one year after the appearance of the first skin lesion. An autopsy revealed that tumor was infiltrating the lungs, pleura, mediastinum, adrenals, liver, and nerve roots. The clinical course in the other patients with Kaposi's sarcoma was similar, except in the oldest two patients. These were men, 59 and 68 years old, who presented with lesions involving the lower extremities. They remained well, without evidence of disseminated disease, but were lost to follow-up three months after diagnosis. Generalized lymphadenopathy was present in 13 of the other 14 patients with Kaposi's sarcoma. Death occurred within three months of diagnosis in 11 patients. Autopsies performed on three of these patients revealed the presence of extensive visceral and lymph-node involvement by tumor.

The 21 practicing dermatologists and pathologists in Haiti were surveyed about their experience in that country with Kaposi's sarcoma. Before 1979, the only case recognized by these physicians occurred in a 54-year-old man with Kaposi's sarcoma documented by biopsy in 1972. The course of his illness is not known. A review of records of cancer biopsies from three private hospitals in Port-au-Prince with a combined total of 180 beds revealed that no cases of Kaposi's sarcoma were recorded during the period from 1968 to May 1983 (at the Canape Vert, Français, and St. François hospitals). A similar review of the records of over 1000 cancer biopsies at the Albert Schweitzer Hospital in Deschapelles, Haiti, revealed that no cases of Kaposi's sarcoma were recorded during the same period. This hospital serves a rural population of 115,000 persons.[10] A review of its autopsy records from 1978 to July 1982 also failed to reveal any cases of Kaposi's sarcoma. Hospital records did include those of a previously healthy 20-year-old man who had generalized seizures in July 1978 and died two weeks later. At autopsy he was found to have central nervous system toxoplasmosis without evidence of underlying cancer. He had not received immunosuppressive therapy. He is the earliest patient with possible AIDS in Haiti known to our group.

Demographic Information

Patients with opportunistic infections and Kaposi's sarcoma were asked their current place of residence. Men with opportunistic infections indicated the following residences: Port-au-Prince, 41 percent; Carrefour, 33 percent; elsewhere in Haiti, 13 percent; and outside Haiti, 13 percent (New York, 2 patients; Miami, 1; Belgium, 1; and the Bahamas, 1). All six female patients with opportunistic infections were from Port-au-Prince. Patients with Kaposi's sarcoma were from diverse regions of Haiti, with 38 percent from Port-au-Prince, 13 percent from Carrefour, and 49 percent from the rest of the country. Census figures for 1982 from the Haitian Institute of Statistics showed a total Haitian population of 5,053,792, of which 48.4 percent were male. The population of Port-au-Prince includes 189,117 male and 253,712 female residents, and the Carrefour population includes 55,986 male and 73,484 female residents. The prevalence rate of men with opportunistic infections in Carrefour was significantly higher than that of men in Port-au-Prince ($P<0.001$ by the chi-square test). This is of interest since Carrefour, a suburb of Port-au-Prince, is recognized as the principal center of male and female prostitution in Haiti.

Information concerning sexual practices, previous illnesses, blood-transfusion history, annual income, and educational and vocational backgrounds was obtained by the patient's physician. Eight of 30 patients (27 percent) for whom this information was available had a history of malaria. Twenty-two of 31 (71 percent) reported a history of venereal disease, with the following diseases noted: gonorrhea, 20 patients; syphilis, 7 patients; herpes genital infection, 4 patients; and nonspecific urethritis and lymphogranuloma venereum, 1 patient each. Sexual activity with both men and women was reported by 2 of 12 men (17 percent) with Kaposi's sarcoma, by 3 of 24 men (13 percent) with confirmed opportunistic infections, and by 2 of 10 men (20 percent) with probable opportunistic infections. No information was available on six men with confirmed or probable opportunistic infections. Five of the 21 men (24 percent) questioned about sexual activity by a Haitian Study Group clinician said they were bisexual. In contrast, only 2 of 31 men (6 percent) on whom such information was obtained from physicians' records from before August 1982 reported bisexuality. None of the nine female patients with either opportunistic infections or Kaposi's sarcoma reported being a prostitute. Illicit drug use was denied by all patients.

Travel and residence histories of the seven bisexual men indicated that they lived either in Carrefour (four men) or in the United States (three). Three had had sexual relations with American men in both Haiti and the United States, and two had had sexual relations with Haitian men with opportunistic infections. Ten of 21 heterosexual men who were questioned said that they had either lived or traveled outside Haiti.

A history of blood transfusion was obtained in 5 of 25 patients (20 percent) with confirmed opportunistic infections. This included two women who had received transfusions 1½ and 6 years before becoming ill and three men who had received transfusions two, three, and five years before their opportunistic infections. One of the men who had received a blood transfusion was also bisexual. No information was available on six patients with confirmed and six with probable opportunistic infections. None of the other patients with either probable AIDS or Kaposi's sarcoma had received transfusions before their illness.

Patients with opportunistic infections or Kaposi's sarcoma were from all strata of Haitian society, as judged by annual income, vocation, and educational experience. The annual incomes reported by 48 patients were as follows: less than \$150, 32 percent; \$150-\$1,000, 33 percent; \$1,000 to \$5,000, 23 percent; \$5,000 to \$10,000, 6 percent; and over \$10,000, 6 percent. Income data were not available for 13 patients. The estimated per capita income in Haiti is \$200 to \$300 per year, according to the Haitian Institute of Statistics. Ten percent of patients had no formal education, 38 percent had attended primary school, 42 percent had attended secondary school, and 10 percent were university graduates. At the time of diagnosis, 28 percent of the patients were unemployed. The occupations of the others were as follows: laborer, 28 percent; farmer, 10 percent; and professional or office worker, 34 percent.

Discussion

The 61 cases described here document the occurrence of opportunistic infections and Kaposi's sarcoma in Haiti. The patients were previously healthy and had no evidence of prior cancer or immunosuppressive therapy. The median age of 32 years, the male predominance (85 percent), and the high mortality (89 percent) are comparable to those reported for AIDS in the United States.[9,11] The findings of lymphopenia in 86 percent of the patients with opportunistic infections and of skin-test anergy in all the patients tested are consistent with an immunodeficiency state. Six of these patients (four with opportunistic infections and two with Kaposi's sarcoma) also had a decrease in the numbers and activity of helper T cells, with normal or increased populations of suppressor T cells. T-cell studies were performed at the Centers for Disease Control through the collaboration of Drs. T. Spira, P. Drotman, and A. Roisin.

The spectrum of opportunistic infections we encountered included diseases in which cellular immunity has a major role in host defense. Esophageal candidiasis and thrush were seen in 93 percent of the patients with opportunistic infections. That is higher than the 30 to 50 percent incidence in Haitians with AIDS in New York and Miami[6,7] and may in part reflect the fact that two of the five clinicians in our group are endoscopists. Tuberculosis was present in 33 percent of the patients with opportunistic infections and usually antedated other infections, as previously reported.[7] Tuberculosis is common in Haiti, but frequency data are not available. All our healthy controls had positive results on the tuberculin test. The prevalence of tuberculosis in Haitian immigrants to the United States in this age group is 8 per 1000 population.[12] The other diagnoses in the 46 cases of opportunistic infections included *P. carinii* pneumonia, 26 percent; disseminated cytomegalovirus infection, 13 percent; anogenital herpesvirus infection, 11 percent; cryptosporidiosis, central nervous system toxoplasmosis, and disseminated cryptococcosis, 4 percent each; and aspergillosis, 2 percent. The treating physicians used personal resources to pay for diagnostic procedures, medications, and autopsies, because most of the patients were indigent (annual income <$1,000). This limited the extent of diagnostic and autopsy evaluations and may have resulted in missed diagnoses in some patients.

The clinical features of Kaposi's sarcoma in 14 of 16 patients were similar to those reported in the United States.[13,14] Although all patients presented with lesions on the lower extremities, lesions subsequently developed on the head, neck, and trunk, with extensive visceral and lymph-node involvement. The patients with opportunistic infections were similar to previously described patients with AIDS in the incidence of lymphadenopathy but had a higher incidence of severe diarrhea.[14] Enteric pathogens were identified in 24 percent of the patients with opportunistic infections. This figure underestimates the prevalence, since diagnostic evaluations were incomplete in some patients. Furthermore, the pathogen identified may not have been responsible for the protracted diarrhea. Specific therapy for giardiasis, amebiasis, shigellosis, salmonellosis, and trichuriasis did not improve the patients' symptoms. The frequency of these enteric pathogens in control populations in Haiti is unknown.

The recognition of Kaposi's sarcoma and opportunistic infections in Haiti is temporally related to the appearance of AIDS in the United States. The earliest possible case of opportunistic infection in Haiti that is known to our group occurred in July 1978, and the first case of fulminant Kaposi's sarcoma was diagnosed in June 1979. The first cases of Kaposi's sarcoma and opportunistic infections in homosexual men in the United States were documented in early 1978.[11] We do not believe that AIDS was present in Haiti before 1978. This contention is supported by the clinical experience of the practicing pathologists and dermatologists in Haiti and by our inability to identify earlier cases through examination of autopsy and biopsy records. It also seems likely that Haitians would have presented to U.S. hospitals sooner if AIDS had been occurring in Haiti before 1978.

Some of the risk factors for AIDS in the United States were present in our patients with opportunistic infections and Kaposi's sarcoma in Haiti. Bisexual activity was reported by 15 percent of the men with Kaposi's sarcoma or opportunistic infections for whom such information was available and by 24 percent of the men prospectively questioned by a clinician in the Haitian Study Group. The identification of bisexual Haitian patients who had had sexual relations with American homosexuals in New York and Miami also provides a link between the two populations. There is a very strong bias against homosexuality in Haiti, and our data may underestimate this risk factor. A correlation between sexual activity and the development of opportunistic infections and Kaposi's sarcoma in Haiti is also suggested by the prevalence of venereal disease (71 percent) in our patients. Residence in Carrefour, a center of prostitution, was reported by 33 percent of the men with opportunistic infections. This was markedly higher than expected and indicates a 2.7-fold greater prevalence of opportunistic infections in men from Carrefour than in men from Port-au-Prince. Blood transfusions had been received by five of our patients, and blood products have been implicated in the transmission of AIDS in the United States.[15,16]

No segment of Haitian society appears to be free of opportunistic infections or Kaposi's sarcoma. These diseases have been diagnosed in the indigent and the wealthy, the illiterate and the educated, and in people with diverse occupations. The number of cases of opportunistic infections and of Kaposi's sarcoma recognized annually is increasing, as in the United States.[9] The clinical course in patients with opportunistic infections or Kaposi's sarcoma in Haiti is similar in most respects to that in patients with AIDS in the United States. Risk factors such as bisexuality and blood transfusions have also been identified in some Haitians.

We are indebted to Drs. George Hensley and Lee Moskowitz (Jackson Memorial Hospital, Miami), Dr. Jose Costa (National Institutes of Health), Dr. Henry Falk (Centers for Disease Control), Dr. J. Civatte (Faculte de Medecine de Paris), and Dr. Janet Mouradian (The New York Hospital–Cornell Medical Center) for histologic review of clinical materials; to Dr. Decatrel Mirville (State University Hospital of Haiti) for administrative support; to Dr. Rosemary Soave (Cornell University Medical College) for assistance in cryptosporidia identification; to the Haitian physicians who referred patients to us; to Drs. Jean Duvivier and Claude Pean-Guichard for allowing us to report on the patients with Kaposi's sarcoma whom they have studied; and to Ms. Jennifer Rayhill for assistance in the preparation of the manuscript.

References

1. Pneumocystis pneumonia — Los Angeles. MMWR 1981; 30:250-2.
2. Gottlieb MS, Schroff R, Schanker HM, et al. *Pneumocystis carinii* pneumonia and mucosal candidiasis in previously healthy homosexual men: evidence of a new acquired cellular immunodeficiency. N Engl J Med 1981; 305:1425-31.
3. Masur H, Michelis MA, Greene JB, et al. An outbreak of community-acquired *Pneumocystis carinii* pneumonia: initial manifestation of cellular immune dysfunction. N Engl J Med 1981; 305:1431-8.
4. Siegal FP, Lopez C, Hammer GS, et al. Severe acquired immunodeficiency in male homosexuals, manifested by chronic perianal ulcerative herpes simplex lesions. N Engl J Med 1981; 305:1439-44.
5. Update on acquired immune deficiency syndrome (AIDS) — United States. MMWR 1982; 31:507-8, 513-4.
6. Vieira J, Frank E, Spira TJ, Landesman SH. Acquired immune deficiency in Haitians: opportunistic infections in previously healthy Haitian immigrants. N Engl J Med 1983; 308:125-9.

7. Pitchenik AE, Fischl MA, Dickinson GM, et al. Opportunistic infections and Kaposi's sarcoma among Haitians: evidence of a new acquired immunodeficiency state. Ann Intern Med 1983; 98:277-84.
8. Opportunistic infections and Kaposi's sarcoma among Haitians in the United States. MMWR 1982; 31:353-4, 360-1.
9. Prevention of acquired immune deficiency syndrome (AIDS): report of inter-agency recommendations. MMWR 1983; 32:101-3.
10. Berggren WL, Ewbank DC, Berggren GG. Reduction of mortality in rural Haiti through a primary-health-care program. N Engl J Med 1981; 304: 1324-30.
11. Update on Kaposi's sarcoma and opportunistic infections in previously healthy persons — United States. MMWR 1982; 31:294, 300-1.
12. Pitchenik AE, Russell BW, Cleary T, Pejovic I, Cole C, Snider DE Jr. The prevalence of tuberculosis and drug resistance among Haitians. N Engl J Med 1982; 307:162-5.
13. Friedman-Kien AE, Laubenstein LJ, Rubinstein P, et al. Disseminated Kaposi's sarcoma in homosexual men. Ann Intern Med 1982; 96:693-700.
14. Centers for Disease Control Task Force on Kaposi's Sarcoma and Opportunistic Infections. Epidemiologic aspects of the current outbreak of Kaposi's sarcoma and opportunistic infections. N Engl J Med 1982; 306:248-52.
15. Possible transfusion-associated acquired immune deficiency syndrome (AIDS) — California. MMWR 1982; 31:652-4.
16. White GC II, Lesesne HR. Hemophilia, hepatitis, and the acquired immunodeficiency syndrome. Ann Intern Med 1983; 98:403-4.

ORIGINAL ARTICLE

AIDS VIRUS INFECTION IN NAIROBI PROSTITUTES

Spread of the Epidemic to East Africa

JOAN K. KREISS, M.D., M.S.P.H., DAVY KOECH, PH.D., FRANCIS A. PLUMMER, M.D., KING K. HOLMES, M.D., PH.D., MARILYN LIGHTFOOTE, PH.D., PETER PIOT, M.D., PH.D., ALLAN R. RONALD, M.D., J.O. NDINYA-ACHOLA, M.B., CH.B., LOURDES J. D'COSTA, M.B., CH.B., PACITA ROBERTS, M.S., ELIZABETH N. NGUGI, AND THOMAS C. QUINN, M.D.

Abstract The acquired immunodeficiency syndrome (AIDS) is epidemic in Central Africa. To determine the prevalence of AIDS virus infection in East Africa, we studied 90 female prostitutes, 40 men treated at a clinic for sexually transmitted diseases, and 42 medical personnel in Nairobi, Kenya. Antibody to human T-cell lymphotropic virus Type III (HTLV-III) was detected in the serum of 66 percent of prostitutes of low socioeconomic status, 31 percent of prostitutes of higher socioeconomic status, 8 percent of the clinic patients, and 2 percent of the medical personnel. The presence of the antibody was associated with both immunologic and clinical abnormalities. The mean T-cell helper/suppressor ratio was 0.92 in seropositive prostitutes and 1.82 in seronegative prostitutes ($P<0.0001$). Generalized lymphadenopathy was present in 54 percent of seropositive prostitutes and 10 percent of seronegative prostitutes ($P<0.0001$). No constitutional symptoms, opportunistic infections, or cases of Kaposi's sarcoma were present.

Our results indicate that the epidemic of AIDS virus infection has, unfortunately, spread extensively among urban prostitutes in Nairobi, Kenya. Sexual exposure to men from Central Africa was significantly associated with HTLV-III antibody among prostitutes, suggesting transcontinental spread of the epidemic.

THE acquired immunodeficiency syndrome (AIDS) has been occurring in epidemic form in Central Africa since the late 1970s.[1-4] The epidemiology of AIDS in Africa differs from that of AIDS in the United States. Whereas homosexual activity and parenteral transmission account for the majority of cases in the United States, transmission through heterosexual activity appears to predominate in Africa.[2,5]

The occurrence of AIDS in Zaire and Rwanda is well documented, but the boundaries of the epidemic in Africa have not yet been determined.[2,3] Because of the high prevalence of AIDS virus infection in Central African prostitutes, we hypothesized that the virus might be spread to other African countries by travelers who frequent prostitutes.[6] We therefore surveyed the prevalence of serum antibody to human T-cell lymphotropic virus Type III (HTLV-III) among prostitutes in Nairobi, where only a few cases of AIDS had been seen by early 1985.[7]

METHODS

Study participants were recruited between February and April 1985 from prostitutes registering at the Pumwami Research Clinic, prostitutes treated at a specially established clinic for AIDS research, and men presenting to the Nairobi City Commission Special Treatment Clinic for sexually transmitted diseases. From previous studies, these groups were known to have high prevalences of sexually transmitted diseases.[8] Medical students and research personnel were invited to volunteer as healthy controls. After informed consent was obtained, a standard questionnaire was administered to all participants, a physical examination was performed, and 25 ml of blood was drawn. The prostitutes underwent pelvic examination, during which swabs were applied to the cervix for isolation of *Neisseria gonorrhoeae* and to any genital ulcer for isolation of *Hemophilus ducreyi*.

Laboratory tests included peripheral-blood total and differential white-cell counts, the rapid plasma reagin test, and the *Treponema pallidum* hemagglutination assay. Peripheral-blood lymphocytes were separated by means of Ficoll–Hypaque gradient-density centrifugation, after which T-cell subsets were quantitated by means of Leu-2 (T suppressor/cytotoxic cells), Leu-3 (T helper/inducer cells), and Leu-4 (total T cells) monoclonal antibodies (Becton-Dickinson, Mountain View, Calif.). Serum was tested for antibody to HTLV-III by two commercially available enzyme-linked immunosorbent assays (Litton-Bionetics, Charleston, S.C., and Electro-Nucleonics, Columbia, Md.) and by Western (immune) blot. Western blots were prepared by electrophoresis of lysates of virus-infected 3.01 (Leu-3^+) cells onto 3 to 27 percent sodium dodecyl sulfate gels (Integration Sciences, Newton, Mass.), transfer of proteins to nitrocellulose filters, and incubation of the filters with serum diluted to 1:1000. Antibodies to viral proteins were detected with the use of ^{125}I-labeled protein A and autoradiographic film. A specimen was considered positive if a p24 protein band was present.

Student's one-tailed and two-tailed t-tests, Mann–Whitney rank-sum tests, chi-square analyses, and Fisher's exact tests were used for comparisons of means and proportions between groups. Multivariate logistic regression was used to determine the extent of association between HTLV-III antibody and selected potential risk factors and coinfections.

From the Division of Infectious Diseases, Department of Medicine, and the Department of Biostatistics, University of Washington, Seattle; the Kenya Medical Research Institute, the Nairobi City Commission Special Treatment Clinic, the Ministry of Health, and the Department of Medical Microbiology, University of Nairobi, Nairobi, Kenya; the Department of Medical Microbiology, University of Manitoba, Winnipeg; the Laboratory of Immunoregulation, National Institute of Allergy and Infectious Diseases, Bethesda, Md.; and the Department of Microbiology, Institute of Tropical Medicine, Antwerp.

RESULTS

Characteristics of the Study Participants

Sixty-four prostitutes from an economically depressed neighborhood in Nairobi were enrolled in the study. This group included 52 Tanzanians, 7 Ugandans, and 5 Kenyans. The average length of residence in Nairobi was six years. The mean age of the group was 29 years, and the mean duration of prostitution was 5 years. These women had an average of 963 sexual encounters per year. Their clients were largely of Kenyan nationality and paid the equivalent of about 50 cents per encounter. These prostitutes performed only vaginal intercourse without oral or anal sex, and none used barrier forms of contraception. The prevalence of sexually transmitted diseases in this group with low socioeconomic status was extremely high: 55 percent had a positive serologic test for syphilis, 45 percent had gonorrhea, and 42 percent had genital ulcers. Of 22 such ulcers, 11 (50 percent) were positive for *H. ducreyi*.

Twenty-six prostitutes of a higher socioeconomic status were recruited from the bar of a tourist hotel. The mean age of this group was 24 years, and the mean duration of prostitution was three years. This group included 15 women from Uganda, 7 from Kenya, and 4 from other African countries. The average length of residence in Nairobi was five years. These women catered to tourists and traveling businessmen from Africa, Europe, and North America, as well as well-to-do Kenyans. They charged each client the equivalent of $5 to $15 and had an average of 124 paid sexual encounters per year. Seven women performed active oral sex in addition to vaginal intercourse, but none practiced anal intercourse. No barrier forms of contraception were used. Eight (31 percent) of these prostitutes had serum samples that were reactive for syphilis, five (19 percent) had gonorrhea, and none had genital ulcers.

Forty men presenting to the Nairobi Special Treatment Clinic with genitourinary symptoms were also enrolled as study participants. Thirty-eight men were from Kenya, and two were from other African countries. Their mean age was 29 years. On average, during the previous year these men had had 17 sexual partners, and 23 (58 percent) had had intercourse with one or more prostitutes. One man was bisexual. None used condoms. Nine (23 percent) of the 40 men had a positive serologic test for syphilis.

Forty-two medical students, laboratory technicians, and other medical personnel were enrolled to serve as controls. This group comprised 18 women and 24 men; 40 were from Kenya, and 2 from other African countries. Their mean age was 26 years. Only one (2 percent) of the controls had a serologic test reactive for syphilis.

Prevalence of Antibody to HTLV-III

All serum samples were tested for HTLV-III antibody by the two enzyme-linked immunosorbent assays and by Western blot analysis. A subject was considered seropositive for HTLV-III if both an immunoassay and the Western blot test were positive. According to these criteria, antibody to HTLV-III was detected in the serum of 42 (66 percent) of 64 of the prostitutes of low socioeconomic status, 8 (31 percent) of 26 of the prostitutes of higher status, 3 (8 percent) of the 40 male clinic patients, and 1 (2 percent) of the 42 controls (Table 1).

Of the 172 serum samples tested, 4 gave positive results on one enzyme-linked immunosorbent assay and negative results on the other; 2 of these 4 gave positive results on the Western blot assay, and 2 gave negative results. All 52 samples that were positive on both immunoassays were also positive on the Western blot assay. Of the 116 serum samples that were negative on both immunoassays, none were positive on Western blot assay.

Correlation of Antibody to HTLV-III with Immunologic Abnormalities

Among the two groups of prostitutes and the group of male patients from the clinic for sexually transmitted diseases, immunologic abnormalities characteristic of AIDS virus infection were associated with seropositivity for HTLV-III. In all three groups, the mean T-cell helper/suppressor ratios were significantly lower in the seropositive than in the seronegative subjects (Table 2). In both groups of prostitutes, the mean percentages of lymphocytes identified as T helper cells were significantly lower, and the percentages of those identified as T suppressor cells significantly higher, in the seropositive than in the seronegative women. Similar differences were noted in the clinic patients. The only seropositive subject in the control group had a reversed helper/suppressor ratio (0.58), a diminished T-helper-cell level (21 percent), and an elevated T-suppressor-cell level (36 percent).

Correlation of Antibody to HTLV-III with Lymphadenopathy and Other Clinical Findings

None of the subjects studied had opportunistic infections or Kaposi's sarcoma, nor did any have constitutional symptoms such as persistent fever, chronic diarrhea, weight loss, or fatigue. However, generalized lymphadenopathy (defined by the presence of lymph nodes at least 1 cm in diameter in two or more extrainguinal chains) was detected in over half the seropositive subjects (Table 2) — i.e., 22 (52 percent) of the seropositive low-status prostitutes, 5 (63 percent) of the seropositive higher-status prostitutes, and 2 (67 percent) of the seropositive male clinic patients. These prevalences of lymphadenopathy were all significantly

Table 1. Prevalence of Serum Antibody to HTLV-III, According to Enzyme-Linked Immunosorbent (ELISA) and Western Blot Assays.*

	ELISA 1	ELISA 2	Western Blot	ELISA and Western Blot
	number positive/number tested (% positive)			
Study groups				
Prostitutes				
Low socioeconomic status	41/64	42/64	42/64	42/64 (66)†
Higher socioeconomic status	8/26	8/26	8/26	8/26 (31)‡
Male clinic patients	3/40	3/40	3/40	3/40 (8)
Control group	2/42	1/42	1/42	1/42 (2)

*All serum samples were tested by three assays; ELISA 1 denotes the assay kit of Electro-Nucleonics, and ELISA 2 that of Litton-Bionetics. A subject was considered seropositive if one ELISA and the Western blot assay were positive.

†Significantly different from control value ($P<0.0001$).

‡Significantly different from control value ($P<0.001$).

Table 2. Clinical and Immunologic Characteristics of the Study Groups, According to Seropositivity or Seronegativity for HTLV-III.

Study Group	Generalized Lymphadenopathy	Absolute Lymphocyte Count	T-Cell Subsets: Helper	Suppressor	Helper: Suppressor Ratio
	affected/total(%)	*cells/mm³*	*% lymphocytes**		
Prostitutes					
Low socioeconomic status					
Seropositive	22/42 (52)	3852	25	31	0.93
	P = 0.001		*P = 0.0004*	*P = 0.01*	*P = 0.0001*
Seronegative	2/22 (9)	3851	34	23	1.79
Higher socioeconomic status					
Seropositive	5/8 (63)	5286	23	37	0.87
	P = 0.01		*P = 0.03*	*P = 0.01*	*P = 0.005*
Seronegative	2/18 (11)	4329	32	19	1.86
Male clinic patients					
Seropositive	2/3 (67)	4055	21	30	0.71
	P = 0.02			*P = 0.04*	*P = 0.05*
Seronegative	2/37 (5)	3249	24	21	1.45

*Percentage of T cells identified as helper cells by Leu-3 monoclonal antibody, and percentage of T cells identified as suppressor cells by Leu-2 monoclonal antibody.

higher than the background prevalences in the corresponding seronegative groups.

Correlation of HTLV-III Antibody with Potential Risk Factors and with Coinfections

A number of variables determined from the interview, physical examination, and laboratory results were evaluated as possible correlates of HTLV-III seropositivity among the groups of prostitutes (Table 3). No significant association was found between HTLV-III antibody and age, duration of prostitution, number of sexual encounters per year, nationality, history of immunizations, injections of medication within the past five years, transfusions, scarification, operations, induced abortions, or dental extractions. Sexual exposure to men of different nationalities, however, was associated with different rates of antibody to HTLV-III. According to logistic-regression analysis, after controlling for socioeconomic status the relative risk (RR) of HTLV-III antibody associated with sexual exposure to partners from Rwanda was 8.73 (P = 0.01). Similar trends were noted for the relation between HTLV-III antibody and sexual exposure to men from Burundi (RR = 5.00, P = 0.08), Uganda (RR = 4.76, P = 0.11), or Kenya (RR = 4.72, P = 0.08), although these differences were not statistically significant. In contrast, the relative risk of HTLV-III antibody associated with sexual exposure to North Americans or Europeans was only 0.80 (P not significant).

Seropositive prostitutes tended to have a higher prevalence of sexually transmitted diseases (gonorrhea, genital ulcers, and syphilis) than did seronegative prostitutes. According to multivariate logistic-regression analysis, after control for socioeconomic status the relative risk of antibody to HTLV-III associated with gonorrhea was 3.80 (P<0.01); with genital ulcers, 3.31 (P<0.05); and with a reactive serologic test to syphilis, 2.52 (P<0.07).

The number of HTLV-III–seropositive men from the clinic was too small for analysis of risk factors. However, all three seropositive men had had one or more contacts with prostitutes. One of these men was bisexual.

Discussion

In this study, we detected AIDS virus infection in over half the Nairobi prostitutes whom we evaluated,

Table 3. Characteristics of Prostitutes with Respect to Potential Risk Factors and Coinfections.

	Low-Status Prostitutes: Seropositive	Low-Status Prostitutes: Seronegative	Higher-Status Prostitutes: Seropositive	Higher-Status Prostitutes: Seronegative
Risk factors				
Age	28 yr	32 yr	23 yr	24 yr
Duration of prostitution	4 yr	5 yr	2 yr	3 yr
Sex acts/year	922	1042	143	116
	percent of group		*percent of group*	
Origin of sex partners				
Kenya	100	100	75	39
Rwanda	5	0	75 *P<0.05*	28
Uganda	2	5	100	61
Burundi	0	0	50	17
Zaire	0	0	50	39
Tanzania	2	5	38	22
North America or Europe	0	0	50	56
Immunizations	100	91	100	94
Injections of medicine	95	96	100	100
Transfusions	14	4	0	11
Scarification*	55	46	75	61
Operations	26	32	13	39
Induced abortions	5	9	13	22
Dental extractions	17	14	50	28
Current infections				
Gonorrhea	55 *P<0.05*	27	38	11
Genital ulcer	50	27	0	0
Syphilis				
By rapid plasma reagin	24	23	38	17
By *T. pallidum* hemagglutination	52	36	25	11

*Ritual practice of making small incisions in the skin for beautification or healing purposes.

as well as in a small number of men who had had sexual encounters with prostitutes. In keeping with investigations in Kinshasa (Zaire) and Kigali (Rwanda), our results provide support for a role for heterosexual contact in transmitting AIDS.[2,3] Homosexuality is uncommon in Kenya. One bisexual man was included in our study population and was seropositive for HTLV-III; he claimed to have had only one homosexual encounter. None of the subjects whom we studied used intravenous drugs. A history of intramuscular injections of medications was virtually universal among the prostitutes, raising the possibility of parenteral transmission of AIDS through contaminated needles and syringes. However, a history of injections was also obtained from nearly all male patients from the clinic for sexually transmitted diseases, who had a much lower prevalence of HTLV-III antibody. More quantitative data on the actual number of recent injections were not obtained in this study.

The associations between certain sexually transmitted diseases and HTLV-III antibody in the prostitutes are of interest. These results are consistent with those of a case–control study, which identified a significant correlation between AIDS in homosexual men and a history of syphilis or a reactive microhemagglutination assay for *T. pallidum*.[9,10] It may be that epithelial integrity is an important barrier to viral transmission and that diseases such as gonorrhea, chancroid, or syphilis, which cause mucosal or squamous epithelial discontinuity or bleeding, are risk factors for AIDS virus infection. Alternatively, factors increasing the risk of AIDS virus infection may coincidentally increase the risk of other sexually transmitted diseases, although we did not find any correlation between the presence of antibody to HTLV-III and the total number of sex partners. A third possibility is that the cellular immune dysfunction that results from AIDS virus infection may predispose to susceptibility to or chronicity of other sexually transmitted diseases.

The high prevalence of HTLV-III antibody among the prostitutes was a surprising finding in view of the paucity of cases of overt AIDS diagnosed in Kenya.[7] The population of Greater Nairobi is approximately 1 million. The total number of prostitutes in Nairobi is not known, but is certainly several thousand. It is possible that some persons with AIDS have not come to medical attention, but given the fairly sophisticated level of medical care in Nairobi, it is unlikely that a substantial number of cases are unrecognized. The prostitutes whom we interviewed did not describe any deaths within the prostitute community during the past five years that were suggestive of AIDS.

An alternative explanation for the scarcity of cases of full-blown AIDS in Kenya is that the virulence of the retrovirus has diminished. However, over half the HTLV-III–seropositive subjects in our study had generalized lymphadenopathy, often with serious immunologic abnormalities, suggesting that in Kenya the AIDS virus induces a pattern of pathologic response similar to that of strains in North America and Central Africa.

We have evidence from stored serum samples of prostitutes of both low and higher socioeconomic classes, collected over the past five years, that AIDS virus infection has been introduced into this community since 1980 (Piot P: unpublished data). Given the long incubation period of the disease, we suspect that overt cases of AIDS may begin appearing within the prostitute population in the near future, and prospective follow-up of our cohort for the natural history of disease progression is under way.

The source of the AIDS virus epidemic in Nairobi must remain speculative, but our data support the hypothesis of transcontinental spread from Central Africa rather than introduction of the virus by visitors from Europe or North America. None of the prostitutes in the low socioeconomic class had had sexual contact with a non-African. Among the prostitutes as a whole, sexual contact with men from Rwanda, Uganda, and Burundi was associated with HTLV-III seropositivity. Many of the prostitutes were from Tanzania or Uganda, and it is possible that some women acquired AIDS virus infection in their countries of origin. However, we found no association between HTLV-III antibody and nationality.

The implications of an epidemic of AIDS virus infection in Kenya are sobering. If urban prostitutes constitute a major reservoir of AIDS virus in such African capitals as Nairobi, Kigali, and Kinshasa, we may expect that the virus will continue to be spread throughout the African continent by heterosexual men serving as vectors of infection from one community of urban prostitutes to another.[2,3,6] Cultural patterns of sexual behavior, along with urban migration of a male work force and attendant disruption of family units, are factors that may facilitate heterosexual transmission of disease in urban centers, with subsequent spread to rural areas. In addition, the relatively high female:male ratio of cases of AIDS in Africa (1:1 in Zaire, compared with 1:16 in the United States), coupled with a high birth rate, raises the possibility that perinatal transmission may result in high rates of the infection among infants and children.[2,5] To limit the spread of this serious disease in Africa, there is an urgent need to initiate public health education programs directed at modifying sexual behavior and limiting sexual contact with persons in high-risk populations.

We are indebted to the participants who volunteered for this study; to Jane Rahedi for her interpretive skills; to Mwaniki Kagai, David Iha, and Darrel Allen for their laboratory support; to Daniel Nganga for assistance; to Dr. Alexander Saunders (Becton-Dickinson, Mountain View, Calif.) for generously providing Leu monoclonal antibodies; and to Ferne Beier for helping in manuscript preparation.

References

1. Clumeck N, Sonnet J, Taelman H, et al. Acquired immunodeficiency syndrome in African patients. N Engl J Med 1984; 310:492-7.

2. Piot P, Quinn TC, Taelman H, et al. Acquired immunodeficiency syndrome in a heterosexual population in Zaire. Lancet 1984; 2:65-9.
3. Van de Perre P, Rouvroy D, Lepage P, et al. Acquired immunodeficiency syndrome in Rwanda. Lancet 1984; 2:62-5.
4. Brun-Vézinet F, Rouzioux C, Montagnier L, et al. Prevalence of antibodies to lymphadenopathy-associated retrovirus in African patients with AIDS. Science 1984; 226:453-6.
5. Update: acquired immunodeficiency syndrome — United States. MMWR 1985; 34:245-8.
6. Van de Perre P, Clumeck N, Carael M, et al. Female prostitutes: a risk group for infection with human T-cell lymphotropic virus type III. Lancet 1985; 2:524-7.
7. Obel AOK, Sharif SK, McLigeyo SO, Gitonga E, Shah MV, Gitau W. Acquired immunodeficiency syndrome in an African. E Afr Med J 1984; 61:724-6.
8. D'Costa LJ, Plummer FA, Bowmer I, et al. Prostitutes are a major reservoir of sexually transmitted diseases in Nairobi, Kenya. Sex Transm Dis 1985; 12:64-7.
9. Jaffe HW, Choi K, Thomas PA, et al. National case-control study of Kaposi's sarcoma and *Pneumocystis carinii* pneumonia in homosexual men: I. Epidemiologic results. Ann Intern Med 1983; 99:145-51.
10. Rogers MF, Morens DM, Stewart JA, et al. National case-control study of Kaposi's sarcoma and *Pneumocystis carinii* pneumonia in homosexual men. 2. Laboratory results. Ann Intern Med 1983; 99:151-8.

ORIGINAL ARTICLE

ANTIBODIES TO HTLV-III IN SWISS PATIENTS WITH AIDS AND PRE-AIDS AND IN GROUPS AT RISK FOR AIDS

Jörg Schüpbach, M.D., Otto Haller, M.D., Markus Vogt, M.D., Rudolf Lüthy, M.D., Helen Joller, M.D., Oswald Oelz, M.D., Mikulas Popovic, M.D., M.G. Sarngadharan, Ph.D., and Robert C. Gallo, M.D.

Abstract We tested serum samples from Swiss subjects by three different assays based on enzyme-linked immunosorbent assay (ELISA) and Western blot techniques for antibodies to proteins associated with the recently discovered human T-cell leukemia/lymphoma virus HTLV-III, the putative etiologic agent for the acquired immunodeficiency syndrome (AIDS). Of 10 patients with AIDS and 10 with pre-AIDS, all were antibody-positive. Furthermore, 37 of 103 intravenous-drug addicts (36 percent), 4 of 40 healthy homosexual men (10 percent), 7 of 83 patients with various types of hepatitis (8.4 percent), but none of 83 healthy blood donors or 10 other controls were antibody-positive. Antibodies to the major viral protein p24 were found consistently and at high titers in the seropositive members of the groups at risk and in those with pre-AIDS but were dramatically reduced in patients with AIDS. In contrast, antibodies to another virus-associated protein, p41, were present in all cases of AIDS and pre-AIDS but were absent in nearly 10 percent of seropositive persons at risk. Whereas p41 and p24 thus appear to be the targets of choice for future screening tests, the ELISA test that is currently available is a useful screening tool.

EPIDEMIOLOGIC data strongly suggest that the acquired immunodeficiency syndrome (AIDS) is caused by an infectious agent, most likely a virus, which is transmitted horizontally through intimate contact or by blood products.[1] The agent, human T-cell leukemia/lymphoma virus (or human T-cell lymphotropic retrovirus) subgroup III (HTLV-III) has recently been isolated.[2-5] HTLV-III belongs to a family of human retroviruses that possess a magnesium-dependent reverse transcriptase of high molecular weight and a major core protein of about 24,000 daltons (p24) and that replicate preferentially in the OKT4-positive (helper) lymphocyte population. In vitro, all subgroups of HTLV have cytopathogenic effects,[2,3,6,7] but such effects are most prominent in HTLV-III. The loss of OKT4-positive cells is a crucial feature of AIDS. Precisely, these cells are the principal target of HTLV-III, and they are destroyed in vitro within a few days after infection.[2,3] Antibodies against HTLV-III indicating present or past infection have been found in up to 100 percent of AIDS cases and in up to 85 percent of cases of pre-AIDS, which is a condition involving a number of nonspecific symptoms occurring in persons at risk for AIDS.[5,8] Antibody prevalences of about 25 percent or higher have been found in the risk groups of healthy homosexual men and intravenous-drug abusers, respectively.[5,8] Virus has been isolated in many of these cases[2,3] and with the improved techniques now in use can be isolated in almost all cases of AIDS and pre-AIDS (Redfield R, et al.: unpublished data). Of particular importance are the cases in which blood or other biologic materials were transmitted from one person to another in whom AIDS later developed. Antibodies to HTLV-III were found in 100 percent of the cases of transfusion-related AIDS, both in the donors and the recipients (Jaffe HW, et al.: unpublished data). HTLV-III was also isolated from a high percentage of mothers of children with AIDS, and both the children and the mothers had antibodies to the virus[3,4] (and Salahuddin SZ, et al.: unpublished data). Altogether, these findings indicate strongly that HTLV-III is the etiologic agent for AIDS. Other human T-cell lymphotropic retroviruses, designated lymphadenopathy-associated virus[9] and immunodeficiency-associated virus,[10] have been isolated from patients with lymphadenopathy syndrome and AIDS. The relation between these viruses and HTLV-III is under study.

In Switzerland, 29 cases of AIDS had been recorded as of July 1984[11] (and Somaini B: personal communication). Most of the patients had traveled to or lived in the United States, Haiti, or equatorial Africa. Most of the cases were diagnosed in the larger urban areas, about half of them in Zurich. In this report we present a seroepidemiologic study of the presence of HTLV-III infection in Zurich patients with AIDS or pre-AIDS, as well as in healthy homosexual men, intravenous-drug addicts, and appropriate controls from the same region. Antibodies to a variety of HTLV-III-associated proteins were specifically identified by three different tests, and their usefulness in screening assays was assessed.

Methods

Serum Samples

AIDS was diagnosed in 10 patients and pre-AIDS in 10 others at the Department of Medicine, University Hospital, Zurich, on the basis of the following criteria: Patients with AIDS were identified clinically as persons presenting with opportunistic infection or Kaposi's sarcoma or both, in accordance with the definition of the Centers for Disease Control (CDC). Patients with pre-AIDS included eight members of groups at risk for AIDS who presented with unexplained lymphadenopathy in two or more extrainguinal sites that lasted for more than three months. Also included in this group were two patients with multiple symptoms or laboratory signs listed in the definition of the AIDS-related complex.[12] Though their signs and symptoms did not meet the definition of the AIDS-related

From the Laboratory of Tumor Cell Biology, National Cancer Institute, Bethesda, Md.; the Institute for Immunology and Virology, University of Zurich, and the Department of Medicine and Institute for Clinical Immunology, University Hospital, Zurich, Switzerland; and the Department of Cell Biology, Litton Bionetics, Inc., Kensington, Md.

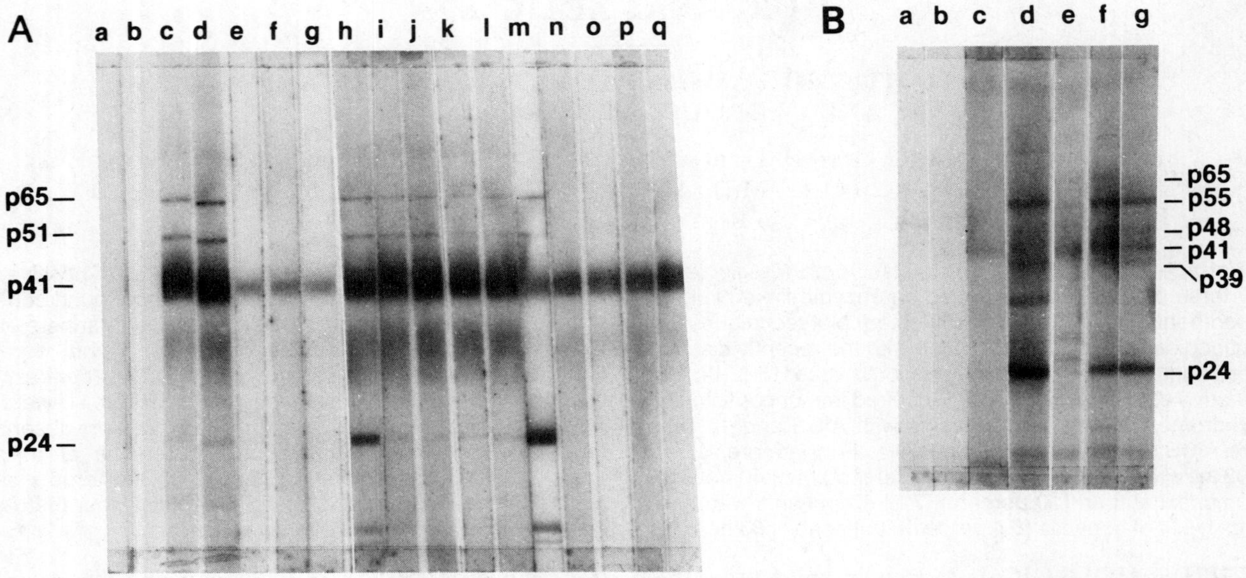

Figure 1. Results of Virus-Strip Radioimmunoassay (A) and Cell-Strip Radioimmunoassay (B) in Representative Serum Samples. Tests were performed as described in the Methods section. The samples in Panel A were from, a, a patient with acute pancreatitis (control); b, a healthy carrier of HTLV-I (control); c and d, AIDS Case A1, serum samples obtained 9.5 months apart; e through g, AIDS Case A2, serum samples obtained at two-month intervals; h through j, pre-AIDS Case B1, serum samples obtained at 4.5-month intervals; k and l, a healthy sex partner of patient A4 with AIDS, samples obtained three months apart; m, pre-AIDS Case B2; n through q, AIDS Case A3, samples obtained at four-month intervals.

The samples in Panel B were from, a and b, heterosexual controls; c, AIDS Case A6; d, pre-AIDS Case B4; e, AIDS Case A7; f, pre-AIDS Case B5; and g, pre-AIDS Case B6.

complex completely (the presence of at least two clinical symptoms and two laboratory signs) it was thought that they were AIDS-related, since both patients were at risk for AIDS. Serum samples were obtained from healthy homosexual controls and from intravenous-drug addicts, all from Zurich, who were participating in a free program of vaccination against hepatitis B virus. Serum samples were collected under sterile conditions and stored at −20°C. Some of the serum samples had already been used in other tests and had undergone repeated freezing and thawing. The assays were done under code with use of the enzyme-linked immunosorbent assay (ELISA) and Western blot techniques as described below.

ELISA

The assay was performed essentially as described by Saxinger and Gallo.[13] HTLV was purified as described elsewhere[2,3] from the mediums of the HTLV-III-producing cell clone H9.[2] HTLV-III was made soluble in a medium containing 0.5 percent Nonidet P40 and 0.5 M sodium chloride, and the extract was diluted with 50 mM sodium bicarbonate (pH 9.6) to a concentration of 5 μg per milliliter. The wells of Immulon I microtiter plates were filled with 0.1 ml of the virus extract and incubated overnight at 4°C. The plates were washed with water and incubated for 20 minutes with 200 μl of 5 percent bovine serum albumin in phosphate-buffered saline. The wells were washed with phosphate-buffered saline and filled with 100 μl of 20 percent normal goat serum in phosphate-buffered saline, followed by 10 μl of the test serums. After incubation for two hours at room temperature, the wells were washed three times with phosphate-buffered saline containing 0.05 percent Tween 20. The wells were incubated for one hour at room temperature with 100 μl of peroxidase-coupled goat antihuman IgG diluted to a strength of 1:2000 in phosphate-buffered saline containing 1 percent normal goat serum. The wells were washed four times with phosphate-buffered saline–Tween and four times with phosphate-buffered saline and exposed for 20 minutes to 100 μl of a substrate mixture containing 0.05 percent orthophenylene-diamine and 0.005 percent hydrogen peroxide in phosphate citrate buffer (pH 5.0). The reaction was stopped by the addition of 50 μl of 4*N* sulfuric acid, and the color yield was measured with a Dynatech ELISA plate reader. Assays were performed in duplicate, and the absorbance readings were scored as follows: more than twice the average of four normal negative controls, score 1; more than three times the normal average, score 2 (clearly positive); more than five times the normal average, score 3; and more than six times the normal average, score 4.

Virus-Strip Radioimmunoassays

HTLV-III was lysed and 200 μg of protein was fractionated by electrophoresis on a 12 percent polyacrylamide slab gel in the presence of sodium dodecyl sulfate according to the method of Laemmli.[14] The protein bands in the gel were electrophoretically transferred to a nitrocellulose sheet as described by Towbin et al.[15] Strip solid-phase radioimmunoassays were then performed as previously described.[5] The sheet was incubated at 37°C for two hours with 5 percent bovine serum albumin in 10 mM TRIS–hydrochloric acid (pH 7.5) containing 0.9 percent sodium chloride and cut into 0.5-cm strips. Each strip was incubated for two hours at 37°C and two hours at room temperature in a screw-cap tube containing 2.5 ml of buffer 1 (20 mM TRIS–hydrochloric acid [pH 7.5], 1 mM EDTA, 0.2 M sodium chloride, 0.3 percent Triton X-100, and 2 mg of bovine serum albumin per milliliter) with a 1:25 dilution of normal goat serum and 0.2 mg of human Fab per milliliter. Test serum samples (25 μl) were then added to individual tubes containing the strips, and incubation was continued for one hour at room temperature and overnight in the cold. The strips were washed three times with a solution containing 0.5 percent sodium deoxycholate, 0.1 M sodium chloride, 0.5 percent Triton X-100, 1 mM phenylmethylsulfonyl fluoride, and 10 mM sodium phosphate, pH 7.5. The strips were incubated for one hour at room temperature with 2.4 ml of buffer 1 and 0.1 ml of normal goat serum.

Affinity-purified and ^{125}I-labeled goat antihuman immunoglobulins (μ chain and Fc fragment-specific) (1.25×10^6 cpm of each) were added to the reaction mixture, and the incubation was continued for 30 minutes at room temperature. The strips were washed as described, dried, mounted, and exposed to x-ray film. The intensity

Table 1. Antibodies to HTLV-III in Homosexual Men with AIDS.

Patient No.	Age	Disorders*	Intensity Scores for Antibodies to HTLV-III†										
			ELISA	virus-strip RIA				cell-strip RIA					
				p65	p51	p41	p24	p65	p55	p48	p41	p39	p24
A1	39	PC, HS	2	2	2	4	2	2	0	0	0	0	0
A2	30	KS, PC, CS, CMV	1	0	0	3	1	2	0	0	0	0	0
A3	57	KS, C	2	0	1	4	0	0	0	0	2	0	0
A4	42	KS, PC, C, M, HS, CMV	2	1	1	3	2	2	0	0	0	0	0
A5	41	KS, HS	0	1	1	3	2	3	0	0	0	0	0
A6	48	KS, LY, HZ	2	1	1	4	0	0	0	0	3	3	1
A7	38	KS	2	2	2	3	3	0	2	2	2	0	1
A8	46	HS, TCP	3	1	1	3	0	0	0	0	2	0	0
A9	30	PC, HZ	2	2	2	4	3	0	3	2	2	2	3
A10	40	KS, C	0	0	2	2	2	0	1	0	0	0	0
Prevalence (%)			*80*	*70*	*90*	*100*	*70*	*40*	*30*	*20*	*50*	*20*	*30*
Mean intensity score			*1.6*	*1*	*1.3*	*3.3*	*1.5*	*0.9*	*0.6*	*0.4*	*1.1*	*0.5*	*0.5*

*PC denotes *Pneumocystis carinii*, HS herpes simplex virus, KS Kaposi's sarcoma, CS cryptosporidiosis, CMV cytomegalovirus, C candida esophagitis, M atypical mycobacterium pneumonia, LY disseminated B-lymphoma, HZ herpes zoster, and TCP thrombocytopenia.

†Tests were performed and the results scored as described in the Methods section. HTLV-III denotes human T-cell leukemia/lymphoma virus III, and RIA radioimmunoassay.

of specific antigen–antibody reactions was assessed visually and assigned a score ranging from 0 to 4, with 0 indicating no reaction; 1, barely detectable; 2, clearly detectable; 3, strong; and 4, very strong.

Cell-Strip Radioimmunoassays

Lysates of the HTLV-III-producing cell clone[2] H4 were used for the production of nitrocellulose strips coated with fractionated cellular lysate and were processed as described above for the virus strips.

Results

Serum samples from patients with AIDS or pre-AIDS, from persons at risk for AIDS, and from various controls were tested for the presence of antibodies to HTLV-III by three different assays: an ELISA based on disrupted HTLV-III and two strip radioimmunoassays based on the Western blot technique, with use of either purified HTLV-III or extracts of cells producing HTLV-III. The results are shown in Tables 1 through 3 and Figure 1. All the subjects were from the metropolitan Zurich area, which has substantial populations of homosexual men and drug addicts.

Among the 10 patients with AIDS (Table 1), samples from 8 were positive according to the ELISA, with an average intensity score of 1.6 (see Methods). Samples from all 10 were positive on the very sensitive virus-strip radioimmunoassay and on the less sensitive cell-strip radioimmunoassay. Representative results of both tests are shown in Figure 1. Interpretation of the cell-strip radioimmunoassay was difficult, especially when specific antibodies were present at low titers. This made it necessary to work at low serum dilutions (1:100), and consequently the nonspecific background was quite high. The most marked reaction in the virus-strip radioimmunoassay was with an antigen of 41,000 daltons, which copurifies with the virus and may represent an envelope component.[4] The majority of the serum samples also recognized an antigen of 65,000 daltons that possibly represents the viral-envelope precursor, which may be analogous to a protein of similar size (p61 to 65) in cells infected by HTLV-I.[16,17] Low-titer antibodies to HTLV-I p61 to 65 have been found by others in a large proportion of patients with AIDS and pre-AIDS and in persons at risk for AIDS.[18-20] When such serum samples were tested by the Western blot technique on strips made from cells producing HTLV-III, a

Table 2. Antibodies to HTLV-III in Patients with Pre-AIDS.

Patient No.	Age	Sex	Risk Group *	Symptoms †	Intensity Score for Antibodies to HTLV-III ‡										
					ELISA	virus-strip RIA				cell-strip RIA					
						p65	p51	p41	p24	p65	p55	p48	p41	p39	p24
B1	25	M	Homosexual, addict	ITP, A, ITR	3	2	2	4	3	2	2	0	0	0	2
B2	29	M	Addict	LAP, ITP	4	2	2	4	4	2	3	2	2	2	4
B3	22	M	Addict	LAP, F, A LP, ITP, An	3	2	1	2	4	1	2	1	2	2	4
B4	51	M	Homosexual	F, LP, A	4	2	2	4	4	2	3	2	2	2	3
B5	38	M	Homosexual	LAP	4	2	2	3	3	2	3	2	2	2	3
B6	19	M	Homosexual	LAP	4	2	1	3	3	0	3	2	2	2	3
B7	35	M	Homosexual	LAP	2	2	1	3	2	2	2	1	2	2	0
B8	24	F	Addict	LAP	3	0	0	2	2	3	3	0	2	2	3
B9	27	M	Homosexual	LAP	4	2	2	4	3	0	3	2	2	2	4
B10	21	M	Homosexual	LAP	2	0	0	3	1	1	2	1	0	0	0
Prevalence (%)					*100*	*80*	*80*	*100*	*100*	*80*	*100*	*80*	*80*	*80*	*80*
Mean intensity score					*3.3*	*1.6*	*1.3*	*3.2*	*2.9*	*1.5*	*2.6*	*1.3*	*1.6*	*1.6*	*2.6*

*Addict denotes intravenous-drug addict.

†ITP denotes idiopathic thrombocytopenic purpura, A cutaneous anergy, ITR inverse T-cell subset ratio, LAP persistent lymphadenopathy, F fever, LP lymphopenia, and An anemia.

‡Tests were performed as described in the Methods section. RIA denotes radioimmunoassay.

Table 3. Antibodies to HTLV-III in Risk Groups and Controls.*

POPULATION	NO. TESTED	NO. POSITIVE †	PREVALENCE	INTENSITY SCORE ON ELISA ‡	PREVALENCE AND INTENSITY SCORE ON VIRUS-STRIP RIA ‡			
					p65	p51	p41	p24
			%		*prevalence (%)/average intensity score*			
Intravenous-drug addicts	103	37	36	3.0	72/2.5	65/2.3	92/2.7	100/2.9
Healthy homosexual men	40	4	10	3.0				
Patients with hepatitis	83	7	8.4	3.1				
Patients with other disorders §	10	0	0	NA	NA	NA	NA	NA
Healthy blood donors of both sexes and of unknown sexual preference	83	0	0	NA	NA	NA	NA	NA

*ELISA denotes enzyme-linked immunosorbent assay, RIA radioimmunoassay, and NA not applicable.

†Number includes only the serum samples that were positive on both ELISA and virus-strip radioimmunoassay.

‡Among those with positive results only.

§Other disorders include lupus erythematosus, Sézary syndrome, polyarthritis, and pancreatitis.

strong reaction with p65 was seen in all cases. In contrast, testing with strips from cells producing HTLV-I resulted in only weak detection of p61 to 65 (data not shown). A reaction was also found with p51, which may also be related to the viral envelope as shown in HTLV-I,[16,17] and less frequently with p24, which is a viral protein coded for by the *gag* gene.[21] The average intensity score (representing the titer) was very high for antibodies to p41: 3.3 out of a possible 4. Average scores for the other antibodies were less than 2 in all cases. These results indicate that p41 is the crucial protein for the serologic diagnosis of HTLV-III infections in AIDS.

Samples from all 10 of the patients with pre-AIDS (Table 2) were clearly positive according to the ELISA, with an average score of 3.3. Antibodies to both p41 and p24 in virus were found in all cases and with average scores of 3.2 and 2.9, respectively. On cell strips p55, which is the precursor of p24 and other *gag*-encoded proteins,[4,22] was detected in all cases (score, 2.6), whereas p24 itself was detected by eight serum samples only, but with a high score of 2.6. In one of the patients, a drop in the titer of antibody to p24 was observed (Fig. 1A, strips h through j). This drop may predict progression to manifest AIDS, since the scores of antibodies to p24 in AIDS are much lower than in pre-AIDS. In contrast to the serum samples of the patients with AIDS, those of the patients with pre-AIDS also frequently reacted with antigens with molecular weights of 48,000 and 39,000. The affiliation of these antigens is unclear at the moment. However, their recognition appears not to correlate with the recognition of p65, and they may instead be related to *gag*. Altogether, the patients with pre-AIDS had considerably higher titers and higher prevalences of antibodies to *gag*-related antigens than the patients with AIDS.

The results of tests in risk groups and controls are shown in Table 3. Serum samples from 103 intravenous-drug addicts were tested by both ELISA and strip-virus radioimmunoassay. None of 61 of these serum samples scoring 0 and none of 5 scoring 1 on ELISA were positive according to virus-strip radioimmunoassay. Therefore, the serum samples of the homosexuals, patients with hepatitis, and controls were tested by virus-strip radioimmunoassay only if the score on ELISA was 1 or higher. Serum samples that were negative according to virus-strip radioimmunoassay were rated negative even if the ELISA was positive. Such false positive or borderline positive ELISA results were found in 19 of the 83 normal blood donors (23 percent) and in 17 of the 83 patients with hepatitis (20 percent). Two (6 percent) of these 36 false positive serum samples had an ELISA score of 4, three (8 percent) a score of 3, 13 (36 percent) a score of 2, and 18 (50 percent) a score of 1. The serum samples of 40 healthy homosexual men and of the 103 drug addicts were free of false positive results. We believe that at least some of the false positive results may have been due to improper handling and storage of serum samples — for example, repeated freezing and thawing.

Antibodies to HTLV-III (all verified by virus-strip radioimmunoassay) were found in 37 of the 103 intravenous-drug addicts (36 percent). Among 40 serum samples obtained in healthy homosexual men before vaccination with hepatitis B virus, 4 were found to be positive. No antibody-positive cases were found among 83 healthy donors of blood or among 10 patients with various diseases, including systemic lupus erythematosus, polyarthritis, and Sézary syndrome. However, 7 antibody-positive cases (8.4 percent) were detected among 83 patients with hepatitis. They included four cases of acute A hepatitis, one case of acute B hepatitis, one case of acute non-A,non-B hepatitis, and one patient with a history of A and B hepatitis. The 48 infected persons with no symptoms had high titers of antibodies to HTLV-III, as shown by the average scores of 3 and higher in the ELISA. The virus-strip radioimmunoassay showed a predominance of antibodies to p24, with a prevalence of 100 percent and an average intensity score of 2.9. Antibodies to p41 were detected less consistently, with a prevalence of 92 percent and a score of 2.7. Antibodies to p24 alone were found in four persons, including three of the seven seropositive patients with hepatitis and one intravenous-drug addict.

Discussion

The 100 percent prevalence of antibodies to HTLV-III among Zurich patients with AIDS and pre-AIDS confirms the results obtained earlier in American patients[5,16] and indicates that AIDS and pre-AIDS in Europe are also associated with infection by this newly discovered member of the family of human T-cell leukemia/lymphoma viruses. Moreover, our results indicate a high prevalence of antibodies to HTLV-III in the Zurich population of healthy homosexual men and an even higher prevalence among the intravenous-drug addicts. In addition, nearly 10 percent of the patients with various types of hepatitis had signs of infection with HTLV-III. This is probably because the principal populations at risk for AIDS are also prone to infection with hepatitis viruses.

The Western blot techniques used in this study allow one to determine the specificity of the antibodies detected. The comparison by virus-strip radioimmunoassay of patients with AIDS, patients with pre-AIDS, and infected persons without symptoms shows that p41 and p24 are the crucial proteins in the serologic diagnosis of HTLV-III infection. Antibodies to p24 are consistently found in asymptomatic seropositive subjects and in patients with pre-AIDS, but decline dramatically in patients with AIDS. In contrast, antibodies to p41 are consistently present in patients with AIDS[8] and pre-AIDS but are absent in about 10 percent of asymptomatic seropositive subjects. This changing pattern suggests that the monitoring of these antibodies may be of prognostic relevance. In one case of pre-AIDS (Fig. 1A, strips h through j) we found a strong drop in titer of antibodies to p24, whereas antibodies to p41 remained unchanged. The drop suggests that the patient may have been in a stage of transition from pre-AIDS to AIDS.

The ELISA is inferior to the virus-strip radioimmunoassay in detecting antibody-positive patients with AIDS (prevalence, 80 percent; mean score, 1.6). However, the ELISA appears to be similarly sensitive in the cases of pre-AIDS and in groups at risk for AIDS. This is suggested by the demonstration that none of 61 serum samples from intravenous-drug addicts that had scores of 0 in the ELISA were positive in the Western blot assay. The four samples with antibodies to p24 alone all had scores of at least 1 in the ELISA. Finally, the high average ELISA scores in these subjects indicate that there are only a few borderline positive persons in these groups. If handled rigorously (i.e., if samples with ELISA scores of 1 or higher are defined as being positive), this test should prevent the transfusion of the vast majority of infected blood donations. Persons with frank AIDS frequently have negative results on ELISA but should presumably not be present among the donors. The ELISA should not be used for purposes other than screening, since it may carry a high rate of false positive results, possibly in part because of improper handling and storage of serum. The identification of HTLV-III in a person should thus never depend on the ELISA alone but should always be confirmed by a virus-strip assay. In the long run, tests based on purified p41 and p24 should prove more satisfactory.

We are indebted to J. Ahmad, K. Arnett, L. Bruch, and R. Bhushan for careful technical assistance.

References

1. Centers for Disease Control Task Force on Kaposi's Sarcoma and Opportunistic Infections. Epidemiologic aspects of the current outbreak of Kaposi's sarcoma and opportunistic infections. N Engl J Med 1982; 306: 248-52.
2. Popovic M, Sarngadharan MG, Read E, Gallo RC. Detection, isolation, and continuous production of cytopathic retroviruses (HTLV-III) from patients with AIDS and pre-AIDS. Science 1984; 224:497-500.
3. Gallo RC, Salahuddin SZ, Popovic M, et al. Frequent detection and isolation of cytopathic retroviruses (HTLV-III) from patients with AIDS and at risk for AIDS. Science 1984; 224:500-3.
4. Schüpbach J, Popovic M, Gilden RV, Gonda MA, Sarngadharan MG, Gallo RC. Serological analysis of a subgroup of human T-lymphotropic retroviruses (HTLV-III) associated with AIDS. Science 1984; 224:503-5.
5. Sarngadharan MG, Popovic M, Bruch L, Schüpbach J, Gallo RC. Antibodies reactive with a human T-lymphotropic retrovirus (HTLV-III) in the serum of patients with AIDS. Science 1984; 224:506-8.
6. Popovic M, Wong-Staal F, Sarin P, Gallo RC. Biology of human T-cell leukemia/lymphoma virus: transformation of human T-cells *in vivo* and *in vitro*. In: Klein G, ed. Advances in viral oncology. Vol. 4. New York: Raven Press, 1984:45-70.
7. Nagy K, Clapham P, Cheingsong-Popov R, Weiss RA. Human T-cell leukemia virus type I: induction of syncytia and inhibition by patient's sera. Int J Cancer 1983; 32:321-8.
8. Safai B, Sarngadharan MG, Groopman JE, et al. Seroepidemiological studies of human T-lymphotropic retrovirus type III in acquired immunodeficiency syndrome. Lancet 1984; 1:1438-40.
9. Barré-Sinoussi F, Chermann JC, Rey F, et al. Isolation of a T-lymphotropic retrovirus from a patient at risk for acquired immune deficiency syndrome (AIDS). Science 1983; 220:868-71.
10. Vilmer E, Barré-Sinoussi F, Rouzioux C, et al. Isolation of a new lymphotropic retrovirus from two siblings with haemophilia B, one with AIDS. Lancet 1984; 1:753-7.
11. Somaini B. AIDS in der Schweiz. Schweiz Med Wochenschr 1984; 114:538-44.
12. AIDS in Europe, status quo 1983 — recommendations: report of a meeting co-sponsored by the Danish Cancer Society, the World Health Organization and the European Organizations for Cooperation in Cancer Prevention Studies, Aarhus, Denmark, October, 1983. Eur J Cancer Clin Oncol 1984; 20:169-73.
13. Saxinger C, Gallo RC. Application of the indirect enzyme-linked immunosorbent assay microtest to the detection and surveillance of human T cell leukemia-lymphoma virus. Lab Invest 1983; 49:371-7.
14. Laemmli UK. Cleavage of structural proteins during the assembly of the head of bacteriophage T4. Nature 1970; 227:680-5.
15. Towbin H, Staehelin T, Gordon J. Electrophoretic transfer of proteins from polyacrylamide gels to nitrocellulose sheets: procedure and some applications. Proc Natl Acad Sci USA 1979; 76:4350-4.
16. Schüpbach J, Sarngadharan MG, Gallo RC. Antigens on HTLV-infected cells recognized by leukemia and AIDS sera are related to HTLV viral glycoprotein. Science 1984; 224:607-10.
17. Lee TH, Coligan JE, Homma T, McLane MF, Tachibana N, Essex M. Human T-cell leukemia virus-associated membrane antigens: identity of the major antigens recognized after virus infection. Proc Natl Acad Sci USA 1984; 81:3856-60.
18. Essex M, McLane MF, Lee TH, et al. Antibodies to cell membrane antigens associated with human T-cell leukemia virus in patients with AIDS. Science 1983; 220:859-62.
19. Downing RG, Eglin RP, Bayley AC. African Kaposi's sarcoma and AIDS. Lancet 1984; 1:478-80.
20. Essex M, McLane MF, Lee TH, et al. Antibodies to human T-cell leukemia virus membrane antigens (HTLV-MA) in hemophiliacs. Science 1983; 221:1061-4.
21. Kalyanaraman VS, Sarngadharan MG, Nakao Y, Ito Y, Aoki T, Gallo RC. Natural antibodies to the structural core protein (p24) of the human T-cell leukemia (lymphoma) retrovirus found in sera of leukemia patients in Japan. Proc Natl Acad Sci USA 1982; 79:1653-7.
22. Hattori S, Kiyokawa T, Imagawa K-I, et al. Identification of *gag* and *env* gene products of human T-cell leukemia virus (HTLV). Virology 1984; 136:338-47.

Epidemiology and Public Health Issues

AIDS Transmission via Transfusion and Dialysis

ORIGINAL ARTICLE

ACQUIRED IMMUNODEFICIENCY SYNDROME (AIDS) ASSOCIATED WITH TRANSFUSIONS

JAMES W. CURRAN, M.D., DALE N. LAWRENCE, M.D., HAROLD JAFFE, M.D., JONATHAN E. KAPLAN, M.D., LAWRENCE D. ZYLA, M.P.H., MARY CHAMBERLAND, M.D., ROBERT WEINSTEIN, M.D., KUNG-JONG LUI, PH.D., LAWRENCE B. SCHONBERGER, M.D., THOMAS J. SPIRA, M.D., W. JAMES ALEXANDER, M.D., GARY SWINGER, D.V.M., ARTHUR AMMANN, M.D., STEVEN SOLOMON, M.D., DAVID AUERBACH, M.D., DONNA MILDVAN, M.D., RAND STONEBURNER, M.D., JANINE M. JASON, M.D., HARRY W. HAVERKOS, M.D., AND BRUCE L. EVATT, M.D.

Abstract Of 2157 patients with the acquired immunodeficiency syndrome (AIDS) whose cases were reported to the Centers for Disease Control by August 22, 1983, 64 (3 percent) with AIDS and *Pneumocystis carinii* pneumonia had no recognized risk factors for AIDS. Eighteen of these (28 percent) had received blood components within five years before the onset of illness. These patients with transfusion-associated AIDS were more likely to be white (P = 0.00008) and older (P = 0.0013) than other patients with no known risk factors. They had received blood 15 to 57 months (median, 27.5) before the diagnosis of AIDS, from 2 to 48 donors (median, 14). At least one high-risk donor was identified by interview or T-cell–subset analysis in each of the seven cases in which investigation of the donors was complete; five of the six high-risk donors identified during interview also had low T-cell helper/suppressor ratios, and four had generalized lymphadenopathy according to history or examination. These findings strengthen the evidence that AIDS may be transmitted in blood.

CASES of the acquired immunodeficiency syndrome (AIDS) were first recognized in homosexual men and in persons who abused drugs intravenously, suggesting a pattern of occurrence similar to that of hepatitis B in the United States.[1-6] Reports of cases of AIDS in men with hemophilia further confirmed this pattern.[7-12] As with hepatitis B, epidemiologic evidence suggests that AIDS is caused by an agent that can be sexually transmitted between homosexual men[13,14] as well as from heterosexual men to their female partners.[15,16] The sharing of contaminated needles is the presumed mode of transmission between drug addicts. The most likely source of transmission of the putative "AIDS agent" to persons with hemophilia is thought to be clotting-factor concentrates (Evatt BL, et al.: unpublished data).[17]

An infant who received multiple transfusions at birth for erythroblastosis fetalis subsequently acquired severe cellular immunodeficiency and multiple opportunistic infections, ultimately dying from *Pneumocystis carinii* pneumonia.[18,19] One of the blood donors was a man who was subsequently diagnosed as having AIDS and who died of it. Other cases of AIDS have been reported to the Centers for Disease Control (CDC) as occurring in persons who did not belong to groups with an increased incidence of AIDS and who had received blood components within five years before the diagnosis of their illness. Below is a summary of these cases and the results of the completed investigations of the blood donors.

From the Centers for Disease Control, Atlanta, Ga.; the Department of Internal Medicine, Michael Reese Hospital, Chicago; the New York City Department of Health, New York; the Beth Israel Medical Center, New York; the Tennessee Department of Public Health, Nashville; the Jefferson County (Alabama) Department of Public Health, Birmingham; and the University of California–San Francisco Medical Center, San Francisco.

METHODS

Case Definition and Surveillance

The CDC surveillance definition of AIDS includes reliably diagnosed diseases indicative of underlying cellular immunodeficiency in the absence of any other cause of reduced resistance or increased susceptibility to that disease. These illnesses include opportunistic infections such as *P. carinii* pneumonia, Kaposi's sarcoma in persons under 60 years of age, and lymphoma limited to the brain.[20] The retrospective-surveillance methods for AIDS have been described elsewhere.[21] Current reporting is supplemented by active surveillance through city and state health departments as well as investigation of all requests to the CDC for pentamidine isethionate for the treatment of *P. carinii* pneumonia.

Investigation of Patients with a History of Previous Transfusion

Patients with AIDS who did not fit into one of the groups known to have an increased incidence of AIDS were investigated. The medical and social histories obtained included information on receipt of blood or blood products during the five years preceding the diagnosis of AIDS. If no other potential risk factors were identified and the patient had previously received transfusions, he or she was classified as having transfusion-associated AIDS. Detailed information was obtained about the dates and reasons for transfusion and the types of blood products received. With the cooperation of blood-collection centers, investigators contacted the donors for a personal confidential interview and physical examination and, when possible, to obtain heparinized blood for T-cell-subset analyses and other immunologic studies as previously described.[22] Public-health officials checked the donor names against a list of patients with reported cases of AIDS. Information from the interview was collected before testing, and the interview results were unknown to the technicians. Donors with symptoms or physical findings suggestive of illness were referred to local health facilities. When the results of immunologic studies were abnormal, new specimens were drawn and the studies were repeated. Donors with persistently abnormal immunologic findings were advised to return for further evaluation in three months. An investigation was considered complete when all available donors had been examined and interviewed and the immunologic studies had been completed.

Since all patients with transfusion-associated AIDS had a diagnosis of *P. carinii* pneumonia, their characteristics were compared with those of other patients without known risk factors who were reported to have such pneumonia. Three representative case histories are included from among the completed investigations.

Analyses of Investigations of Donors

If AIDS resulted from transmission of an agent through transfusion, presumably at least one donor would have been affected by the agent in each case. Donors may or may not experience symptoms or have signs associated with AIDS, but most donors transmitting the disease would be expected to come from populations previously recognized as having an increased incidence of AIDS (i.e., homosexual men with multiple partners, abusers of intravenous drugs, persons born in Haiti, or patients with hemophilia). Using the definition of a high-risk donor (a person belonging to a group at increased risk for AIDS or having a reversed ratio [<1.00] of T-helper to T-suppressor lymphocytes), we identified a single high-risk donor during each of the initial investigations, regardless of the number of donors. To test the statistical significance of these findings, we used the binomial model as described below in an analysis of the distributions of high-risk donors in the seven completed investigations.

Analysis of the Distribution of High-Risk Donors in Cases of Transfusion-Associated AIDS

In using the binomial model to analyze the high-risk-donor distributions, we assumed that (1) the seven completed investigations were representative of all cases of transfusion-associated AIDS; (2) the true prevalence of high-risk donors in the overall donor population was no higher than our prevalence estimates (we used the total number of high-risk donors identified in the donor investigations as an estimate of the prevalence of high-risk donors in the overall donor populations); (3) the prevalence estimates could be considered constant for the various cases of transfusion-associated AIDS and the relevant donor populations; and (4) the probability of identifying one high-risk donor was independent of identifying others.

The null hypothesis states that the number of patients with transfusion-associated AIDS exposed to a high-risk donor is not greater than that expected by chance on the basis of the total number of donors to which each patient was exposed and the estimated prevalence of high-risk donors in the overall donor population.

The probability of finding x high-risk donors [f(x)] among an individual patient's set of n donors is determined by using the binomial distribution:

$$f(x) = \frac{n!}{x!\,(n-x)!}\,p^x q^{n-x},$$

where $x = 0,1,2, \ldots n$, $p =$ the prevalence of high-risk donors in the overall donor population, and $q = 1-p$. Hence, the probability of finding no high-risk donors in a set of n donors is

$$f(0) = \frac{n!}{0!\,(n-0)!}\,p^0 q^{n-0} = q^n.$$

The probability of finding one or more high-risk donors in the same set of donors is $1-f(0)$ or $1-q^n$.

Results

By August 22, 1983, 2157 cases of AIDS had been reported to the CDC from the United States. When broken down into mutually exclusive categories, this figure included 2033 persons reported to be either homosexual or bisexual men (71.6 percent), past or present abusers of intravenous drugs (16.8 percent), persons born in Haiti and currently living in the United States (5.1 percent), or persons with hemophilia (0.8 percent). One hundred twenty-four persons (5.8 percent) belonged to none of the above high-incidence groups. Of these 124 patients, 82 had a diagnosis of *P. carinii* pneumonia, 23 had opportunistic infections other than *P. carinii* pneumonia, and 19 had Kaposi's sarcoma.

Adequate histories on transfusion were available for 13 of the 19 patients with Kaposi's sarcoma and 22 of the 23 patients with opportunistic infections other than *P. carinii* pneumonia. Of these, only one man with Kaposi's sarcoma had received a transfusion within the previous five years. Since the results of his immunologic tests were normal and his physician considered his course more typical of classic Kaposi's sarcoma, donor investigation was not undertaken and his case was excluded from the analyses.

Of the 82 patients with *P. carinii* pneumonia who were not identified with a high-incidence group, 18 were sexual partners of men or women in high-incidence groups. Of the remaining 64, 18 (28 percent) gave a history of having received a transfusion within five years before diagnosis and were classified as having transfusion-associated AIDS. Table 1 compares these 18 patients with the remaining 46 patients with *P. carinii* pneumonia who were among persons who were not identified with a high-incidence group. Patients with transfusion-associated AIDS were significantly older and more likely to be white than the other patients with *P. carinii* pneumonia.

Table 1. Characteristics of Reported Cases of AIDS and *Pneumocystis carinii* Pneumonia in 64 Persons Not Identified as Belonging to a Group at Increased Risk for AIDS.*

	Cases Associated with Transfusion within 5 Years	Cases Not Associated with Transfusion
Number of cases	18	46
Sex		
Female	8 (44)	17 (37)
Male	10 (56)	29 (63)
Ethnic group		
White	16 (89)†	14 (30)
Black	0	18 (39)
Hispanic	1 (6)	13 (28)
American Indian	0	1 (2)
Asian	1 (6)	0
Age (yr)		
Range	19–67‡	24–72
Median	54	42
Mean	52.1	41.5
Current status		
Alive	8 (44)	19 (41)
Dead	10 (56)	27 (60)
State of residence		
New York	6 (33)	21 (46)
California	3 (17)	1 (2)
New Jersey	1 (6)	5 (11)
Florida	1 (6)	7 (15)
Other	7 (39)	12 (26)
Year of diagnosis		
Before 1981	0	1 (2)
1981	0	3 (6)
1982	6 (33)	15 (33)
1983 (Jan–Aug)	12 (67)	27 (59)

*Values in parentheses represent rounded-off percentages.

†Patients with transfusion-associated AIDS were significantly more likely to be white than the other 46 patients (chi-square = 15.48; P = 0.00008).

‡Patients with transfusion-associated AIDS were significantly different in age distribution from the other 46 patients (Wilcoxon two-sample test, P = 0.0013).

Table 2. Transfusion Histories of 18 Adults with *P. carinii* Pneumonia and Transfusion-Associated AIDS.

Case No.	Age/Sex; Ethnic Group	Date of Diagnosis of Pneumonia	Date of Transfusion	Reasons for Transfusion	No. of Units (Type)*	Months from Transfusion to Onset of Illness	Months from Transfusion to Pneumonia Diagnosis	Status of Donor Investigation
1	52/M; white	6/82	3/81	Exploratory laparotomy, peritonitis	4 (2 PC, 2 FFP)	15	15	In progress
2	64/M; Hispanic	7/82	1/81	Cardiac surgery (coronary bypass)	20 (8 PC, 2 FFP, 10 PL)	15	18	Completed
3	56/F; white	8/82	11/77 4/80†	Mastectomy Hysterectomy	3 (1 PC, 2 WB)	14–43†	28–57†	Completed
4	19/M; white	10/82	12/79	Trauma	2 (PC)	34	34	Completed
5	49/F; white	12/82	2/80	Thrombocytopenia	6 (PL)	27	34	Completed
6	45/F; white	12/82	2/79 7/79 6/81‡	Cardiac surgery (valvular)	28 (4 PC, 3 FFP, 15 WB, 6?)	10–38‡	18–46‡	Completed
7	53/M; white	3/83	11/80	Cardiac surgery (coronary bypass)	16 (7 WB, 4 FFP, 5 PL)	26	28	In progress
8	52/F; white	3/83	10/80	Mastectomy	4 (PC)	24	27	Unable to be completed
9	33/F; Asian	4/83	9/81	Cardiac surgery (aortic-valve replacement)	34 (7 PC, 2 WB, 10 FFP, 15 PL)	17	19	Completed
10	62/M; white	4/83	1/82	Vascular surgery (aortofemoral bypass)	31 (6 PC, 18 WB, 7 FFP)	12	15	In progress
11	61/M; white	5/83	12/80	Cardiac surgery (coronary bypass)	23 (5 PC, 8 WB, 7 FFP, 1 PL, 2 Alb)	26	29	In progress
12	55/F; white	5/83	3/80	Cardiac surgery (coronary bypass)	4 (2 PC, 2 FFP)	33	38	In progress
13	66/M; white	5/83	8/81	Cardiac surgery (coronary bypass)	6 (3 PC, 1 WB, 2 FFP)	17	21	Completed
14	60/M; white	6/83	4–6/81§	Bleeding ulcers	12 (including PC)	24–26§	24–26§	In progress
15	67/F; white	7/83	3/80§ 7/81§	Intestinal polyps Cardiac surgery (aortic-valve replacement)	20 (2 PC, 5 PC, 4 FFP, 9 PL)	18–34§	24–40§	In progress
16	44/M; white	6/83	5–6/82§	Trauma, surgery	48 (7 PC, 20 WB, 2 FFP, 19 PL)	11–12§	12–13§	In progress
17	40/M; white	7/83	5/80	Cardiac surgery (coronary bypass)	22 (9 PC, 2 WB, 1 FFP, 10 PL)	37	38	In progress
18	60/F; white	8/83	8/79	Hysterectomy	4 (2 PC, 2?)	39	48	In progress

*PC denotes packed cells, WB whole blood, FFP fresh-frozen plasma, PL platelets, and Alb albumin.

†The later surgery (shorter duration) is considered more likely to be associated with AIDS in this case. One of the two donors for the latter surgery currently has unexplained generalized lymphadenopathy and a persistently reversed helper/suppressor ratio. The shorter duration was used to compute the interval between transfusion and onset of diagnosis.

‡One of the donors during 1981 was a homosexual man with generalized lymphadenopathy and a transiently reversed helper/suppressor ratio. The shorter duration was used to compute the interval between transfusion and onset of diagnosis.

§Because of the absence of complete information, the midpoint between the transfusions was used to compute the intervals between transfusions and onset or diagnosis.

Table 2 describes the transfusion histories of the 18 patients with transfusion-associated AIDS. Fifteen of the 18 patients (83 percent) received transfusions in association with surgery, 9 of whom had cardiac surgery. Although two patients had had mastectomies for breast carcinoma, neither had evidence of persistent or recurrent disease, nor had they received chemotherapy or radiotherapy within one year before the onset of their current illness. The time between transfusion and onset of illness ranged from 10 to 43 months (median, 24.5 months; mean, 22.7), with 15 to 57 months lapsing between transfusion and the diagnosis of *P. carinii* pneumonia (median, 27.5 months; mean, 26.6). The 18 patients received transfusions from as few as 2 to as many as 48 donors (median, 14; mean, 15.9). No single type of blood product was received by all 18 patients: 16 received packed cells, 12 received fresh-frozen plasma, 9 received whole blood, and 8 received platelets.

The first reported case of transfusion-associated

AIDS was diagnosed in June 1982, and 12 of the 18 cases were diagnosed after March 1983. The dates of transfusions were much earlier; 14 patients received transfusions before the first cases of AIDS were reported to the CDC in June 1981.

Donor Investigations

Results of the seven completed donor investigations are summarized in Table 3. Altogether, eight high-risk donors were identified by history or immunologic evaluation. None of the donors identified in this series were reported to have AIDS. Six of the seven patients with AIDS were exposed to at least one donor from a group at increased risk for AIDS, and all seven were exposed to a donor with a decreased helper/suppressor ratio. Five of the six high-risk donors identified by history also had decreased helper/suppressor ratios. The blood components donated by the eight high-risk donors to patients with transfusion-associated AIDS included platelets (three patients), whole blood (two patients), fresh-frozen plasma (two patients), and packed cells (one patient).

The probability that at least the observed number of patients with AIDS had been exposed to one or more high-risk donors by chance alone was 0.014. This probability remained significant when the definition of high-risk donor was changed to include only donors in a group at increased risk of AIDS (P = 0.028) or those with a reversed helper/suppressor ratio (P = 0.007), depending on which definition of high-risk donor was used. Thus, the null hypothesis is rejected, and patients with transfusion-associated AIDS were more likely to be exposed to a high-risk donor than would be expected on the basis of the number of donors to whom each patient was exposed and the prevalence estimates of high-risk donors in the overall donor population.

Among the first 13 cases of transfusion-associated AIDS reported, donor investigations were completed in 7. The blood-donor records for Case 8 were destroyed in a fire. Interviews and examinations of donors have been initiated in three additional cases; a single high-risk donor has been identified thus far in two of these cases.

Selected Case Histories (Also See Table 2)

Case 4

A 19-year-old man had been in good health until he received multiple fractures and a renal contusion in an automobile accident in December 1979. After therapy, including receipt of two units of packed red cells, he was discharged from the hospital on February 21, 1980, and recovered completely from his injuries. In September 1981 he had a thoracic condition (diagnosed as herpes zoster), which resolved shortly. In October 1982 he was hospitalized with respiratory distress, and a bilateral diffuse infiltrate was noted on a chest film. At an open-lung biopsy *P. carinii* was found. The patient responded to therapy with trimethoprim-sulfamethoxazole. He was readmitted on March 7, 1983, for recurrent pneumonia, and *P. carinii* was again isolated. Laboratory studies indicated elevated levels of IgG and IgA in October 1982 and a decreased helper/suppressor ratio (0.7) in March 1983. Despite therapy with trimethoprim-sulfamethoxazole and pentamidine isethionate, he died on March 20, 1983.

The patient had no history of homosexual contact, intravenous drug abuse, or other known or suspected risk factors for AIDS. Although no autopsy was performed, there was no evidence of a concomitant immunosuppressive disease. The two donors were interviewed and examined. One was a healthy married man with no risk factors for AIDS and with normal results on immunologic studies. The second donor, a 32-year-old homosexual man with multiple

Table 3. Prevalence of High-Risk Donors among Donors to Seven Patients with Transfusion-Associated AIDS.

Case No.	All Donors*	High-Risk Donors		
		Belonging to Group at High Risk for AIDS†	Having T_H/T_S Ratio <1.00†	Other Characteristics
2	14 (6)	1 (13)	1 (12)	One man was an asymptomatic former intravenous-drug abuser with a normal T_H/T_S ratio (1.5); a second man had a decreased ratio (0.9) but denied AIDS risk factors
3	3	0 (3)	1 (3)	A man with a persistently decreased T_H/T_S ratio (0.64, 0.71), lymphadenopathy, and a history of syphilis and hepatisis B who denied risk factors for AIDS
4	2	1 (2)	1 (2)	A homosexual man with multiple partners, lymphadenopathy, and a decreased T_H/T_S ratio (0.7)
5	6	1 (6)	1 (6)	A homosexual man with multiple partners, a history of lymphadenopathy, and a currently decreased T_H/T_S ratio (0.8)
6	24 (4)	1 (19)	1 (18)	A homosexual man with multiple partners, lymphadenopathy, and a decreased T_H/T_S ratio (0.8)
9	34	1 (30)	1 (5)	A homosexual man with multiple partners and a decreased T_H/T_S ratio (0.6)
13	6	1 (5)	1 (2)	A homosexual man with multiple partners and a decreased T_H/T_S ratio (0.7)
	89 (10)‡	6 (78)‡	7 (48)	

*U.S. donations within five years before diagnosis of AIDS (additional donations obtained from Europe are in parentheses).

†Figures in parentheses indicate number of donors on whom information was available. T_H/T_S denotes T helper/T suppressor.

‡The 78 donors who were interviewed and examined included 52 men and 26 women. Six of the 11 American donors not interviewed were women.

sexual partners, gave a history of unexplained generalized lymphadenopathy that had persisted since 1979; a lymph-node biopsy specimen demonstrated benign hyperplasia. In April 1983 he had generalized lymphadenopathy and a helper/suppressor ratio of 0.69.

Case 6

A 45-year-old married woman had congenital heart disease that had required a pulmonary valvulotomy in 1957, repair of an atrial septal defect in 1970, and placement of a pacemaker in 1977. She received blood during her procedures in 1957 and 1970, but not in 1977. She remained well until 1979, when she underwent a hysterectomy for benign disease. During that hospitalization, she had hemorrhage and was treated for septic shock and endocarditis. Surgery was required later that year to replace her tricuspid valve. She was hospitalized in July 1981 for replacement of her tricuspid and pulmonic valves and placement of a permanent pacemaker. In April 1982 she was hospitalized for evaluation of unexplained fever. She was discharged without a specific diagnosis or therapy, but was readmitted in August 1982 for persistent fever, dyspnea, diarrhea, unexplained weight loss, and oral candidiasis. In December 1982, a gallium scan of the lungs demonstrated increased radiotracer uptake, chest films revealed progressive diffuse interstitial infiltrates, and *P. carinii* was detected in material obtained by transbronchial biopsy. The results of scalene-node and bone-marrow biopsies were normal. In February 1983 the patient's neurologic status declined. On CT scanning, findings in several areas were compatible with a diagnosis of central-nervous-system toxoplasmosis, although a brain biopsy showed no pathologic process. The indirect fluorescent antibody titer to toxoplasma antigen was 1:128. The patient's neurologic status and CT-scan findings improved after therapy with pyrimethamine, sulfadiazine, dexamethasone, and folinic acid, and she was discharged in June 1983. In December 1982 the peripheral-blood white-cell count was 2400 with 9 percent lymphocytes, and the OKT4/OKT8 ratio was 0.04. In June 1983 she remained leukopenic and lymphopenic (white-cell count, 1700 with 7 percent lymphocytes). Currently she remains chronically ill.

The patient and her husband of more than 23 years denied having risk factors for AIDS. Although she was hospitalized in a center caring for patients with AIDS, since she had no previously recognized risk factors, this diagnosis was not seriously considered during her first admission.

During her hospitalizations in 1979 and 1981, she received blood components from 28 donors. Nineteen of the 24 American donors were interviewed and examined, and T-cell subsets were analyzed on heparinized blood from 18. Three donors refused testing, one was living outside the United States, and one could not be located. One of the 12 male donors examined was a 28-year-old homosexual man with multiple sexual partners and cervical, axillary, epitrochlear, and inguinal lymphadenopathy noted at the time of examination. His OKT4/OKT8 ratio was 0.8.

Case 9

A 33-year-old unmarried woman had immigrated to the United States from Hong Kong in 1969. In September 1981 she underwent surgery to replace her aortic valve and received blood products from 34 donors. She remained well until February 1983, when she presented with fever and was found to have acute sinusitis and thrush. In April 1983 she was hospitalized for recurrent fever and cough; a chest film demonstrated bilateral pulmonary infiltrates, and *P. carinii*, *Cryptococcus neoformans*, and cytomegalovirus were found in an open-lung-biopsy specimen. She was profoundly lymphopenic, with a helper/suppressor ratio of 0.75. She denied having sexual contact with members of groups with an increased incidence of AIDS and had no history of intravenous-drug abuse. Thirty of the 34 donors were located and examined, including a healthy homosexual man who had had multiple sexual partners, no abnormalities on physical examination, but a helper/suppressor ratio of 0.60.

Discussion

Epidemiologic data suggest that AIDS is caused by an infectious agent that may be transmitted through sexual contact, through sharing contaminated needles, or through the concentrates used to treat hemophilia. Our description of 18 adults without other risk factors in whom AIDS developed after transfusion indicates that other blood components may transmit AIDS. Furthermore, the seven completed donor investigations provide circumstantial evidence that exposure to as little as one unit may result in transmission. The failure to identify definite cases of AIDS or even severe symptoms among the donors examined suggests that affected donors with only mild or inapparent illness account for the majority of cases of transfusion-associated AIDS.

The clinical and immunologic pattern observed in these 18 adults is essentially identical to that described in other patients with AIDS. These 18 cases represent nearly 30 percent of the 64 cases of *P. carinii* pneumonia without identified risk factors. In contrast, only 1.5 percent of the U.S. population receives transfusions each year, although the transfusion rate for persons over 65 is three to four times this figure.[23-24] The 30 percent proportion associated with transfusion is probably an underestimate since the epidemiologic information is incomplete on many of the remaining 46 patients without a history of transfusions (Table 1). Some of these 46 patients probably had undetected risk factors, since many died before adequate histories were obtained.

Over 60 percent of cases of transfusion-associated AIDS were reported from New York, California, New Jersey, and Florida — the four states with the largest number of reported cases of AIDS. This is consistent with the observation that most blood used for transfusion is obtained in the region in which it is used.

The profiles of the patients with transfusion-associated AIDS closely resemble those of other recipients of transfusions in the United States, although they were older and more likely to be female than other groups with AIDS. Nearly 40 percent were 60 years of age or older. In 1980, 57 percent of the more than 3 million transfusion recipients in the United States were women, and the 11 percent of the population over 65 years of age accounted for 44 percent of the transfusion recipients.[24] Patients with AIDS had most often received their transfusions in association with surgical procedures, often coronary-bypass surgery, or for other conditions not known to be associated with severe clinical immunosuppression. In comparison, 62 percent of the transfusions in the United States are associated with surgical procedures, with malignant neoplasms and cardiovascular disorders the two most common disease categories listed for transfusion recipients.[24]

All 18 patients with transfusion-associated AIDS had a diagnosis of *P. carinii* pneumonia, the most common serious opportunistic infection among other groups of patients with AIDS. Since the surveillance definition of AIDS excluded cases of Kaposi's sarcoma in persons over 60 years of age, a reported case of disseminated Kaposi's sarcoma associated with transfusion in a 69-year-old man was not included above. When the sarcoma was diagnosed in late 1982, the patient's immunologic test results and rapidly fatal course were more typical of the Kaposi's sarcoma seen in AIDS than of the classic form of the disease seen in elderly men. Sixteen months before the onset of symptoms the patient had received three units of blood during coronary-bypass surgery. One of the two donors who were located and examined was a homosexual man with multiple sexual partners, a recent history of zoster, and an OKT4/OKT8 ratio of 1.1.

The mean number of units received by patients with transfusion-associated AIDS (16) was five times greater than the slightly more than three units per patient reported in national surveys of transfusions.[23-24] Receipt of a larger number of units would increase one's risk of exposure to a rare agent, but there may be additional factors related to multiple transfusions.

The finding of a suspect donor associated with each case of transfusion-associated AIDS was unlikely to have occurred by chance. Only 6 of 78 donors interviewed were identified as belonging to groups with an increased incidence of AIDS, and these 6 men accounted for 5 of the 7 with decreased helper/suppressor ratios. The validity of the use of the binomial model to analyze the distribution of high-risk donors in the completed investigations required certain assumptions to be valid. The representative cases investigated involved no known selection bias. Although all unknown bias cannot be ruled out, the prevalence estimates used in the analyses were conservative. The true prevalence of homosexual men with multiple partners and of past or present abusers of intravenous drugs in the donor population is unlikely to exceed the 8 percent estimate substantially. The 15 percent prevalence estimate for decreased helper/suppressor ratios is very conservative, since it is six times greater than normal control values in the CDC laboratory.

Investigation of transfusion-associated cases may provide insight into the natural history of AIDS. The mean period between transfusion and diagnosis (27 months) in the cases of transfusion-associated AIDS was even longer than that noted in a cluster of sexually linked cases among homosexual men.[14-25] Four of the high-risk donors were noted to have generalized lymphadenopathy, a condition often associated with AIDS. The donors themselves were often unaware of the lymphadenopathy, which was sometimes documented months to years after donation. Compliance with current guidelines for prevention of AIDS would now result in the exclusion from donating blood of the five homosexual men with multiple partners and the man with a history of drug abuse.[26]

The pattern observed in the investigation of transfusion-associated AIDS in adults is consistent with the case of acquired immunodeficiency after transfusion in an infant.[18-19] Additional cases of unexplained immunodeficiency and severe opportunistic infections have been reported in infants.[27-29] Of 28 infants whose cases were reported to the CDC, 17 were born to parents who belonged to a group with an increased incidence of AIDS. Two of these 17 infants and 6 of the other 11 infants had received transfusions shortly after birth. Further investigation of these cases and of the pediatric acquired immunodeficiency syndrome are needed to clarify the meaning of transfusion-associated disease in infants.

The current number of cases of AIDS associated with transfusion is small, representing about 1 percent of the reported cases of AIDS in the United States. These 18 cases were diagnosed during approximately 12 months, a period when over 3 million persons in the United States received transfusions. However, most of these patients received their transfusions between 1979 and early 1982, a time when the prevalence of AIDS — and presumably of donors affected by the putative AIDS agent — was much lower than during late 1982 and early 1983.

In March 1983 the Public Health Service recommended that persons with symptoms suggestive of AIDS and members of groups at increased risk for AIDS refrain from donating blood or plasma.[26] Several other organizations, including the American Red Cross, the American Association of Blood Banks, the National Hemophilia Foundation, the American Association of Physicians for Human Rights, and the Council of Community Blood Centers, have issued similar recommendations, and the Food and Drug Administration has issued specific guidelines for blood- and plasma-collection centers. Although it will not be possible to evaluate the effectiveness of these measures immediately, compliance with them should decrease the number of blood donations potentially associated with the transmission of AIDS.

Note added in proof: By December 12, 1983, 2952 cases of AIDS had been reported to the CDC. Among these, 31 adults are under investigation as having received blood transfusions within five years before diagnosis and having no other identified risk factors.

We are indebted to the following people for assisting in the evaluation and investigation of cases and donors: Pauline Thomas, M.D., Stephen Friedman, M.D., Meredith Smith, James Monroe, Rebecca Reiss, and Armondo Hermoso, M.D., New York City Department of Health; Johannah Pindyck, M.D., New York Blood Center; Shelley Gordon, M.D., and Robert Holtzman, M.D., Bellevue Hospital, New York; Carol Harris, M.D., and Neil Steigbigel, M.D., Montefiore Medical Center, New York; Donald Kaminsky, M.D., and Patricia Wexler, M.D., Beth Israel Medical Center, New York; Selma Dritz, M.D., San Francisco Department of Health; Stanley Deresinski, M.D., and Richard Miller, M.D., Stanford University Medical Center; Herbert Perkins, M.D., Irwin Memorial Blood Bank, San Francisco; Toby Kircher, M.D., Connecticut Department of Health; Joseph Lossick, D.O., Columbus (Ohio) Department of Health; Robert Thompson, M.D., University of Virginia Medical Center; Leroy Harris, M.D., University of Alabama Medical Center, Huntsville, Ala.; Robert C. Rendtorff, M.D., Memphis- Shelby County Health Department; Emmel Golden, Jr., M.D., and William Potter, M.D., Baptist Memorial Hospital, Memphis, Tenn.; Armando Orlina, M.D., Antonio Chan, M.D., Mark Levin, M.D., and Sherwin Kabins, M.D., Michael Reese Medical Center, Chicago; and Kenneth Debeneditis, M.D., Redding Hospital Medical Center, Redding, Pa.; to Lewellys Barker, M.D., Joseph Bove, M.D., George Grady, M.D., Martin Hirsch, M.D., Leon Hoyer, M.D., and Cladd Stevens, M.D., for reviewing the cases and the manuscript; to Frances Porcher and Walter Dowdle, Ph.D., for editorial assistance; and to Quo Vadis Harris for help in preparing the manuscript.

References

1. *Pneumocystis pneumonia* — Los Angeles. MMWR 1981; 30:250-2.
2. Kaposi's sarcoma and *Pneumocystis* pneumonia among homosexual men — New York City and California. MMWR 1981; 30:305-8.
3. Gottlieb MS, Schroff R, Schanker HM, et al. *Pneumocystis carinii* pneumonia and mucosal candidiasis in previously healthy homosexual men: evidence of a new acquired cellular immunodeficiency. N Engl J Med 1981; 305:1425-31.
4. Masur H, Michelis MA, Greene JB, et al. An outbreak of community-acquired *Pneumocystis carinii* pneumonia: initial manifestation of cellular immune dysfunction. N Engl J Med 1981; 305:1431-8.
5. Siegal FP, Lopez C, Hammer GS, et al. Severe acquired immunodeficiency in male homosexuals, manifested by chronic perianal ulcerative herpes simplex lesions. N Engl J Med 1981; 305:1439-44.
6. Hymes KB, Cheung T, Greene JB, et al. Kaposi's sarcoma in homosexual men — a report of eight cases. Lancet 1981; 2:598-600.
7. *Pneumocystic carinii* pneumonia among persons with hemophilia A. MMWR 1982: 31:365-7.
8. Update on acquired immune deficiency syndrome among patients with hemophilia A. MMWR 1982; 31:644-52.
9. Ehrenkranz NJ, Rubini JR. Pneumocystis carinii pneumonia complicating hemophilia-A. J Fla Med Assoc 1983; 70:116-8.
10. Davis KC, Horsburgh CR Jr, Hasiba V, Shocket AL, Kirkpatrick CH. Acquired immunodeficiency syndrome in a patient with hemophilia. Ann Intern Med 1983; 98:284-6.
11. Elliott JL, Hoppes WL, Platt MS, et al. The acquired immunodeficiency syndrome and *Mycobacterium avium-intracellulare* bacteremia in a patient with hemophilia. Ann Intern Med 1983; 98:290-3.
12. Poon M-C, Landay A, Prasthofer EF, Stagno S. Acquired immunodeficiency syndrome with *Pneumocystis carinii* pneumonia and *Mycobacterium avium-intracellulare* infection in a previously healthy patient with classic hemophilia: clinical, immunologic, and virologic findings. Ann Intern Med 1983; 98:287-90.
13. Jaffe HW, Choi K, Thomas PA, et al. National case-control study of Kaposi's sarcoma and *Pneumocystis carinii* pneumonia in homosexual men. I. Epidemiologic results. Ann Intern Med 1983; 99:145-51.
14. A cluster of Kaposi's sarcoma and *Pneumocystis carinii* pneumonia among homosexual male residents of Los Angeles and Orange Counties, California. MMWR 1982; 31:305-7.
15. Immunodeficiency among female sexual partners of males with acquired immunodeficiency syndrome — New York. MMWR 1983; 31:697-8.
16. Harris C, Small CB, Klein RS, et al. Immunodeficiency in female sexual partners of men with the acquired immunodeficiency syndrome. N Engl J Med 1983; 308:1181-4.
17. Curran JW, Evatt BL, Lawrence DN. Acquired immune deficiency syndrome: the past as prologue. Ann Intern Med 1983; 98:401-3.
18. Possible transfusion-associated acquired immune deficiency syndrome — California. MMWR 1982; 31:652-4.
19. Ammann AJ, Cowan MJ, Wara DW, et al. Acquired immunodeficiency in an infant: possible transmission by means of blood products. Lancet 1983; 1:956-8.
20. Update on acquired immune deficiency syndrome — United States. MMWR 1982; 31:507-14.
21. Centers for Disease Control Task Force on Kaposi's Sarcoma and Opportunistic Infections. Epidemiologic aspects of the current outbreak of Kaposi's sarcoma and opportunistic infections. N Engl J Med 1982; 306: 248-52.
22. Vieira J, Frank E, Spira TJ, Landesman SH. Acquired immune deficiency in Haitians: opportunistic infections in previously healthy Haitian immigrants. N Engl J Med 1983; 308:125-9.
23. Surgenor D, Schnitzer SS. Summary report: 1979 National Blood Data Center Survey of U.S. Blood Services. American Blood Commission report to the National Heart, Lung, and Blood Institute, 1980.
24. Surgenor D, Schnitzer SS. The nation's blood resource 1979 and 1980. American Blood Commission draft report to the National Heart, Lung, and Blood Institute, 1981.
25. Auerbach D, Darrow W, Jaffe H, Curran J. A cluster of the acquired immune deficiency syndrome: patients linked by sexual contact. Am J Med (in press).
26. Prevention of acquired immune deficiency syndrome: report of inter-agency recommendations. MMWR 1983; 32:101-3.
27. Oleske J, Minnefor A, Cooper R Jr, et al. Immune deficiency syndrome in children. JAMA 1983; 249:2345-9.
28. Rubinstein A, Sicklick M, Gupta A, et al. Acquired immunodeficiency with reversed T_4/T_8 ratios in infants born to promiscuous and drug-addicted mothers. JAMA 1983; 249:2350-6.
29. Joncas JH, Delage G, Chad Z, Lapointe N. Acquired (or congenital) immunodeficiency syndrome in infants born of Haitian mothers. N Engl J Med 1983; 308:842.

MEDICAL INTELLIGENCE

COINCIDENTAL APPEARANCE OF LAV/HTLV-III ANTIBODIES IN HEMOPHILIACS AND THE ONSET OF THE AIDS EPIDEMIC

BRUCE L. EVATT, M.D., EDWARD D. GOMPERTS, M.D., J. STEVEN McDOUGAL, M.D., AND ROSEMARY B. RAMSEY, M.S.

THE acquired immunodeficiency syndrome (AIDS) may be caused by a human T-cell lymphotropic retrovirus, termed "lymphadenopathy-associated virus" (LAV) by Institut Pasteur scientists in France[1,2] and "human T-cell lymphotropic virus type III" (HTLV-III) by scientists at the National Institutes of Health in the United States.[3,4] These retroviruses are antigenically indistinguishable[5]; they have been isolated from a large number of patients with AIDS or AIDS-related conditions in France and the United States,[1-6] and in one instance from a blood donor and the recipient of the donor's blood, both of whom contracted AIDS.[7]

Patients with AIDS or the lymphadenopathy syndrome and other groups at risk for AIDS have a higher incidence of antibody to LAV/HTLV-III than controls.[2,8-10] In recent studies in Denmark[11] and the United States,[12] prevalence rates of 64 and 72 percent, respectively, were reported for populations with asymptomatic hemophilia.

To determine when antibody to LAV emerged in the hemophilia population, we obtained samples from the Centers for Disease Control serum bank that had been collected in 1968 and between 1978 and 1984 from hemophiliacs residing in California, Georgia, New York, and Texas, and tested them for antibody to viral proteins p25 and p41 of LAV. Antibody to LAV first appeared at the same time that cases of AIDS began to be reported.

METHODS

Serum Samples

Serum samples from 15 persons with mild hemophilia A had been stored in the Centers for Disease Control serum bank since their collection in 1968 and 1969 in New York, California, and Texas. The clinical histories of the 15 patients were not available.

Blood samples from 21 patients with hemophilia A, 6 with hemophilia B, 1 with von Willebrand's disease, and 1 with factor VII deficiency were collected between 1978 and 1984. All these patients had been enrolled in a hemophilia comprehensive-care program at Children's Hospital of Los Angeles, and clinical histories were available. Commercial factor concentrates were the primary treatment for bleeding in all 29 patients. Charts were reviewed with respect to the patient's present health status, the transfusion history, and the use of concentrate. None of the 21 patients had any epidemiologically recognized risk factors for AIDS other than hemophilia. Lymphocyte subpopulations were quantitated by indirect immunofluorescence, with T-cell monoclonal antibodies (against Leu-1, Leu-2, Leu-3, Leu-4, and Leu-5; Becton–Dickinson Monoclonal Antibody Center, Mountain View, Calif.) on recent blood specimens (1983 to 1984) collected in California.

From the Division of Host Factors, Center for Infectious Diseases, Centers for Disease Control, Atlanta, and the Children's Hospital of Los Angeles.

Also available for testing were serum samples from patients with hemophilia A who resided in Georgia (collected from 14 patients in 1981 and from 8 in 1984). These patients had severe hemophilia A and were treated with factor VIII concentrates.

Antibody to LAV

All serum samples were tested blindly at the Centers for Disease Control. Results were reported to the patients' attending physicians, who provided medical counsel to patients who were seropositive for LAV antibody.

LAV was obtained from Dr. J.C. Chermann, Institut Pasteur, Paris, and propagated in primary fetal cord lymphocytes, as previously described.[2] The virus was separated from supernatant fluids by ultracentrifugation (80,000×g for 60 minutes) through a 30 percent (wt/wt) sucrose cushion.[13] LAV was suspended in 0.01 M TRIS buffer, pH 8.0, containing 1 percent sodium dodecyl sulfate, 0.25 mg of bromophenol blue per milliliter, 10 percent (vol/vol) glycerol, and 5 percent (vol/vol) 2-mercaptoethanol, and was heated at 65°C for 30 minutes. Western blots were performed by the method of Tsang et al.[14] Serum samples were tested at a 1:100 dilution. Banding patterns of antibody to p25 and p41 were compared with those of a serum known to be positive, diluted 1:4000 (Fig. 1).

RESULTS

Antibody to LAV was not detected in the serum samples collected in 1968 and 1969 from 15 patients with mild hemophilia A. Before 1980 it was present in only 1 (5 percent) of 21 patients with hemophilia A in California (Table 1). In 1978 the single seropositive patient was a two-year-old child who had received blood transfusions as well as factor VIII concentrate. Among most of the 21 patients with hemophilia A in California, seroconversion did not occur until 1982, and then rapidly increased in 1983. By 1984, more than 85 percent of the group had antibody to LAV.

When stored serum samples obtained in 1981 and 1984 from patients with hemophilia A living in Georgia were tested, 8 of 14 (57 percent) were positive in 1981 and 8 of 8 (100 percent) were positive in 1984 (data not shown). There was a selection bias in the Georgia serum samples in that they were from patients who had more severe hemophilia and who, as a group, had received more concentrates than average. However, the trend was toward increased seropositivity (P = 0.04, Fisher's exact test) from 1981 to 1984, like the trend in California.

The extent of seroconversion among patients with hemophilia B was not as great as among those with hemophilia A (Table 1). None of six patients with hemophilia B were seropositive in 1978 or 1979; two patients (33 percent) had antibody to LAV by 1984. One of the two has been on renal dialysis and has received repeated transfusions of erythrocytes and

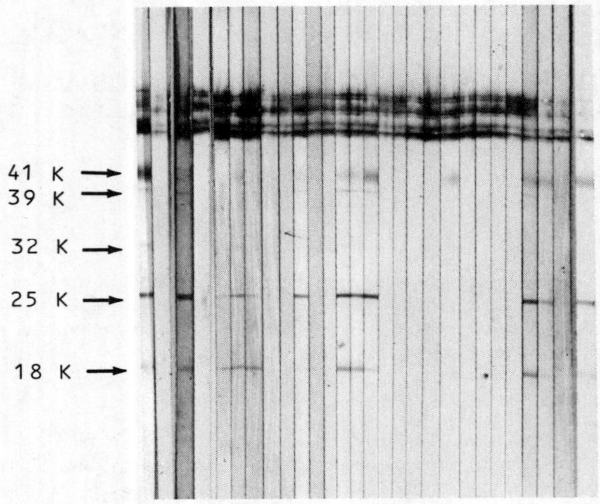

Figure 1. Representative Banding Patterns Showing Antibody to p25 and p41 Antigens of Lymphadenopathy-Associated Virus, Determined by the Western Blot Technique.

The strips on the right and left show banding patterns of a serum known to be positive. The banding patterns of normal serum are shown in the second strip from the right and the second from the left. The remainder are patterns of serum samples from representative seropositive and seronegative patients with hemophilia.

other blood products. The other patient received factor IX concentrates about once a month for minor bleeding episodes. One factor VII–deficient patient was treated only with factor IX concentrates and has remained seronegative for LAV.

None of the patients with antibody to LAV have contracted AIDS. Of the 22 patients receiving factor VIII concentrates (21 with hemophilia A and 1 with von Willebrand's disease), 6 with hemophilia A and the 1 with von Willebrand's disease (32 percent) have had mild lymphadenopathy; 1 patient had thrombocytopenia necessitating splenectomy. Helper/suppressor T-cell ratios below 1.0 were found in 7 (50 percent) of 14 patients tested; all 7 were seropositive for LAV antibody. Of the seven patients receiving factor IX concentrates (six with hemophilia B and one with a factor VII deficiency) only one had lymphadenopathy; this patient had antibody to LAV. One of the seven had a reduced helper/suppressor T-cell ratio (0.51). All seronegative patients were free of lymphadenopathy and immune abnormalities.

Discussion

More than 85 percent of 21 patients with hemophilia A in a California clinic had antibody to LAV in 1981, 1982, or 1983. Among patients in Georgia who had the same form of hemophilia, a similar development of seropositivity occurred from 1981 through 1984. No data before 1981 were available for the patients in Georgia, so the beginning of seroconversion in this group could not be determined. Georgia was among the first states to report AIDS in a patient with hemophilia (1983); California did not report a case until one year later.

If the data from our studies are extrapolated to the U.S. hemophiliac population, seroconversion in hemophiliacs began shortly after the beginning of the AIDS epidemic among homosexual men and intravenous drug users (1979 to 1980), and the timing of seroconversion correlates well with the first cases of AIDS in hemophiliacs,[15] in late 1981 and early 1982. The temporal relationship between seroconversion and the epidemic among hemophiliac patients strongly supports the hypothesis that LAV is the etiologic agent of AIDS.

Studies initially performed with the HTLV membrane-antigen assay provided the first evidence of retrovirus seropositivity in hemophiliacs,[16,17] but the prevalence was low (5 to 19 percent). Antibodies to HTLV-I (measured by the Western blot technique) have subsequently been found in only 1 of 169 patients with hemophilia.[18] Since the HTLV membrane-antigen test measures antibodies to membrane antigens induced by HTLV-I infection of the assay cells, seropositivity in these early studies could have been caused, in part, by cross-reactivity between HTLV-III/LAV and HTLV-I.

Table 1. Antibody to Lymphadenopathy-Associated Virus (LAV) p25 and p41 Proteins in Patients with Hemophilia in California, by Year Plasma Was Collected.*

Patient No.	1978	1979	1980	1981	1982	1983	1984
Hemophilia A							
1	+		+	+	+	+	+
2		–	–		+	+	+
3	–	–	–				+
4	–	–				+	+
5	–		–			+	
6	–		–			+	+
7	–	–	–			+	
8		–				+	
9		–	–			+	+
10	–			–			+
11	–					+	
12	–			–		+	+
13	–		–				+
14	–	–	–		+	+	
15	–						+
16	–		–			+	+
17	–					+	+
18		–					+
19	–				–		
20		–				–	
21		–				–	
von Willebrand's disease							
1	–					+	+
Hemophilia B							
1	–						+
2	–						+
3	–					–	
4	–						–
5		–					–
6		–					–
Factor VII deficiency							
1	–					–	

*A plus sign denotes positive, a minus sign negative, and a blank not done.

The high prevalence of antibody to LAV in this study and in two other recent studies in Georgia and Denmark[11,12] suggests that exposure to LAV is widespread among patients receiving factor VIII concentrates. The rapidity with which the seroconversion took place, the widespread geographic location of seropositive patients (i.e., California, Georgia, and Denmark), and the fact that a positive serologic response to LAV is related to the amount of factor VIII used[12] suggest that factor VIII concentrate is a vehicle for the spread of LAV and that the concentrate may have contained LAV during the years 1980 to 1983. Since factor VIII and factor IX concentrates are manufactured from pooled plasma and each lot is distributed to many geographic locations, seroconversion in patients receiving clotting factor would be expected to be nearly simultaneous in various locations.

The low incidence of LAV seroconversion in patients with hemophilia B who were treated with factor IX concentrates suggests that if LAV is transmitted in factor concentrates, the frequency of transmission may be lower with factor IX than with factor VIII concentrates. Another study of patients with hemophilia B in Georgia[12] has also reported a low incidence of antibody to LAV. In both studies the number of patients with hemophilia B was too small to draw conclusions concerning the factor IX–deficient population. In both Georgia and California, the frequency of treatment, and thus the number of exposures to a potential agent, was about the same for patients with hemophilia A and for those with hemophilia B. Patients with hemophilia B, like those with hemophilia A, receive other blood products as well as factor concentrate, and these may also be vehicles for the transmission of LAV. In fact, antibody to LAV has been found at slightly higher rates than expected in some patients who are regularly given blood products other than factor VIII concentrates (Jason JM, et al.: unpublished data). Further studies may clarify the relative risk associated with factor VIII and factor IX concentrates.

The implications of LAV seropositivity for an individual hemophiliac are unknown, since the immune abnormalities associated with seropositivity suggest a wide spectrum of responses to infection with LAV.[12] Seropositivity may mean that the patient is infected with the virus and will contract the AIDS syndrome or is immune to AIDS. The incubation period for AIDS is thought to range from one to five years, and most patients who have had seroconversion have been followed for only one to two years. The prognosis for seropositive persons with mild or no symptoms of the disease will require longitudinal evaluation.

It is possible that antibody to LAV is acquired passively from immunoglobulins found in factor VIII concentrates. However, this seems unlikely, because the patients with hemophilia had widely varying treatment schedules and received different lots of factor concentrate, yet the appearance of seropositivity was uniform in time. Likewise, it is possible that seropositivity is caused not by infectious virus but by immunization with noninfectious LAV or LAV proteins derived from virus disrupted during the processing of plasma into factor VIII concentrate. However, this explanation does not account for all cases of seroconversion, because infectious LAV has been isolated from some patients with hemophilia[6] (and unpublished data from the Centers for Disease Control).

We are indebted to Michael Parvin, M.S., Debra W. Jackson, B.S., and Susan Kennedy, B.S., for technical assistance; to V.S. Kalyanaraman, Ph.D., and Donald P. Francis, M.D., for advice and support concerning the LAV testing; to Walter R. Dowdle, Ph.D., John V. Bennett, M.D., and James W. Curran, M.D., for guidance; to Frances Porcher for editorial assistance; and to Patsy Bellamy for assistance in manuscript preparation.

References

1. Barré-Sinoussi F, Cherman JC, Rey F, et al. Isolation of a T-lymphotropic retrovirus from a patient at risk for acquired immune deficiency syndrome (AIDS). Science 1983; 220:868-71.
2. Montagnier L, Chermann JC, Barré-Sinoussi F, et al. A new human T-lymphotropic retrovirus: characterization and possible role in lymphadenopathy and acquired immune deficiency syndrome. In: Gallo RC, Essex M, Gross L, eds. Human T-cell leukemia/lymphoma virus 1984. Cold Spring Harbor, N.Y.: Cold Spring Harbor Laboratory, 1984:363-79.
3. Gallo RC, Salahuddin SZ, Popovic M, et al. Frequent detection and isolation of cytopathic retroviruses (HTLV-III) from patients with AIDS and at risk for AIDS. Science 1984; 224:500-2.
4. Popovic M, Sarngadharan MG, Read E, Gallo RC. Detection, isolation, and continuous production of cytopathic retroviruses (HTLV-III) from patients with AIDS and pre-AIDS. Science 1983; 224:497-500.
5. Broder S, Gallo RC. A pathogenic retrovirus (HTLV-III) linked to AIDS. N Engl J Med 1984; 311:1292-7.
6. Vilmer E, Barré-Sinoussi F, Rouzioux C, et al. Isolation of a new lymphotropic retrovirus in two hemophiliac B siblings, one presenting with acquired immunodeficiency syndrome. Lancet 1984; 1:753-7.
7. Feorino PM, Kalyanaraman VS, Haverkos HW, et al. Lymphadenopathy associated virus infection of a blood donor–recipient pair with acquired immunodeficiency syndrome. Science 1984; 225:69-72.
8. Schüpbach J, Popovic M, Gilden RV, Gonda MA, Sarngadharan MG, Gallo RC. Serological analysis of a subgroup of human T-lymphotropic retroviruses (HTLV-III) associated with AIDS. Science 1984; 224: 503-5.
9. Sarngadharan MG, Popovic M, Bruch L, Schüpbach J, Gallo RC. Antibodies reactive with human T-lymphotropic retroviruses (HTLV-III) in the serum of patients with AIDS. Science 1984; 224:506-8.
10. Kalyanaraman VS, Cabradilla CD, Getchell JP, et al. Antibodies to the core proteins of lymphadenopathy-associated virus (LAV) in patients with AIDS. Science 1984; 225:321-3.
11. Melbye M, Biggar RJ, Chermann JC, Montagnier L, Stenbjerg S, Ebbesen P. High prevalence of lymphadenopathy virus (LAV) in European hemophiliacs. Lancet 1984; 2:40-1.
12. Ramsey RB, Palmer EL, McDougal JS, et al. Antibody to lymphadenopathy-associated virus in haemophiliacs with and without AIDS. Lancet 1984; 2:397-8.
13. Kalyanaraman VS, Sarngadharan MG, Poiesz B, Ruscetti FW, Gallo RC. Immunological properties of a type C retrovirus isolated from cultured human T-lymphoma cells and comparison to other mammalian retroviruses. J Virol 1981; 38:906-15.
14. Tsang VCW, Peralta JM, Simons AR. Enzyme-linked immunoelectrotransfer blot techniques (EITB) for studying the specificities of antigens and antibodies separated by gel electrophoresis. Methods Enzymol 1983; 92:377-91.
15. Evatt BL, Ramsey RB, Lawrence DN, Zyla LD, Curran JW. The acquired immunodeficiency syndrome in patients with hemophilia. Ann Intern Med 1984; 100:499-504.
16. Essex M, McLane MF, Lee TH, Falk L, Howe CWS, Mullins JI. Antibodies to cell membrane antigens associated with human T-cell leukemia virus in patients with AIDS. Science 1983; 220:859-62.
17. Evatt BL, Stein SF, Francis DP, et al. Antibodies to human T cell leukaemia virus-associated membrane antigens in haemophiliacs: evidence for infection before 1980. Lancet 1983; 2:698-701.
18. Chorba TL, Jason JM, Ramsey RB, et al. HTLV-I antibody status in hemophilia patients treated with factor concentrates prepared from U.S. plasma sources and in hemophilia patients with AIDS. Thromb Haemostas (in press).

SOUNDING BOARD

SCREENING DONATED BLOOD AND PLASMA FOR HTLV-III ANTIBODY

Facing More than One Crisis?

Michael T. Osterholm, Ph.D., M.P.H., Robert J. Bowman, M.D., Michael W. Chopek, M.D., J. Jeffrey McCullough, M.D., Jack A. Korlath, M.P.H., and Herbert F. Polesky, M.D.

Little question remains that the causative agent of the acquired immunodeficiency syndrome (AIDS) is the newly recognized retrovirus, human T-cell lymphotropic virus Type III (HTLV-III).[1-5] AIDS, the AIDS-related complex, and asymptomatic HTLV-III infection have been associated with several well-defined high-risk groups, including recipients of blood and blood products.[6-8] Protection of our nation's blood and plasma supply from HTLV-III contamination has been one of the highest public health priorities related to the AIDS epidemic.

Studies of symptomatic and asymptomatic members of high-risk groups indicate that those who are infected with HTLV-III are also likely to be positive for HTLV-III antibody[3,9-11] Tests to detect HTLV-III antibody, including an enzyme-linked immunosorbent assay (ELISA), have been described; the sensitivity and specificity of these tests in correctly identifying a person who has been exposed to HTLV-III appear to be very high (>93 percent).[12] Despite the high specificity of the newly licensed tests for HTLV-III antibody, each year thousands of volunteer blood donors will be falsely identified as positive for HTLV-III antibody if the recently issued U.S. Public Health Service (PHS) interagency recommendations for blood and plasma screening are implemented.[8] We fear that efforts to alleviate the crisis of HTLV-III contamination of the blood and plasma supply will create a second, equally critical crisis: that of major blood and plasma shortages.

In the light of the need to protect the quality of the blood and plasma supply, it is not ethically justifiable at this time to withhold HTLV-III antibody screening; however, we believe that the implications of the PHS interagency recommendations for individual donors and the blood supply in general have not been adequately addressed. The personal trauma for a donor who receives a false positive test report and the inevitable adverse and widespread publicity that will be associated with this problem, in conjunction with the already volatile atmosphere of the AIDS epidemic, may well result in a marked decrease in the pool of volunteer blood donors. This decrease in the donor pool could result in potential life-threatening shortages of blood and plasma. In Minnesota and other states where there have been no confirmed cases of transfusion-associated AIDS, such shortages pose a much more serious problem than the risk of transfusion-associated AIDS.

We review here the pros and cons of HTLV-III antibody screening and donor notification, and the ramifications for Minnesota's blood and plasma supply. In addition, we provide recommendations that we believe will protect blood and plasma from HTLV-III contamination and minimize the risk of a major disruption in the supply.

Background

Screening for HTLV-III antibody, in combination with the previous recommendation that members of high-risk groups voluntarily refrain from donating blood, is hailed by many in the blood banking and public health communities as necessary to reduce the "crisis" associated with HTLV-III contamination of blood and plasma.[12]

On the basis of initial HTLV-III antibody studies conducted by five companies seeking licensure to market their ELISA test kits, the Food and Drug Administration has licensed two manufacturers as of March 20, 1985 (Petricciani J: personal communication). These tests were licensed for purposes of screening donor samples so that potentially infectious units of blood and plasma can be eliminated from the supply available for transfusion or manufacture into injectable products. These tests are not currently intended for diagnostic purposes.

The PHS interagency recommendations state that "if the repeat ELISA test is positive or if other tests are positive, it is the responsibility of the collection facility to ensure that the donor is notified." Other test methods used in HTLV-III antibody research include the Western blot technique immunofluorescence, and radioimmunoprecipitation.[8-11,13-15] However, most are currently available only in research laboratories. Thus, it is likely that in many situations the "test of choice" for repeat testing will be the same ELISA test.

The Pros and Cons of Screening and Donor Notification

Pros

The reasons for implementing a nationwide screening program for HTLV-III antibody in blood banks and plasma centers are clear. After the first reports of the occurence of AIDS among persons with hemophilia and those who had a history of transfusion, it was evident that a serologic screening test for the etiologic agent or a surrogate marker in blood and plasma was needed.

Data presented by the five companies seeking test-kit licensure indicate that the antibody tests are both sensitive and specific.[12] Abbott Laboratories and

Electro-Nucleonics, the first manufacturers to receive licenses, demonstrated during initial studies that their tests have a sensitivity of 93.4 and 99.6 percent and a specificity of 99.8 and 99.2 percent, respectively (according to the manufacturers' package inserts).

Routine use of the screening test will also reduce the anxiety among blood-component recipients who are concerned about the risk of HTLV-III infection from transfusion. Finally, if a healthy donor has a reactive test and is in fact infected with HTLV-III, appropriate medical care can be initiated, and counseling provided to minimize the risk of HTLV-III transmission.

The reasons for screening blood and plasma for HTLV-III antibody are laudable, and convincing scientific evidence has been presented that such screening should be initiated.

Cons

Despite the impressive sensitivity and specificity of the ELISA test, its use among the more than 7 million annual blood donors will mean that some blood and plasma units that are not reactive will be contaminated with HTLV-III.[16] These represent false negative test results. Also, thousands of donors will have repeatedly reactive tests without actually having HTLV-III antibody present. Theoretical estimates from the ELISA test-kit package inserts indicate that if the seroprevalence of HTLV-III antibody in the donor population is 0.1 percent, 68 to 89 percent of all repeatedly reactive ELISA tests are likely to represent false positive results.

What will repeatedly reactive ELISA tests mean for the donor? According to the PHS interagency recommendations, such a donor should be questioned about possible exposure to the virus or risk factors for AIDS with respect to his or her sexual contacts. Additional laboratory studies "might" include tests for sexually transmitted diseases, for immune function, and where available, for the presence of HTLV-III. One can only speculate about the total cost of this medical evaluation. Moreover, who will be responsible for it: the donor, the blood center, or blood recipients? The recommendations also suggest that the donor's sexual contacts "might" be tested for HTLV-III antibody; with the number of contacts likely to be tested, additional false positive results will inevitably occur.

It will be difficult to determine conclusively whether a person is infected with HTLV-III by his of her life style of history alone. However, if a donor is considered likely to have an HTLV-III infection, the PHS interagency recommendations state that the following considerations should be kept in mind: The long-term prognosis for a person who is infected is not known; asymptomatic persons may transmit HTLV-III to others; regular medical evaluation is advisable; there is a risk of infecting others by sexual intercourse or intimate kissing, toothbrushes, razors, and other such implements should not be shared; women who are seropositive or whose sexual partners are seropositive may transmit infection to their offspring; when seeking medical or dental care for illness, such persons should inform their physicians of their antibody status; and finally, antibody testing should be available to persons who "may have been infected" through their contact with a seropositive person. Questions have also been raised about discrimination, insurability, and employability of persons identified as antibody-positive.

Thus, there are substantial social and psychological implications for donors who are informed that their blood sample is reactive for HTLV-III antibody. These issues are confounded by the lack of information regarding the prognostic implications of a true positive test.The presence of HTLV-III antibody indicates a prior infection with the virus but does not necessarily mean that the person is currently infectious or will contract AIDS. For the person who is truly positive for HTLV-III antibody, the recommendations are unfortunately appropriate. However, for donors falsely labeled as antibody-positive, these results will probably do needless harm to their social and personal relationships.

On the basis of the manufacturers' estimates of the ELISA test's sensitivity and specificity, the chance of a repeatedly reactive HTLV-III antibody test ranges from 2 to 8 per 1000 donors. As donors become better informed about the likelihood of a reactive test, they may begin to view a donation as a major risk to their well-being. Our experience indicates that the more informed a person is about the implications of HTLV-III antibody testing, the greater the likelihood that he or she will consider withholding donations at this time.

Thus, it is also imperative to consider the impact of HTLV-III antibody screening on the availability of blood and plasma. With the screening of donors for HTLV-III antibody and removal of reactive units from the blood and plasma supply, less than 1 percent of units will be eliminated. Even this level of reduction will require compensation, but no one can deny that it is necessary.

In Minnesota, less than 3 percent of current red-cell products will become outdated. Therefore, a shortage of even 10 percent of the blood and plasma supply, resulting from donations being withheld, could seriously affect the availability of blood. Such a shortage might be compensated for by more conservative transfusion therapy. However, since 1983, blood-component usage has remained constant in many parts of the United States, suggesting that physicians may have already become more conservative in their approach to transfusion therapy. One might also expect blood banks to try to collect more blood to compensate for losses, but this could be costly and unsuccessful if the basis for the shortage is the loss of public support.

Minnesota HTLV-III Antibody Screening

For a better appreciation of the implications of donor screening and notification, we have projected the results of the implementation of the interagency recommendations for screening in Minnesota. Our situation will be similar to that in most states.

As of March 18, 1985, 126 cases of transfusion-associated AIDS and 68 cases of AIDS in persons with hemophilia have been reported in the United States (Statistical Surveillance Section, AIDS Branch, Centers for Disease Control: unpublished data). However, 83 (66 percent) of the 126 transfusion-associated cases have occurred in persons in only five states (New York, California, Florida, New Jersey, and Texas). The other cases have occurred in 19 other states, suggesting that the incidence of transfusion-associated AIDS reflects the incidence of AIDS in the general population. In Minnesota there have been 23 confirmed cases of AIDS; none have been related to transfusion. In addition, 26 states have not documented a single transfusion-associated case of AIDS. Therefore, it is unlikely that the same problem of transfusion-associated AIDS seen in New York, San Francisco, and other "high-risk" geographic areas is imminent in Minnesota or other "low-risk" areas.

There are five primary blood banks in Minnesota, which collect 266,000 blood units annually from 190,000 volunteer donors. The average annual number of units donated per person is 1.4. We estimate that each year plasma centers in the state collect approximately 303,000 plasma units and that the average person donates plasma 5.2 times a year. From this information and that in the manufacturers' package inserts, we have calculated the estimated annual number of blood and plasma donors in Minnesota who will be repeatedly reactive for HTLV-III antibody by ELISA, assuming a 0.1 percent seropositive rate. The rate of repeatedly true positive results will be 0.7 to 0.8 per 1000 donors, and the rate of repeatedly false positive results will be 1.5 to 7 per 1000 donors. Thus, each year we might expect to find 175 to 209 truly antibody-positive donors and between 371 and 1701 falsely positive donors among those who have repeatedly positive screening tests. The test-performance values provided by the manufacturers are ascertained under prelicensure study conditions and may vary with large-scale screening. This is notable, since a difference of only 0.6 percent in the predicted specificity between the two licensed tests — a difference that might be statistically insignificant — would result in a 450 percent increase in the number of repeatedly false positive results.

Documenting false positive tests in an average of seven donors in our state every working day and informing the donors of the results will have an indirect impact on our state's blood and plasma supply as the medical, social, and economic implications of being positive for HTLV-III antibody become known.

The number of false positive results could be reduced if the ELISA were used in combination with another test method, such as the Western blot test, immunofluorescence, or radioimmunoprecipitation. However, since the sensitivity and specificity of these tests vary, it is difficult to predict the frequency of positive results for both the ELISA and one of the other tests.[10,11,13] It appears to be possible for at least one of these tests to have a higher specificity than the ELISA. For example, the viral specificity of the Western blot technique can be substantiated by reactivity with specific HTLV-III polypeptides (p24 and gp41). The use of such tests could substantially reduce the number of donors inappropriately notified of false positive ELISA results. However, these other methods have yet to be standardized, particularly with an emphasis on specificity.

Recommendations

Blood recipients have a right to expect that all efforts have been made to ensure that the blood units they receive have been tested by the most technologically advanced methods in order to minimize the risk of transmission of infectious agents. At the same time, donors have a right to expect consideration and protection so that their generous gift does not lead to a personal disaster. We believe that a reasonable middle ground can be reached.

First of all, we agree with previous recommendations that members of high-risk groups should eliminate themselves as donors in spite of the implementation of screening tests. One recent report suggests that self-elimination of high-risk group members has taken place since the PHS recommendations of March 1983.[17] However, because of the one-year to five-year incubation period for transfusion-associated AIDS, the impact of this policy will not be realized for several years.[18]

Secondly, blood and plasma centers should implement screening for HTLV-III antibody, using the currently licensed ELISA test kits, as soon as possible. All blood and plasma units found to be repeatedly reactive should be removed from the distribution system.

Thirdly, units found to be reactive on repeat ELISA testing should then be tested by another method. Whichever method is employed to confirm the repeatedly reactive ELISA results, it should be standardized, it should be readily available to all blood banks and plasma centers, and it should have a very high specificity, even at the risk of a considerable decrease in sensitivity. The donor should be informed of a positive blood sample only if it is repeatedly reactive by ELISA and is also positive by another standardized method of testing conducted in a laboratory that has demonstrated proficiency with that method. We realize that implementation of this recommendation could delay donor notification by many months. However, we believe that this extra measure of protection against notification of a false positive result is a price that must be paid if we are to ensure that the volunteer donor system remains intact.

Finally, alternative sites for HTLV-III antibody testing in members of high-risk groups need to be established concurrently with the donor-notification process. Until donor notification begins, members of high-risk groups will not donate blood or plasma in order to learn of their HTLV-III antibody status, and alternative test sites will be unnecessary.

References

1. Barré-Sinoussi F, Chermann JC, Rey F, et al. Isolation of a T-lymphotropic retrovirus from a patient at risk for acquired immune deficiency syndrome (AIDS). Science 1983; 220:868-71.
2. Popovic M, Sarngadharan MG, Read E, Gallo RC. Detection, isolation, and continuous production of cytopathic retroviruses (HTLV-III) from patients with AIDS and pre-AIDS. Science 1984; 224:497-500.
3. Gallo RC, Salahuddin SZ, Popovic M, et al. Frequent detection and isolation of cytopathic retroviruses (HTLV-III) from patients with AIDS and at risk for AIDS. Science 1984; 224:500-3.
4. Levy JA, Hoffman AD, Kramer SM, Landis JA, Shimabukuro JM, Oshiro LS. Isolation of lymphocytopathic retroviruses from San Francisco patients with AIDS. Science 1984; 225:840-2.
5. Barré-Sinoussi F, Mathur-Wagh U, Rey F, et al. Isolation of lymphadenopathy-associated virus (LAV) and detection of LAV antibodies from US patients with AIDS. JAMA 1985; 253:1737-9.
6. Curran JW, Lawrence DN, Jaffe H, et al. Acquired immunodeficiency syndrome (AIDS) associated with transfusions. N Engl J Med 1984; 310:69-75.
7. Landesman SH, Ginzburg HM, Weiss SH. The AIDS epidemic. N Engl J Med 1985; 312:521-5.
8. Provisional Public Health Service inter-agency recommendations for screening donated blood and plasma for antibody to the virus causing acquired immunodeficiency syndrome. MMWR 1985; 34:1-5.
9. Sarngadharan MG, Popovic M, Bruch L, Schüpbach J, Gallo RC. Antibodies reactive with a human T-lymphotropic retrovirus (HTLV-III) in the serum of patients with AIDS. Science 1984; 224:506-8.
10. Weiss SH, Goedert JJ, Sarngadharan MG, et al. Screening test for HTLV-III (AIDS agent) antibodies: specificity, sensitivity and applications. JAMA 1985; 253:221-5.
11. Schüpbach J, Haller O, Vogt M, et al. Antibodies to HTLV-III in Swiss patients with AIDS and pre-AIDS and in groups at risk for AIDS. N Engl J Med 1985; 312:265-70.
12. Marwick C. Use of AIDS antibody test may provide more answers. JAMA 1985; 253:1694-9.
13. Carlson J, Hinrichs S, Bryant M, et al. HTLV-III antibody screening of blood bank donors. Lancet 1985; 1:523-4.
14. Schüpbach J, Popovic M, Gilden RJ, Gonda MA, Sarngadharan MG, Gallo RC. Serological analysis of a subgroup of human T-lymphotropic retroviruses (HTLV-III) associated with AIDS. Science 1984; 224:503-5.
15. Antibodies to a retrovirus etiologically associated with acquired immunodeficiency syndrome (AIDS) in populations with increased incidences of the syndrome. MMWR 1984; 33:377-9
16. Salahuddin SZ, Groopman JE, Markham PD, et al. HTLV-III in symptom-free seronegative persons. Lancet 1984; 2:1418-20.
17. Pindyck J, Waldman A, Zang E, Oleszko W, Lowy M, Bianco C. Measures to decrease the risk of acquired immunodeficiency syndrome transmission by blood transfusion. Transfusion 1985; 25:3-9.
18. Prevention of acquired immune deficiency syndrome (AIDS): report of inter-agency recommendations. MMWR 1983; 32:101-3.

ORIGINAL ARTICLE

TRANSFUSION-ASSOCIATED ACQUIRED IMMUNODEFICIENCY SYNDROME

Evidence for Persistent Infection in Blood Donors

Paul M. Feorino, Ph.D., Harold W. Jaffe, M.D., Erskine Palmer, Ph.D., Thomas A. Peterman, M.D., Donald P. Francis, M.D., V.S. Kalyanaraman, Ph.D., Robert A. Weinstein, M.D., Rand L. Stoneburner, M.D., W. James Alexander, M.D., Cathy Raevsky, Jane P. Getchell, Dr.P.H., Donna Warfield, Harry W. Haverkos, M.D., Barbara W. Kilbourne, M.P.H., J.K.A. Nicholson, Ph.D., and James W. Curran, M.D.

Abstract To investigate whether infection with human T-cell lymphotropic virus/lymphadenopathy-associated virus (HTLV-III/LAV) may be persistent in asymptomatic persons and to correlate infection with seropositivity, we performed virologic and serologic studies in 25 of 30 persons who were identified as being at high risk for the acquired immunodeficiency syndrome (AIDS) and who had donated blood to patients who later contracted transfusion-associated AIDS. High-risk donors were those who belonged to a high-risk population, had AIDS or a closely related condition, or had a low ratio of helper to suppressor T lymphocytes. We performed similar studies in 6 of the 24 patients with AIDS who had received donations from this group. HTLV-III/LAV was isolated from 22 of the 25 donors, between 12 and 52 months (mean, 28) after they had donated blood, and from all 6 recipients, between 14 and 37 months (mean, 26) after they had received blood.

Of the 22 virus-positive donors, 2 have contracted AIDS, 5 have generalized lymphadenopathy, and 15 (68 percent) remain asymptomatic. Antibodies to HTLV-III/LAV were detectable by the enzyme-linked immunosorbent assay in serum samples obtained from each person at the time the virus was isolated.

We conclude that infection with HTLV-III/LAV may be persistent and asymptomatic for years. This demonstration that viremic patients may be asymptomatic supports the use of serologic screening of donated blood to supplement current procedures for the prevention of transfusion-associated AIDS.

The acquired immunodeficiency syndrome (AIDS) was first reported in 1981 in homosexual men and intravenous drug abusers.[1-5] Subsequent cases in persons with hemophilia[6-9] and recipients of blood transfusions[10,11] confirmed a pattern of occurrence suggesting that the cause was a transmissible infectious agent. Convincing evidence has recently been provided that a retrovirus, termed "human T-cell lymphotropic virus Type III" (HTLV-III), "lymphadenopathy-associated virus" (LAV), or "AIDS-associated retrovirus" (ARV), is the cause of AIDS.[12-15] Contributing to the etiologic association was the isolation of this virus from a blood donor and recipient, each of whom contracted AIDS.[16]

By April 1985, 9760 cases of AIDS had been reported in the United States, with the incidence continuing to increase in all high-risk groups. A total of 214 cases were reported (2.2 percent) either in persons with no other risk factors who had received blood transfusions (143 cases) or in persons with hemophilia who had received clotting-factor concentrates (71 cases). Interviews or T-cell subset analyses confirmed that patients with transfusion-associated AIDS had previously received a unit of blood obtained from a donor at high risk for AIDS.[10] In each completed investigation of transfusion-associated AIDS, at least one donor was found to have detectable antibodies to HTLV-III/LAV (Jaffe HW, et al.: unpublished data). To determine how long infection persists in high-risk donors and to correlate infection with seropositivity, we attempted to isolate HTLV-III/LAV from patients with transfusion-associated AIDS and high-risk donors identified in these investigations.

From the Centers for Disease Control, Atlanta; the Department of Internal Medicine, Michael Reese Hospital, Chicago; the New York City Department of Health, New York; the Jefferson County (Alabama) Department of Health, Birmingham; and the Colorado Department of Health, Denver.

Methods

Classification of Cases and Donors

Cases meeting the Centers for Disease Control surveillance definition of adult or pediatric AIDS[17,18] were classified as transfusion-associated if the patient had received blood or blood components between 1978 and the onset of illness and no other potential risk factors were identified in an interview. Donors were interviewed confidentially and underwent physical examination, blood specimens were obtained, and T-cell subset analyses were performed as previously described.[10,19] Donors were classified as "high risk" if they belonged to a group with a recognized increased incidence of AIDS, had AIDS or a closely related condition (e.g., unexplained generalized lymphadenopathy), or had a ratio of helper to suppressor T lymphocytes that was less than 1.00. Specimens were available from 7 patients with AIDS and 27 high-risk donors identified in 24 completed investigations.

Specimen Collection and Storage

Heparinized venous blood obtained from study participants was shipped to the Centers for Disease Control, where it was separated by Ficoll–Hypaque density centrifugation. Serum was collected from clotted blood samples by low-speed centrifugation. Lymphocytes and serum were frozen at −70°C and −20°C, respectively, until testing. The interval from specimen collection to isolation attempts ranged from 0 to 16 months (median, 9) for the 7 patients with AIDS and from 0 to 30 months (median, 11) for the 27 donors. Lymphocytes from five normal controls were interspersed with those from study participants, and all specimens were examined under code.

Virus Isolation and Serologic Methods

The virus-isolation techniques we used have been described previously.[16] Briefly, thawed lymphocytes were cocultivated with three-day-old phytohemagglutinin-stimulated normal human lymphocytes in RPMI-1640 medium containing 5 percent interleukin-2. Normal human lymphocytes were added every four to five days. The cultures were monitored for virus replication by immunofluorescence and particulate reverse transcriptase assays performed at intervals for 28 days. Concentrated culture fluids were assayed for particulate reverse transcriptase activity with the synthetic template primer $(A)_n\ (dt)_{12\text{-}18}$ and either 7.5 nmol of magnesium per liter or 0.1 nmol of manganese per liter as a cation.[15] The direct immunofluorescence test was performed with human serum containing a high titer of antibody to HTLV-III/LAV.[16] All cultures were examined by thin-section electron microscopy. Cells that were positive for reverse transcriptase activity and controls were fixed with 2.5 percent glutaraldehyde, postfixed with osmium tetroxide, embedded in Epon–Araldite, and stained with lead citrate and uranyl acetate. Cultured cells were considered to be infected if they met each of the following criteria: (1) produced reverse transcriptase in the supernatant fluid, (2) expressed antigens that were specific for HTLV-III/LAV, and (3) contained HTLV-III/LAV–like virus particles when examined by electron microscopy.[16] Primary cultures of eight different batches of normal human lymphocytes used for cocultivation were monitored similarly to ensure that there was no primary infection or laboratory contamination. Cultures were performed from August to October 1984.

An enzyme-linked immunosorbent assay (ELISA) was performed with whole disrupted HTLV-III/LAV (CDC-451; Jaffe HW, et al.: unpublished data). Competitive radioimmunoassays were used to compare the major core proteins of selected isolates with HTLV-III/LAV (CDC-451 or LAV), as described previously.[16]

Table 1. Laboratory Results and Interval from Transfusion or Donation to Specimen Collection in Patients with Transfusion-Associated AIDS and in High-Risk Donors.*

Subject No.	Diagnosis at Examination (Date of Diagnosis)	Date of Donation/ Transfusion	Date of Specimen Collection	T_H/T_S Ratio†	ELISA Results	Virus Isolation‡
Donor 1	Healthy	10/80	9/83	0.3	+	+
Recipient 1	AIDS (3/83)	10/80	11/83	0.2	+	+
Donor 2	Healthy	11/80	9/83	0.6	+	+
Recipient 2	AIDS (4/83)	11/80	4/83	0.8	+	+
Donor 3	Healthy	8/81	7/83	0.7	+	+
Recipient 3	AIDS (5/83)	8/81	8/83	0.3	+	+
Donor 4	Healthy	11/80	10/83	0.9	+	+
Recipient 4	AIDS (7/83)	11/80	11/83	0.4	+	+
Donor 5	Healthy	10/82	8/84	0.02	+	+
Recipient 5	AIDS (4/84)	10/82	5/84	0.1	+	+
Donor 6	AIDS (12/82)	11/82	1/84	0.02	+	+
Recipient 6	AIDS (12/83)	11/82	1/84	0.5	+	+
Donor 7	Lymphadenopathy (6/83)	3/82	6/83	0.5	+	+
Recipient 7	AIDS (4/83)	3/82	4/83	0.4	+	UTE
Donor 8	Lymphadenopathy (8/82)	4/80	11/82	0.6	+	+
Donor 9	Lymphadenopathy (1980)	10/81	2/83	1.3	+	+
Donor 10	AIDS (11/81)	3/81	3/82	0.1	+	+
Donor 11	Healthy	2/80	3/83	0.5	+	+
Donor 12	Lymphadenopathy (1/83)	7/81	1/83	0.8	+	+
Donor 13	Healthy	12/80	7/83	0.8	+	+
Donor 14	Healthy	3/80	7/83	0.6	+	+
Donor 15A	Healthy	6/82	11/83	1.5	+	+
Donor 15B	Healthy	6/82	12/83	0.1	+	+
Donor 15C	Healthy	6/82	12/83	1.9	−	−
Donor 15D	Healthy	6/82	ND	2.1	−	ND
Donor 16	Healthy	6/81	4/83	0.7	+	+
Donor 17	Healthy	10/82	7/84	0.4	+	+
Donor 18	Healthy	9/80	2/84	0.4	+	+
Donor 19	Healthy	1/83	8/84	0.3	+	+
Donor 20A	Lymphadenopathy (2/84)	10/79	2/84	0.9	+	+
Donor 20B	Healthy	10/79	2/84	1.1	+	+
Donor 21A	Healthy	1/81	12/82	1.8	+	−
Donor 21B	Healthy	1/81	ND	0.9	−	ND
Donor 22A	Healthy	7/81	10/83	1.2	−	−
Donor 22B	AIDS (6/84)	7/81	ND	0.2	+	ND
Donor 23	Lymphadenopathy (1979)	7/79	10/83	1.5	+	UTE
Donor 24	AIDS (2/84)	3/82	4/84	0.2	+	UTE

*UTE denotes unable to evaluate, and ND not done.

†T_H/T_S denotes helper to suppressor T lymphocytes; a ratio under 1.0 was considered abnormal.

‡A culture was considered positive if inoculated cells demonstrated reverse transcriptase activity, were positive on direct immunofluorescence for HTLV-III/LAV antigens, and contained HTLV-III virus particles by electron microscopy. All three criteria were required. Negative cultures were negative by all three criteria.

Results

As of April 1985, the Centers for Disease Control had received reports of 143 cases meeting the criteria for transfusion-associated AIDS: 129 in adults and 14 in infants. The patients had received blood components from an average of 15 different donors. The median time from transfusion to the diagnosis of AIDS was 29 months for adults and 14 months for infants.

Donor investigations were completed for 24 cases (6 in infants and 18 in adults). Of the 296 donors identified in these investigations, 30 were classified as high risk according to the criteria listed above. At least one high-risk donor was identified in each investigation, and more than one was identified in each of four investigations (Table 1). Twenty-five donors (83 percent) were classified as high risk because they reported belonging to a group with an increased incidence of AIDS. One donor had generalized lymphadenopathy and a decreased ratio of helper to suppressor T lymphocytes, and the other four had persistently abnormal ratios of helper to suppressor T lymphocytes. All 30 high-risk donors were men. Twenty-eight (93 percent) were reportedly without symptoms at the time of blood donation. Two (Donors 9 and 23, Table 1) reported a history of enlarged lymph nodes but were otherwise in good health. Serum samples obtained at the time of physical examination from 26 (87 percent) of the 30 high-risk donors and from 7 patients with transfusion-associated AIDS contained antibodies to HTLV-III/LAV as detected by ELISA (Table 1).

Lymphocyte cultures from 6 patients and 25 high-risk donors (identified in 22 of the 24 investigations) could be adequately evaluated. Virus was detected by reverse transcriptase activity, expression of viral antigens detectable by immunofluorescence, and electron microscopy in cultures from all 6 patients with transfusion-associated AIDS and from 22 of the 25 high-risk donors (Table 1). Virus was isolated from one high-risk donor identified in each of 20 investigations, and from two donors identified in each of 2 investigations (Donors 15 and 20, Table 1). Although no lymphocyte specimen was available from Donor 22B, he was seropositive for HTLV-III/LAV by ELISA and has subsequently contracted AIDS. Of the three high-risk donors in whom virus could not be detected, two had no detectable antibodies. The major core proteins of six of the virus isolates were examined by competitive radioimmunoassay and found to be antigenically identical to each other and to the major core protein (p24) of HTLV-III/LAV.

Specimens were obtained an average of 28 months (range, 12 to 52) after the 22 virus-positive high-risk donors had given blood and 26 months (range, 14 to 37) after the six patients with transfusion-associated AIDS had received blood. At the time of examination, 15 (68 percent) of the virus-positive donors were healthy, 2 had been diagnosed as having AIDS, and 5 had generalized lymphadenopathy. The ratio of helper to suppressor T lymphocytes was decreased in 19 of the 22 donors. There appeared to be no relation between the time of lymphocyte storage and the isolation of virus. Virus was isolated from frozen specimens from 0 to 30 months (mean, 11) after storage at −70°C. Lymphocyte specimens from Donors 23 and 24 and Recipient 7 could not be adequately evaluated because of interference with cell growth or measurement of reverse transcriptase activity or both. Such interference is regularly found to be due to bacterial, viral, or yeast contamination of the cell culture. This problem is encountered more frequently in specimens from patients with AIDS (Recipient 7 and Donor 24) or lymphadenopathy (Donor 23) than in specimens from asymptomatic persons. There was no evidence of HTLV-III/LAV infection in coded cultures of lymphocytes from controls or in batches of normal human lymphocytes.

Discussion

In over 90 percent of the completed investigations of transfusion-associated AIDS, HTLV-III/LAV was recovered from peripheral lymphocytes collected from the high-risk donor 12 to 52 months after the blood donation had taken place. In 18 of these investigations, only one high-risk donor was identified; serum samples from the other donors were found to be negative for HTLV-III/LAV by ELISA and Western blot assays performed in two laboratories (Jaffe HW, et al.: unpublished data). Therefore, it is likely that the identified high-risk donors transmitted HTLV-III/LAV at the time of their donation. The virologic data demonstrate that infection generally persisted for two years or more in these persons. Most of the infected donors have remained asymptomatic (15 of 22) or have had generalized lymphadenopathy (5 of 22). Two of the donors from whom virus was isolated had been diagnosed as having AIDS by the time of the physical examination.

The isolation of HTLV-III/LAV from both donors and recipients in six investigations provides further evidence of the etiologic role of HTLV-III/LAV in AIDS. In our first report[16] both the donor and recipient contracted AIDS before the virus was isolated, raising the question whether HTLV-III/LAV might represent an opportunistic infection in both. We now report on five additional donor–recipient pairs from whom virus was isolated; in all five the donor was apparently an asymptomatic carrier of HTLV-III, and the recipient contracted AIDS. Molecular comparisons between these isolate pairs and prototype viruses are under way to establish their precise identity and to detect any changes in their genomes over time.

These data suggest that most high-risk blood donors implicated in the transmission of HTLV-III/LAV are chronic carriers of the virus who have minimal or no symptoms. It is not yet clear whether such prolonged infection is typical of all persons infected with the virus. Nonetheless, these observations underline the importance of identifying high-risk donors in cases of transfusion-associated AIDS in order to prevent future blood donations from them. Virus isolation correlated well with ELISA positivity at the time of specimen collection. The failure to isolate HTLV-III/LAV from two seronegative high-risk donors does not rule out the possibility that a donor can be seronegative yet infectious, since isolation of HTLV-III has recently been reported in four homosexual men without detectable antibody.[20] A virus-positive seronegative person would appear to be the exception, however, since only 4 of 96 virus-positive subjects in that study lacked detectable antibody. It is reassuring that serum specimens from each of 28 persons from whom HTLV-III/LAV was isolated were positive by ELISA. In addition, we have recently isolated HTLV-III/LAV from 8 of 12 asymptomatic homosexual men who had undergone seroconversion 4 to 69 months (median, 33) previously.[21] Serologic tests to detect antibody to HTLV-III/LAV by techniques similar to ours are now available for the screening of blood and plasma collected in the United States. The persistence of infection with HTLV-III/LAV in asymptomatic donors supports the use of serologic screening to supplement current procedures for the identification of blood donors from populations with an increased incidence of AIDS.[22]

We are indebted to Stephen McDougal, M.D., and Thomas Spira, M.D., for assisting in the immunologic studies; to Ava Wilhite, Walter Dowdle, Ph.D., and Frederick Murphy, D.V.M., Ph.D., for editorial assistance; and to Quo Vadis Harris for preparing the manuscript.

References

1. *Pneumocystis* pneumonia — Los Angeles. MMWR 1981; 30:250-2.
2. Gottlieb MS, Schroff R, Schanker HM, et al. *Pneumocystis carinii* pneumonia and mucosal candidiasis in previously healthy homosexual men: evidence of a new acquired cellular immunodeficiency. N Engl J Med 1981; 305:1425-31.

3. Masur H, Michelis MA, Greene JB, et al. An outbreak of community-acquired *Pneumocystis carinii* pneumonia: initial manifestation of cellular immune dysfunction. N Engl J Med 1981; 305:1431-8.
4. Siegal FP, Lopez C, Hammer GS, et al. Severe acquired immunodeficiency in male homosexuals, manifested by chronic perianal ulcerative herpes simplex lesions. N Engl J Med 1981; 305:1439-44.
5. Hymes KB, Cheung T, Greene JB, et al. Kaposi's sarcoma in homosexual men — a report of eight cases. Lancet 1981; 2:598-600.
6. *Pneumocystis carinii* pneumonia among persons with hemophilia A. MMWR 1982; 31:365-7.
7. Davis KC, Horsburgh CR, Hasiba U, Schocket AL, Kirkpatrick CH. Acquired immunodeficiency syndrome in a patient with hemophilia. Ann Intern Med 1983; 98:284-6.
8. Elliott JL, Hoppes WL, Platt MS, Thomas JG, Patel IP, Gansar A. The acquired immunodeficiency syndrome and *Mycobacterium avium-intracellulare* bacteremia in a patient with hemophilia. Ann Intern Med 1983; 98:290-3.
9. Poon M-C, Landay A, Prasthofer EF, Stagno S. Acquired immunodeficiency syndrome with *Pneumocystis carinii* pneumonia and *Mycobacterium avium-intracellulare* infection in a previously healthy patient with classic hemophilia. Ann Intern Med 1983; 98:287-90.
10. Curran JW, Lawrence DN, Jaffe H, et al. Acquired immunodeficiency syndrome (AIDS) associated with transfusions. N Engl J Med 1984; 310:69-75.
11. Ammann AJ, Cowan MJ, Wara DW, et al. Acquired immunodeficiency in an infant: possible transmission by means of blood products. Lancet 1983; 1:956-8.
12. Barré-Sinoussi F, Chermann JC, Rey F, et al. Isolation of a T-lymphotropic retrovirus from a patient at risk for acquired immune deficiency syndrome (AIDS). Science 1983; 220:868-71.
13. Gallo RC, Salahuddin SZ, Popovic M, et al. Frequent detection and isolation of cytopathic retroviruses (HTLV-III) from patients with AIDS and at risk for AIDS. Science 1984; 224:500-3.
14. Sarngadharan MG, Popovic M, Bruch L, Schüpbach J, Gallo RC. Antibodies reactive with human T-lymphotropic retroviruses (HTLV-III) in the serum of patients with AIDS. Science 1984; 224:506-8.
15. Levy JA, Hoffman AD, Kramer SM, Landis JA, Shimabukuro JM, Oshiro LS. Isolation of lymphocytopathic retroviruses from San Francisco patients with AIDS. Science 1984; 225:840-2.
16. Feorino PM, Kalyanaraman VS, Haverkos HW, et al. Lymphadenopathy associated virus infection of a blood donor-recipient pair with acquired immunodeficiency syndrome. Science 1984; 225:69-72.
17. Update on acquired immune deficiency syndrome (AIDS) — United States. MMWR 1982; 31:507-14.
18. Update: acquired immunodeficiency syndrome (AIDS) — United States. MMWR 1984; 32:688-91.
19. Vieira J, Frank E, Spira TJ, Landesman SH. Acquired immune deficiency in Haitians: opportunistic infections in previously healthy Haitian immigrants. N Engl J Med 1983; 308:125-9.
20. Salahuddin SZ, Groopman JE, Mardham PD, et al. HTLV-III in symptom-free seronegative persons. Lancet 1984; 2:1418-20.
21. Jaffe HW, Feorino PM, Darrow WW, et al. Persistent infection with HTLV-III/LAV in apparently healthy homosexual men. Ann Intern Med (in press).
22. Prevention of acquired immune deficiency syndrome (AIDS): report of inter-agency recommendations. MMWR 1983; 32:101-3.

CORRESPONDENCE

NO AIDS AMONG PATIENTS ON DIALYSIS?

To the Editor: I have been intrigued by the apparent rarity of the acquired immunodeficiency syndrome (AIDS) in the dialysis population. One would expect that in such a population — whose members have been invaded by needles and frequent transfusions for many years and have been in a chronic state of immunosuppression — the incidence of AIDS would be much higher than in the general population. The incidence of hepatitis — classic and other forms — is as well documented as those of other viruses — e.g., cytomegalovirus — and all patients on dialysis seem to be susceptible to almost every other infection possible.

I have asked many of my nephrologist colleagues about their experience, and they agree that AIDS is almost unheard of in this population. Is there something special about renal failure that protects its victims? It would be interesting to determine the incidence of AIDS in the dialysis population.

DAVID N. EDELBAUM, M.D., F.A.C.P.
8540 S. Sepulveda Blvd., Suite 1100
Los Angeles, CA 90045

LACK OF CORRELATION BETWEEN PROMISCUITY AND SEROPOSITIVITY TO HTLV-III FROM A LOW-INCIDENCE AREA FOR AIDS

To the Editor: Early studies of homosexual men in high-incidence areas for AIDS revealed an association between numbers of sexual partners and risk of the disease.[1,2] More recent studies, also in high-incidence areas, have also shown a significant correlation between the numbers of sexual partners and seropositivity to HTLV-III.[3] These data have been interpreted by many homosexual men to mean that a lack of sexual promiscuity is protective against the disease. These findings may not be relevant to regions of low disease incidence.

In January 1984, 320 homosexual residents of northeastern Ohio, a low-incidence area, were recruited by advertisement to participate in a survey designed to evaluate sexual practices and risk factors for the development of AIDS. Each participant underwent a brief history and physical examination, completed an epidemiologic questionnaire, and had serum drawn. Ninety-eight serum samples were then tested for antibody to HTLV-III by enzyme-linked immunosorbent assay, yielding an estimated rate of seropositivity of 23.6 percent for the study group. Seropositive and seronegative men did not differ when number of sexual partners, frequency of travel, and drug abuse were compared. When sexual practices were compared, however, seropositive subjects were more likely to have engaged in passive anal intercourse ($P<0.05$). In addition, 6 of the first 10 homosexual men with AIDS who represented local or endemic cases treated at the Cleveland Clinic Foundation admitted to five or fewer sexual contacts in the preceding two years.

It is not apparent why promiscuity does not appear to be a significant risk factor for seropositivity to HTLV-III in our area, or why a high proportion of our patients with AIDS have had relatively few sexual partners. One possible explanation is that in an area where the virus is not widespread, the risk of infection and subsequent disease may be more a function of the nature of one's sexual contacts than of the number. An important factor may be whether a person has sexual contact with members of the segment of the homosexual community that has a high incidence of sexually transmitted disease. This "core population" represents a minority of community members, but its recognition leads to an important concept in understanding the epidemiologic factors in the spread of various sexually transmitted diseases[4] and now possibly AIDS. If this observation is substantiated in other low-incidence areas, then homosexual men from these regions will have to be further cautioned regarding their risks.

LEONARD H. CALABRESE, D.O.
MAX R. PROFFITT, PH.D.
SUSAN REHM, M.D.
Cleveland Clinic Foundation

MICHAEL LEDERMAN, M.D., JOHN T. CAREY, M.D.,
HAROLD B. HOUSER, M.D., KAY EDMONDS, M.S.,
AND JERROLD J. ELLNER, M.D.
Case Western Reserve University
School of Medicine
Cleveland, OH 44106

REFERENCES

1. Kornfeld H, Stowe RAV, Lange M, Reddy MM, Grieco MH. T-lymphocyte subpopulations in homosexual men. N Engl J Med 1982; 307:729-31.
2. Stahl RE, Friedman-Kien A, Dubin R, Marmor M, Zolla-Pazner S. Immunologic abnormalities in homosexual men: relationship to Kaposi's sarcoma. Am J Med 1982; 73:171-8.
3. Anderson R, Levy J. Prevalence of antibodies to AIDS-associated retrovirus in single men in San Francisco. Lancet 1985; 2:217.
4. Williams D. The changing life style of homosexual men in the last fifteen years. In: Friedman-Kien AE, Laubenstein LJ, eds. AIDS: the epidemic of Kaposi's sarcoma and opportunistic infections. New York: Masson, 1983.

AIDS IN A CHILD 5½ YEARS AFTER A TRANSFUSION

To the Editor: We wish to report a case of acquired immunodeficiency syndrome (AIDS) presenting after 5½ years in a child who had received a single blood transfusion.

A white boy was referred at 5½ years of age for chronic oral candidiasis, later proved to be secondary to AIDS. He had weighed 7 lb, 13 oz (3.5 kg) at birth, after a normal full-term gestation, and had received 75 ml of packed red cells shortly after delivery, the indication being a fetal–maternal transfusion. He was subsequently healthy (there was an uncomplicated episode of varicella at 5 years) until the age of 5½ years, when he had oral candidiasis unresponsive to nystatin. Three months later he had *Pneumocystis carinii* pneumonia, treated successfully with trimethoprim–sulfamethoxazole.

Immunologic studies showed absolute lymphopenia (lymphocyte count, 665 per cubic millimeter) and increased levels of IgA (741 mg per deciliter); studies of lymphocyte subpopulations revealed normal levels of OKT3 (pan-T-cell marker) and OKT8 (T suppressor), markedly low levels of OKT4 (T helper), a low T4/T8 ratio (0.2), and depressed responses to stimulation with the mitogens phytohemagglutinin and concanavalin A. Titers of antibody to human T-cell lymphotropic virus Type III were positive in the patient and negative in other family members. His blood donor was an asymptomatic homosexual with a history of intravenous drug abuse, who has a positive HTLV-III antibody titer. The donor's blood has been given to many recipients since our patient's transfusion.

Our patient has the longest latency period of transfusion-related AIDS reported to the Centers for Disease Control.

Physicians should be aware that patients are at risk from even a single blood transfusion, and the latency period may be as long as 5½ years.

Michael J. Maloney, M.D.,
Frederick Cox, M.D.,
Betty B. Wray, M.D.,
Margaret F. Guill, M.D.,
and Jennifer Hagler, M.D.
Medical College of Georgia
Augusta, GA 30912

David Williams, M.D.
Department of Human Resources
Atlanta, GA 30909

Epidemiology and Public Health Issues

Heterosexual Transmission, Intravenous Drug Use, and Other Transmission Concerns

ORIGINAL ARTICLE

IMMUNODEFICIENCY IN FEMALE SEXUAL PARTNERS OF MEN WITH THE ACQUIRED IMMUNODEFICIENCY SYNDROME

CAROL HARRIS, M.D., CATHERINE BUTKUS SMALL, M.D., ROBERT S. KLEIN, M.D., GERALD H. FRIEDLAND, M.D., BERNICE MOLL, PH.D., EUGENE E. EMESON, M.D., ILYA SPIGLAND, M.D., AND NEAL H. STEIGBIGEL, M.D.

Abstract Because the current outbreak of acquired immunodeficiency syndrome (AIDS) among previously healthy adults may be caused by a transmissible biologic agent, and because it may be preceded by immunologic abnormalities with or without a prodromal illness, we studied seven female sexual partners of male patients with the syndrome. The male patients were all drug abusers. One of the seven women was found to have the full-blown syndrome, a second had an illness consistent with the prodrome of AIDS (generalized lymphadenopathy, lymphopenia, and a decreased ratio of helper to suppressor T cells), and four others had generalized lymphadenopathy or lymphopenia, with or without a decreased ratio of helper to suppressor T cells. Only one woman had no abnormalities. These findings suggest that AIDS may be transmitted between heterosexual men and women.

An unusual occurrence of opportunistic infections or Kaposi's sarcoma (or both) associated with the acquired immunodeficiency syndrome (AIDS) in previously healthy persons has recently been reported.[1-11] The initial description of patients with this syndrome included predominantly white male homosexuals living in urban areas.[1] Subsequently, it became clear that heterosexual intravenous-drug abusers, a disproportionate number of Haitian immigrants, and a small number of hemophiliacs were also affected.[3,9,12,13] A prodromal illness including fever, weight loss, diarrhea, oral thrush, and lymphadenopathy has occurred in many of these patients.[2,3,5,9] Although the exact cause remains unknown, environmental and host factors, including viral or other transmissible agents, illicit drug use, and genetic factors, have been postulated as contributory, possibly in association with one another. The distribution of the syndrome best fits the hypothesis that AIDS is caused by a biologic agent transmissible by a variety of routes, including sexual contact and intravenous injection.

To define further the populations affected with this syndrome and explore the possible role and routes of transmission of a biologic agent, we studied the regular female sexual partners of our male patients with the syndrome. Seven women were available for investigation. Their seven male partners were all drug abusers. In this paper we describe the demographic, clinical, virologic, and immunologic characteristics of these seven women. One of the seven had AIDS, one had an illness consistent with the prodrome of AIDS, and four had clinical or laboratory abnormalities associated with the syndrome. One woman had no abnormalities.

METHODS

Subjects

In July 1982 we began to evaluate the regular sexual partners of the 17 heterosexual male patients with AIDS who had been treated at Montefiore Medical Center, North Central Bronx Hospital, or the Bronx Municipal Hospital Center. The patients were all previously healthy men below the age of 60 years who had evidence of cellular immunodeficiency and of severe opportunistic infections or Kaposi's sarcoma (or both). Nine of them have been described elsewhere.[9] We were able to identify 12 regular sexual partners of these men, of whom 7 were available for study, 4 could not be located and 1 refused to participate. The seven women gave informed consent and were interviewed in detail by the investigators, with special attention to sexual practices and drug use. All of the male index cases had been carefully and repeatedly questioned in detail about sexual contacts and drug abuse. All seven subjects received a physical examination. Historical data for each subject were confirmed by means of a personal interview conducted by members of the Centers for Disease Control (CDC) Task Force on the Acquired Immune Deficiency Syndrome or by personnel from the New York City Department of Health (or both). Each interview lasted about 90 minutes and involved the use of a detailed standardized CDC questionnaire administered by the expert interviewer. Generalized lymphadenopathy was defined as the presence of palpable lymph nodes larger than 1 cm at two or more extrainguinal sites. At the beginning of this study, none of the subjects had sought medical attention. All abnormalities that were found and their potential association with AIDS were discussed with the subjects; however, no specific recommendations were made regarding the continuation of relations with the male index cases.

Routine Studies

Standard techniques were used to determine absolute lymphocyte counts. Routine chemistries and serologic tests for syphilis were performed.

Immunologic Studies

Intradermal injections of candida, mumps, trichophytin, and tuberculin purified-protein-derivative antigens were used to test for cutaneous anergy. In vitro studies included identification of all peripheral T cells, helper/inducer T cells, and suppressor/cytotoxic T cells, with use of the monoclonal antibodies OKT3, OKT4, and OKT8, respectively, in an indirect immunofluorescence assay, as previously described.[14] Serum immunoglobulins were evaluated by routine methods.

Viral and Other Studies

All these studies were performed in the Diagnostic Virology Laboratory of Montefiore Medical Center under the direction of one of us (I.S.). Throat, rectal, and urinary viral cultures were performed as previously described.[9] For each patient, serum IgG antibody titers to the following were determined: Epstein–Barr viral capsid antigen (by indirect immunofluorescence), cytomegalovirus (by complement fixation), and *Toxoplasma gondii* (by indirect fluorescence). Hepatitis B surface antigen, antibody to hepatitis B surface antigen, and IgG antibody to hepatitis A virus were measured by

From the Division of Infectious Diseases, Department of Medicine, and the Divisions of Immunopathology and Virology, Department of Pathology, Montefiore Medical Center, the Bronx; the Department of Medicine, North Central Bronx Hospital; and the Departments of Medicine and Pathology, Albert Einstein College of Medicine, the Bronx.

Dr. Harris and Dr. Butkus Small are supported by a training grant (5-T32-AI070183-03) from the National Institute of Allergy and Infectious Diseases.

radioimmunoassay. The methods used in these determinations have been reported elsewhere.[9] Antibody titers to herpes simplex virus and the chlamydia group were measured by complement fixation. Monosticon Dri-Dot (Organon Diagnostics, West Orange N.J.) and ox-cell hemolysis were done routinely.

RESULTS

Clinical and laboratory values are shown in Table 1.

Demographic Data

Of the seven women, five were Hispanic (of Puerto Rican background), one was black, and one was white. Their ages ranged from 23 to 39 years (mean, 31). All were long-term residents of New York City, and none had a history of previous serious, recurrent, venereal, or opportunistic infections. The information given by all seven women was considered to be reliable. All the women stated that they had maintained exclusively heterosexual relations. Upon repeated questioning, all seven women denied the use of intravenous drugs or inhalants (cocaine or nitrites). All denied any contact with drug-using paraphernalia except for one accidental needle puncture in Subject 4. One woman had a history of moderate alcohol intake. Four of the women were employed, and one was a student. The women all claimed that they had had sexual relations only with their partners (the index cases) throughout the relationship. Subjects 2, 5, 6, and 7 occasionally engaged in anal intercourse; this practice was specifically denied by the other women. Six of the women lived in the same household as the corresponding index case.

All the male partners had had opportunistic infections and cellular immunodeficiency diagnosed within the past 18 months. All had a history of intravenous drug abuse (heroin or heroin and cocaine), except for cocaine snorting only in the partner of Subject 2. All were strictly heterosexual, except for the partner of Subject 2, who had had homosexual encounters two to four years earlier. He denied having had any homosexual experience after the beginning of his sexual relationship with Subject 2. For each couple, the temporal association between onset of symptoms in the index cases and onset of symptoms in the women, as well as the onset of sexual relations between the partners, is shown in Table 1.

Clinical Features

Subject 1 (the female partner in Couple 1) began losing weight and had malaise in June 1982 but did not seek medical care at that time. At her initial evaluation one month later she was noted to have oral candidiasis, and over the next three days fever, a nonproductive cough, hypoxemia, and diffuse pulmonary interstitial infiltrates developed. She responded to a course of trimethoprim–sulfamethoxazole and then to pentamidine — a change necessitated by the development of granulocytopenia. A transbronchial lung biopsy performed after five days of therapy revealed *Pneumocystis carinii* by methenamine-silver stain and by electron microscopy. She continued to have generalized lymphadenopathy and oral thrush. Subjects 2, 3, and 6 also had generalized lymphadenopathy. Subjects 2 and 3 reported that the duration of adenopathy was 5 and 12 months, respectively. Subject 3 had been taking phenytoin for two years because of a seizure disorder. Adenopathy had not been noted by Subject 6 but was found on physical examination. A lymph-node biopsy performed on Subject 2 revealed lymphoid hyperplasia. The other subjects had no signs or symptoms.

Subject 2 had mild thrombocytopenia (the platelet count ranged between 68,000 and 121,000). A bone-

Table 1. Demographic, Clinical, and Laboratory Characteristics of the Seven Women and Their Male Partners with AIDS.

	COUPLE 1	COUPLE 2	COUPLE 3
Male index cases			
Onset of prodrome	1/82	6/81	1/80
Opportunistic infections (date)	Oral thrush (3/82); *P. carinii* (6/82, 10/82)*	Oral thrush (6/82); *P. carinii* (6/82); disseminated *M. avium–intracellulare* (12/82)	Oral thrush (9/81); *P. carinii* (9/82, 2/83)
Kaposi's sarcoma	No	Yes	No
Female subjects			
Age (yr)	37	23	32
Ethnic group	Black	Hispanic	White
Drug abuse	Ethanol	None	None
Start of sexual relations with index case	1976	June 1981	1977
Prodromal symptoms (date)	Weight loss (6/82); generalized lymphadenopathy	Generalized lymphadenopathy (2/82)	Generalized lymphadenopathy (8/81)
Opportunistic infections (date)	*P. carinii* (7/82); oral thrush (7/82)	None	None
Cutaneous anergy‡	Yes	No	No
Lymphopenia (cells/mm^3)	500§	1120	None
Helper/suppressor T cells¶	0.0	0.82	3.1
Viral culture	Cytomegalovirus (urine); adenovirus (urine); herpes simplex (throat)	Neg.	Neg.
Epstein–Barr virus antibody titer	1:5120	1:2560	1:1280
Cytomegalovirus antibody titer	1:32	1:16	<1:4
Serum immunoglobulins (mg/dl) ‖			
IgG	2050	1950	1320
IgA	1470	280	183
IgM	232	210	225

*Died.

†Not noted by subject but detected on physical examination.

‡Subjects 2, 3, 5, 6, and 7 reacted only to mumps antigen, with erythema at 48 hours; Subject 4 reacted only to tuberculin purified protein derivative (1 tu).

marrow examination performed when the platelet count was 120,000 revealed normal megakaryocytes.

Immunology, Virology, and Serology

Subject 1 had manifestations of cutaneous anergy. The other six women responded to one of the skin tests. Four of the women had lymphopenia on at least one determination. Subjects 1 and 2 had a low percentage of helper T cells and a ratio of helper to suppressor T cells that was lower than normal. Subject 5 also had a low ratio of helper to suppressor T cells, although the percentages of helper and suppressor T cells were within the normal range.

Two subjects had markedly increased levels of IgG, and one of them (Subject 1) also had a markedly increased level of IgA. The other five patients had high normal or slightly elevated levels of IgG.

None of the women had clinical signs of infectious mononucleosis, atypical lymphocytosis, positive Monosticon tests, or positive ox-cell-hemolysis tests. However, five had high titers of Epstein–Barr viral antibody (1:1280 to 1:10,240). Two had cytomegalovirus titers of 1:32. None of the toxoplasma, herpes simplex, or chlamydia-group titers were elevated above the normal values. None of the women had hepatitis B surface antigen, but Subject 2 had antibody to it, and Subject 6 had antibody to hepatitis A virus. All viral cultures were negative, except for those of Subject 1. Adenovirus and cytomegalovirus were simultaneously isolated from her urine, and herpes simplex was isolated from her throat. Serologic tests for syphilis were all negative.

Table 1 (Continued).

Couple 4	Couple 5	Couple 6	Couple 7
4/82	9/81	8/81	12/80
Oral thrush (7/82); *P. carinii* (7/82)*	Oral thrush (10/81); *P. carinii* (11/81); disseminated *M. gordonae* (11/82)	Oral thrush (10/81); disseminated histoplasmosis (12/81)*	Oral thrush (4/82); *P. carinii* (4.82); disseminated *M. avium–intracellulare* (12/82)
Yes	No	No	No
39	26	37	25
Hispanic	Hispanic	Hispanic	Hispanic
None	None	None	None
1977	1977	1966	1972
None	None	Generalized lymphadenopathy†	None
None	None	None	None
No	No	No	No
1430	1220	None	None
1.75	1.1	2.0	2.1
Neg.	Neg.	Neg.	Neg.
1:10,240	1:1280	1:320	1:320
1:8	1:32	1:16	<1:4
1200 180 298	1400 167 159	1250 231 198	1340 154 194

§Lowest lymphocyte count (normal value, ≥1500).

¶Normal range, 1.4 to 3.6.

‖Normal ranges: IgG, 639–1349; IgA, 70–312; IgM, 56–352.

Discussion

This study suggests that subjects who are sexual partners of heterosexual men with AIDS are at risk of acquiring the syndrome. The previously described risk factors of promiscuous male homosexuality[1-9,11,15,16] and illicit drug use[3,9,10] were absent in the seven women in this study. None were Haitian[12] and none had hemophilia[13]. The only common risk factor we could identify in all the subjects was prolonged monogamous contact with a male patient who had documented AIDS.

In one woman AIDS was manifested by weight loss, generalized lymphadenopathy, oral thrush, *P. carinii* pneumonia, and immunologic abnormalities associated with the syndrome.

Another had persistent generalized lymphadenopathy (hyperplastic on biopsy), lymphopenia, a decreased ratio of helper to suppressor T cells with a decreased percentage of helper T cells, and an elevated level of IgG. Although this woman was clinically well, the constellation of features was consistent with the prodrome frequently described in patients with AIDS. In a previous report, 44 percent of 73 patients with Kaposi's sarcoma and 23 percent of 61 patients with *P. carinii* pneumonia had lymphadenopathy.[5] In addition, persistent generalized lymphadenopathy has been detected in a group of 51 homosexual men, some of whom also had anergy or reversed ratios of helper to suppressor T cells. Kaposi's sarcoma subsequently developed in one of these patients.[17]

Four of the five other subjects in our study had some of the clinical, immunologic, or viral features associated with AIDS. Two (Subjects 3 and 6) had generalized lymphadenopathy. It should be noted that Subject 3 was taking phenytoin, which may have been responsible for the lymphadenopathy.[18] Two women (Subjects 4 and 5) had lymphopenia, one with markedly elevated titers of antibody to Epstein–Barr virus and one with an associated reduced ratio of helper to suppressor T cells. High titers of antibody to Epstein–Barr virus have been described in patients with AIDS and disseminated Kaposi's sarcoma[6] or opportunistic infections.[9]

These abnormalities, previously described in patients with AIDS and found in five of the six women in this study without fully expressed AIDS, may represent early or subclinical AIDS. Whether opportunistic infections or Kaposi's sarcoma will eventually develop in these women can be determined only by continued observation. It is unlikely that the fully expressed AIDS in one woman, the prodrome in another, and the various abnormalities associated with the syndrome in four of the other five were due to chance. Investigation of a larger series of patients and a suitable control group will be necessary to prove the postulate that this syndrome is transmissible from men to their female sexual contacts. Transmission of AIDS in heterosexual couples is supported by the recent report of AIDS in a non-drug-abusing female sexual contact of a male heroin abuser.[10]

The hypothesis that an agent transmissible to sexual contacts may be responsible for the abnormalities in cellular immunity present in this syndrome is supported by the recent report of a cluster of homosexual men in California with Kaposi's sarcoma and *P. carinii* pneumonia. Nine of these patients had had sexual contact with other known cases within five years of acquiring the illness.[15] In this cluster an incubation period of 9 to 22 months was postulated. However, all patients had a homosexual life style and had had many sexual partners. In contrast, our subjects denied having had sexual contact with anyone other than the index case for 2 to 17 years (mean, 7.9). Because of the prolonged and repetitive sexual relations in our couples, a defined incubation period cannot be determined. Subject 2 had prodromal symptoms within eight months after beginning to have sexual relations with the index case. This is consistent with the postulated incubation period in the California cluster.[15]

This study suggests that AIDS may be sexually transmitted between heterosexual men and women.

We are indebted to William Darrow, Ph.D., of the Centers for Disease Control Task Force on AIDS and to Rebecca Reiss, M.P.H., of the New York City Department of Health for performing patient interviews; to Michela Catalano, M.D., for assisting in the evaluation of Subjects 5 and 7; to Stephen Baum, M.D., for performing the electron microscopy; and to Mrs. Joyce Sloman for assistance in preparing the manuscript.

References

1. Pneumocystis pneumonia — Los Angeles. MMWR 1981; 30:250-2.
2. Gottlieb MS, Schroff R, Schanker HM, et al. *Pneumocystis carinii* pneumonia and mucosal candidiasis in previously healthy homosexual men: evidence of a new acquired cellular immunodeficiency. N Engl J Med 1981; 305:1425-31.
3. Masur H, Michelis MA, Greene JB, et al. An outbreak of community-acquired *Pneumocystis carinii* pneumonia: initial manifestation of cellular immune dysfunction. N Engl J Med 1981; 305:1431-8.
4. Siegal FP, Lopez D, Hammer GS, et al. Severe acquired immunodeficiency in male homosexuals, manifested by chronic perianal ulcerative herpes simplex lesions. N Engl J Med 1981; 305:1439-44.
5. Centers for Disease Control Task Force on Kaposi's Sarcoma and Opportunistic Infections. Epidemiologic aspects of the current outbreak of Kaposi's sarcoma and opportunistic infections. N Engl J Med 1982; 306:248-52.
6. Friedman-Kien AE, Laubenstein LJ, Rubinstein P, et al. Disseminated Kaposi's sarcoma in homosexual men. Ann Intern Med 1982; 96:693-700.
7. Mildvan D, Mathur U, Enlow RW, et al. Opportunistic infections and immune deficiency in homosexual men. Ann Intern Med 1982; 96:700-4.
8. Follansbee SE, Busch DF, Wofsy CB, et al. An outbreak of *Pneumocystis carinii* pneumonia in homosexual men. Ann Intern Med 1982; 96:705-13.
9. Small CB, Klein RS, Friedland GH, Moll B, Emeson EE, Spigland I. Community-acquired opportunistic infections and defective cellular immunity in heterosexual drug abusers and homosexual men. Am J Med 1983; 74:433-41.
10. Masur H, Michelis MA, Wormser GP, et al. Opportunistic infection in previously healthy women: initial manifestations of a community-acquired cellular immunodeficiency. Ann Intern Med 1982; 97:533-9.
11. Greene JB, Sidhu GS, Lewin S, et al. *Mycobacterium avium-intracellulare:* a cause of disseminated life-threatening infection in homosexuals and drug abusers. Ann Inter Med 1982; 97:539-46.
12. Vieira J, Frank E, Spira TJ, Landesman SH. Acquired immune deficiency in Haitians: opportunistic infections in previously healthy Haitian immigrants. N Engl J Med 1983; 308:125-9.
13. *Pneumocystic carinii* pneumonia among persons with hemophilia A. MMWR 1982; 31:365-7.
14. Moll B, Emeson EE, Small CB, Friedland GH, Klein RS, Spigland I. Inverted ratio of inducer to suppressor T-lymphocyte subsets in drug abusers with opportunistic infections. Clin Immunol Immunopathol 1982; 25:417-23.
15. A cluster of Kaposi's sarcoma and *Pneumocystis carinii* pneumonia among homosexual male residents of Los Angeles and Orange Counties, California. MMWR 1982; 31:305-7.
16. Durack DT. Opportunistic infections and Kaposi's sarcoma in homosexual men. N Engl J Med 1981; 305:1465-7.
17. Persistent, generalized lymphadenopathy among homosexual males. MMWR 1982; 31:249-51.
18. Sparberg M. Diagnostically confusing complications of diphenylhydantoin therapy: a review. Ann Intern Med 1963; 59:914-30.

SPECIAL REPORT

INFECTION-CONTROL GUIDELINES FOR PATIENTS WITH THE ACQUIRED IMMUNODEFICIENCY SYNDROME (AIDS)

John E. Conte, Jr., M.D., W. Keith Hadley, M.D., Merle Sande, M.D., and The University of California, San Francisco, Task Force on the Acquired Immunodeficiency Syndrome

A TASK force* at the University of California, San Francisco, has developed infection-control guidelines for patients with the acquired immunodeficiency syndrome (AIDS). The task force included representatives of the University of California, San Francisco, and the city and county of San Francisco; administrators from various San Francisco hospitals; and other health-care workers with a special interest in AIDS. It also considered guidelines that had been developed by the infection-control committees at both University of California Moffitt Hospital† and San Francisco General Hospital.‡

The purpose of this report is to present the findings of the task force and, recognizing that a scientific basis for many of the decisions is currently lacking, to point out the areas of disagreement. We hope that airing these issues will serve a useful purpose by encouraging further discussion and investigation.

The first case of AIDS in San Francisco was recognized in 1981. By December of that year, 35 cases had been reported in California, mostly from San Francisco and Los Angeles.[1] As of June 1, 1983, a total of 1508 cases, of which 575 had been fatal, had been reported to the Centers for Disease Control (CDC) from 35 states, and 109 cases had been reported from 17 other countries. The CDC is receiving reports of four to five new cases per day, and present estimates are that the number of cases is doubling every six months (Starcher T, CDC public-health advisor: personal communication).

AIDS principally affects male members of certain groups, including homosexuals, intravenous-drug abusers, patients with hemophilia who are receiving factor VIII concentrate, and Haitians. AIDS has also been reported in some recipients of blood transfusions, in infants born into families with risk factors for AIDS,[2-4] and in women who use intravenous drugs or who are sexual partners of men who use intravenous drugs or have the syndrome.[5-7] There are no identifiable risk factors present in 5.7 percent of patients with AIDS (Starcher T: personal communication).

AIDS is characterized by variable, often severe suppression of the cellular immune system and a marked reduction in the helper-to-suppressor T-cell ratio.[8] Patients are susceptible to the development of Kaposi's sarcoma and some other cancers and to a variety of opportunistic infections, including *Candida albicans, Pneumocystis carinii,* cytomegalovirus, herpes simplex, *Cryptococcus neoformans, Histoplasma capsulatum, Mycobacterium avium-intracellulare, Toxoplasma gondii,* legionella, cryptosporidium, and isospora.

The cause of AIDS is unknown, but epidemiologic data suggest a transmissible agent, probably a virus. Several viruses have been suggested, including cytomegalovirus,[8,9] Epstein–Barr virus,[4,10] herpes simplex virus,[11] and human T-cell leukemia virus.[12-17]

Transmission of the disease appears to have an epidemiologic pattern similar to that of hepatitis B, and for this reason, precautions appropriate for hepatitis B should be used as a guide in implementing infection-control procedures.[2,18] This suggests that the disease may be transmitted by blood, tissue, and secretions or excretions that may contain blood (or the virus), such as semen, urine, and stool, and that precautions should be directed at reducing exposure to these body fluids. The incubation period has not been well defined but ranges possibly from a few months to 24 months or more (Starcher T: personal communication). To date, health-care workers do not appear to have a high risk for contracting AIDS, with most (but not all) cases in health-care workers occurring in members of high-risk groups. There has been no evidence of person-to-person transmission through casual contact.[2]

The guidelines were developed to address two main concerns: the potential transmissibility of a putative AIDS agent and the transmissibility of opportunistic pathogens.

The Definition of AIDS as Applied to Infection-Control Measures

The CDC has defined persons for whom precautions should be taken[18] as "persons with: opportunistic infections that are not associated with other underlying immunosuppressive disease or therapy; Kaposi's sarcoma (patients under 60 years of age); chronic gen-

*Members of the task force were Merle A. Sande, M.D., chairman, Paul Volberding, M.D., co-chairman, Arthur Ammann, M.D., Robert Brody, M.D., Marcus Conant, M.D., John E. Conte, Jr., M.D., Donald Fink, M.D., Stephen Follansbee, M.D., Jeffrey Golden, M.D., Moses Grossman, M.D., Keith Hadley, M.D., Philip Hopewell, M.D., Richard Jacobs, M.D., Peter Jenson, M.D., Leslie Lingaas, Ronald Lipsy, Grace Lusby, R.N., Jacqueline Octavio, R.N., Jerry Rankin, Michela Reichman, Linda Rosendorf, M.S., Mervyn Silverman, M.D., Richard Sweet, M.D., Pearl Toy, M.D., Constance Wofsy, M.D., and Mary Anne Johnson, M.D.

†Members of the Ad Hoc Advisory Committee for AIDS at Moffitt Hospital were John E. Conte, Jr., M.D., chairman, Donald Abrams, M.D., David Altman, M.D., Arthur Ammann, M.D., Stephen Cohen, M.D., Marcus Conant, M.D., Stephen Follansbee, M.D., Jeffrey Golden, M.D., Jane Hirsch, R.N., Jay Levy, M.D., Ronald Lipsy, Jacqueline Octavio, R.N., Linda Rosendorf, M.S., Helen Schietinger, R.N., Gwynn Simon, M.D., Daniel Stites, M.D., Carol Viele, R.N., William West, and Betty Wimberly, R.N.

‡Members of the San Francisco General Hospital Infection Control Committee were Keith Hadley, M.D., co-chair, Mary Anne Johnson, co-chair, June Fisher, M.D., Moses Grossman, M.D., Grace Lusby, R.N., Mary Anne McGuire, R.N., Anthony Meyers, M.D., Richard Sweet, M.D., and Constance Wofsy, M.D.

eralized lymphadenopathy, unexplained weight loss and/or prolonged unexplained fever in persons who belong to groups with apparently increased risks of AIDS (homosexual males, intravenous drug abusers, Haitian entrants, hemophiliacs); and possible AIDS (hospitalized for evaluation)."

Comment: There was no important dissent among members of the task force regarding this definition of AIDS for the purpose of infection control. It is reasonable to include hospitalized patients for whom the diagnosis is being considered but is not yet established. Although the relation of the chronic lymphadenopathy syndrome to AIDS is not understood, some patients with AIDS have had opportunistic pathogens, such as *Mycobacterium avium-intracellulare,* isolated from lymph nodes. Also, the full syndrome of AIDS has developed in some patients with adenopathy, and in a number of cases, patients with Kaposi's sarcoma have presented with only lymph-node involvement. For these reasons, this group of patients is included in the definition.

Identifying the Patient

The attending physician has the following responsibilities: (1) to identify the patient who falls into one of the above categories in order that appropriate procedures can be instituted; (2) to report the diagnosis to the state health department, since in California AIDS is now a reportable disease (for purposes of reporting, the state of California and the CDC use the following case definition: an instance of a reliably diagnosed disease that is at least moderately indicative of an underlying cellular immune deficiency in a patient who has had no known underlying cause of cellular immune deficiency nor any other cause of reduced resistance reported to be associated with that disease[19]); and (3) to determine, in consultation with the Infection Control Unit, when appropriate precautions or isolation measures can be discontinued.

Comment: The purpose of this guideline is to establish clearly the responsibility for identification of patients with AIDS or possible AIDS. False labeling of patients as having the syndrome leads to undue anxiety, and failure to identify patients with AIDS could have serious medical consequences. It was the consensus that these responsibilities rest with the primary-care physician.

Precautions

In general, measures consistent with those suggested for the prevention of hepatitis B should be followed.[2,18] Specimens from patients should have a warning label of the biohazard type that does not mention a specific disease, and should be placed in a waterproof bag or container for transport. Gloves should be worn by persons who are in contact with blood, blood specimens, tissue, any body fluids, or excretions or articles or surfaces potentially contaminated by them. After such contact, hands should be washed immediately with soap and water. Thorough hand-washing is mandatory before contact with patients suspected of having or known to have AIDS and before leaving the patient's room. Gowns are recommended for those likely to have direct contact with the patient's secretions, excretions, or blood. Environmental surfaces contaminated with blood or other body fluids should be cleaned immediately with a disinfectant, such as a 1:10 dilution of 5.25 percent sodium hypochlorite solution.

Comment: Each of the committees supported the concept that the epidemiology of AIDS parallels that of hepatitis B and that control measures appropriate to that infection should be used. There was general agreement that there is no evidence for airborne transmission and that spread of the disease through casual contact is unlikely.

The task force recommended that specimens being sent to the laboratory should be labeled "H/A (a code abbreviation for hepatitis/AIDS) precautions."

Masks

Masks are not routinely necessary for patients with AIDS. They should be worn by patients who are coughing when it is necessary for them to leave the hospital room. Masks should be worn by visitors and health-care workers who have direct and sustained contact with a coughing patient or an intubated patient whose throat is being suctioned.

Comment: There was considerable disagreement between committees and among committee members regarding this guideline. One view was that the routine use of masks was not necessary except for a coughing patient in whom the diagnosis of tuberculosis had not yet been ruled out. In this situation, health-care personnel in the patient's room should wear masks, and the patient should wear a mask when leaving the room for any reason. Thus, "mask precautions" for patients with AIDS should be followed as for patients with tuberculosis, only if tuberculosis has not been ruled out. This policy is currently followed by some metropolitan hospitals involved with the care of AIDS patients (Otten J, infection control coordinator, Jackson Memorial Hospital, University of Miami, Fla., and Ehrenkrantz J, director, South Florida Hospital Consortium for Infection Control, Miami: personal communications).

The final recommendations of the task force were more conservative. They are based on the potential for the transmission of opportunistic pathogens, not just tuberculosis, to other patients, perhaps because of high levels of inocula in the patients with AIDS. The task force concluded that masks should be worn by any coughing patient who leaves the hospital room and by health-care workers and visitors who have "direct and sustained contact" with any coughing patients with AIDS. This position is supported by animal studies[20] that suggest that *P. carinii* pneumonia is transmitted through the air. A similar mask policy is followed in some hospitals in Los Angeles (Parrish N, infection-control practitioner, University of California, Los Angeles: personal communication) and New York (Gilligan N, nurse epidemiologist, St. Luke's–Roosevelt Hospital, New York: personal communication).

Protective Eyewear

Protective eyewear (goggles) should be worn in situations in which splatter with blood, bloody secretions, or body fluids is expected.

Comment: This guideline is intended for physicians, dentists, technicians, nurses, and other health-care workers directly involved in the performance of such procedures as bronchoscopy, endoscopy, or oral surgery, which are likely to produce aerosols. It is based on the "conjunctival splash" type of exposure that is described for hepatitis B. Other procedures, such as endotracheal intubation, endotracheal-tube or tracheotomy manipulations, and other surgical procedures, must be judged on an individual basis. We are not requiring nurses to wear protective eyewear when they attend intubated patients in the intensive-care unit.

Needles and Syringes

Needles and syringes should be disposed of in rigid-wall, puncture-resistant containers. Needles should not be resheathed after use, and disposable equipment should be used whenever possible.

Employees with needle-stick injuries should report to the employee health service and be treated according to the needle-stick protocol[21] at their hospital.

Comment: Considerable debate arose over the necessity or wisdom of follow-up studies after AIDS-related needle-stick injuries. At present, the task force does not recommend follow-up lymphocyte studies unless they are done on a research basis, since a variety of illnesses — such as cytomegalovirus-induced mononucleosis,[22] influenza, Epstein–Barr virus infection, hepatitis B infection, and biliary cirrhosis[23,24] — have been shown to reverse the helper-to-suppressor ratio. Thus, information so derived may produce untoward anxiety, while not accurately predicting or identifying the disease.

Linen and Fomites

All contaminated disposable items (visibly soiled with potentially infectious material) should be considered "infectious waste" and identified as such. Contaminated linen should be double-bagged.

Comment: In our hospitals, as in many others, "infectious waste" requires special transport and disposal and is identified by "red bagging." Laundry is double-bagged and washed as usual in the hospital laundry. Because of the difficulty of refurbishing and decontaminating "Clinitron" beds after use by patients with AIDS, these devices are not recommended.

Private versus Multiple-Bed Rooms

A private room is not necessary if the patient is cooperative, is not coughing, and can be adequately instructed in personal hygiene. However, it may be prudent to admit patients with AIDS to private rooms, when available. When a double room is used, the other patient should not be an impaired host who is susceptible to opportunistic infection or someone who might harbor potential opportunistic infections that could be transmitted to the patient with AIDS.

Comment: Considerable controversy arose over this guideline. Some members thought that private rooms were not necessary since there is no evidence for casual transmission of AIDS, but they agreed that the roommate of a patient with AIDS should not be a patient who is immunosuppressed or clinically infected with potentially transmissible pathogens.

The recommendations of the task force were more cautious. Although it stated that strict-isolation rooms were not necessary for patients with AIDS, the task force added that it may be "prudent" to admit patients to private rooms. This was thought not to be essential for the cooperative patient. The final wording of the guideline attempts to reflect both these points of view.

Refusal to Care for Patients with AIDS

There is no scientific reason for healthy personnel to be excused from delivering care to patients with AIDS. Those who believe they are at high risk for infection because of their own immune status should be encouraged to discuss their work responsibilities with their personal physician. If the physician determines that there are certain assignments the employee should not accept, this fact should be communicated in writing to the employing department for appropriate action, according to the institution's policies and procedures. Pregnant employees should not engage in the direct care of patients with AIDS, because of the potential for birth defects from cytomegalovirus and the potentially large amounts of this virus that may be disseminated from such patients.

Comment: It is our experience that some health-care workers, including physicians, are reluctant to care for patients with AIDS. Both committees believed that there were risks associated with caring for all sick persons and that, providing appropriate precautions were taken, care should not be denied to patients with AIDS on grounds that lacked scientific merit. In cases in which the employee refuses outright to perform his or her duties, the issue is an ethical, legal, and administrative problem that must be handled on an individual basis.

Cardiopulmonary Resuscitation in the Hospital Setting

Resuscitation bags, or disposable devices for mouth-to-mouth cardiopulmonary resuscitation (CPR) should be available for every patient and should be used for resuscitation. Such devices should be kept at the bedside of patients with AIDS and other patients with potentially transmissible infections — for example, hepatitis B infection or tuberculosis. When such a CPR device is available, the employee is obligated to administer CPR. The decision to withhold direct mouth-to-mouth resuscitation from a patient with AIDS when a CPR device is not available is solely that of the individual employee.

CPR training should include instruction in the use of disposable devices to prevent mouth-to-mouth contact between the resuscitator and the patient. Hospital employees with documented AIDS should be excused from participating in the two-person manikin phase of the CPR training program. Consideration should be given to revising the recertification procedures to eliminate mouth-to-mouth contact with the manikin during the two-person training phase for all persons undergoing CPR recertification. Employees with AIDS should not, however, be excused from other phases of the training program, nor should they be discouraged from becoming recertified in CPR.

Comment: Although there are good epidemiologic data to support the occurrence of a transmissible agent of AIDS in blood, there is no current evidence for its presence in saliva. In performing cardiopulmonary resuscitation the resuscitator may come into contact with saliva containing blood or vomitus or both. This exposure to blood may serve as a way of transmitting the AIDS agent. For these reasons, the task force members felt strongly that these issues should be addressed in the guidelines.

The decision to delay or withhold mouth-to-mouth resuscitation from a patient with possible or documented AIDS in the hospital setting involves moral and ethical considerations. One must balance the universal right of all patients to be resuscitated, if they so desire, against the right of health-care workers to protect themselves from contracting a serious infectious illness, however remote that risk may be.

The task force members also expressed concern that exposure to bloody saliva may take place during the two-person manikin training for CPR recertification. Thus, although the possibility that an AIDS agent may be transmitted by this route was thought to be extremely low, this concern was considered valid.

Direct Patient-Care Responsibilities for Employees with AIDS

Because the task force was unable to reach a consensus on this issue, two alternatives were offered. The first was that a hospital could decide to make an effort to reassign asymptomatic employees with AIDS to positions not involving patient care in order to protect the employee from nosocomial pathogens and to protect high-risk patients from opportunistic pathogens possibly carried by the employee. The second alternative was that a hospital could consider each asymptomatic employee with AIDS on a case-by-case basis. The employee health service, in conjunction with the employee's personal physician, would have to determine that the employee was both free from transmissible infection and not at risk for contracting an infectious disease in the course of performing his or her patient-care duties. Patient-care responsibilities could then be assigned according to the results of a continuing clinical evaluation of the employee's health status.

Comment: This issue led to the sharpest differences of opinion between the committees and among members of the task force. The ad hoc advisory committee concluded that there were no epidemiologic grounds for recommending the removal from direct patient contact of employees with AIDS who were asymptomatic, except perhaps when the patient was immunosuppressed and would be at risk of acquiring an opportunistic infection. The task force was more cautious and concluded that an individual hospital could elect to advise employees with AIDS to accept non-patient-care positions.

The final report of the task force deals with this issue in a noncommittal way by offering both alternatives.

Disinfection of Instruments

Lensed instruments should be sterilized with ethylene oxide or glutaraldehyde after each use.[25] Respiratory-therapy tubing must be thoroughly washed and at least pasteurized after each use in a patient. Any instrument that comes into contact with blood, secretions, excretions, or tissue must be sterilized before reuse; this includes such anesthesia equipment as laryngoscopes and endotracheal tubes.

Outpatients

These guidelines should also apply to the outpatient and emergency settings. Separate examining rooms are not necessary and are in many situations not practical or feasible. Efforts should be made, however, to minimize direct contact between patients with AIDS and other severely immunocompromised patients. Specimen labeling, equipment sterilization, and disposition of equipment should be performed as for hospitalized patients. Outpatients with AIDS may use common waiting areas and bathroom facilities.

References

1. California State Department of Health, Infectious Disease Section. Kaposi's sarcoma and *Pneumocystis carinii* pneumonia — update. Calif Morbid 1981; December 4(47).
2. Prevention of acquired immune deficiency syndrome (AIDS): report of inter-agency recommendations. MMWR 1983; 32:101-3.
3. Oleske J, Minnefor A, Cooper R Jr, et al. Immune deficiency syndrome in children. JAMA 1983; 249:2345-9.
4. Rubinstein A, Sicklick M, Gupta A, et al. Acquired immunodeficiency with reversed T_4/T_8 ratios in infants born to promiscuous and drug-addicted mothers. JAMA 1983; 249:2350-6.
5. Masur H, Michelis MA, Wormser GP, et al. Opportunistic infection in previously healthy women: initial manifestations of a community-acquired cellular immunodeficiency. Ann Intern Med 1982; 97:533-9.
6. Immunodeficiency among female sexual partners of males with acquired immune deficiency syndrome (AIDS) — New York. MMWR 1983; 31:697-8.
7. Harris C, Small CB, Klein RS, et al. Immunodeficiency in female sexual partners of men with the acquired immunodeficiency syndrome. N Engl J Med 1983; 308:1181-4.
8. Gottlieb MS, Schroff R, Schanker HM, et al. *Pneumocystis carinii* pneumonia and mucosal candidiasis in previously healthy homosexual men: evidence of a new acquired cellular immunodeficiency. N Engl J Med 1981; 305:1425-31.
9. Kaposi's sarcoma and *pneumocystis* pneumonia among homosexual men — New York and California. MMWR 1981; 30:305-8.

10. Sonnabend J, Witkin SS, Purtilo DT. Acquired immunodeficiency syndrome, opportunistic infections, and malignancies in male homosexuals: a hypothesis of etiologic factors in pathogenesis. JAMA 1983; 249: 2370-4.
11. Siegal FP, Lopez C, Hammer GS, et al. Severe acquired immunodeficiency in male homosexuals, manifested by chronic perianal ulcerative herpes simplex lesions. N Engl J Med 1981; 305:1439-44.
12. Human T-cell leukemia virus infection in patients with acquired immune deficiency syndrome: preliminary observations. MMWR 1983; 32:233-4.
13. Marx JL. Human T-cell leukemia virus linked to AIDS. Science 1983; 220:806-9.
14. Barré-Sinoussi F, Chermann JC, Rey F, et al. Isolation of a T-lymphotropic retrovirus from a patient at risk for acquired immune deficiency syndrome (AIDS). Science 1983; 220:868-71.
15. Essex M, McLane MF, Lee TH, et al. Antibodies to cell membrane antigens associated with human T-cell leukemia virus in patients with AIDS. Science 1983; 220:859-62.
16. Gelmann EP, Popovic M, et al. Proviral DNA of a retrovirus, human T-cell leukemia virus, in two patients with AIDS. Science 1983; 220: 862-5.
17. Gallo RC, Sarin PS, Gelmann EP, et al. Isolation of human T-cell leukemia virus in acquired immune deficiency syndrome (AIDS). Science 1983; 220:865-7.
18. Acquired immune deficiency syndrome (AIDS): precautions for clinical and laboratory staffs. MMWR 1982; 31:577-9.
19. Chin J. The reporting of AIDS cases in California. California Department of Health Services, March 23, 1983.
20. Hughes WT. Natural mode of acquisition for de novo infection with *Pneumocystis carinii*. J Infect Dis 1982; 145:842-8.
21. Conte JE Jr, Barriere S. Manual of antibiotics and infectious diseases. 5th ed. Philadelphia: Lea & Febiger. (in press).
22. Carney WP, Rubin RH, Hoffman RA, Hansen WP, Healey K, Hirsch MS. Analysis of T lymphocyte subsets in cytomegalovirus mononucleosis. J Immunol 1981; 126:2114-6.
23. Rubin RH, Carney WP, Schooley RT, et al. The effect of infection on T lymphocyte subpopulations: a preliminary report. Int J Immunopharmacol 1981; 3:307-12.
24. Thomas HC. T cell subsets in patients with acute and chronic HBV infection, primary biliary cirrhosis and alcohol induced liver disease. Int J Immunopharmacol 1981; 3:301-5.
25. Simmons BP. Guidelines for hospital environmental control. Atlanta: Centers for Disease Control, February 1981.

SPECIAL REPORT

OCCUPATIONAL RISK OF THE ACQUIRED IMMUNODEFICIENCY SYNDROME AMONG HEALTH CARE WORKERS

EUGENE MCCRAY, M.D. AND THE COOPERATIVE NEEDLESTICK SURVEILLANCE GROUP

Abstract In August 1983, we initiated nationwide prospective surveillance of health care workers with documented parenteral or mucous-membrane exposures to blood or other body fluids of patients with the acquired immunodeficiency syndrome (AIDS) or AIDS-related illnesses. The purpose of the surveillance project is to quantitate prospectively the risk to health care workers of acquiring the AIDS virus, human T-cell lymphotropic virus Type III/lymphadenopathy-associated virus (HTLV-III/LAV), as a result of occupational exposures. By December 31, 1985, 938 health care workers were being followed in the surveillance project. The mean length of follow-up was 15 months (range, 0 to 56) and 531 health care workers (57 percent) had been followed for more than one year. Needlestick injuries and cuts with sharp instruments accounted for 76 percent of the exposures. Over 85 percent of all exposures were to blood or serum.

None of the health care workers have acquired signs or symptoms of AIDS. Analyses of T-lymphocyte subsets were performed for 341 (36 percent) of the exposed health care workers, and tests for antibody to HTLV-III/LAV were performed for 451 (48 percent). Seven health care workers who had low helper/suppressor T-lymphocyte ratios on initial testing were retested; only three had persistently low ratios. Only two health care workers tested were seropositive for antibody to HTLV-III/LAV.

The results of this surveillance project, thus far, suggest that the risk to health care workers of occupational transmission of HTLV-III/LAV is low (the upper bound of the 95 percent confidence interval for the seroprevalence rate among workers with ≥3 months of follow-up with HTLV-III/LAV antibody testing is 1.65 percent) and appears to be related to parenteral exposure to blood.

THE acquired immunodeficiency syndrome (AIDS) is caused by a human retrovirus known as human T-cell lymphotropic virus Type III (HTLV-III), also called lymphadenopathy-associated virus (LAV) and AIDS-associated retrovirus.[1-7] Serologic tests can detect antibody to HTLV-III/LAV, thereby providing an indicator of past or present infection with the virus.[8-16] Serologic evidence of exposure to HTLV-III/LAV is seen in 70 to 100 percent of patients with AIDS[8,17-20] and in up to 70 percent of asymptomatic persons in certain populations with an increased risk of AIDS.[8-14,17-26] However, preliminary data suggest that the prevalence of antibody to HTLV-III/LAV is less than 1 percent among persons who are not in identified risk groups for the disease (e.g., blood donors).[9,14,19,21,22]

Early in the AIDS epidemic, it became apparent that some persons with an increased risk of acquiring hepatitis B infection (i.e., homosexual men, intravenous drug users, and transfusion recipients) also had an increased risk of acquiring AIDS or HTLV-III/LAV infection. Because health care workers have an increased risk of hepatitis B infection, we were concerned that those taking care of patients with AIDS might face an increased risk of acquiring AIDS or AIDS-related illnesses. To evaluate this possibility, in August 1983 we initiated nationwide prospective surveillance of health care workers with parenteral or mucous-membrane exposure to blood or other body fluids from patients with AIDS or illnesses considered to be part of the AIDS spectrum (e.g., chronic generalized lymphadenopathy and wasting syndrome). This report presents the results of surveillance of health care workers enrolled from August 15, 1983, to December 31, 1985.

The Cooperative Needlestick Surveillance Group consists of cooperating investigators from 283 participating centers in the United States and 10 cooperating investigators at the Centers for Disease Control. Names of participating centers and cooperating investigators can be obtained upon request from Dr. McCray at the Epidemiology Branch, Hospital Infections Program 1-5044, Center for Infectious Diseases, 1600 Clifton Rd., Centers for Disease Control, Atlanta, GA 30333.

METHODS

Project Design

Health care workers were eligible for enrollment in the surveillance project if they had been exposed to blood or other body fluids of a patient with AIDS or an AIDS-related illness as a result of a needlestick, a cut with a sharp object, contamination of an open wound, or contamination of a mucous membrane (e.g., a splash in the eye of blood or other fluid). In this surveillance project, the case definition for AIDS was the Centers for Disease Control (CDC) surveillance definition.[23] Illnesses considered part of the AIDS spectrum are unexplained chronic generalized lymphadenopathy[24,25] and other combinations of signs and symptoms that are included in the term "AIDS-related complex."[26]

The following evaluations were performed for each health-care worker upon enrollment and at each follow-up visit (every six months): a history was taken and a physical examination was performed by a physician or nurse practitioner; laboratory studies, including a white-cell count with a differential cell count and a platelet count, were performed at the cooperating institution; and serum and whole-blood specimens were obtained and sent to the CDC within 24 hours of collection. The serum specimens were banked for future testing; phenotypic T-cell subset analyses were performed on the specimens of whole blood.

Upon enrollment, each health care worker completed a confidential questionnaire about nonoccupational risk factors for AIDS (e.g., a history of possible sexual exposure and intravenous drug use). All data were submitted on coded forms, and codes could be broken only by the cooperating investigator at each institution. Thus, no identifying information on enrolled health care workers was available to the CDC. In addition, a case-report form was completed on the patient to whom the health care worker was exposed, if the case had not previously been reported to the CDC.

The surveillance project was initially designed to enroll, over a three-year period, 500 health care workers with documented parenteral or mucous-membrane exposure to clinically diagnosed patients with AIDS or illnesses within the AIDS spectrum. Since more than 900 health care workers were enrolled during the first 28 months of the project, we decided to limit new enrollments to health care workers who had parenteral exposures to blood from patients with asymptomatic or symptomatic infection with HTLV-III/LAV and from whom an "acute" (≤30 days from the exposure) serum sample was available.

Immunologic Testing

Immunologic testing for lymphocyte subpopulations was performed at the CDC by indirect immunofluorescence on a fluorescence-activated cell sorter (Becton Dickinson, Sunnyvale, Calif.) with use of commercially available monoclonal antibodies (OKT3 for T cells, OKT4a for T helper cells, and OKT8 for T suppressor cells) (Ortho Pharmaceuticals, Raritan, N.J.) and a fluorescein-conjugated antimouse immunoglobulin (prepared at the CDC by methods described previously[27,28]).

Testing for HTLV-III/LAV Antibody

Testing of banked serum samples for HTLV-III/LAV antibody was begun shortly after the procedure became available at the CDC, one year after the surveillance project was initiated. Before the HTLV-III/LAV antibody test was performed, written informed consent was obtained from the health care worker. Consent forms were maintained at participating institutions.

Antibody to HTLV-III/LAV was measured with the Abbott HTLV-III enzyme immunoassay (Abbott Laboratories, North Chicago).[29] A serum specimen was retested if, according to the criteria for interpretation of this assay, it was reactive on initial testing. If the serum sample was reactive on repeat testing, the sample was interpreted as positive for antibody to HTLV-III/LAV. Any health care worker with a positive test for HTLV-III/LAV antibody by the Abbott assay was contacted by the institutional investigator for collection of additional serum and whole-blood samples for follow-up testing. All positive tests for HTLV-III/LAV antibody by the Abbott assay were confirmed by the enzyme-linked immunoelectro-transfer blot (Western blot) technique.[15]

A test for antibody to HTLV-III/LAV by the Abbott assay was considered a "true positive" if the assay was performed on initial and follow-up serum samples and both tests were positive, and the Western blot assay was positive on initial and follow-up serum samples. A positive test for antibody to HTLV-III/LAV that did not meet these criteria was considered "false positive." "False positive" tests were interpreted as negative in the case definition of HTLV-III/LAV infection (see below).

Virus isolation from fresh lymphocytes (≤24 hours after collection of the whole-blood sample) was attempted for all subjects with a true or false positive test for antibody to HTLV-III/LAV by the Abbott assay.[7]

Case Definition of HTLV-III/LAV Infection

The following criteria were used to define the serologic status of exposed health care workers: seronegativity (i.e., all serum specimens obtained on or after the date of exposure were negative for antibody to HTLV-III/LAV by the Abbott assay); seropositivity (i.e., an initial serum specimen obtained on or after the date of exposure was positive for antibody to HTLV-III/LAV by the Abbott assay, and positivity was confirmed by the Western blot assay [a seropositive health care worker was considered to have had HTLV-III/LAV infection]); and seroconversion (i.e., an initial serum specimen obtained on or after the date of exposure was negative for antibody to HTLV-III/LAV by the Abbott and Western blot assays, but follow-up serum specimens were positive for antibody to HTLV-III/LAV by both assays).

Statistical Analysis

Confidence limits for the true rate of seropositivity were calculated for the number of health care workers tested for HTLV-III/LAV antibody and the number found to have a positive test.[30]

Results

Enrollees

As of December 31, 1985, 966 health care workers had been enrolled in the surveillance project; 938 are being followed. Twenty-eight health care workers who left the institutions at which they had been enrolled were lost to follow-up and were not included in subsequent analyses. Exposure of health care workers was reported from hospitals, clinics, and state and local health departments in 40 states, the District of Columbia, and Puerto Rico. Eight states reported on approximately two thirds of the exposed health care workers: New York, 159 (17 percent); California, 111 (12 percent); New Jersey, 74 (8 percent); Pennsylvania, 67 (7 percent); Florida, 59 (6 percent); Ohio, 55 (6 percent); Massachusetts, 52 (6 percent); and Texas, 41 (4 percent). Enrolled subjects ranged in age from 18 to 76 years (mean ±SD, 33.5±9.0); 85 percent were white and 78 percent were female. The enrolled subjects included 572 nurses (61 percent), 155 physicians or medical students (17 percent), 97 laboratory workers (10 percent), 52 phlebotomists (6 percent), and 41 respiratory therapists (4 percent). The remaining 21 health care workers (2 percent) had less direct contact with patients or laboratory specimens. As of December 31, 1985, the mean length of follow-up for enrolled subjects was 15 months (median, 13; range 0 to 56); 805 (86 percent) had been followed for more than six months and 531 (57 percent) for more than one year.

Circumstances of the Exposures

Most exposures occurred in direct patient care areas: 528 (56 percent) occurred in a patient's room or on the wards, 207 (22 percent) in intensive care units, and 33 (4 percent) in emergency clinics. One hundred two (11 percent) occurred in operating or procedure rooms or morgues, and 68 (7 percent) took place in laboratories. Eighty-six percent of the subjects were exposed to blood or serum, 8 percent to saliva, 2 percent to urine, and 4 percent to other body fluids or unknown sources (Table 1). If recommended precau-

Table 1. Route of Exposure and Type of Potentially Infective Body Fluid to Which Enrolled Health Care Workers Were Exposed.

Route of Exposure	Body Fluid				
	Blood	Saliva	Urine	Other/Unknown	Total
	no. of health care workers (%)				
Needlestick	612	2	1	22	637 (68)
Mucous membrane	57	64	7	4	132 (14)
Contamination of an open wound	70	4	8	11	93 (10)
Cut with a sharp object	72	1	1	2	76 (8)
Total (%)	811 (86)	71 (8)	17 (2)	39 (4)	938 (100) (100)

Table 2. Circumstances of Exposure among 373 Health Care Workers with Preventable Exposures to Body Fluids of Patients with AIDS or AIDS-Related Illnesses.

Circumstance of Exposure	No. of Health Care Workers (%)*
Recapping a used needle	152 (16)
Injury from a needle improperly disposed of or a sharp object	119 (13)
Contamination of an open wound	93 (10)
Using needle-cutting device	9 (1)
Total	373 (40)

*Number (%) of exposed health care workers in the enrolled group (n = 938) with exposures that were probably preventable.

tions had been followed,[31-33] 40 percent of the exposures could probably have been prevented (Table 2).

Patients to Whom Health Care Workers Were Exposed

In several instances, more than one health care worker at a particular institution had a documented exposure to the same patient; the 938 subjects had exposures to the blood or other body fluids of 666 patients with AIDS or AIDS-related illness. Information is available on 598 (90 percent) of these 666 patients. Of these 598 patients, 88 percent (527) met the CDC surveillance definition for AIDS, and 12 percent (71) had AIDS-related illnesses. The group of 527 patients with AIDS consisted of 356 homosexual or bisexual men (68 percent), 92 intravenous drug users (17 percent), 13 patients with hemophilia (2 percent), 14 blood-transfusion recipients (3 percent), 9 heterosexual contacts of persons in risk groups (2 percent), 9 children with at least one parent in a risk group for AIDS (2 percent), and 34 persons with no identified risk factor for AIDS (6 percent) (including 14 persons born in countries in which most cases of the disease have not been associated with known risk factors). Of the 71 patients with AIDS-related illnesses, 59 (83 percent) were in a group known to have an increased risk of contracting AIDS.

Immunologic Testing

For 341 health care workers, analyses of T-lymphocyte subsets in whole blood were performed on specimens received at the CDC by December 15, 1984. On initial testing, 328 subjects (96 percent) had normal T helper/T suppressor cell ratios. These blood specimens were obtained at a mean period after exposure (±SD) of 123±165 days (median, 54; range, 0 to 1084). Of the 12 health care workers whose initial specimens showed abnormally low ratios, 7 submitted follow-up whole-blood specimens for determination of T helper/T suppressor cell ratios. Three of these seven had a persistent ratio below 1.0 (normal range, 1.0 to 3.9). None of the three have had clinical manifestations of HTLV-III/LAV infection. One of the three had an initial ratio of 0.77 and follow-up ratios of 1.36, 0.94, and 0.78, respectively. This subject has not consented to HTLV-III/LAV antibody testing. One of the remaining two was seronegative (the T helper/T suppressor cell ratio was initially 0.40 and a follow-up ratio was 0.45) for antibody to HTLV-III/LAV, and the other was seropositive (see below).

Testing for HTLV-III/LAV Antibody

Of the 938 health care workers, 451 have had 1016 serum samples tested for antibody to HTLV-III/LAV. Of these 451, 85 percent (386) were exposed to blood or serum (79 percent through needlesticks) and 15 percent (65) were exposed to other body fluids (23 percent through needlesticks) (Table 3). The mean period from exposure to collection of the first serum specimen was 112 days (median, 41; range, 0 to 1027); 41 percent of the subjects (185) had the first specimen collected within 30 days after the exposure. The mean number of days from exposure to collection of the last serum sample for antibody determination was 380 days (median, 364; range, 0 to 1304). Of the 451 health care workers whose serum was tested for antibody, 21 percent (96) have not yet had a follow-up serum sample tested, 78 percent (350) have had tests on at least two serum samples obtained more than 90 days apart, and 61 percent (275) have had tests on at least two serum samples obtained at least 6 months apart. Eighty-four percent (378) have had at least one serologic test performed more than 90 days after the date of exposure, and 79 percent (356) have had at least one serologic test performed more than 180 days after the date of exposure (Table 4).

Two health care workers were seropositive for antibody to HTLV-III/LAV (Table 3). Both had parenteral exposure to blood from a patient with AIDS. The first seropositive health care worker (Subject 1) was positive for the antibody when first tested nine months after exposure. Subject 1 is a female nurse who sustained a puncture wound from a colonic biopsy needle that was used on a patient with AIDS. The needle was visibly contaminated with blood and feces.

Table 3. Results of Testing Health Care Workers for Antibody to HTLV-III/LAV, According to Route of Exposure and Type of Body Fluid.

Route of Exposure	Body Fluid				No. Positive for Antibody
	Blood	Saliva	Other	Total	
Needlestick	305	2	13	320	2*
Contamination of mucous membrane	25	29	10	64	0
Contamination of an open wound	23	4	5	32	0
Cut with a sharp object	33	0	2	35	0
Total	386	35	30	451	2
(%)	(85)	(8)	(7)	(100)	

*Both needlestick exposures were to blood from a patient with AIDS.

Table 4. Number of Health Care Workers Tested for Antibodies to HTLV-III/LAV, According to Number of Days from Exposure to Collection of First Specimen and Number of Days from Exposure to Collection of Last Specimen.

Days from Exposure to First Specimen	Days from Exposure to Last Specimen*			
	1–30	31–90	91–180	>180
	no. of workers			
0–30 (n = 185)	43	3	7	132
31–60 (n = 86)	0	18	4	64
61–90 (n = 45)	0	9	0	36
>90 (n = 135)	0	0	11	124
Total	43	30	22	356

*The mean number of days from exposure to collection of the last serum sample was 380 (range, 1 to 1304; median, 364).

The nurse was treated with hepatitis B immune globulin after exposure. Her initial serum specimen was drawn upon enrollment in the surveillance project (287 days after the exposure); the specimen was positive for HTLV-III/LAV antibody. Follow-up serum samples, obtained 476 and 617 days after the date of exposure, were also positive. The serum sample obtained on day 287 was positive by Western blot assay for antibodies to p24 and p41 antigens. The serum samples obtained on days 476 and 617 were equivocal on Western blot assays for antibodies to the p24 and p41 antigens. The T helper/T suppressor cell ratios in whole blood obtained on days 287, 476, and 617 were 0.67, 0.82, and 0.06, respectively (normal range, 1.0 to 3.9). The results of viral culture for HTLV-III/LAV performed on the nurse's blood were negative. When interviewed by health officials, she denied known risk factors for infection with HTLV-III/LAV. Her sexual partner was seropositive for antibody to HTLV-III/LAV but declined to be interviewed by health officials; therefore, heterosexual transmission could not be excluded as the source of the health care worker's infection.[34]

The second seropositive health care worker (Subject 2) had an "acute" serum specimen (within 30 days of exposure) that was negative for antibody to HTLV-III/LAV and a six-month follow-up specimen that was positive. The results of viral culture for HTLV-III/LAV in blood were negative. The case history of Subject 2 is presented in a Letter to the Editor in this issue of the *Journal*.[35]

Discussion

The epidemiology of AIDS is similar in some respects to that of hepatitis B virus infection. Both hepatitis B and HTLV-III/LAV infection can be transmitted through sexual contact, through blood transfusions, and through contaminated needles shared by intravenous drug users. However, the epidemiology of HTLV-III/LAV infection appears to differ markedly from that of hepatitis B infection in the health care setting. Whereas acquisition of hepatitis B infection is an occupational hazard for health care workers,[36] with an incidence of seroconversion of 19 to 27 percent after accidental percutaneous injection of blood or serum from patients who are positive for hepatitis B e antigen,[37,38] the risk of HTLV-III/LAV infection to health care workers exposed to patients with AIDS appears to be extremely low.

Two of the health care workers enrolled in this surveillance project had antibody to HTLV-III/LAV. One was seropositive on initial testing and on all subsequent testing. However, no serum specimens obtained before her enrollment in the project, more than nine months after the exposure, were available for testing. The investigation of this health care worker for other possible risk factors for HTLV-III/LAV infection is incomplete because her sexual partner has declined to participate in the follow-up. Thus, a clear interpretation of the epidemiology of this subject's infection is not possible.

The second seropositive health care worker was negative for antibody to HTLV-III/LAV when first tested shortly after her exposure but was positive approximately six months after the exposure.[35] An epidemiologic investigation conducted by state and federal public health officials did not identify other risk factors for HTLV-III/LAV infection in this subject or her husband. Therefore, this health care worker has a documented case of occupationally acquired HTLV-III/LAV infection.

There are two reports in the medical literature in which a total of four health care workers were believed to have contracted HTLV-III/LAV infection as a result of occupational exposure. The first report describes a nurse in England who had seroconversion, acquiring antibody to HTLV-III/LAV as measured by enzyme immunoassay, indirect immunofluorescence, and a Western blot assay performed at the CDC, after an accidental needlestick exposure to blood from a patient with AIDS.[39] The nurse apparently had none of the recognized risk factors for AIDS. At the time of publication of that report, three months after the exposure, the nurse had no signs or symptoms of AIDS.

The second report describes three health care workers who were found to have antibody to HTLV-III/LAV, as measured by enzyme and Western blot assays, when first tested more than six months after parenteral exposure to blood.[34] Two of these three subjects have also been described in the *Morbidity and Mortality Weekly Report*.[40] The third subject in that report is the same as Subject 1 in this article. These three health care workers denied belonging to known risk groups for AIDS. However, their HTLV-III/LAV infections cannot be definitely ascribed to occupational transmission because serum specimens from the time of the exposure or within 30 days of it are unavailable, making it impossible to determine when they actually became infected. In addition, no information is available concerning the health status of the donors of the pooled blood products to which one of the three health care workers was exposed.

The absence of signs and symptoms of AIDS and the low prevalence of antibody to HTLV-III/LAV in health care workers in this surveillance project, along with results from other studies,[34,41,42] suggest that the risk to health care workers of occupational transmission of HTLV-III/LAV is low. In this project, the observed seroconversion rate among all health care workers with both an acute serum specimen (≤30 days after exposure) and at least one follow-up specimen (>90 days after exposure) tested is 0.72 percent (1 of 139 [upper bound of the 95 percent confidence interval, 3.34 percent]); among those with parenteral exposure to blood, the seroconversion rate is 0.94 percent (1 of 106 [upper bound of the confidence interval, 4.36 percent]). The seroprevalence rate among all health care workers with at least one serum sample tested more than 90 days after exposure is 0.53 percent (2 of 378 [upper bound, 1.65 percent]); and among the cohort with parenteral exposures to blood, the seroprevalence rate is 0.72 percent (2 of 278 [upper bound, 2.24 percent]).

The low incidence of seroconversion resulting from exposure to patients with AIDS is reassuring. However, fewer than 15 percent of the health care workers in the surveillance project have been exposed to patients who do not meet the CDC surveillance definition of AIDS (i.e., they are not either asymptomatic persons or persons with illnesses within the AIDS spectrum who are positive for antibody to HTLV-III/LAV), and such patients, who may have higher levels of circulating T lymphocytes than patients with AIDS as defined by the CDC, may have higher circulating titers of virus and may therefore be more likely to transmit HTLV-III/LAV infection. Thus, the data from this surveillance project do not permit conclusions about the risk to health care workers of acquiring HTLV-III/LAV infection from patients infected with HTLV-III/LAV who do not meet the CDC surveillance definition of AIDS. Future efforts to define the occupational risk of HTLV-III/LAV infection in health care workers will focus on prospective studies of those with parenteral exposures to potentially infectious material from patients with HTLV-III/LAV infection who do not meet the CDC definition of AIDS.

Recommendations for preventing AIDS in health care workers are designed to minimize the risk of mucosal or parenteral exposure to potentially infectious material from patients with asymptomatic or symptomatic infection with HTLV-III/LAV.[30-32,43-45] In this surveillance project, 40 percent of the exposures could probably have been prevented if the workers had followed recommended precautions. Despite the low incidence of documented transmission of HTLV-III/LAV infection from patients to health care workers, these precautions remain valid because they emphasize infection-control practices that may reduce the risk of acquiring other infections, such as hepatitis B virus. Health care workers should become familiar with and follow the recommended precautions when caring for or handling specimens from persons with AIDS or AIDS-related illnesses.

References

1. Essex M, McLane MF, Lee TH, et al. Antibodies to cell membrane antigens associated with human T-cell leukemia virus in patients with AIDS. Science 1983; 220:859-62.
2. Barré-Sinoussi F, Chermann JC, Rey F, et al. Isolation of a T-lymphotropic retrovirus from a patient at risk for acquired immune deficiency syndrome (AIDS). Science 1983; 220:868-71.
3. Popovic M, Sarngadharan MG, Read E, Gallo RC. Detection, isolation, and continuous production of cytopathic retroviruses (HTLV-III) from patients with AIDS and pre-AIDS. Science 1984; 224:497-500.
4. Gallo RC, Salahuddin SZ, Popovic M, et al. Frequent detection and isolation of cytopathic retroviruses (HTLV-III) from patients with AIDS and at risk for AIDS. Science 1984; 224:500-3.
5. Schüpbach J, Popovic M, Gilden RV, Gonda MA, Sarngadharan MG, Gallo RC. Serological analysis of a subgroup of human T-lymphotropic retroviruses (HTLV-III) associated with AIDS. Science 1984; 224:503-5.
6. Feorino PM, Kalyanaraman VS, Haverkos HW, et al. Lymphadenopathy associated virus infection of a blood donor–recipient pair with acquired immunodeficiency syndrome. Science 1984; 225:69-72.
7. Levy JA, Hoffman AD, Kramer SM, Landis JA, Shimabukuro JM, Oshiro LS. Isolation of lymphocytopathic retroviruses from San Francisco patients with AIDS. Science 1984; 225:840-2.
8. Sarngadharan MG, Popovic M, Bruch L, Schüpbach J, Gallo RC. Antibodies reactive with human T-lymphotropic retroviruses (HTLV-III) in the serum of patients with AIDS. Science 1984; 224:506-8.
9. Brun-Vezinet F, Rouzioux C, Barre-Sinoussi F, et al. Detection of IgG antibodies to lymphadenopathy-associated virus in patients with AIDS or lymphadenopathy syndrome. Lancet 1984; 1:1253-6.
10. Laurence J, Brun-Vezinet F, Schutzer SE, et al. Lymphadenopathy-associated viral antibody in AIDS: immune correlations and definition of a carrier state. N Engl J Med 1984; 311:1269-73.
11. Safai B, Sarngadharan MG, Groopman JE, et al. Seroepidemiological studies of human T-lymphotropic retrovirus type III in acquired immunodeficiency syndrome. Lancet 1984; 1:1438-40.
12. Antibodies to a retrovirus etiologically associated with acquired immunodeficiency syndrome (AIDS) in populations with increased incidences of the syndrome. MMWR 1984; 33:377-9.
13. Saxinger C, Gallo RC. Applications of the indirect enzyme-linked immunosorbent assay microtest to the detection and surveillance of human T cell leukemia-lymphoma virus. Lab Invest 1983; 49:371-7.
14. Kalyanaraman VS, Cabradilla CD, Getchell JP, et al. Antibodies to the core protein of lymphadenopathy-associated virus (LAV) in patients with AIDS. Science 1984; 225:321-3.
15. Tsang VCW, Peralta JM, Simons AR. Enzyme-linked immunoelectrotransfer blot techniques (EITB) for studying the specificities of antigens and antibodies separated by gel electrophoresis. Methods Enzymol 1983; 92:377-91.
16. Barré-Sinoussi F, Mathur-Wagh U, Rey F, et al. Isolation of lymphadenopathy-associated virus (LAV) and detection of LAV antibodies from US patients with AIDS. JAMA 1985; 253:1737-9.
17. Ramsey RB, Palmer EL, McDougal JS, et al. Antibody to lymphadenopathy-associated virus in haemophiliacs with and without AIDS. Lancet 1984; 2:397-8.
18. Goedert JJ, Sarngadharan MG, Biggar RJ, et al. Determinants of retrovirus (HTLV-III) antibody and immunodeficiency conditions in homosexual men. Lancet 1984; 2:711-6.
19. Gazzard BG, Shanson DC, Farthing C, et al. Clinical findings and serological evidence of HTLV-III infection in homosexual contacts of patients with AIDS and persistent generalised lymphadenopathy in London. Lancet 1984; 2:480-3.
20. Tsoukas C, Gervais F, Shuster J, et al. Association of HTLV-III antibodies and cellular immune status of hemophiliacs. N Engl J Med 1984; 311:1514-5.
21. Schüpbach J, Haller O, Vogt M, et al. Antibodies to HTLV-III in Swiss patients with AIDS and pre-AIDS and in groups at risk for AIDS. N Engl J Med 1985; 312:265-70.
22. Cheingsong-Popov R, Weiss RA, Dalgleish A, et al. Prevalence of antibody to human T-lymphotropic virus type III in AIDS and AIDS-risk patients in Britain. Lancet 1984; 2:477-80.
23. Update on acquired immune deficiency syndrome (AIDS) — United States. MMWR 1982; 31:507-14.
24. Persistent, generalized lymphadenopathy among homosexual males. MMWR 1982; 31:249-51.
25. Gottlieb MS, Schroff R, Schanker HM, et al. *Pneumocystis carinii* pneumonia and mucosal candidiasis in previously healthy homosexual men: evidence of a new acquired cellular immunodeficiency. N Engl J Med 1981; 305:1425-31.

26. Krause RM. Koch's postulates and the search for the AIDS agent. Rev Infect Dis 1984; 6:270-9.
27. Nicholson JKA, McDougal JS, Spira TJ, Cross GD, Jones BM, Reinherz EL. Immunoregulatory subsets of the T helper and T suppressor cell populations in homosexual men with chronic unexplained lymphadenopathy. J Clin Invest 1984; 73:191-201.
28. Nicholson JKA, Jones BM, Cross GD, McDougal JS. Comparison of T and B cell analyses on fresh and aged blood. J Immunol Methods 1984; 73:29-40.
29. Enzyme immunoassay for the detection of antibody to human T-lymphotropic virus type III (HTLV-III) in human serum or plasma. North Chicago: Abbott Laboratories, 1985:1-16.
30. Cox DR, Hinkley DV. Theoretical statistics. London: Chapman & Hall, 1974.
31. Acquired immune deficiency syndrome (AIDS): precautions for clinical and laboratory staffs. MMWR 1982; 31:577-80.
32. Acquired immunodeficiency syndrome (AIDS): precautions for health-care workers and allied professionals. MMWR 1983; 32:450-1.
33. Williams WW. CDC guideline for infection control in hospital personnel. Infect Control 1983; 4:326-49.
34. Weiss SH, Saxinger WC, Rechtman D, et al. HTLV-III infection among health care workers: association with needle-stick injuries. JAMA 1985; 254:2089-93.
35. Stricof RL, Morse DL. HTLV-III/LAV seroconversion following a deep intramuscular needlestick injury. N Engl J Med 1986; 314:1115.
36. Hadler SC, Doto IL, Maynard JE, et al. Occupational risk of hepatitis B infection in hospital workers. Infect Control 1985; 6:24-31.
37. Werner BG, Grady GF. Accidental hepatitis-B-surface-antigen-positive inoculations: use of e antigen to estimate infectivity. Ann Intern Med 1982; 97:367-9.
38. Seeff LB, Wright EC, Zimmerman HJ, et al. Type B hepatitis after needle-stick exposure: prevention with hepatitis B immune globulin: final report of the Veterans Administration Cooperative Study. Ann Intern Med 1978; 88:285-93.
39. Needlestick transmission of HTLV-III from a patient infected in Africa. Lancet 1984; 2:1376-7.
40. Update: Evaluation of human T-lymphotropic virus type III/lymphadenopathy-associated virus infection in health-care personnel — United States. MMWR 1985; 34:575-8.
41. Hirsch MS, Wormser GP, Schooley RT, et al. Risk of nosocomial infection with human T-cell lymphotropic virus III (HTLV-III). N Engl J Med 1985; 312:1-4.
42. Weiss SH, Goedert JJ, Sarngadharan MG, et al. Screening test for HTLV-III (AIDS agent) antibodies: specificity, sensitivity, and applications. JAMA 1985; 253:221-5.
43. Conte JE Jr, Hadley WK, Sande M, et al. Infection-control guidelines for patients with the acquired immunodeficiency syndrome (AIDS). N Engl J Med 1983; 309:740-4.
44. A hospitalwide approach to AIDS: recommendations of the advisory committee on infections within hospitals — American Hospital Association. Infect Control 1984; 5:242-8.
45. Recommendations for preventing transmission of infection with human T-lymphotropic virus type III/lymphadenopathy-associated virus in the workplace. MMWR 1985; 34:682-95.

ORIGINAL ARTICLE

LACK OF TRANSMISSION OF HTLV-III/LAV INFECTION TO HOUSEHOLD CONTACTS OF PATIENTS WITH AIDS OR AIDS-RELATED COMPLEX WITH ORAL CANDIDIASIS

Gerald H. Friedland, M.D., Brian R. Saltzman, M.D., Martha F. Rogers, M.D., Patricia A. Kahl, R.N., Martin L. Lesser, Ph.D., Marguerite M. Mayers, M.D., and Robert S. Klein, M.D.

Abstract To determine the risk of transmission of human T-cell lymphotropic virus Type III/lymphadenopathy-associated virus (HTLV-III/LAV) to close but nonsexual contacts of patients with the acquired immunodeficiency syndrome (AIDS), we studied the nonsexual household contacts of patients with AIDS or the AIDS-related complex with oral candidiasis. Detailed interviews, physical examinations, and tests for serum antibody to HTLV-III/LAV were performed on 101 household contacts of 39 AIDS patients (68 children and 33 adults), all of whom had lived in the same household with an index patient for at least three months. These contacts had shared household items and facilities and had close personal interaction with the patient for a median of 22 months (range, 3 to 48) during the period of presumed infectivity.

Only 1 of 101 household contacts — a five-year-old child — had evidence of infection with the virus, which had probably been acquired perinatally rather than through horizontal transmission.

This study indicates that household contacts who are not sexual partners of, or born to, patients with AIDS are at minimal or no risk of infection with HTLV-III/LAV.

SINCE the recognition of the epidemic of the acquired immunodeficiency syndrome (AIDS) in 1981, several populations have been described that are at increased risk of infection with the human T-cell lymphotropic virus Type III/lymphadenopathy-associated virus (HTLV-III/LAV) and disease due to it. These include homosexual men,[1] intravenous drug abusers,[2] and recipients of transfusions of blood and blood products.[3,4] In addition, transmission of HTLV-III/LAV infection to heterosexual partners of patients with AIDS[5] and children born to mothers with AIDS or in high-risk groups has been described.[6]

The major routes of transmission of HTLV-III/LAV infection have been well established. Bloodborne transmission is supported by the presence of AIDS and HTLV-III/LAV infection in transfusion recipients and hemophiliacs, as well as in intravenous drug abusers, among whom sharing of needles is common.[7] HTLV-III/LAV has been isolated from peripheral blood in both symptomatic and asymptomatic cases of infections.[8] Transmission also appears to occur by means of intimate sexual contact, both homosexual and heterosexual,[5,9] and the virus has been isolated from semen.[10] Isolation of HTLV-III/LAV from saliva has been accomplished,[10,11] but there is no direct evidence for transmission by means of this fluid. The risk of transmission by less intimate contact is believed to be low or nonexistent. In support of this view is the indirect evidence that AIDS has remained confined almost exclusively to the risk groups initially described, in which close to 95 percent of all cases occur.[12] Except for sexual partners and children born to infected mothers, none of the family members in more than 12,000 cases reported to the Centers for Disease Control (CDC) are known to have contracted AIDS (CDC: unpublished data). In addition, hospital workers in frequent contact with patients and patients' blood have been found to be seronegative for antibody to HTLV-III/LAV.[13] Finally, most children in whom AIDS has developed have belonged to an age group in which perinatal transmission has been strongly suggested.[12] Nonetheless, the possible risk of transmission of HTLV-III/LAV infection to close contacts of infected persons remains of great concern. To address this issue directly, we identified and studied a large number of close but nonsexual household contacts of patients with AIDS or the AIDS-related complex with oral candidiasis.

From the Division of Infectious Diseases, the Department of Medicine, and the Departments of Pediatrics, Biostatistics, and Epidemiology, Montefiore Medical Center, North Central Bronx Hospital, and Albert Einstein College of Medicine, Bronx, N.Y., and the AIDS Branch, Centers for Disease Control, Atlanta, Ga.

Supported under a Cooperative Agreement (U62/CCU200741-01) with the Centers for Disease Control, and by a grant A0-2O8 with the New York State AIDS Institute. Dr. Saltzman was supported by a Training Grant (5-T32-AI-070183-06) from the National Institute of Allergy and Infectious Diseases.

Methods

Definition of Index Patients and Household Contacts

AIDS was defined according to criteria established by the CDC.[14,15] In adults (persons over the age of 18), AIDS-related complex was defined as the presence of (1) unexplained generalized lymphadenopathy (at least one lymph node of more than 1 cm) involving two or more extrainguinal node-bearing areas and persisting for at least three months, or unexplained oral candidiasis, confirmed by microscopy, and (2) two laboratory abnormalities — a low absolute number of helper T cells (<408 cells per cubic millimeter) and a low T-helper/T-suppressor (T4/T8) ratio (<1.0).

A diagnosis of AIDS-related complex was made in children less than 13 years of age if at least one of the following major clinical criteria or at least three minor clinical criteria, plus at least one laboratory criterion, were all present for at least two months. The major clinical criteria were interstitial pneumonitis, parotid-gland enlargement, and oral candidiasis in the absence of antibiotic therapy. The minor criteria were recurrent bacterial infections, generalized lymphadenopathy, hepatomegaly, diarrhea, and failure to thrive. Laboratory criteria included an elevated concentration of one or more serum immunoglobulins, lymphopenia, a low absolute number of T lymphocytes, a low absolute number of T-helper lymphocytes, and a low T-helper/T-suppressor ratio (<1.0).

Household contacts were defined as persons who were not sexual partners but who lived in the same household as the AIDS patient for at least 3 months in the period starting 18 months before the onset of symptoms in the patient and ending at the time of contact screening.

Subject Recruitment and Evaluation

Evaluation of household contacts began in October 1984 and was carried out through April 1985. Household contacts were derived from three populations: (1) available contacts of patients who had been cared for and died at our institution within one year before the initiation of the study, (2) contacts of living patients treated at our institution from October 1984 to April 1985, and (3) contacts of patients referred from other New York City medical institutions between October 1984 and April 1985. Beginning in October 1984, all living patients with AIDS who were treated at our institution were interviewed to determine the constellation of their households and families. With the patients' consent, eligible household members were invited to participate in the study. If the patients had died before the initiation of screening, their known household contacts were invited to participate. If household members had been referred from other institutions, the diagnosis of AIDS in the index case was confirmed by our review of the medical records.

After informed consent was obtained, each household member was screened by means of a detailed, standardized interview, a physical examination, and laboratory testing. The interview included recording of demographic variables and the medical history (including birth history for children), an assessment of possible risk factors for AIDS, a complete history of sexual activity and drug use, and a detailed assessment of the duration and type of household exposure to the patient with AIDS. Subjects 13 years of age and older were interviewed directly. The parents or guardians of subjects under 13 years were interviewed instead of the subjects themselves. Complete physical examinations were performed, with particular attention to the presence of lymphadenopathy, oral candidiasis, weight loss, and failure to thrive.

Laboratory Evaluation

Laboratory evaluation included complete blood count and measurement of immunoglobulins, T-cell subsets, and antibodies to HTLV-III/LAV by enzyme immunoassay. Complete blood counts were performed according to standard methods. Lymphopenia was defined as the presence of fewer than 1200 lymphocytes per cubic millimeter. IgG was measured by radial immunodiffusion (normal range, 564 to 1765 mg per deciliter for adults and 269 to 1641 for children). Serum and heparinized venous blood obtained from study participants were shipped overnight to the CDC, where studies of T-cell subsets, serologic testing for HTLV-III/LAV, and viral isolation were performed. T-cell subsets were measured in whole blood (children under two years) or in lymphocytes separated from whole blood by Ficoll–Hypaque gradient as previously described.[16] Absolute T-cell counts were calculated from percentages of T-cell subsets and lymphocyte counts (the normal range for absolute T4-cell counts was 408 to 1583 per cubic millimeter; the normal T4/T8 ratio was 1.0 to 4.0). Antibodies to HTLV-III/LAV were determined by an enzyme immunoassay (Abbott Laboratories, North Chicago). All serum samples were tested twice. A single positive result in any sample was confirmed with the Western blot assay.[17] Cultures for HTLV-III/LAV were performed as previously described.[18]

Statistical Analysis

Summary statistics for continuous-type variables (i.e., time intervals) are expressed in terms of medians, ranges, and quartiles. The term "interquartile range" refers to the range in which the middle 50 percent of the sample lies. We determined exact confidence intervals for the binomial proportions.

Results

From October 1984 to April 1985, 41 living patients with AIDS or the AIDS-related complex with oral candidiasis were available for interview and agreed to participate in the study. We identified 140 household contacts through this group, and 63 additional contacts of 12 patients who had died of AIDS from September 1983 through September 1984 at our institution. Thirty household contacts of seven patients were referred from other institutions. Of the 233 household contacts of 60 patients, 36 were sexual partners of index cases. Since sexual transmission of HTLV-III/LAV has been well documented, these subjects were evaluated separately and were not included in the present study. Eighty-nine (45 percent) of the remaining household contacts declined to participate in the study: 55 percent were "too busy" with work or school or "not interested" in the issue, or felt that screening was "unnecessary"; an additional 15 percent were "opposed to research," 16 percent could not be located, and 15 percent could not be screened because the index patient did not consent to participation of his or her family.

Thus, a total of 108 nonsexual household contacts of 41 patients were evaluated. Seven were excluded from analysis — three because of the presence of risk factors for AIDS (one intravenous drug abuser and two homosexual men), one because blood was not obtained, one because household contact lasted less than three months, and two because review of hospital records of the index case failed to confirm the diagnosis of AIDS. The remaining 101 household contacts of 39 patients constituted the study population. Of the 39 index patients, 37 had AIDS and two had AIDS-related complex with oral candidiasis. There were 27 males and 12 females. Twenty-eight patients were heterosexual intravenous drug abusers (72 percent), one patient was a homosexual intravenous drug abuser (3 percent), three patients were homosexual or bisexual (8 percent), three were sexual partners of persons known to belong to risk groups (8 percent), and four had no documented risk factor for AIDS (10 percent). None of the household contacts had sexual contact with a patient with AIDS or had any other risk factors for AIDS.

Of the 101 household contacts, 72 (71 percent) were Hispanic, 18 (18 percent) were black, 7 (7 percent) were white, and 4 (4 percent) were in other ethnic groups. Of 77 contacts reporting household income, 50 (65 percent) had an income below \$10,000, 19 (25 percent) had incomes of \$10,000 to \$20,000, and 8 (10 percent) had incomes above \$20,000; 80 percent of the study subjects belonged to households in which three or more people were supported by such incomes. The 33 adult contacts had completed a mean of 9.5 years of education (median, 10; range, 0 to 16). Forty-five of the contacts were male and 56 were female. Their mean age was 19.4 years (median, 13; range, 0.8 to 78). The 101 contacts included 68 children under the age of 18 (50 were the biologic children of AIDS patients, and 18 were not), 3 offspring over the age of 18, 10 siblings, 11 parents (2 fathers and 9 mothers), and 9 other relatives. Thirty-three of the contacts were older than 18 years, 47 were 6 to 18 years old, and 21 were less than 6 years of age at the time of screening.

Table 1. Months of Household Contact with Patients with AIDS among 101 Household Members.*

	Median	Range	Interquartile Range†
From January 1978	37	3–87	16–68
From 18 months before symptoms in patient	22	3–48	9–27
From onset of symptoms in patient	7	0–35	5–13
From diagnosis of AIDS in patient	1	0–21	0–6

*All intervals were calculated to time of evaluation of household member.

†Range in which the middle 50 percent of the sample lies.

Fifteen of these 21 were biologic children of index cases. Six of the 15 children were born to four mothers who contracted AIDS, and 3 others were born to mothers who had serum antibody to HTLV-III/LAV at the time of screening.

The 55 percent of household contacts who participated in the study were of geographic, ethnic, and socioeconomic backgrounds similar to those of the total household-contact population, but differed somewhat in age distribution. The screened population had an identical proportion of children 6 to 18 years old (47 percent) but a lower proportion of adults (33 vs. 41 percent) and a higher proportion of children under 6 years old (21 vs. 12 percent).

Duration of Household Contact

Two variables — the duration of household contact with the index patient, and the amount of time elapsed between initial exposure to the patient and the time of screening — were calculated for several periods.

Of the 101 household contacts, 94 lived with the index patient for at least three months while the patient was symptomatic or after AIDS or AIDS-related complex was diagnosed. Seven lived with the index patient for 3 months or longer during the period 18 months before the onset of symptoms but less than 3 months afterward. Only one contact lived with an index patient only during the 18-month period before the onset of symptoms. The total duration of the household exposure of the contacts to the patients was substantial (Table 1).

Among the 101 household contacts, a median of 31 months elapsed from the time of initial exposure to the patients during the period beginning 18 months before the onset of patients' symptoms to the time of screening (range, 3 to 54 months; interquartile range, 23 to 35).

Seventy-eight household members had their initial contact with a patient during the 18 months before the onset of symptoms. For this group, the median number of months elapsed from initial exposure to screening was 32 (range, 17 to 54; interquartile range, 26 to 38). Eighty-eight household members had initial or continuing contact with the patients after the onset of symptoms but before the diagnosis of AIDS or AIDS-related complex. For this group, the median number of months elapsed to the time of screening was 13 (range, 1 to 36; interquartile range, 8 to 19). Sixty-eight household members had initial or continuing contact with a patient after the diagnosis was established. For this group, the median number of months elapsed to the time of screening was 9 (range, 1 to 32; interquartile range, 3 to 19).

Types of Household Exposure

Among household members, there was substantial sharing of items and facilities with the patients, as well as considerable personal interaction (Table 2). After the diagnosis of AIDS was established, most types of household personal interactions with the index case were reduced substantially. However, a high percentage of household members assisted the patient with bathing, dressing, and eating. These activities were usually increased by parents, siblings, and older children of the patients.

Clinical and Laboratory Findings

No household contact had AIDS; one met the criteria for AIDS-related complex in children. Of the 101 household contacts, 99 (98 percent) were seronegative for HTLV-III/LAV antibodies by enzyme immunoassay and 100 (99 percent) were negative for antibody when Western blot assay was performed for confirmation (Table 3). Both household contacts with HTLV-III/LAV antibodies on immunoassay were children. One child, a two-year-old girl, was positive on enzyme immunoassay but negative on Western blot testing. She had no symptoms suggestive of HTLV-III/LAV

Table 2. Type of Contact with Patients with AIDS among 101 Household Members.

Activity	Percentage of Members in Activity
Sharing of household items	
Razors	9
Toothbrushes	7
Nail clippers	42
Combs	51
Towels	37
Clothes	15
Eating utensils	25
Eating plates	46
Drinking glasses	48
Sharing of household facilities	
Bed	37
Toilet	90
Bath or shower	92
Kitchen	93
Washing items used by patients	
Dishes	65
Toilet	49
Bath	55
Clothes	38
Interacting with patient	
Helping to bathe	10
Helping to dress	16
Helping to eat	13
Shaking hands	21
Hugging	79
Kissing on cheek	83
Kissing on lips	17

Table 3. Antibodies to HTLV-III/LAV among Household Contacts of Patients with AIDS.

Contact Group (in Relation to Patient)	No. Screened	No. Positive (Percent)	
		Enzyme Immunoassay	Western Blot
Children <6 yr	**21**	**2 (10)**	**1*(5)**
Biologic offspring	15	2 (13)	1*(7)
Other	6	0	—
Children 6–18 yr	**47**	0	—
Adults	**33**	0	—
Parents	11		
Siblings	10		
Other	12		
Total	*101*	*2 (2)*	*1*(1)*

*Infection was probably acquired through perinatal transmission (see text).

infection. Her physical examination was normal, and she was in the 5th percentile for height and 37th percentile for weight. Her hematocrit, white-cell count, IgG concentration, T4/T8 ratio, and absolute T4-cell count were all within normal limits. A repeat specimen obtained eight months later was negative on enzyme immunoassay. Lymphocytes cultured at this second screening did not grow HTLV-III/LAV. Immunoassay testing of the child's mother was positive at 31 months after the child's birth but negative at 27 and at 35 months. Western blot testing of the mother's immunoassay-positive specimen was negative, and lymphocytes obtained from her at the same time as well as on a subsequent screening failed to grow virus. The child's father was given a diagnosis of AIDS in September 1984. There was no history of sexual abuse of the girl by her father.

The second child was the five-year-old daughter of two intravenous drug abusers. Her mother was given a diagnosis of AIDS in September 1984. The child was positive on enzyme immunoassay, which was confirmed by Western blot assay. Culture of her peripheral-blood lymphocytes for HTLV-III/LAV, however, was negative. She has been hospitalized three times since birth for bacterial pneumonia and was noted to have oral candidiasis at one year of age. At the time of screening (at the age of five years) the child had generalized lymphadenopathy without oral candidiasis and was in the 62nd percentile for height and 37th percentile for weight. Although the total white-cell and lymphocyte counts were normal, the percentage of T4 cells was low (33 percent) and the percentage of T8 cells high (56 percent), with a consequent T4/T8 ratio of 0.59. IgG was elevated, at 2800 mg per deciliter. On rescreening three months later, the child's T-cell ratio remained low (0.35), and her IgG was elevated (3000 mg per deciliter).

Immunologic testing of the household contacts gave the following results. Of 86 subjects in whom lymphocyte counts were performed, 79 had normal counts and 7 had lymphopenia. Of 94 in whom IgG was measured, 84 (90 percent) had normal levels, 9 had elevated levels (1560 to 2800 mg per deciliter), and 1 had a low level (90 mg per deciliter). Of 100 subjects in whom T-cell subsets were determined, 92 had a normal percentage of T4 cells and 6 had a low percentage; 4 of the 100 had low T4/T8 ratios — 3 because of an increase in the percentage of T8 cells alone and 1 because of both a decrease in T4 cells and an increase in T8 cells. Of 86 subjects in whom absolute T-cell counts were calculated, 83 (96 percent) had normal counts and 3 (4 percent) had low counts (168, 232, and 287 per cubic millimeter, respectively). These three patients had lymphopenia, which accounted for their low T4-cell counts, but had normal T4/T8 ratios and IgG levels. Only one subject, the five-year-old seropositive child, had more than a single immunologic abnormality.

Five additional children in the household-contact population were born after January 1, 1978, to three mothers in whom AIDS subsequently developed. None of the mothers had symptoms of AIDS at the time of delivery. The mean interval between delivery and the onset of symptoms in the mothers was 37 months (range, 16 to 55). The five children were negative for HTLV-III/LAV antibody and healthy, without any major physical or immunologic abnormalities. In addition, three healthy seronegative children under six years of age were born to two mothers who had antibody to HTLV-III/LAV on enzyme and Western blot assays but who did not have AIDS or AIDS-related complex. Two of the children were born 51 and 52 months before screening of the mother. One child was born seven months after her mother was documented as seropositive.

Discussion

In this study, despite prolonged and close contact with patients with AIDS or AIDS-related complex, 100 of 101 household contacts did not contract HTLV-III/LAV infection. The only contact who became infected was a five-year-old child whose mother had AIDS. This infection appeared to have been acquired by perinatal transmission, since the child had had signs and symptoms of HTLV-III/LAV infection since infancy. We interpreted the results of enzyme immunoassay of serum from a two-year-old child as being falsely positive, since the Western blot assay and a repeat enzyme immunoassay were negative. In addition, the child was clinically well and had no immunologic abnormalities. We conclude that nonsexual household contacts of patients with AIDS or AIDS-related complex with oral candidiasis are at minimal or no risk for horizontal transmission of HTLV-III/LAV infection (95 percent confidence interval, 0 to 2 percent).

We were able to screen the majority of household contacts of index patients. They were representative of the total household-contact population except for the larger proportion of children under the age of six — the group that might be expected to be at highest risk for horizontal transmission of HTLV-III/LAV within the household setting. We have no evidence that persons who may have been ill or infected declined to participate in the study. Persons who belonged to risk groups and who did not choose to participate would have been removed from analysis by the study protocol. Thus, we believe that there was no discernible selection bias in the study population that might weaken our conclusions.

The precise period of infectivity of patients with AIDS is not known, but studies of transfusion recipients who contracted AIDS[4,19] clearly indicate that persons with HTLV-III/LAV may be infectious for months to years before the onset of symptoms. For this reason, we arbitrarily chose for study several periods of household exposure before the onset of symptoms of AIDS: from 1978, because this year represents the approximate beginning of the AIDS epidemic, and from 18 months before the onset of symptoms in the index case. The current state of knowledge suggests that a patient with AIDS is likely to be infectious during most or all of the latter period. Support for this view is derived from studies of transfusion-related AIDS in which continued carriage of virus in the blood of implicated donors, even those without symptoms, has been demonstrated over long periods, ranging from 12 to 52 months (mean, 28).[19] In the present study, household members had substantial household exposure to patients with AIDS during the period in which the patients were likely to be carrying virus and to be contagious. Periods of household exposure after the diagnosis of AIDS were briefer for several reasons, including early death or prolonged hospitalization of the index case, early screening of household contacts after the diagnosis of AIDS was documented, and fluidity and changes in household structure after diagnosis. Most of the families in this study were poor and lived in crowded conditions, which would be expected to facilitate horizontal transmission of infection. In addition, substantial sharing of household facilities and items likely to be soiled with body secretions took place during the period of presumed infectivity, as did the close personal interaction and affectionate behavior expected among family members.

Little information exists about the time of seroconversion after exposure to the virus. Limited information suggests that seroconversion occurs within one to four months. In one instance, in which a nurse was stuck with a needle from a patient with AIDS, seroconversion was documented 49 days after exposure.[20] In a longitudinal study of seronegative homosexual men, seroconversion was documented 19 to 56 days after the onset of an acute illness with lymphadenopathy.[21] In recently developed animal models, a similar time course from exposure to seroconversion was noted.[22,23] In the present study, a substantial amount of time elapsed between initial exposure to the patient in the household setting and the time of screening. On the basis of the limited data available, it appears that sufficient time had elapsed for seroconversion to have occurred in most subjects if there was a substantial risk. Follow-up of the household contacts will be necessary to confirm continuing seronegativity, but it is reasonable to assume that seroconversion will be unlikely in those with no further contact with the index cases.

False negative and false positive results on tests for antibody to HTLV-III/LAV are unlikely. Each enzyme immunoassay was repeated, and positive results were tested by Western blot assay and virus culture. Small numbers of household members had immunologic abnormalities that were minor and nonspecific and not associated with HTLV-III/LAV seropositivity. No patient had more than one independent abnormality, except the one HTLV-III/LAV–positive child. It is most likely that this child acquired the infection congenitally or during the perinatal period. However, it is interesting and important to note that she was the only infected child among six children born since 1978 to four women with AIDS and three children born to two HTLV-III/LAV–positive, asymptomatic mothers. The risk of infection with HTLV-III/LAV among children born to infected mothers is not known. These very preliminary findings suggest that it is not substantial; however, large-scale prospective studies are needed to address this issue properly.

Hepatitis B and HTLV-III/LAV infection are quite similar epidemiologically. The populations at greatest risk and the presumed routes of transmission are almost identical. Homosexual men, intravenous drug abusers, transfusion recipients, sexual partners of infected persons, and infants born of infected mothers all have increased rates of infection with both agents. Several studies have found apparent horizontal transmission of hepatitis B infection in households.[24,25] Therefore, despite the fact that HTLV-III/LAV, like hepatitis B, is present in saliva and blood, it is reassuring that horizontal transmission of HTLV-III/LAV appears to be minimal to nonexistent in the household setting.

This study has expanded and confirmed the findings of previous studies of small numbers of household contacts.[26] The absence of horizontal transmission of HTLV-III/LAV infection as determined in this study should serve to alleviate the fears and concerns of the growing number of household members and other close contacts of patients with AIDS, as well as the population at large. Established guidelines for controlling the spread of AIDS both within the hospital and outside it appear to be reasonable and safe. Families of patients appear to be at little or no risk of HTLV-III/LAV infection. This study supports the view that transmission of the infection requires injection of blood or blood products or intimate sexual contact, and that longstanding household exposure to patients with AIDS is associated with little or no risk of transmission of HTLV-III/LAV infection.

We are indebted to Harold Jaffe, M.D., James Curran, M.D., and Neal Steigbigel, M.D., for critically reviewing the manuscript; to Ms. Cheryl Feiner, M.P.H., for performing computer analyses; to Ms. Bonnie Jones and Mr. Charles Schable for performing laboratory tests; and to Ms. Ingrid Symes and Ms. Leticia Vasquez for helping to prepare the manuscript.

References

1. Pneumocystis pneumonia — Los Angeles. MMWR 1981; 30:250-2.
2. Moll B, Emeson EE, Small CB, Friedland GH, Klein RS, Spigland I. Inverted ratio of inducer to suppressor T-lymphocyte subsets in drug abusers with opportunistic infections. Clin Immunol Immunopathol 1982; 25:417-23.
3. *Pneumocystis carinii* pneumonia among persons with hemophilia A. MMWR 1982; 31:365-7.
4. Curran JW, Lawrence DN, Jaffe H, et al. Acquired immunodeficiency syndrome (AIDS) associated with transfusions. N Engl J Med 1984; 310:69-75.
5. Harris C, Small CB, Klein RS, et al. Immunodeficiency in female sexual partners of men with the acquired immunodeficiency syndrome. N Engl J Med 1983; 308:1181-4.
6. Rubinstein A, Sicklick M, Gupta A, et al. Acquired immunodeficiency with reversed T4/T8 ratios in infants born to promiscuous and drug-addicted mothers. JAMA 1983; 249:2350-6.
7. Friedland GH, Harris C, Butkus-Small C, et al. Intravenous drug abusers and the acquired immunodeficiency syndrome (AIDS): demographic, drug use, and needle-sharing patterns. Arch Intern Med 1985; 145: 1413-7.
8. Gallo RC, Salahuddin SZ, Popovic M, et al. Frequent detection and isolation of cytopathic retroviruses (HTLV-III) from patients with AIDS and at risk for AIDS. Science 1984; 224:500-3.
9. Jaffe HW, Choi K, Thomas PA, et al. National case-control study of Kaposi's sarcoma and *Pneumocystis carinii* pneumonia in homosexual men. I. Epidemiologic results. Ann Intern Med 1983; 99:145-51.
10. Zagury D, Bernard J, Leibowitch J, et al. HTLV-III in cells cultured from semen of two patients with AIDS. Science 1984; 226:449-51.
11. Groopman JE, Salahuddin SZ, Sarngadharan MG, et al. HTLV-III in saliva of people with AIDS-related complex and healthy homosexual men at risk for AIDS. Science 1984; 226:447-9.
12. Update: acquired immunodeficiency syndrome — United States. MMWR 1985; 34:245-8.
13. Hirsch MS, Wormser GP, Schooley RT, et al. Risk of nosocomial infection with human T-cell lymphotropic virus III (HTLV-III). N Engl J Med 1985; 312:1-4.
14. Update: acquired immunodeficiency syndrome (AIDS) — United States. MMWR 1982; 32:389-91.
15. Update: acquired immunodeficiency syndrome (AIDS) — United States. MMWR 1984; 32:688-91.
16. Nicholson JKA, Jones BM, Cross GD, McDougal JS. Comparison of T and B cell analyses on fresh and aged blood. J Immunol Methods 1984; 73:29-40.
17. Tsang VCW, Peralta JM, Simmons AR. Enzyme-linked immunoelectrotransfer blot techniques (EITB) for studying the specificities of antigens and antibodies separated by gel electrophoresis. In: Langone JJ, van Vunakis H, eds. Methods in enzymology: immunochemical techniques. New York: Academic Press, 1983:377-91.
18. Feorino PM, Kalyanaraman VS, Haverkos HW, et al. Lymphadenopathy-associated virus infection of a blood donor-recipient pair with acquired immunodeficiency syndrome. Science 1984; 225:69-72.
19. Feorino PM, Jaffe HW, Palmer E, et al. Transfusion-associated acquired immunodeficiency syndrome: evidence for persistent infection in blood donors. N Engl J Med 1985; 312:1293-6.
20. Needlestick transmission of HTLV-III from a patient infected in Africa. Lancet 1984; 2:1376-7.
21. Cooper DA, Gold J, Maclean P, et al. Acute AIDS retrovirus infection: definition of a clinical illness associated with seroconversion. Lancet 1985; 1:537-40.
22. Fultz PN, Francis DP, Droderson JR, et al. Experimental infection of chimpanzees with HTLV-III/LAV as a potential model for AIDS. Presented at the International Conference on Acquired Immunodeficiency Syndrome, Atlanta, April, 1985.
23. Alter HJ, Eichberg JW, Masur H, et al. Transmission of HTLV-III infection from human plasma to chimpanzees: an animal model for AIDS. Science 1984; 226:549-52.
24. Bernier RH, Sampliner R, Gerety R, Tabor E, Hamilton F, Nathanson N. Hepatitis B infection in households of chronic carriers of hepatitis B surface antigen: factors associated with prevalence of infection. Am J Epidemiol 1982; 116:199-211.
25. Szmuness W, Prince AM, Hirsh RL, Brotman B. Familial clustering of hepatitis B infection. N Engl J Med 1973; 289:1162-6.
26. Redfield RR, Markham PD, Salahuddin SZ, et al. Frequent transmission of HTLV-III among spouses of patients with AIDS-related complex and AIDS. JAMA 1985; 253:1571-3.

CORRESPONDENCE

"FREE" NEEDLES FOR INTRAVENOUS DRUG USERS AT RISK FOR AIDS: CURRENT DEVELOPMENTS IN NEW YORK CITY

To the Editor: In the absence of either effective treatment or effective vaccines, reducing transmission-related behavior is the most practical means of trying to control the acquired immunodeficiency syndrome (AIDS) epidemic. Intravenous drug users constitute the second largest group of persons with AIDS in the United States; 2249 of the 13,216 U.S. cases have intravenous drug use as their primary risk factor, and an additional 1144 have both intravenous drug use and male homosexuality as risk factors. Furthermore, in the United States, intravenous drug users are the primary source of transmission to heterosexuals and to children (AIDS Activity, Centers for Disease Control: personal communication).

Human T-cell lymphotropic virus Type III/lymphadenopathy-associated virus, the virus that causes AIDS, is spread among intravenous drug users primarily through the sharing of needles for drug injection.[1,2] In New York, public health authorities are currently considering the lifting of some of the legal restrictions on the availability of sterile needles as a way of preventing AIDS. [3,4] Whether intravenous drug users would use readily available sterile needles is one of the important issues in their considerations. We report here on two recent developments involving "free" sterile needles that are a response to the AIDS epidemic among intravenous drug users in New York City.

The Street Research Unit of the New York State Division of Substance Abuse Services, which is composed primarily of ex-addicts, has been monitoring street-drug activity in New York City for the past decade.[5] Since the spring of 1985, they have observed two types of "free" sterile needles in the city.

The first type involves a modified "two-for-one" sale. Some needle sellers are now including an extra needle with the sale of a complete syringe and needle (the packages are stapled together). A new syringe with needle typically sells for $2 in New York City, but this complete syringe with an extra needle sells for only $2.50. The "extra point" can be used immediately if the first needle becomes clogged when a drug user is preparing to inject. Because it is just before injection that a drug user is most likely to be experiencing withdrawal or craving symptoms and is therefore most likely to use whatever needle is available, the availability of a spare "point" at this particular time may be an important way of keeping an individual drug user from using someone else's needle.

The other source of "free" needles is drug dealers who have been observed to include a "free" needle and syringe with sales of $25 and $50 bags of heroin, although this practice does not appear to be as widespread in the city as the "extra point" sales described above. These two "free needle" marketing tactics indicate an increased demand for clean needles among intravenous drug users in New York City and an effort by present suppliers to meet that increased demand.

These observations are consistent with our previous findings[6] of an increased use of sterile needles among intravenous drug users, and they strengthen the argument that a meaningful reduction in the risk of AIDS is possible in this group.

This work was supported in part through a grant (DA 03574) from the National Institute on Drug Abuse to Narcotic and Drug Research, Inc.

The opinions expressed in this letter do not necessarily reflect official policy of the New York State Division of Substance Abuse Services, the National Institute on Drug Abuse, or Narcotic and Drug Research, Inc.

Don C. Des Jarlais, Ph.D.,
and William Hopkins, M.A.
New York State Division of Substance Abuse Services
New York, NY 10047

References

1. Cohen H, Marmor M, Des Jarlais DC, et al. Behavioral risk factors for HTLV-III/LAV seropositivity among intravenous drug users. Presented at the International Conference on Acquired Immunodeficiency Syndrome (AIDS), Atlanta, April 1985.
2. Weiss S, Ginzburg H, Goeddart J, et al. Risk for HTLV-III exposure and AIDS among parenteral drug abusers in New Jersey. Presented at the International Conference on Acquired Immunodeficiency Syndrome (AIDS), Atlanta, April 1985.
3. Waldholz M. New York City's health unit urges easier syringe rule. Wall Street Journal. September 3, 1985:14.
4. Choosing between two killers. New York Times. September 15, 1985:E20.
5. Frank B. Current drug use trends in New York City. In: Proceedings of the Community Correspondents Group. Rockville, Md.: National Institute on Drug Abuse, 1980:1-5.
6. Des Jarlais DC, Friedman SR, Hopkins W. Risk reduction for the acquired immunodeficiency syndrome among intravenous drug users. Ann Intern Med (in press).

SHARING OF NEEDLES AMONG USERS OF INTRAVENOUS DRUGS

To the Editor: Intravenous drug users are the second largest group at risk for AIDS, accounting for 17 percent of the cases. The transmission of AIDS among intravenous drug users has been associated with the sharing of blood-contaminated needles. Although needle sharing is often responsible for the transmission of AIDS in this group, the prevalence of this behavior is not known.

We investigated needle sharing among 224 male drug abusers admitted to a 30-day inpatient drug-treatment program over a 19-month period (September 1983 through March 1985). Of the 224 subjects, 193 (86 percent) reported intravenous drug use. Their average frequency of drug use was once daily, and drugs were taken intravenously more than 75 percent of the time. Among these intravenous users, 68 percent (131) engaged in needle sharing, and they did so during 40 percent of their drug-use episodes. Among the needle sharers, 77 percent (101) reported sharing with relatives and close friends only, and the other 23 percent (30) reported sharing with casual acquaintances and strangers.

The drugs primarily used by the subjects were heroin (24 percent), amphetamines (23 percent), cocaine (22 percent), heroin and cocaine in combination (11 percent), and pentazocine (8 percent). Needle sharing was reported by over 50 percent of the subjects in each primary-drug group. These data indicate that needle sharing is common and frequently practiced among intravenous drug users. A recent study[1] found that street addicts were aware of the risk of AIDS associated with needle sharing and showed an increased interest in using new needles. The latter finding suggests a decrease in needle sharing. We found that the majority of sharers did so with those well known to them, such as relatives and close friends, which may indicate that they are showing some caution in needle sharing. These results suggest that intravenous drug users may be responsive to public-information campaigns addressing the health risks of needle sharing. Merely increasing the availability of needles without undertaking educational interventions might have a limited effect, since needle sharing has been found to be associated with socialization, communal feeling, and protection in the drug culture,[2] not merely with shortages of needles.

Further research is needed to identify effective procedures for reducing the risk of AIDS among intravenous drug users. Rapid implementation of risk-reduction procedures is critical, especially in geographic areas where drug abuse is prevalent but the AIDS epidemic is still limited.

John L. Black, Ph.D., Michael P. Dolar, Ph.D.,
Horace A. DeFord, M.D.,
Jody A. Rubenstein, M.S.,
Walter E. Penk, Ph.D.,
Ralph Robinowitz, Ph.D.,
and John R. Skinner, B.S.
Dallas Veterans Administration Medical Center
Dallas, TX 75216

References

1. Howard J, Borges P. Needle sharing in the Haight: some social and psychological functions. J Health Soc Behav 1970; 11:220-30.
2. Des Jarlais DC, Friedman SR, Hopkins W. Risk reduction for the acquired immunodeficiency syndrome among intravenous drug users. Ann Intern Med 1985; 103:755-9.

HIV INFECTION WITH SEROCONVERSION AFTER A SUPERFICIAL NEEDLESTICK INJURY TO THE FINGER

To the Editor: In the April 24 issue of the *Journal*, Stricof and Morse reported a well-documented case of HIV (HTLV-III/LAV) seroconversion in a health care worker after a needlestick injury.[1] A Special Report evaluating the occupational risk of acquired immunodeficiency syndrome (AIDS) appeared in the same issue.[2] We have recently investigated a case of HIV seroconversion after an occupational needlestick injury.

During a thoracentesis a nurse received a superficial self-inflicted needlestick injury to the finger while recapping the needle, which was contaminated by the bloody pleural fluid of a patient with persistent generalized lymphadenopathy, pleural effusion, seropositivity for HIV, and hepatitis B surface antigen. She immediately received specific immunoglobulins and the hepatitis B vaccine. Twenty-five days after the injury, fatigue, fever, and vomiting developed. On day 26, her temperature was 39.4°C; the physical examination was normal. The white-cell count was 3000, with 40 percent neutrophils, 24 percent lymphocytes, and 2 percent plasma cells. On day 53, acute anicteric hepatitis developed. The serum aspartate aminotransferase level rose to 418 mU per milliliter on day 68 and returned to a normal level within two months. Viral titers and blood cultures ruled out acute cytomegalovirus and Epstein–Barr virus infection. Serologic tests for hepatitis A and B were still negative on day 181.

Serum samples were studied for HIV antibody by both enzyme-linked immunosorbent assay and Western blotting. The samples were negative on days 1 and 13, but were positive on days 68, 82, and 151, with a protein specificity for p18, p25, p55, and gp110. Blood viral cultures for HIV were negative on days 103 and 181. The physical examination was persistently normal. Peripheral-blood mononuclear cells were studied with similar results on days 110 and 181; there were 680 lymphocytes per cubic millimeter, 105 T4 cells, and 195 T8 cells. A skin test for tuberculin was positive.

Detailed epidemiologic investigation of the nurse and her husband did not identify any risk factors for HIV infection. In addition, the husband was negative for HIV antibody when tested 110 days after the injury.

In two previously described cases of HIV seroconversion in health care workers, contamination occurred after parenteral exposure to blood.[1,3] In the case reported here, the infective medium was pleural fluid and the wound was superficial. This type of contamination emphasizes the need for strict precautions regarding the handling of needles and of any body fluids from patients infected with HIV. Another notable feature of this case was the occurrence of acute hepatitis without proof of involvement of the usual viral agents. The hepatitis was therefore possibly related to the primary infection by HIV.

Eric Oksenhendler, M.D.,
Martine Harzic, M.D.,
Jeanne-Marie Le Roux, M.D.,
Claire Rabian, M.D.,
and Jean Pierre Clauvel, M.D.
Saint-Louis Hospital
75475 Paris Cedex 10, France

References

1. Stricof RL, Morse DL. HTLV-III/LAV seroconversion following a deep intramuscular needlestick injury. N Engl J Med 1986; 314:1115.
2. McCray E, the Cooperative Needlestick Surveillance Group. Occupational risk of the acquired immunodeficiency syndrome among health care workers. N Engl J Med 1986; 314:1127-32.
3. Needlestick transmission of HTLV-III from a patient infected in Africa. Lancet 1984; 2:1376-7.

INFREQUENCY OF ISOLATION OF HTLV-III VIRUS FROM SALIVA IN AIDS

To the Editor: The acquired immunodeficiency syndrome (AIDS) is a sexually transmitted disease that can also be transmitted through contaminated blood or blood products. This fact is supported in part by the recovery of human T-cell lymphotropic virus Type III (HTLV-III), the etiologic agent of AIDS, from blood and semen.[1,2] However, the report of HTLV-III isolation from the saliva of infected patients[3] has raised concern about the possible casual transmission of this virus, although epidemiologic studies have not supported casual contagion.

In the past 12 months, we have attempted to isolate HTLV-III from 83 saliva samples from 71 homosexual men seropositive for HTLV-III, who were studied at the Massachusetts General Hospital. All saliva specimens were cultured within 60 minutes after collection. In addition, blood was also obtained from 50 of the 71 men for virus isolation. Our results are summarized in Table 1. One of 83 saliva specimens (1 percent) was positive for HTLV-III, whereas 28 of 50 blood cultures (56 percent) yielded the virus. The virus-positive saliva (unfiltered) was obtained from a patient with AIDS who had pneumocystis pneumonia, candidal esophagitis, and thrush. His saliva culture demonstrated reverse transcriptase activity only after 21 days in culture. In contrast, his blood culture showed reverse transcriptase activity on day 3. This suggests that the HTLV-III titer of this patient's saliva was substantially less than that of his blood.

The infrequent isolation of HTLV-III from saliva reported here is unlikely to be due to improper methods, because our isolation rate from the blood of infected persons is comparable to those reported by other laboratories.[5] In addition, we have had little difficulty in recovering the virus from the cerebrospinal fluid and neural tissues of HTLV-III-infected patients with neurologic dysfunction.[6] Therefore, we conclude that HTLV-III is present infrequently in the saliva of infected persons. When it was detected in the saliva of one patient with intraoral disease, the amount of virus present was small. These findings are consistent with epidemiologic data indicating that casual transmission of HTLV-III does not occur, even among household members exposed to the saliva of infected persons.[7] These results may be useful in allaying public concern regarding the casual spread of AIDS and HTLV-III infection.

Table 1. Isolation of HTLV-III from 83 Saliva and 50 Blood Samples from 71 Seropositive Homosexual Men.*

Patient Group (No.)	Saliva†	Blood‡
	no. positive/no. tested	
Healthy seropositive (20)	0/20	7/17
AIDS-related complex (32)	0/38	14/21
AIDS (19)	1/25	7/12
Total (71)	1/83	28/50

*HTLV-III denotes human T-cell lymphotropic virus Type III, and AIDS acquired immunodeficiency syndrome.

†Fifty of the saliva specimens were cultured as described by Groopman et al.[3]; 24 specimens were similarly cultured except without prior filtering of the saliva through a 0.45-μm filter (Millipore); 9 specimens were cultured with use of H9 cells as targets as previously described.[2]

‡Blood was cultured for HTLV-III as described by Feorino et al.[4]

David D. Ho, M.D., Roy E. Byington, B.S., Robert T. Schooley, M.D., Theresa Flynn, R.N., Teresa R. Rota, M.A., and Martin S. Hirsch, M.D.
Massachusetts General Hospital
Boston, MA 02114

References

1. Gallo RC, Salahuddin SZ, Popovic M, et al. Frequent detection and isolation of cytopathic retroviruses (HTLV-III) from patients with AIDS and at risk for AIDS. Science 1984; 224:500-3.
2. Ho DD, Schooley RT, Rota TR, et al. HTLV-III in the semen and blood of a healthy homosexual man. Science 1984; 226:451-3.
3. Groopman JE, Salahuddin SZ, Sarngadharan MG, et al. HTLV-III in saliva of people with AIDS-related complex and healthy homosexual men at risk for AIDS. Science 1984; 226:447-9.
4. Feorino PM, Kalyanaraman VS, Haverkos HW, et al. Lymphadenopathy associated virus infection of a blood donor-recipient pair with acquired immunodeficiency syndrome. Science 1984; 225:69-72.
5. Markham PD, Salahuddin SZ, Popovic M, et al. Advances in the isolation of HTLV-III from patients with AIDS and AIDS-related complex and from donors at risk. Cancer Res 1985; 45:Suppl:4588S-91S.
6. Ho DD, Rota TR, Schooley RT, et al. Isolation of HTLV-III from cerebrospinal fluid and neural tissues of patients with neurologic syndromes related to the acquired immunodeficiency syndrome. N Engl J Med 1985; 313:1493-7.
7. Education and foster care of children infected with HTLV-III/LAV. MMWR 1985; 34:517-21.

Epidemiology and Public Health Issues

General Public Health Issues Related to AIDS

SPECIAL REPORT

THE AIDS EPIDEMIC

Sheldon H. Landesman, M.D., Harold M. Ginzburg, M.D., M.P.H., and Stanley H. Weiss, M.D.

During 1984 several important developments advanced our understanding of the acquired immunodeficiency syndrome (AIDS). A retrovirus known as human T-cell leukemia (lymphotropic) virus type III (HTLV-III),[1] also called lymphadenopathy-associated virus, was identified as the probable cause of AIDS.[2] AIDS-associated retrovirus[3] is also probably the same agent. An enzyme-linked immunosorbent assay (ELISA) has been developed to detect antibodies to HTLV-III,[4] thereby providing an indicator of whether or not a person has been exposed to the virus. Clinical researchers have identified various therapeutic agents that appear to inhibit viral replication in vitro.[5,6] Although the ultimate goal of all these research activities is a better understanding of the pathogenesis of diseases related to HTLV-III and the development of definitive preventive and therapeutic measures, no therapeutic intervention has permanently reversed the HTLV-III–associated immunodeficiency, nor has the full meaning of HTLV-III seropositivity been elucidated. In spite of the extraordinarily rapid scientific progress to date, AIDS remains an epidemic disease whose natural history and cure are unknown.

Seroepidemiologic information gathered in recent months indicates that the extent of HTLV-III infection is more serious and complex than was originally anticipated. We review here the magnitude of HTLV-III exposure, the outcome of such exposure, the economic burden of HTLV-III–related disease, and the social, ethical, and public implications of this epidemic for the future.

HTLV-III Seropositivity — Extent of Exposure

The ELISA serum antibody test for HTLV-III is useful for screening purposes and in epidemiologic AIDS research.[7] When it is used for diagnostic purposes, an additional confirmatory test is recommended to rule out false positive results.[7-9] A confirmed positive test indicates that a person has been exposed to the virus and has mounted an immunologic response (serum antibodies). However, this test does not indicate whether the person currently harbors the virus (i.e., is an HTLV-III carrier), although HTLV-III has been isolated from antibody-positive subjects.[1] Furthermore, additional studies are required to demonstrate that there are not antibodies to other viruses that cross-react in the test. In this issue of the *Journal*, Evatt et al. present data indicating that there had been extensive exposure to HTLV-III among patients with hemophilia by 1981-1982. They also found that by 1984 virtually all the hemophiliac patients they studied were antibody positive.[10] Similar studies by Goedert et al.,[11] Melbye et al.,[12] and Eyster et al.[13] also document the recent and nearly total HTLV-III seroconversion of patients with hemophilia — a process linked to the use of factor VIII concentrates prepared in the United States.

Seroepidemiologic studies have been conducted among other high-risk populations. In San Francisco, the prevalence of HTLV-III antibodies among homosexual men attending a clinic for treatment of sexually transmitted diseases rose from 1 percent in 1978 to 25 percent in 1980 and to 65 percent in 1984.[14] Homosexual communities in nonepidemic cities are also experiencing rising rates of HTLV-III seropositivity. For example, seropositivity for lymphadenopathy-associated virus rose from less than 10 percent in 1978 to 49 percent in 1984 among unselected homosexual men attending a clinic for sexually transmitted diseases in Denver (Judson F, et al.: unpublished data). In a prospective cohort of homosexual men from Pittsburgh, HTLV-III antibody seropositivity rose from 10 percent in 1983 to 28 percent in 1984 (Rinaldo C: personal communication).

An analogous situation exists among users of parenteral drugs. In Queens, New York, 29 percent of parenteral-drug users admitted to a methadone detoxification treatment program in 1981-1982 were positive for HTLV-III antibodies (Robert-Guroff M: personal communication), and 87 percent of the patients admitted to a Manhattan methadone detoxification program were antibody positive in 1984.[14] Fifty percent of parenteral-drug users in Newark and Jersey City, New Jersey, who were in drug-treatment programs were positive for antibodies to HTLV-III in 1984 (Weiss SH, et al.: unpublished data).

The difference between the high rates of HTLV-III seropositivity noted in some major urban coastal cities over the past several years (based on ELISA testing of previously stored samples) and the lower seropositivity rates in inland cities and suburban areas is narrowing as the virus continues to spread. Similarly, HTLV-III–related disease is being reported more frequently from less densely populated regions of this country.

Surprisingly, the rate of HTLV-III seropositivity among Haitian immigrants was found to be less than 5 percent in a survey conducted in New York City.[15] This relatively low seroprevalence rate is in marked contrast to the rates observed among asymptomatic patients with hemophilia and among homosexual men and parenteral-drug users in the New York City area.[7] From these data, it does not appear that being of Haitian extraction by itself, in isolation from other risk factors, increases the relative risk of being exposed to HTLV-III.

Seropositivity is extremely low among heterosexual men and women who are not members of known high-risk groups.[4,7] This does not mean, however, that heterosexual people are not at risk for AIDS. AIDS is a sexually transmissible disease, and thus any sexual partner of a person exposed to the virus may contract the virus. The extent of intimate sexual contact needed to transmit the virus from one partner to another is unknown. Sexual contact with prostitutes previously exposed to the virus may explain some of the cases currently classified by the Centers for Disease Control as being in the "no known risk" category.[16] A link between prostitutes who use nonparenteral drugs and HTLV-III seropositivity is also suggested from studies in Africa and Haiti. In the United States, approximately one third of all women entering treatment for narcotic addiction have at some time engaged in prostitution to earn money to buy drugs.[17] Therefore, the HTLV-III seroprevalence rate may be high among prostitutes, with obvious potential risk for their clients as well.

At present it is impossible to give an accurate figure for the total number of persons in this country who are positive for HTLV-III antibodies. On the basis of the above data, however, one can estimate the total to be at least 400,000 persons. The potential pool of people at increased risk of exposure to the virus is larger. The population of parenteral-drug users is approximately 400,000.[18] In addition, more than a million people may occasionally use parenteral drugs (cocaine and heroin).[18] If one uses Kinsey's historical estimate that 10 percent of the adult male population are homosexual,[19,20] then on the basis of the estimate of 159 million persons in the United States ages 18 and older,[21] there are approximately 8 million homosexual men in the United States. Given what is already known about the high risk groups and the potential for spread to other populations, the implications of the presence of this virus in a community are staggering.

Although seroconversion has been documented in both human beings and chimpanzees between two and eight weeks after inoculation with material from persons positive for HTLV-III or from patients with AIDS,[22,23] detectable antibodies have not developed in some asymptomatic, immunologicaly normal persons infected with HTLV-III virus for more than six months.[9,24] These virus-positive, antibody-negative persons may represent the earliest stage of HTLV-III infection, with active viral replication and very little or no antibody response — possibly a stage of antigen excess. The unknown number of such serologically negative but virologically positive persons further complicates the AIDS picture.

Outcome in Persons Positive for HTLV-III Antibody

The complete clinical spectrum of HTLV-III–related disease is unknown.[7,25] There are numerous prospective, retrospective, and cross-sectional studies that are attempting to provide sufficient information about the viral infection and its sequelae. These studies will assist clinicians in developing therapeutic interventions and public health officials in developing primary prevention programs.

Information from some of these studies is sobering. In each of six different studies, the proportion of HTLV-III seropositive persons in whom full-blown AIDS developed during follow-up periods of one to five years ranged from 4 to 19 percent[9,13,26,27] (and Marmor M: personal communication; Weiss SH, et al.: unpublished data). In several of these studies nonspecific symptoms suggesting early stages of AIDS-related illnesses have developed in up to an additional 25 percent of those exposed to the virus. These symptoms have included weight loss, chronic unexplained fever or diarrhea, oral candidiasis, generalized lymphadenopathy, and thrombocytopenia. We do not know the proportion of these persons who will subsequently have full-blown AIDS.

An emerging concern about those being exposed to HTLV-III is that they may eventually acquire lymphomas,[25] such as Burkitt's-like lymphomas.[28] Both Hodgkin's and non-Hodgkin's lymphomas may also be associated with AIDS.[29-31] Iatrogenic and congenital immunodeficiency syndromes are associated with an excess of lymphoid-type malignant conditions,[32] such as the non-Hodgkin's lymphomas that develop at an increased rate among recipients of renal allografts after several years of immunosuppressive therapy.[33] HTLV-III is associated with chronic immunosuppression. It has been reported to share properties of both known leukemia-associated retroviruses and slow viruses (lentiviruses).[34] Both slow viruses and HTLV-III have been associated with neurologic disorders.[35] Therefore, it is not unreasonable to anticipate an increase during the next two decades in the number of lymphomas and perhaps other long-term sequelae among persons currently exposed to HTLV-III.

The Centers for Disease Control currently estimates that 8000 new cases of AIDS will be reported for the 12-month period ending in October 1985 (Curran JW: unpublished data). Because the epidemic has not yet peaked, the total number of cases for all of 1985 will exceed 8000. Quinn,[36] using data from the work of Hardy et al.,[20] recently estimated that there will be 40,000 new cases of AIDS in the next two years. AIDS is not on the wane.

Economic Considerations

An epidemic of this magnitude severely stresses the health care system in terms of its financial cost, use of resources, and effect on medical and support personnel. A recent study of hospitalized patients with AIDS indicates that they have an average life span of 224 days after being hospitalized for their first opportunistic infection (Bienstock J: personal communication). The average direct lifetime hospital cost for the care of such patients is calculated to be $42,000. If there are at least 8000 new cases of AIDS in 1985, then the estimated cost of inpatient care for patients with newly diagnosed disease will be approximately $336 million. This is an underestimate of the total medical care costs, since it does not include the costs of outpatient care or medication. It also fails to consider the other elements of social cost, such as lost employment, reduced productivity, shortened life expectancy, and social-welfare services. In this country there are approximately 12 million units of blood products collected each year.[37] The cost of the ELISA antibody test and associated expenses for the replacement of suspect blood products, notification of donors, and counseling of donors when necessary would add approximately another $100 million per year.[37] Therefore, it is not unreasonable to estimate that AIDS will cost our society more than half a billion dollars during the next calendar year.

The less tangible costs of the AIDS epidemic can be viewed on any ward providing medical care to patients with the disease. The psychological strain on the patients, their friends and relatives, and the medical and nursing staff is great. For several decades, medical practitioners have not had to face an epidemic of a fatal infectious disease among previously healthy persons.

Implications of HTLV-III Antibody Testing

The anticipated widespread introduction of tests for HTLV-III antibodies in the near future has sparked controversy among certain segments of the population. The current major clinical application of the HTLV-III antibody ELISA is to screen blood products, thereby helping to minimize the risk of transfusion-associated AIDS. However, it is clear that the ELISA and its confirmatory tests will be used for other clinical and diagnostic applications. All the uses of this test pose complex legal, medical, social, and ethical issues. False positive and false negative results are to be expected, as with all screening tests.[7] The adverse consequences of a false positive test are obvious. Those of a false negative test, especially when the test is being used to screen donated blood products, are clear as well. The successful implementation of these tests in the setting of the blood-collection agency is contingent on the continuation of self-exclusion guidelines. Donors who are members of high-risk groups or at potential risk of HTLV-III exposure (e.g., sexual contacts of risk-group members) must not donate. If self-exclusion is not continued, it is possible that contaminated blood products could slip through the screening net and lead to an increased risk of transfusion-associated AIDS.

Persons who are tested by blood-collection agencies for the presence of antibodies to HTLV-III will be notified of the results of the test.[9] How intrusive may blood-collection agencies be in attempting to notify people of the results of their tests? Issues like this surrounding the use of the test are being addressed by a number of governmental and private panels; guidelines will be forthcoming when the new test is approved by the Food and Drug Administration.

The implication of a true positive HTLV-III test for an apparently healthy person are evident. It is possible that in the future health and life insurance could be denied or employment could be terminated. States may require compulsory reporting of HTLV-III–positive results to their health departments for surveillance purposes. States may require HTLV-III testing before issuing a marriage license. Some people may consider a positive result as presumptive evidence that a never-married man 30 years of age or older is homosexual or that a minority person from the inner city is a narcotics addict.

Social, Ethical, and Public Health Considerations

The complexities associated with AIDS transcend the medical diagnosis and treatment of the disease. The great social and economic burden associated with AIDS and the more subtle personal effects of a positive ELISA test create a multitude of difficulties that cannot be resolved in isolation or piecemeal.

Adequate financial resources for research dealing with this catastrophic and ultimately fatal illness must continue. Resources for the treatment of patients with full-blown AIDS and other HTLV-III–related diseases are also necessary, as are companion funds for needed social services for the patients, their friends, and service providers. The health dollars currently allocated to treat HTLV-III–related illnesses are at the expense of other health programs. Given the finite resources of our economy, any decisions either to commit new resources or to reallocate existing ones must be made consciously, and the consequences acknowledged. Private and public funding sources will be needed. The feasibility of creating a national catastrophic fund for HTLV-III–related disease, modeled after the end-stage-renal-disease program, needs to be considered.

Hospitals in cities with large numbers of patients with AIDS have either already established AIDS wards or are considering doing so. There are ample historical precedents for the development of disease-specific wards (wards for fever, diabetes, tuberculosis, and poliomyelitis have all existed in the past). Current medical practice has permitted the establishment of oncology wards. Such an approach may enhance patient care by permitting better coordination of inpatient services, improving follow-up of patients, and allowing the more efficient use of social services. Because the medical and nursing staffs of these wards are likely to be knowledgeable about the medical, social, and emotional aspects of the disease, they will become a major educational and emotional resource for patients and their families. Supportive services for the health care providers will also be easier to maintain. AIDS wards will also facilitate clinical trials of new chemotherapeutic agents and diagnostic techniques.

However, the establishment of AIDS wards could

provoke controversy. Members of high-risk groups may fear the stigma associated with their overrepresentation on such wards. Nonetheless, the practicality and efficiency of such specialized wards or hospitals may justify their existence.

The licensing of the HTLV-III antibody test is imminent. There are conflicting and legitimate interests surrounding HTLV-III testing that must be addressed at this time. It is not enough to say that neither medical management nor public health policies can rationally be based on seropositivity.[37] Confidentiality is a central issue in HTLV-III testing; many persons and organizations may want or demand to see certain people's test results. Access to this private medical information will vary with the circumstances under which the test is performed. The person being tested should be aware of who may have access to the results. Therefore, the general use of an informed-consent procedure before the HTLV-III test is performed by either clinicians or blood-collection agencies should be considered. Such a consent form would place the patient on notice about what would happen to the assay results and how he or she could obtain the results, with adequate explanation.

As outlined above, current seroprevalence and seroconversion estimates indicate that large numbers of persons are or will become infected with HTLV-III; tens of thousands will contract AIDS and subsequently die.[36] The need for a nationally coordinated health program managed by the states and the cities and towns has been recognized. The initial steps have been taken in this cooperative effort to minimize morbidity and mortality from AIDS and to address the related social and economic burdens. However, it is important to recognize that as far as we have come in understanding HTLV-III exposure and related diseases this year, there needs to be a continued commitment of resources, because we have a great deal more to learn and to do.

References

1. Gallo RC, Salahuddin SZ, Popovic M, et al. Frequent detection and isolation of cytopathic retroviruses (HTLV-III) from patients with AIDS and at risk for AIDS. Science 1984; 224:500-3.
2. Barré-Sinoussi F, Chermann JC, Rey F, et al. Isolation of a T-lymphotropic retrovirus from a patient at risk for acquired immune deficiency syndrome (AIDS). Science 1983; 220:868-71.
3. Levy JA, Hoffman AD, Kramer SM, Landis JA, Shimabukuro JM, Oshiro LS. Isolation of lymphocytopathic retroviruses from San Francisco patients with AIDS. Science 1983; 255:840-2.
4. Sarngadharan MG, Popovic M, Bruch L, Schüpbach J, Gallo RC. Antibodies reactive with human T-lymphotropic retrovirus (HTLV-III) in the serum of patients with AIDS. Science 1984; 224:506-8.
5. Mitsuya H, Popovic M, Yarchoan R, et al. Suramin protection of T-cells in vitro against infectivity and cytopathic effect of HTLV-III. Science 1984; 226:172-4.
6. McCormick JB, Getchell J, Mitchell S, Hicks DR. Ribavirin suppresses replication of lymphadenopathy associated virus in cultures of human adult T-lymphocytes. Lancet 1984; 2:1367-9.
7. Weiss SH, Goedert JJ, Sarngadharan MG, et al. Screening test for HTLV-III (AIDS agent) antibodies: specificity, sensitivity, and applications. JAMA 1985; 253:221-5.
8. Schüpbach J, Haller O, Vogt M, et al. Antibodies to HTLV-III in Swiss patients with AIDS and pre-AIDS and in groups at risk for AIDS. N Engl J Med 1985; 312:265-70.
9. Provisional Public Health Service inter-agency recommendations for screening donated blood and plasma for antibody to the virus causing AIDS. MMWR 1985; 34:1-5.
10. Evatt BL, Gomperts ED, McDougal JS, Ramsey RB. Coincidental appearance of LAV/HTLV-III antibodies in hemophiliacs and the onset of the AIDS epidemic. N Engl J Med 1985; 312:483-6.
11. Goedert JJ, Eyster ME, Sarngadharan MG, et al. Antibodies reactive with human T-cell leukemia viruses in the serum of hemophiliacs receiving factor VIII concentrate. Blood 1985; 65:492-5.
12. Melbye M, Froebel KS, Madhok R, et al. HTLV-III seropositivity in European haemophiliacs exposed to factor VIII concentrate imported from the USA. Lancet 1984; 2:1444-6.
13. Eyster ME, Goedert JJ, Sarngadharan MG, Weiss SH, Gallo RC, Blattner WA. Development and early natural history of HTLV-III antibodies in persons with hemophilia. JAMA (in press).
14. Antibodies to a retrovirus etiologically associated with acquired immunodeficiency syndrome (AIDS) in populations with increased incidences of the syndrome. MMWR 1984; 33:377-9.
15. Frank E, Weiss SH, Compas JC, et al. AIDS in Haitian-Americans, a reassessment. Cancer Res (in press).
16. Chamberland ME, Castro KG, Haverkos HW, et al. Acquired immunodeficiency syndrome in the United States: an analysis of cases outside high-incidence groups. Ann Intern Med 1984; 101:617-23.
17. Ginzburg HM, Weiss SH, MacDonald MG, Hubbard RL. HTLV-III exposure among drug users. Cancer Res (in press).
18. Ginzburg HM. Intravenous drug users and the acquired immune deficiency syndrome. Public Health Rep 1984; 99:206-11.
19. Kinsey AC, Pomeroy WB, Martin CE. Sexual behavior in the human male. Philadelphia: WB Saunders, 1948.
20. Hardy AM, Allen JR, Morgan WM, Curran JW. The incidence rate of acquired immunodeficiency syndrome in selected populations. JAMA 1985; 253:215-20.
21. United States Bureau of the Census. Population estimates and projections. Current Population Rep. July 1982 (series P-25, No. 917).
22. Gajdusek DC, Amyx HL, Gibbs CJ Jr, et al. Infection of chimpanzees by human T-lymphotropic retroviruses in brain and other tissues from AIDS patients. Lancet 1985; 1:55-6.
23. Needlestick transmission of HTLV-III from a patient infected in Africa. Lancet 1984; 2:1376-7.
24. Salahuddin SZ, Groopman JE, Markham PD, et al. HTLV-III in symptom-free seronegative persons. Lancet 1984; 2:1418-20.
25. Goerdert J, Blattner W. The epidemiology of the acquired immunodeficiency syndrome. In: DeVita VT, Hellman S, Rosenberg SA, eds. AIDS. Philadelphia: JB Lippincott (in press).
26. Goerdert J, Sarngadharan MG, Biggar RJ, et al. Determinants of retrovirus (HTLV-III) antibody and immunodeficiency conditions in homosexual men. Lancet 1984; 2:711-6.
27. Melbye M, Biggar RJ, Ebbesen P, et al. Seroepidemiology of HTLV-III antibody in Danish homosexual men: prevalence, transmission, and disease outcome. Br Med J 1984; 289:573-5.
28. Biggar RJ, Horm J, Lubin JH, Goerdert JJ, Greene MH, Fraumeni JF Jr. Cancer trends in a population at risk of AIDS. JNCI (in press).
29. Ziegler JL, Beckstead JA, Volberding PA, et al. Non-Hodgkin's lymphoma in 90 homosexual men: relation to generalized lymphadenopathy and the acquired immunodeficiency syndrome. N Engl J Med 1984; 311: 565-70.
30. Metroka CE, Cunningham-Rundles S, Pollack MS, et al. Generalized lymphadenopathy in homosexual men. Ann Intern Med 1983; 99:585-91.
31. Schoeppel SL, Hoppe RT, Dorfman RF, et al. Hodgkin's disease in homosexual men with generalized lymphadenopathy. Ann Intern Med 1985; 102:68-70.
32. Blattner WA, Hoover RN. Cancer in the immunosuppressed host. In: DeVita VT, Helman S, Rosenberg SA, eds. Cancer: principles and practice of oncology. Philadelphia: JB Lippincott (in press).
33. Hanto DW, Frizzera G, Purtilo DT, et al. Clinical spectrum of lymphoproliferative disorders in renal transplant recipients and evidence for the role of Epstein–Barr virus. Cancer Res 1981; 41:4253-61.
34. Gonda MA, Wong-Stall F, Gallo RC, Clements JE, Naryan O, Gilden RV. Sequence homology and morphologic similarity of HTLV-III and visna virus, a pathogenic lentivirus. Science 1985; 227:173-7.
35. Shaw GM, Harper ME, Hahn BH, et al. HTLV-III infection in brains of children and adults with AIDS encephalopathy. Science 1985; 227:177-82.
36. Quinn TC. Perspectives on the future of AIDS. JAMA 1985; 253:247-9.
37. Goldsmith MF. Medical news. JAMA 1985; 253:173-81.

SPECIAL REPORT

THE ACQUIRED IMMUNODEFICIENCY SYNDROME

Infection Control and Public Health Law

Michael Mills, J.D., Constance B. Wofsy, M.D., and John Mills, M.D.

BECAUSE they can be transmitted to others, infectious diseases of all kinds have for many years been the subject of statutes, regulations, and court decisions imposing special constraints on both the patient's freedom and the physician's practice. The acquired immunodeficiency syndrome (AIDS) is now known to be an infectious disease. Three laboratories have recovered from patients with AIDS unique T-lymphocyte–associated retroviruses (the so-called AIDS retroviruses) that are almost certainly the etiologic agent.[1-3] Serologic studies have confirmed the relation between AIDS retrovirus infection, AIDS, and the AIDS-related complex.[2,3]

The legality of measures to control the spread of infectious diseases is determined under principles of constitutional law that require the individual's interest in liberty and privacy to be balanced against the public's interest in health and safety. Balancing these interests in the context of AIDS is particularly difficult, because the interests on each side are so fundamental and so strongly affected by the nature of the infection. For the individual, measures to control the spread of AIDS may invade privacy, constrain sexual conduct and procreation, and limit liberty. For the public, AIDS retrovirus infection continues to spread, especially among high-risk groups, and is often fatal; no vaccine or chemotherapeutic agent has been proved to prevent infection, reduce infectivity, or ameliorate the disease. We therefore believe that AIDS poses the most profound issues of constitutional law and public health since the Supreme Court approved compulsory immunization in 1905.[4] In this report, we discuss the legal principles that should guide those concerned with AIDS — physicians, patients, public health officials, and the courts. Since few cases concerning AIDS have been decided and only one statute has been passed, we draw on precedents in statutes, regulations, and court decisions concerning other potentially fatal or incurable communicable diseases.[5]

We also draw on currently accepted medical knowledge about the disease. The transmission of AIDS generally follows the epidemiologic pattern of the hepatitis B virus.[6-8] More specifically, it is transmitted chiefly through the exchange of blood, semen, and perhaps other fluids through sexual intercourse, the sharing of hypodermic needles, and transfusion.[9] AIDS occurs most often in populations frequently ostracized — homosexual men and intravenous drug users.[9] Beyond those who have AIDS as defined by the Centers for Disease Control, as many as 1 million other people may be infected with the AIDS retroviruses.[10] They include patients with the AIDS-related complex, asymptomatic persons identified epidemiologically as the likely sources of infection for patients with AIDS (e.g., through transfusion), and asymptomatic persons identified only by laboratory testing. These people are likely to be the main epidemiologic reservoir for AIDS, because they may be infectious for years, perhaps decades, with few or no symptoms and because until recently there was no test to detect the carrier state.[1-3,11,12]

Legal principles applicable to patients with AIDS should therefore apply equally to other persons if their infectiousness is confirmed by the best available testing methods. Among those with a known risk of exposure to AIDS — homosexual men and intravenous drug users, for example — detection of antibody to human T-cell lymphotropic virus Type III (HTLV-III), using the recently licensed enzyme-linked immunosorbent assay, is 99 percent predictive of prior AIDS retrovirus infection.[13] Among other groups, the predictive value of the test is much lower; positive results must therefore be confirmed by Western blot or another reliable confirmatory test.[13] The presence of antibody definitely directed against AIDS retroviruses appears virtually 100 percent predictive of prior infection and potential infectiousness.[13]

The Responsibilities of Physicians and Patients

The Duty to Report AIDS

Cases of AIDS, as defined by the Centers for Disease Control, are reportable to the public health authorities everywhere in the United States and in many other countries as well.[14] Because reporting requirements are set by each state separately and may change, the relevant state's law should be reviewed.

Physicians, hospitals, laboratories, and indeed, "any other person knowing of or attending a case" are all required by law to report cases of communicable diseases such as AIDS. For failure to do so, the laws set fines ranging from $5 to $1,000, and in a few states jail sentences up to 90 days are possible. Prosecutorial attention is rarely given to enforcement of the reporting laws,[15] and we know of no one who has been fined or imprisoned for failure to report a case of AIDS or another communicable disease. Nevertheless, if a physician's failure to report a case of AIDS is clearly responsible for secondary cases, his or her license may be in jeopardy.[16]

Precedents set in cases of other infectious diseases point to a possible civil action for damages if preventable morbidity or mortality results from a physician's failure to report a case of AIDS.[17-19] In 1974, in the case of *Derrick* v. *Ontario Community Hospital*,[18] for example, the neighbor of a patient with a staphylococcal infection sued the treating hospital for failure to report the disease, claiming that the hospital's lapse prevented the public health officer from doing his duty under California law to "prevent the spread of the disease." The court accepted the neighbor's legal theory and permitted a trial to determine the facts, although it noted the need to prove a causal link between the failure to report and the neighbor's illness. In the case of AIDS, the known modes of transmission suggest that the defendant might claim that the patient with the secondary infection had assumed the risk of the infection or had contributed to its development. Moreover, the usefulness of the infection-control measures taken by public health authorities, once notified, is uncertain, and the activity resulting in transmission is likely to have been unwitnessed. Proving a causal link in the transmission of AIDS would therefore be difficult.

Cases of infection with the AIDS retroviruses in people who do not have AIDS need not be reported, except in Colorado.[20] Because such people are infectious,[3,11] however, reporting could legally be required. A registry of typhoid carriers, defined as persons with typhoid bacilli in their feces or urine on two separate examinations at least 48 hours apart, has been maintained in California for many years. Similarly, because of the severity of the risks of AIDS, the public health authorities may consider requiring the reporting of patients with the AIDS-related complex and those who are asymptomatic but infectious. The Colorado Board of Health, for example, has recently adopted regulations that would require doctors and laboratories to report the names and addresses of those persons with positive results on the HTLV-III antibody test. California, in contrast, has recently enacted a statute that forbids disclosure of the results of HTLV-III antibody tests without written authorization by the person tested.

Although reporting of those who are infected but not sick would increase the epidemiologic information available for use in infection control and would be constitutionally permissible, two problems remain. First, without a comprehensive and compulsory screening program, the people reported would be a self-selected group and probably a small fraction of those infected. Second, since there is no generally accepted means of controlling the spread of AIDS other than education, the usefulness of reporting identifying information to public health authorities would not outweigh the adverse social and economic consequences to the infected person of possible disclosure of his or her infectiousness.

The Patient's Right to Confidentiality

Having accepted responsibility for treating a patient, the physician and hospital have a duty to keep confidential all facts about the patient's diagnosis and treatment except those they are required to report.[5] Public health departments have a similar duty.[21] AIDS has provoked so much fear, and the groups most at risk are so likely for other reasons to be stigmatized, that physicians must pay particular attention to maintaining confidentiality. Improper disclosure of the illness may have serious, unjustified adverse consequences for the patient with AIDS, who may, in turn, have cause to make a civil claim for damages against the person making the wrongful disclosure.[22-24]

Nevertheless, some disclosure is proper — to those unequivocally at risk.[25-29] In California, for example, "[i]t shall be the duty of the physician in attendance on a case considered to be an infectious or communicable disease, to give detailed instructions to members of the household in regard to precautionary measures to be taken for preventing the spread of the disease" (California Administrative Code, Title 17, Section 2514). Contact tracing for syphilis and gonorrhea may require disclosure of the patient's illness. In cases of AIDS, disclosures of a similar narrow scope — to the patient's spouse or lover, for example — would not be unlawful on the part of physicians or public health officers.

Confidentiality is also very important for people with confirmed laboratory evidence of AIDS retrovirus infection who do not have AIDS. California's recently enacted statute forbidding disclosure of the results of tests for HTLV-III antibody is in direct conflict, however, with the legal rules, mentioned above, that permit narrow disclosure in cases of diseases other than AIDS, as well as with the California statutes that require such disclosure. Until this conflict in the law is resolved, California physicians who believe that the patient's contacts would be jeopardized if there were no disclosure should seek the assistance of the public health authorities, who may more easily accept the risk of acting in the face of a conflict in the law. If that assistance is unavailable or unavailing, disclosure after careful consideration and consultation, in our view, would be morally and legally defensible.

Instructing Patients

Physicians must explain fully to patients with AIDS the currently accepted view of the best infection-control measures. (Because patients infected with the AIDS retrovirus who do not have AIDS are also infectious, the principles discussed in this and the next two sections apply to them as well.) By statute, some states require such instructions for the traditional sexually transmitted diseases. Since prevention is the only generally accepted means of controlling infection, we believe this requirement should apply to AIDS. If such instructions are not given and the patient subsequently engages in an activity shown to result in transmission of the infection, the physician may risk civil liability for damages to another person who becomes ill as a result.[17,25] Recommended instructions have been adopted by the U.S. Public Health Service.[30] Although we are aware of differences of opinion within the medical community on a few details of what a patient with AIDS should or should not do, legal prudence and medical uncertainty about the disease suggest making stricter rather than more lenient recommendations.

Patients' Legal Risks

Failure to adhere to accepted measures to avoid infecting others can subject patients to criminal charges as well as civil liability for damages. In California, as in many other states, "any person afflicted with any contagious, infectious, or communicable disease who willfully exposes" another person to the disease is guilty of a misdemeanor (California Health and Safety Code, Section 3353). Penalties are a fine of $25 to $50, 90 days in jail, or both. Other states have similar statutes, although most are limited to sexually transmitted diseases, "venereal diseases," or specific diseases such as syphilis and gonorrhea.

No cases imposing civil liability for transmission of AIDS are known to us, but cases concerning other sexually transmitted diseases demonstrate the legal risk.[31-35] In the important recent case of *Kathleen K.* v. *Robert B.*, for example, a woman claimed that she had contracted genital herpes simplex infection during sexual intercourse with a man "at a time when he knew, or in the exercise of reasonable care should have known, that he was a carrier of venereal disease" but did not disclose that fact.[31] Guided by the precedent of earlier decisions awarding damages against persons who had intentionally or carelessly exposed others to syphilis, the court held that Kathleen K.'s legal theories were sound and that she could go forward at trial to prove that the facts were as she claimed. On November 12, 1985, a man who said he had been Rock Hudson's lover filed suit against Hudson's estate, his former secretary, and two physicians.[36] The suit alleges that Hudson, the secretary, and the physicians concealed from the plaintiff the fact that Hudson had AIDS at a time when he and Hudson were known to be sexually involved. The claims against the physicians raise the issue of liability for failure to report a case of AIDS or to disclose to those at risk, as well as the issue in *Kathleen K.* v. *Robert B.*

The Physician's Responsibility for Recalcitrant Patients

If a patient with AIDS will not modify his or her behavior to avoid further spread of the disease, then the physician may directly warn those who are at risk (e.g., the patient's spouse or lover).[5] Indeed, the physician has a duty to do so,[25,27,28,37] but that duty would be fulfilled by reporting the patient's recalcitrance to the public health authorities, who have the responsibility for notifying contacts and other epidemiologic tasks.

We know of no case in which a physician who reported a communicable disease to public health authorities has subsequently been held liable for failing personally to warn those he or she knew or should have known were exposed to the patient. Of course, notifying the health department does not guarantee that contacts will be traced and notified in the case of every communicable disease, because health departments allocate limited resources in the way that they judge will be most effective. The San Francisco Health Department, for example, has not undertaken routine tracing of the sexual contacts of homosexual men with AIDS because there is no evidence that such tracing would slow the spread of the disease. Patients with AIDS may be infectious for a long time before being diagnosed,[1-3,12] the infection is incurable, and up to 50 percent of those in high-risk groups may already be infected.[2,38] The most seriously affected groups — the male homosexual communities in New York and San Francisco — have undertaken thoughtful educational and counseling programs. These, together with the educational efforts of the public health authorities, are a more effective means of preventing additional cases than tracing of contacts when so many are already infected. The prevalence of infection among heterosexuals is much lower, education is more sporadic, and the perception of risk is much less; thus, case-finding efforts in that group have been warranted.[2,3,39]

The Powers of the Public Health Authorities

Even with the counseling and reporting measures we have recommended for physicians, there are still some patients so irresponsible or mentally incompetent that no voluntary measure is adequate to protect the public health. Isolation and other compulsory measures of infection control have therefore been considered[40,41] and are likely to be considered again.

In many states, patients with tuberculosis who do not follow the infection-control instructions of public health officers may be isolated at home or in an institution. Persons with salmonellosis may not work in occupations involving food handling or direct care of children, the elderly, or patients in hospitals. Local health departments regularly inspect public swimming pools and may close those that are a hazard to health. These and many other similar public health measures are widely used and broadly accepted for the control of diseases other than AIDS. Carefully applied, they should also serve for AIDS.

Public health officials have broad powers to conduct epidemiologic investigations of infectious diseases for well-defined purposes: informing those exposed about the risks of the disease, testing to determine whether exposure has led to infection, and treating patients and contacts to prevent further transmission of disease. Diseases that may affect minors and newborns and diseases with especially severe consequences are given particular attention — whether or not specific preventive measures or treatments are available. Nevertheless, when the prevalence of a pathogen, such as gonorrhea, is very high, the public health authorities may not uniformly trace contacts and intervene, despite the severe risks — such as the risk of gonococcal arthritis or endocarditis and neonatal blindness — to those unsuspectingly exposed. Lacking unlimited resources, the authorities may use other strategies. For example, the statutes mandating treatment of all neonates to prevent ophthalmia neonatorum tacitly acknowledge that epidemiologic measures will not detect all cases of maternal gonorrhea.

Quarantine as a strategy for infection control has generally been used only in individual cases for narrow purposes: to enforce the treatment of a noncompliant patient infected with tuberculosis, to segregate a patient with an untreatable but self-limited disease such as smallpox, or to control the spread of a severe and highly communicable disease such as plague. Quarantine has been used only rarely for patients with sexually transmitted diseases. Long-term quarantine of large populations in isolated communities has been invoked in the 20th century only for leprosy, and that use is now widely thought to have been unjustified.[42]

California's statutory scheme of compulsory measures to protect the public health is typical. Health officers have comprehensive authority to take whatever measures are necessary to prevent the spread of disease, and they have specific authority to order isolation or quarantine of places or persons, including the contacts of a patient. Violation of an order for isolation or quarantine is a misdemeanor.

Although public health officers have in the past been able to order confinement without explanation or review, courts today can be expected to impose the requirements for due process applied to the involuntary commitment of the mentally ill.[43] Los Angeles County, for example, now requires that there be an administrative hearing immediately after confinement if a patient with tuberculosis asks for one.[44] If the authorities want to continue confinement beyond 60 days, they must prove to 9 of 12 jurors at a trial that the patient is still infectious and is a threat to public health because he or she would not reliably participate in a voluntary treatment program.

We know of only two cases in which public health authorities have sought orders of isolation or quarantine against persons infected with the AIDS retroviruses, although we know of homosexual men whose conduct — continued sexual contact with multiple partners, for example — appears to warrant some limitation on their freedom. Balancing the individual's rights to liberty and privacy against the society's interest in limiting the harm caused by a fatal infectious disease raises extraordinarily difficult questions of constitutional law. Compulsory measures of various kinds may or may not be constitutionally justified, depending on what is known about such epidemiologic variables as the mode of transmission, the degree and duration of infectiousness, and the existence of a symptom-free carrier state. If these variables were to reach the worst values, then the courts would be faced, perhaps for the first time, with deciding whether severe invasions of the individual rights of infected persons are justified to protect against the rapid spread of a fatal and incurable disease through the general population.

Isolation or quarantine, like compulsory antibody testing and other means that may be proposed to control the spread of AIDS, must meet a two-part constitutional standard. First, there must be a rational relation between the proposed means of control and the state's legitimate interest in the health of its citizens.[45] Second, there must be no less restrictive means available to protect the community.[46-49] The application of these principles is illustrated by the case of a Florida prostitute with AIDS who was recently confined to her home and ordered to wear an electronic monitor that signaled the police if she strayed more than 200 ft from her telephone.[50] Prostitutes have often been treated harshly by the courts, more harshly than their customers, and are for that reason more likely to bear the brunt of compulsory measures to control the spread of AIDS than others who may present a greater risk of infecting greater numbers. Nevertheless, assuming the facts to be as reported and recognizing that they have not yet been reviewed by a higher court, this woman — proved infectious and persevering in conduct that exposed others to infection — presented a specific danger. Preventing that conduct by a form of house arrest was less restrictive than imprisonment and achieved the public health interest with reasonable efficacy, although maintaining house arrest for a long period would be difficult. We do not suggest that restrictions of this sort should be imposed generally on people who are infectious with the AIDS retroviruses, whether they are prostitutes, homosexual men, or others. Rather, we describe this unusual case to sharpen the analysis of the legal issues.

Because AIDS is fatal and incurable, we expect that the courts will defer greatly to the judgment of the medical community and would uphold severe measures if shown a medical consensus that the measures were necessary and effective. Given facts less stark than those we assumed in the Florida case, however, a consensus on effectiveness — i.e., the constitutional requirement, first, that there be a rational relation between the means of control (with attendant loss of liberty or privacy) and the legitimate end (slowing the spread of AIDS) and, second, that the means should be tailored to that end — may be difficult to demonstrate. Infection with AIDS retroviruses is often widespread in high-risk groups, so isolation of a few infectious persons might not substantially reduce the transmission of the virus. Infectivity may well be lifelong, so isolation might have to continue for many years. And the activities that lead to transmission are private, so the terms of isolation would be very intrusive. All these factors demand caution in considering isolation or quarantine of those who appear to be irresponsible. Certainly, general measures of isolation or quarantine for those infected with the AIDS retroviruses, without regard to confirmed irresponsible conduct by individuals, would be useless as well as constitutionally suspect.

San Francisco's bathhouses have demonstrated both the argument for compulsory measures to control the spread of AIDS and the complexity of the process of formulating such measures. The bathhouses nominally offer, for the price of admission, relaxation in saunas, steam rooms, and hot tubs; but some of them are widely known to facilitate anonymous sexual contact with multiple partners — an ideal circumstance for the transmission of AIDS. Because the San Francisco director of public health has the authority to close any establishment that is a danger to the health of the community, he considered closing all the bathhouses in the city when he concluded that warnings about unsafe practices had not been heeded.[51] Such a sweeping remedy for the problem of the transmission of AIDS might have been attacked on constitutional grounds as not being the least restrictive means to control the spread of the infection at the time. A quarantine of 10,000 persons, for example, was overturned in 1900 because the court found no reasonable relation between the report of nine deaths from bubonic plague and an order by the San Francisco Board of Health confining 10,000 people to the 12 blocks of Chinatown in which they lived, without restricting their activities within the district.[49] In the case of the bathhouses, a more limited regulation was adopted that forbade sexual contact in the baths and required the posting of educational and warning signs.[52] We believe that these measures would easily have withstood legal challenge.

In October 1984, having found that some of the bathhouses were not following the regulations, the San Francisco Health Department ordered the closing of particular bathhouses in which multiple anonymous sexual activity had continued. When owners of the bathhouses defied the order, the city sought an injunction enforcing it, but the California Superior Court in San Francisco refused. Instead, the court ordered specific measures to inhibit sexual practices likely to transmit AIDS; the owners were to remove all doors on bathhouse booths and cubicles, make public all private areas, hire monitors to inspect the premises every 10 minutes, and expel patrons observed to be engaging in high-risk sexual activity as defined by the San Francisco AIDS Foundation — i.e., sexual acts with multiple partners involving the exchange of bodily fluids.[53] The court's decision was a roundabout and probably an ineffective means to block a known disease vector. We believe that the department's order closing particular bathhouses proved to have ignored or defied the less restrictive regulations was lawful and should have been enforced.

The courts' traditional view of permissible restraints on the freedom of persons who are probable sources of infection is exemplified by the 1973 decision of the U.S. Court of Appeals for the Tenth Circuit in *Reynolds* v. *McNichols*.[54,55] The Denver, Colorado, ordinance challenged in *Reynolds* allowed persons arrested for, but not necessarily convicted of, any "offense related to sex" to be detained for 48 hours for examination and treatment. The Denver regulations also authorized the public health officer to order any other person "reasonably suspected" of having a sexually transmitted disease to "walk in" to the Department of Health and Hospitals, presumably for diagnosis and treatment.

In *Reynolds*, the Court of Appeals dismissed the plaintiff's complaint that her constitutional rights had been violated by repeated detentions and walk-in orders and concluded, first, that 48 hours' detention without bail for examination and treatment was a medically reasonable and constitutionally permissible infringement of liberty in the light of the social costs of sexually transmitted diseases and, second, that a rational presumption could be made that those subject to detention were likely to have a sexually transmitted disease.[54]

We do not believe that the conclusions reached in *Reynolds* v. *McNichols* are supportable, because the restraints on individual liberty and privacy imposed outweigh the social costs of the diseases being controlled. The mode of legal analysis, however, is the correct one for deciding what compulsory measures may be justified to identify unknown vectors of AIDS. We must ask whether groups likely to be infectious can be identified through rational criteria without intrusions on their privacy and liberty that are unreasonable in the light of the dangers of AIDS. Requiring patients with syphilis and other sexually transmitted diseases to identify their sexual contacts to public health authorities is common.[56,57] For the reasons discussed above, tracing of contacts of patients with AIDS is currently of limited usefulness.

Some form of mandatory testing, like that announced for the United States armed forces, may be considered for broader populations. Once again, conclusions about the legality of such measures depend on medical facts. Compulsory testing has long been established for syphilis.[54,55] Issuing a marriage license only after a serologic test for syphilis has been considered a reasonable means of limiting the risk of infection to spouses or children, although no data are available on the current contribution of such tests to the control of syphilis; we suspect that it is small.

An acceptable program of compulsory testing for AIDS, however, is far more difficult to devise, both because the usefulness of the test results for purposes other than protecting the blood supply is unknown and because the risk of unreasonable invasions of individual rights is great. Blood samples are not by themselves troublesome, but deciding from whom to take them certainly is. Tests for syphilis, after all, are not administered to all heterosexual men or women. Risk groups for AIDS have been defined, but identifying the members of some groups — intravenous drug users or homosexual men, for example — would be difficult, and the identification process would itself invade privacy. Moreover, the implications of the presence of antibody to the AIDS retroviruses are unclear; in some cases, it may indicate inactive past infection rather than present infectiousness.[13] Finally, there is no consensus on the actions to be taken toward those who have evidence of active infection. For these reasons, we believe that mandatory testing programs should be rejected until their benefits and costs can be better understood. In the meantime, control of the AIDS epidemic must continue to rely on voluntary measures encouraged by vigorous and widespread counseling and education.

References

1. Broder S, Gallo RC. A pathogenic retrovirus (HTLV-III) linked to AIDS. N Engl J Med 1984; 311:1292-7.
2. Levy JA, Hoffman AD, Kramer SM, Landis JA, Shimabukuro JM, Oshiro LS. Isolation of lymphocytopathic retroviruses from San Francisco patients with AIDS. Science 1984; 225:840-3.
3. Laurence J, Brun-Vezinet F, Schutzer SE, et al. Lymphadenopathy-associated viral antibody in AIDS: immune correlations and definition of a carrier state. N Engl J Med 1984; 311:1269-73.
4. Jacobson v. Massachusetts. US Rep 1905; 197:11-39.
5. Mills M. Legal aspects of infectious disease practice: Typhoid Mary and other hazards. Med Times 1983; 111(8):83-6.
6. Curran JW, Lawrence DN, Jaffe H, et al. Acquired immunodeficiency syndrome (AIDS) associated with transfusions. N Engl J Med 1984; 310: 69-75.
7. Jaffe HW, Choi K, Thomas PA, et al. National case-control study of Kaposi's sarcoma and *Pneumocystis carinii* pneumonia in homosexual men. Part 1. Epidemiologic results. Ann Intern Med 1983; 99:145-51.
8. Chamberland ME, Castro KG, Haverkos HW, et al. Acquired immunodeficiency syndrome in the United States: an analysis of cases outside high-incidence groups. Ann Intern Med 1984; 101:617-23.
9. Fauci AS, Masur H, Gelmann EP, Markham PD, Hahn BH, Lane HC. The acquired immunodeficiency syndrome: an update. Ann Intern Med 1985; 102:800-13.
10. Landesman SH, Ginzburg HM, Weiss SH. The AIDS epidemic. N Engl J Med 1985; 312:521-5.
11. Auerbach DM, Darrow WW, Jaffe HW, Curran JW. Cluster of cases of the acquired immune deficiency syndrome: patients linked by sexual contact. Am J Med 1984; 76:487-92.
12. Groopman JE, Salahuddin SZ, Sarngadharan MG, et al. HTLV-III in saliva of people with AIDS-related complex and healthy homosexual men at risk for AIDS. Science 1984; 226:447-9.
13. Weiss SH, Goedert JJ, Sarngadharan MG, et al. Screening test for HTLV-III (AIDS agent) antibodies: specificity, sensitivity, and applications. JAMA 1985; 253:221-5.
14. Update: acquired immunodeficiency syndrome (AIDS) — United States. MMWR 1984; 33:661-2.
15. Hershey N. Putting teeth into the public health reporting laws. Am J Public Health 1976; 66:399-400.
16. Disciplinary action by Board of Medical Quality Assurance for failure to report a reportable infectious disease. California Morbidity. August 11, 1978.
17. Davis v. Rodman. Southwestern Reporter 1921; 227:612-5. (Arkansas).
18. Derrick v. Ontario Community Hospital. California Reporter 1975; 120: 566-72. (Fourth District Court of Appeal).
19. Jones v. Stanko. Northeastern Reporter 1928; 160:456-8. (Ohio Supreme Court).
20. Colorado. Rules and regulations pertaining to communicable disease control. Board of Health, 1985.
21. Lambda Legal Defense and Education Fund, Inc. *AIDS Legal Guide* 1984.
22. Horne v. Patton. Southern Reporter (2nd series) 1973; 287:824-35. (Alabama Supreme Court).
23. Doe v. Roe. New York Supplement (2nd series) 1977; 400:668-80. (Supreme Court, New York County).
24. Schaffer v. Spicer. Northwestern Reporter (2nd series) 1974; 215:134-41. (South Dakota Supreme Court).
25. Skillings v. Allen. Northwestern Reporter 1919; 173:663-5. (Minnesota Supreme Court).
26. Perkins HS, Jonsen AR. Conflicting duties to patients: the case of a sexually active hepatitis B carrier. Ann Intern Med 1981; 94:523-30.
27. Gill v. Hartford Accident & Indemnity Co. Southern Reporter (2nd series) 1978; 337:420-1. (Florida Second District Court of Appeal).
28. Tarasoff v. Regents of the University of California. California Reporter 1976; 131:14-42. (California Supreme Court).
29. Simonsen v. Swensen. Northwestern Reporter 1920; 177:831-3. (Nebraska Supreme Court).
30. United States Department of Health and Human Services, Public Health Service. AIDS Information Bulletin: the Public Health Service response to AIDS. Washington, D.C.: United States Department of Health and Human Services, 1985.
31. Kathleen K. v. Robert B. California Reporter 1984; 198:273-7. (Court of Appeal, Second District).
32. Crowell v. Crowell. Southeastern Reporter 1920; 105:206-14. (North Carolina Supreme Court).
33. American Law Institute. Restatement (Second) of Torts § 892(B) comment e, illustration 5, 1979.
34. Duke v Housen. Pacific Reporter (2nd Series) 1979; 589:334-58. (Wyoming Supreme Court).
35. Prentice RA, Murray PC. Liability for transmission of herpes: using traditional tort principles to encourage honesty in sexual relationships. J Contemp Law 1984; 11:67-103.
36. McPherson M. Hudson estate sued: alleged former lover says actor hid AIDS. The Washington Post. November 13, 1985:B1.
37. Edwards v. Lamb. Atlantic Reporter 1899; 45:480-1. (New Hampshire Supreme Court).
38. Goedert JJ, Sarngadharan MG, Biggar RJ, et al. Determinants of retrovirus (HTLV-III) antibody and immunodeficiency conditions in homosexual men. Lancet 1984; 2:711-6.
39. Hirsch MS, Wormser GP, Schooley RT, et al. Risk of nosocomial infection with human T-cell lymphotropic virus III (HTLV-III). N Engl J Med 1985; 312:1-4.
40. Nichols CD. AIDS — a new reason to regulate homosexuality? J Contemp Law 1984; 11:315-43.
41. Goldstein R. The other AIDS story: quarantine! Village Voice. May 1, 1984:16.
42. Benenson AS, ed. Control of communicable diseases in man. 13th ed. Washington, D.C.: American Public Health Association, 1980:192.
43. Greene v. Edwards. Southeastern Reporter (2nd series) 1980; 263:661-4. (West Virginia Supreme Court of Appeals).
44. Balderas v. Pitchess. California Superior Court, Los Angeles County. (No. CA 000617).
45. Camara v. Municipal Court. United States Reports 1967; 387:523-40.
46. Rock v. Carney. Michigan Reports 1921; 216:280-91. (Supreme Court).
47. Barmore v. Robertson. Northeastern Reporter 1922; 134:815-21. (Illinois Supreme Court).
48. Rennie v. Klein. Federal Reporter (2nd Series) 1981; 653:836-70. (Third Circuit Court of Appeals).
49. Jew Ho v. Williamson. Federal Reporter 1900; 103:10-27. (Northern District of California Circuit Court).
50. Hooker with AIDS confined. Daily News. September 28, 1985:5.
51. Fain N, Goldstein R. Will San Francisco close the baths? Village Voice. April 10, 1984:18.
52. Collier S. Preventing the spread of AIDS by restricting sexual conduct in gay bathhouses: a Constitutional analysis. Golden Gate L Rev 1985: 301-30.
53. People v. Owen. California Superior Court, San Francisco County, November 28, 1984. (No. 830321).
54. Reynolds v. McNichols. Federal Reporter (2nd Series) 1973; 488:1378-86. (Tenth Circuit Court of Appeals).
55. Curran WJ. Venereal disease detention and treatment: prostitution and civil rights. Am J Public Health 1975; 65:180-1.
56. People v. Strautz. Northeastern Reporter (2nd Series) 1944; 54:441-5. (Illinois Supreme Court).
57. Wragg v. Griffin. Northwestern Reporter. 1919; 170:400-3. (Iowa Supreme Court).

SPECIAL REPORT

PREFERENCES OF HOMOSEXUAL MEN WITH AIDS FOR LIFE-SUSTAINING TREATMENT

Robert Steinbrook, M.D., Bernard Lo, M.D., Jeffrey Moulton, Ph.D., Glenn Saika, M.A., Harry Hollander, M.D., and Paul A. Volberding, M.D.

THE acquired immunodeficiency syndrome (AIDS) raises questions about appropriate care for patients with this incurable and progressive disease. Although individual episodes of infection and malignant disease can be treated, the underlying immune deficit cannot now be reversed. Decisions about whether to undertake life-sustaining treatment, such as mechanical ventilation and cardiopulmonary resuscitation, must frequently be made. Because these decisions require value judgments and informed consent as well as technical expertise, they should be made jointly by physicians and patients.[1-3]

The care of patients with AIDS also illustrates the usefulness of advance directives about life-sustaining treatment. Many patients with AIDS become mentally incompetent and unable to participate in decisions about their care. It has been recommended that patients provide advance directives to guide their care if they become incompetent.[4] These directives may take the form of discussions with physicians, friends, or family members; a living will; or a durable power of attorney for health care, which allows the competent patient to designate a proxy to make decisions about medical care if he or she should become incompetent to make such decisions.

For incompetent patients, the traditional approach is shared decision making by the physician and the family, following the patient's previously expressed wishes.[3] Many patients with AIDS, however, want their partners or friends, not family members, to make the necessary decisions with their physicians. Yet the patient's partner or friend has no legal standing to make decisions unless designated as a proxy through a durable power of attorney for health care.

Little is known about the preferences of patients with AIDS for life-sustaining treatment and their use of advance directives. We surveyed 118 homosexual male outpatients with AIDS in order to answer these questions: (1) Had they thought about life-sustaining treatment? (2) What were their preferences about life-sustaining treatment? (3) How did they react to thinking about life-sustaining treatment? (4) What were their preferences for discussing such treatment with physicians? and (5) Were patients providing advance directives to guide care?

Methods

The study was conducted between January and May 1985 at the outpatient AIDS clinics at San Francisco General Hospital and the University of California, San Francisco. The San Francisco General Hospital clinic cares for approximately 50 percent of homosexual men with AIDS in San Francisco and is a major referral center.

Patients eligible for the study were homosexual men who met the criteria of the Centers for Disease Control for the diagnosis of AIDS[5,6] and who came to the clinics on selected days. Eligible patients were identified through a review of their medical records and by the clinic staff. Patients were excluded if they declined to take part or if they were visiting the clinic for the first time. New patients were asked to participate during a subsequent visit.

After giving informed consent, patients completed a 15-minute self-administered, closed-response questionnaire. The questionnaire asked patients whom they wanted to designate to make decisions about their health care if they became too sick to make decisions themselves and what specific care they would want. The questionnaire is available from the authors upon request. Specific topics included (1) how much patients had thought about life-sustaining treatment; (2) preferences for treatment of *Pneumocystis carinii* pneumonia, the most common opportunistic infection in AIDS and a frequent cause of death (patients were asked about hospitalization, intensive care and mechanical ventilation, and cardiopulmonary resuscitation for both a first and a subsequent episode of *P. carinii* pneumonia); (3) preferences for the treatment of severe *P. carinii* pneumonia and severe memory loss, with "no chance" that their condition would improve; (4) emotional responses to thinking or talking about life-sustaining treatment; (5) preferences for discussions with physicians about life-sustaining treatment and perceptions of physician's interest in such discussions; (6) preferences for substitute decision makers if they were unable to make decisions themselves; (7) whether patients had talked to their physicians, partners, friends, or family members about life-sustaining treatment, completed living wills, or executed durable powers of attorney for health care; (8) estimates of the survival to hospital discharge of patients with *P. carinii* pneumonia who require intubation and mechanical ventilation, both for a first and for a subsequent episode; and (9) the consistency of patient's preferences over time.

The questionnaire also asked about demographic variables, such as education and employment; medical variables, such as previous hospitalizations and functional status; psychological variables, such as depression and social support; and social variables, such as involvement in a primary relationship and the parents' knowledge of and attitudes toward the patient's sexual preference. Information about each patient's age, diagnoses, date of diagnosis of AIDS, and previous hospitalizations was collected from medical records. Participation was voluntary and did not affect patient care. To minimize bias, we worded the questions so that all answers, such as a desire for more or less care, seemed equally acceptable.

The study and the questionnaire were approved by the Committee on Human Research at the University of California, San Francisco. A code was used to maintain the confidentiality of the data. Physicians were unaware of their patients' responses. Student's t-tests and chi-square analyses were used to assess the statistical significance of differences between groups of patients.

In testing for factors associated with dependent variables, we used the following independent variables: demographic variables (time since diagnosis, education, and employment); medical variables (prior hospitalizations, prior hospitalization in the intensive care unit, diagnosis of *P. carinii* pneumonia, and ability to walk one block or climb one flight of stairs); psychological variables (depression, number of close friends and relatives, and number of friends who had been hospitalized or had died from AIDS); and social variables (involvement in a primary relationship and the parents' knowledge of and attitudes toward the patient's sexual preference).

Supported in part by a grant from the University of California Task Force on AIDS.

Results

Patients' Characteristics

Questionnaires were completed by 118 male patients, 112 from San Francisco General Hospital and 6 from the University of California, San Francisco. Three patients declined to participate. The majority of the patients were young, well educated, and severely ill (Table 1). Most of their friends and parents knew they were homosexual.

Consideration of Life-Sustaining Treatment

Seventy-eight percent of the patients had thought a lot or a moderate amount about what care they would want if they had *P. carinii* pneumonia. Sixty-six percent had thought a lot or a moderate amount about whom they wanted to designate to make medical decisions for them if they were unable to do so themselves. Nine percent of patients had changed their minds about life-sustaining treatment, and 22 percent had changed their minds about substitute decision makers.

Table 1. Characteristics of 118 Homosexual Male Patients with AIDS.

Mean age, yr (range)	35 (22–55)
Months since diagnosis (range)	10 (2–39)
Underlying illness (%)	
P. carinii	56
Kaposi's sarcoma	53
Hospitalization (%)	
Within past 12 months	73
In intensive care unit	12
Functional status (%)	
Unemployed or disabled	73
Trouble walking 1 block or climbing 1 flight of stairs	32
Education (%)	
High-school graduate	97
College graduate	55
Parental attitude (%)*	
Definitely knew patient was homosexual	90
Highly or mostly accepting	73
Friends knew patient was homosexual (%)	93
In primary relationship (%)	36
Depressed (%)	35

*Percentage among patients whose parents were living (n = 98).

Preferences for Treatment of Pneumocystis

Ninety-five percent of the patients wanted hospitalization and antibiotic treatment for *P. carinii* pneumonia, 55 percent wanted admission to the intensive care unit and mechanical ventilation, and 46 percent wanted cardiopulmonary resuscitation. There were no significant differences in the preferences of patients for care of first or subsequent episodes of *P. carinii* pneumonia. No demographic, medical, psychological, or social variables predicted patients' preferences for intensive care and mechanical ventilation. If they acquired both severe memory loss and severe *P. carinii* pneumonia, 19 percent of patients wanted intensive care and intubation, and 17 percent wanted cardiopulmonary resuscitation.

Table 2. Emotional Reactions of the 118 Patients to Discussing Life-Sustaining Treatment.

Reaction	Percent*
In control of things	56
Cared for	47
Anxious	44
Sad	40
Relieved	33
"It's all over"	19
Giving up	12

*Most patients gave multiple responses.

One patient poignantly stated his anguish and ambivalence about life-sustaining treatment:

> I switch back and forth in my view. On the one hand, I do not want to die in the hospital and am terrified of dying on a respirator. On the other hand, if there were a chance for recovery, I would equate the decision not to go on with suicide. . . . I don't have any hope anymore that something is going to be found to cure me before I die. . . . I sometimes wish I would get run over by a bus before I have to face these problems.

Emotional Reactions to Discussing Life-Sustaining Treatment

Patients had ambivalent but generally positive reactions to discussing life-sustaining treatment (Table 2). One patient commented, "I hope physicians everywhere will remember they are dealing with real people and not with plastic dolls they can manipulate at whim. I am frightened, but not of death. Rather, I am frightened of being helpless."

Preferences for Discussing Life-Sustaining Treatment with Physicians

Although 73 percent of patients wanted to discuss life-sustaining treatment with their physicians, only one third had done so. No demographic, medical, psychological, or social variables predicted which patients wanted such discussions. In particular, patients with negative emotional reactions to discussing life-sustaining treatment wanted such discussions as often as other patients.

Patients with *P. carinii* pneumonia had discussed life-sustaining treatment more often than patients who did not have the disease (33 percent vs. 13 percent, chi-square = 6.11, $P<0.01$). No other independent variable identified the patients who had had discussed life-sustaining treatment with their physicians.

Of the patients who wanted such discussions, 58 percent said the patient should initiate them and 36 percent said the physician should do so. Sixty-nine percent of these patients wanted to discuss life-sustaining treatment as outpatients, after getting to know their physicians; 54 percent wanted such discussions in the hospital when they were seriously ill; 37 percent, on hospital admission; and 24 percent, when AIDS was diagnosed.

Preferences for Substitute Decision Makers

Forty-seven percent of patients wanted their partners or friends to act as substitute decision makers if they became incompetent, 32 percent wanted family members, and 14 percent wanted their physicians. Patients whose parents were only somewhat or not at all accepting of their homosexuality wanted their partners or friends to be the decision makers more often than patients whose parents were more accepting (73 percent vs. 39 percent; chi-square = 9.39, P<0.01). One patient commented, "I used to feel my parents were always the ones to make decisions if I got really sick. Now I feel my best friend is more qualified because he sees me all the time and knows my wishes better than my parents."

Advance Directives

Two thirds of the patients had provided advance directives to guide care if they became mentally incompetent (Table 3). Patients who had been hospitalized in the past year were more likely to have discussed life-sustaining treatment with their families than those who had not (49 percent vs. 19 percent; chi-square = 7.25, P<0.01) and were more likely to have completed a living will (38 percent vs. 15 percent; chi-square = 4.59, P<0.05).

Of all the patients, 28 percent had executed a durable power of attorney for health care. This group included 42 percent of patients who wanted their partners or friends to act as decision makers, 41 percent of patients who had thought a lot or a moderate amount about substitute decision makers, 40 percent of patients who did not want intensive care for pneumocystis, 37 percent of patients who had pneumocystis, and 34 percent of patients who had been hospitalized during the previous year. Patients who had executed a durable power of attorney were in the minority in all subgroups.

Estimates of Prognosis for *P. carinii* Pneumonia

Patients overestimated the survival of patients with pneumocystis who required intubation (Fig. 1). They gave a mean estimate (±SD) of 53±23 percent for the proportion of patients surviving to discharge after a first episode of *P. carinii* pneumonia requiring intubation, and one of 30±23 percent for the proportion

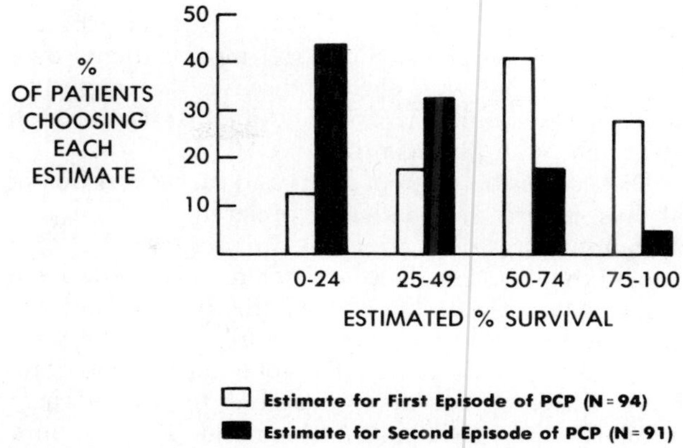

Figure 1. Patients' Estimates of Prognosis in Cases of *P. carinii* Pneumonia (PCP) Requiring Intubation.

surviving a second episode. The reported survival rate is 14 percent.[7] Patients' estimates of survival were not significantly associated with their preferences for life-sustaining treatment or with the diagnosis of *P. carinii* pneumonia.

Discussion

Increasingly, physicians and patients must decide what treatment is appropriate for chronic, progressive, and incurable diseases such as AIDS. Patients with AIDS may have advantages in reaching decisions about life-sustaining treatment, because they are often young, previously healthy, and well educated and because they often take an active role in decisions about their medical care. They are an important group for studying the preferences of patients for life-sustaining treatment and the feasibility of advance directives.

AIDS is a new disease, and knowledge of its pathophysiology is rapidly increasing. When our understanding of a disease is incomplete and alternative treatments seem equally acceptable, the preferences of the patient may be even more important than in the case of diseases for which prognosis and therapy are well established.[8] In *P. carinii* pneumonia, as noted earlier, survival to hospital discharge after intubation is 14 percent.[7] Some patients may consider the possibility of additional weeks or months of life to be worth intensive treatment; other patients may desire only supportive care. Furthermore, some patients with AIDS may want experimental therapy, in the hope that a therapeutic breakthrough will reverse their disease.

Our results refute several common objections to discussing life-sustaining treatment with patients. These objections include the following: (1) patients have not thought about life-sustaining treatment and advance directives; (2) patients do not want such discussions; (3) patients have negative emotional reactions to such discussions; and (4) patients' preferences for care can be predicted without discussions. We found that most patients had thought about care for *P. carinii* pneumo-

Table 3. Advance Directives for Life-Sustaining Treatment among the 118 Patients.

Type of Directive	Percent*
Discussion with family	42
Discussion with partner	69†
Living will	31
Durable power of attorney for health care	27
Discussion with physician	24
No advance directive	33

*Some patients provided more than one form of advance directive.
†Percentage of patients in a primary relationship (n = 42).

nia and advance directives and wanted to discuss them with physicians. Similarly, most patients over the age of 65 or with chronic diseases that might require life-sustaining treatment want to discuss such treatment with physicians.[9]

Discussions between patients and care givers do not always ensure that patients' preferences about life-sustaining treatment are elicited or respected.[10-12] In one study, 4 of 136 decisions not to resuscitate were made against the wishes of the patient or the family.[11] In another study, patients or family members were involved in 83 percent of decisions not to resuscitate but in only 25 percent of decisions to resuscitate.[12] Similarly, living wills are problematic. They are ambiguous, inflexible, and legally binding only in limited situations.

The durable power of attorney for health care has advantages over other advance directives because it is flexible and gives legal sanction to shared decisions by physicians and proxies.[4] Patients with AIDS would particularly benefit from it if they had strong preferences about life-sustaining treatment or wanted their lovers or friends, rather than family members, to make decisions for them. Without the durable power of attorney, partners and friends have no legal standing in sharing decisions with physicians. In our study, however, less than half the patients who wanted their partners or friends to be substitute decision makers had executed durable powers of attorney for health care.

We also found that many patients overestimated the effectiveness of life-sustaining treatments. This finding should not discourage physicians from discussing life-sustaining treatment with patients. Rather, it emphasizes the need for repeated discussions with patients, beginning in the outpatient setting. Physicians can elicit patients' questions, provide counseling and education, and make sure patients' directives are consistent and realistic. Listening to patients, discussing their concerns, and stressing supportive care may be helpful to patients with chronic incurable disease. Physicians may also bring the durable power of attorney for health care to the attention of their patients.

It is unclear why so many patients who wanted to discuss life-sustaining treatment with physicians had not done so. It seems plausible to suggest that some patients were less likely than others to act on their desire to have such discussions — for example, those who perceived their physicians as insensitive, awkward, or too busy, those who did not have pneumocystis, those who had never been hospitalized, or those who had had AIDS for only a short period. Our data, however, do not support these hypotheses, although the number of patients in some analyses was small. The nature of the barriers to discussion is not clear, but several factors may have an effect. Outpatients may deny the gravity of their illness, for instance, or may fear abandonment if care is limited. Another possible barrier is diffusion of responsibility among many care givers.[13] Since patients may find it difficult to change their traditionally passive role,[14] care givers may wish to initiate discussions about these sensitive issues.

Our study has several limitations. First, our conclusions may not be generalizable. San Francisco General Hospital is a major referral center for patients with AIDS. San Francisco has an active homosexual community and special resources for AIDS patients, including volunteer counseling and legal support. Such resources may encourage patients to think about life-sustaining treatment and to provide advance directives for care. Moreover, our conclusions may not apply to patients with AIDS who are not homosexual. Second, our study is based primarily on patients' own reports, which may not always be accurate. For example, patients may have forgotten previous discussions of life-sustaining treatment with their physicians. In further studies, researchers may wish to interview care givers or to observe interactions between doctors and patients. Third, the preferences of patients may change over time — for example, when their disease progresses and they are hospitalized. Our cross-sectional study could not determine how frequently such change occurs. A prospective cohort study could provide information on changes in patients' preferences over time. Fourth, the power of our study to detect associations was limited by the sample size. Fifth, because of multiple comparisons, some associations may appear statistically significant when in fact they are based only on chance.

In conclusion, our study suggests that most patients with this fatal progressive illness have thought about life-sustaining treatment, have preferences about their care, and want to discuss life-sustaining treatment with their physicians. However, many patients have not provided advance directives, including some who might benefit from the durable power of attorney for health care. Many patients also have misconceptions about the effectiveness of life-sustaining treatment, even though they are well educated and live in a city where their illness is widely publicized. We suggest that physicians who care for patients with AIDS and other serious chronic illnesses should take an active role in educating patients about life-sustaining treatment and inviting them to provide advance directives.

References

1. Jonsen AR, Siegler M, Winslade WJ. Clinical ethics. New York: Macmillan, 1982:109-24.
2. Lo B, Steinbrook RL. Deciding whether to resuscitate. Arch Intern Med 1983; 143:1561-3.
3. President's Commission for the Study of Ethical Problems in Medicine and Biomedical and Behavioral Research. Deciding to forego life-sustaining treatment. Washington: U.S. Government Printing Office, 1983.
4. Steinbrook R, Lo B. Decision making for incompetent patients by designated proxy: California's new law. N Engl J Med 1984; 310:1598-601.
5. Update: acquired immune deficiency syndrome (AIDS) — United States. MMWR 1984; 32:688-91.
6. Selik RM, Haverkos HW, Curran JW. Acquired immune deficiency syndrome (AIDS) trends in the United States, 1978-1982. Am J Med 1984; 76:493-500.
7. Murray JF, Felton CP, Garay SM, et al. Pulmonary complications of the acquired immunodeficiency syndrome: report of a National Heart, Lung, and Blood Institute workshop. N Engl J Med 1984; 310:1682-8.

8. Kassirer JP, Pauker SG. The toss-up. N Engl J Med 1981; 305:1467-9.
9. Lo B, McLeod G, Saika G. Patient attitudes to discussing life-sustaining treatment. Clin Res 1985; 33:258A. abstract.
10. Youngner SJ, Lewandowski W, McClish DK, Juknialis BW, Coulton C, Bartlett ET. 'Do not resuscitate' orders: incidence and implications in a medical intensive care unit. JAMA 1985; 253:54-7.
11. Lo B, Saika G, Strull W, Thomas E, Showstack J. 'Do not resuscitate' decisions: a prospective study at three teaching hospitals. Arch Intern Med 1985; 145:1115-7.
12. Evans AL, Brody BA. The do-not-resuscitate order in teaching hospitals. JAMA 1985; 253:2236-9.
13. Lidz CW, Meisel A, Osterweis M, Holden JL, Marx JH, Munetz MR. Barriers to informed consent. Ann Intern Med 1983; 99:539-43.
14. Greenfield S, Kaplan S, Ware JE Jr. Expanding patient involvement in care: effects on patient outcomes. Ann Intern Med 1985; 102:520-8.

SOUNDING BOARD

THE AIDS EPIDEMIC: MULTIDISCIPLINARY TROUBLE*

JUNE E. OSBORN, M.D.

IN this essay I shall try to summarize in mid-course the status of a unique series of events in human history, which involves virtually all facets of modern knowledge but is usually referred to simply as the acquired immunodeficiency syndrome (AIDS) epidemic. Humanity has embarked on a mortal race with a novel pathogen of great subtlety. If this were ancient Greece and I an oracle, my task would be simpler. The fiendishness implicit in the mode of pathogenicity of the AIDS virus could be appreciated as eminently suitable for an instrument of the gods, and the potential inadequacy of society's response to the epidemic would be deemed appropriate punishment for the hubris that allowed the natural sciences to get so far ahead of the social and behavioral sciences. Perhaps the fact that would most amuse the gods is the ostensible ease of preventing further spread: the virus causing AIDS is, for the moment, a pathogenetic weakling that is truly difficult to transmit except by sexual routes.

But, knowing what we know, we cripple ourselves in Sophoclean fashion. The people at greatest risk of becoming infected — homosexual men — have been beleaguered by society to such an extent that they may evade or ignore the efforts to control the spread of AIDS. The members of the second highest risk group — intravenous drug abusers — have already said goodbye to cautious mores and are probably refractory to instructions concerning their own salvation, let alone that of others.

And the people in charge have a truncated vocabulary: the very messages that we must broadcast in order to abort the epidemic and buy time for further scientific advance require the use of words that are taboo in high places. We need urgently to pursue so-called psychosocial research — but we may not be "explicit," and we may not, in fact, send out messages that even seem to condone sexual and other practices that deviate from a governmentally sanctioned norm. No official document should use the phrase "safe sex," even if that currently appears to be the major promising route to safety for an important segment of the population. Well may the gods laugh!

We in the United States have a world-class epidemic on our hands, which we have exported so effectively that the rest of the world is only a little bit behind us. The 14,000 Americans in whom AIDS has been diagnosed to date are only the most unlucky of the more than half a million people in the United States who are already infected with the new virus,[1] and yet the first round of cases has already strained our human and societal resources. Nearly half of those diagnosed as having AIDS are dead, and their deaths have been distinctly unpeaceful. A few of them were unfortunate souls who needed blood transfusions, usually for urgent surgical reasons, which turned out to be the vehicle for viral transmission. Others were embarked on an illegal dash to intravenous chemical suicide, which was only hastened by microbial intervention. But most of them were talented young men who had chosen atypical life styles for their own personal — perhaps biologic — reasons. We should remind ourselves that among the dying may be the Tchaikovskys and Prousts of our time — dying before the flower of their creativity has enjoyed even brief bloom.

The outlines of the economic impact of the epidemic are just beginning to emerge, and the specter is terrible to contemplate. It is useful, in order to appreciate the economic trouble to come, to think of *every single case* of AIDS as costing the same as a heart transplantation, and for roughly the same reasons. By unhappy chance, the health care industry had been launched by Congress into a vigorous effort at cost containment through the vehicle of diagnosis-related groups (DRGs) just before the gods struck! My economist friends tell me that the strategy for creating a DRG for AIDS has yet to be designed and the situation is fairly chaotic at present. If we sense trouble now, however, we should remember that a substantial fraction of the patients who have already been given the diagnosis of AIDS have died, and so the anticipated doubling in numbers of patients diagnosed in the next year will have far more than twice the impact on the health care industry — all the more so, since the majority of cases are concentrated in just a few cities. No tropical storm has the economically devastating potential of the new cases of AIDS expected in the next few years, and yet I have read only an occasional suggestion that disaster funds should be made available for the AIDS hurricane now gathering force.[2]

There is a politically interesting aspect of the epidemic that has thus far been mercifully obscure. Although the virus causing AIDS is surely American by adoption, not by birth (the most likely location of transfer to the human species is in Central Africa[3]), the epidemic is indeed all-American in its initial dissemination. Most of the rest of the world is catching up with us, with a lag time of two or three years,[4] but the exportations from the United States are easily tracked. We are indeed one world in operational — if not in peaceful — terms. A recent paper from Japan, for instance, documented the absence of antibody from a number of Japanese groups, including homosexuals, but reported 27 percent seropositivity among

*An abridged version of a paper read before the Institute of Medicine, National Academy of Sciences, Washington, D.C., on October 16, 1985.

patients with hemophilia, which was directly related to the American source of the factor VIII and IX concentrates used to treat them.[5] The introduction of AIDS into Denmark and Australia was readily traceable to the return of homosexual men from vacations in New York and San Francisco.[6]

Even the presence of the poor Haitians in the high-risk category may reflect the penchant of American homosexual men for vacationing in Haiti, coupled with the dire poverty that makes prostitution a frequent means of subsistence survival for Haitian adolescents of either sex. A recent analysis of the distribution of infection in Haiti showed a typical frequency of human T-cell lymphotropic virus, Type III, antibody in the general population, contrasting with a markedly higher frequency in areas known to be centers for prostitution, male and female alike.[7]

Scientifically, the news is better; in fact, the news would be really good if we were more able to put known facts to use. The progress of biomedical science in the forced march of the AIDS epidemic has been truly spectacular and is worthy of admiration and, I suppose, a bit of international self-congratulation. Extraordinary scientific effort does not always lead to extraordinary progress, but in this case it has. Witness the incredible speed with which the virus was isolated — in three separate laboratories in France and the United States.[8-10] Note also that less than a year elapsed from viral isolation and establishment of a highly productive cell-culture system to systematic and thorough screening of blood on a massive scale.[11] Reassuringly, the entire enterprise was carefully monitored and regulated by a state-of-the-art cadre of scientists at the Food and Drug Administration. Those are scientific and logistic accomplishments of unprecedented magnitude. I think it is safe to say that humankind has never responded so quickly and thus far so effectively to a novel medical challenge.

It is interesting to note that the science leading up to the recognition of the epidemic represented very recent advances in immunology, including definition of lymphocyte subsets, sophisticated analyses of T-cell physiology, and elegant dissection of lymphokines and their roles in response to diverse stimuli and stresses. As it turns out, the immune response is an exquisitely modulated system of checks and balances, and yet without the insights derived from the immunologic advances of the '60s and '70s, we might have failed to identify AIDS for a dangerously long period. A colleague of mine has a little sign on his bulletin board that says, "The first step to solving a problem is to see it clearly." I believe we should all feel some reassurance that the technologic advances of the past two or three decades are at least allowing us to see this problem clearly in scientific terms.

First of all, the AIDS virus is really a poor pathogen in terms of its communicability. The human race would be gone by now if syphilis had been more adept at dissemination, and the AIDS virus is even less effectual in that heterosexual transmission is inefficient.[12] If we could put into action the knowledge we have gained from epidemiologic study, we could forecast an end to the trouble, or at least an end to the further spread of the virus. However, we must keep in mind that the AIDS virus is a new pathogen; although the general trend of new human microbes is thought to be toward settling down and domesticating further, we have almost no experience to justify that theoretical expectation. On evolutionary grounds, it behooves a successful parasite not to "make waves," and with that in mind one could argue that the new virus is likely to become less transmissible and less virulent. But evolution takes a very long time, and humanity has known this virus for less than 30 years.

Turning to virology and immunology, hopes and possible disappointments loom in equal measure. Animal models of retrovirus vaccines have begun to show some promise: with ornate chemical manipulation one can create a subunit vaccine of feline leukemia virus that will protect kittens against future viral challenge.[13] But the virus of AIDS has some nasty properties, even for a retrovirus. Like Kipling's leopard, it changes its antigenic spots at frequent intervals, perhaps enough to evade previously evoked immune responses.[14] That kind of antigenic variation is familiar to students of the parasitic world; many of the pervasive and successful eukaryotic parasites of humans have antigenic variation as a major pathogenetic mechanism. But the public is accustomed to more stable viral threats; the viruses causing measles, mumps, polio, and rabies all vary slightly at the molecular level but, mercifully, have remained in categorically exact array for purposes of vaccines. Not so the new retrovirus, and thus a new variable must be introduced into vaccine parlance.

Another worry lies in the relative difficulty of identifying antibodies that actually neutralize the virus of AIDS (the antibodies measured in the test now used are indicative of viral infection but are very weak in their capacity to render the virus noninfectious). It is possible that monoclonal technology will help to identify epitopes on parts of antigenic molecules that pervade the immune response to many variants and might be more effective in neutralization. There are precedents for those situations in other retrovirus infections, and I have confidence that solutions can be found, but the science isn't easy, to say the least.

Before I leave the topic of potential vaccines, however, I must make two further points, one scientific and one practical. Scientifically, there is a fundamental cause for concern about a vaccine for this virus, since the cellular receptor that the virus requires to initiate infection is in fact the receptor for the T-cell antigen.[15] The reason for the devastation of AIDS is the lethal viral effect on T cells, which are required for an effective immune response to foreign antigens, and one must be careful not to harm those cells in attempting immunization.

On a practical note, there is room for much skepticism about the advent of a vaccine any time soon.

Even if a vaccine were at hand, the logistics of testing it would be hard to imagine. In order to establish protective efficacy, one would need a group of willing, thoroughly informed research subjects at high risk but as yet unexposed. The slowness of the viral infection would make assessment of both efficacy and safety a tremendous challenge, and the liability problems would be vast. Who would want to manufacture such a vaccine? To whom would it be given? High-risk groups? The general public? If we can't cope with pertussis, how can we manage a vaccine for the AIDS virus? Remembering the attempted mass immunization against swine flu, many of us shiver when the possibility of a vaccine is regarded as a panacea.

Let us turn now to hopes for treatment and cure. For those already ill with AIDS, the AIDS-related complex, or the lymphadenopathy syndrome, much of the damage is done. The DNA equivalent of the viral genome is intricately woven into their own cellular DNA, and their immune systems have been wounded, possibly beyond repair. There have been some elegant efforts to reconstitute or augment what is left of these patients' immune responsiveness, but the results have not been encouraging. I believe that the largest hope for intervention lies in understanding the role of various cofactors in determining whether a person remains asymptomatically infected or goes on to the development of lethal disease. From the beginning of the epidemic there have been hints that other infections, drugs, and life-style characteristics have contributed to the occurrence of AIDS in the populations at highest risk, and it will be crucial to understand the importance of such factors in order to counsel the hundreds of thousands of people we believe to be asymptomatically infected at present.

I realize that my remarks are gloomy, but I do believe we are in serious trouble. However, some events of the past few years are sources of optimism. First, the perceived impossibility of behavioral modification has been given the lie by the sharp downturn in indicator infections, such as gonorrhea, in homosexual populations in recent months. Second, assuming that we can get the present epidemic under control, much of the scientific progress made under such urgent conditions is likely to be relevant in other biomedical contexts. Intensive study of the retroviruses has yielded insights about oncogenes, cellular and molecular replication, and malignant change that may have a huge yield in our understanding of cancer and of cellular differentiation. Information gleaned from increasingly fine dissection of the immune response is already proving useful in analyses of aging. Some of the chronic diseases most frustrating to researchers, such as rheumatoid arthritis and lupus erythematosus, may be close to yielding to the advances spinning off from research on AIDS. And finally, the observation that the AIDS virus takes privileged sanctuary in the central nervous system[16] may add insight about the causes of chronic neurologic diseases.

In the meantime, we must communicate patiently and clearly to a frightened public what we know and what we are learning. As always happens in times of panic, fringe groups are arising to raise the level of static and make the message hard to hear, and we will have to shout our message of prevention. The ongoing epidemic of smoking has taught us that prevention as a strategy is peculiarly hard to sell as long as treatment and cure are bandied about as alternatives, so we must be very sure not to dilute the message with false or distant hopes.

Once again, preventive medicine — in its drab and unattractive garb — turns out to be the solution. I often like to point out that, if you "do" preventive medicine and public health exactly right, exactly nothing happens and things are very dull. Let us all pray for a little boredom.

References

1. Curran JW, Morgan WM, Hardy AM, Jaffe HW, Darrow WW, Dowdle WR. The epidemiology of AIDS: current status and future prospects. Science 1985; 229:1352-7.
2. Groopman JE, Detsky AS. Epidemic of the acquired immunodeficiency syndrome: a need for economic and social planning. Ann Intern Med 1982; 99:259-61.
3. Saxinger WC, Levine PH, Dean AG, et al. Evidence for exposure to HTLV-III in Uganda before 1973. Science 1985; 227:1036-8.
4. Update: acquired immunodeficiency syndrome — Europe. MMWR 1985; 34:583-9.
5. Tsuchie H, Kurimura T, Hinuma Y. Survey of the prevalence of AIDS-associated virus (LAV) infection in Japan. J Infect 1985; 10:272-6.
6. Melbye M, Biggar RJ, Ebbesen P, et al. Seroepidemiology of HTLV-III antibody in Danish homosexual men: prevalence, transmission, and disease outcome. Br Med J 1984; 289:573-5.
7. Landesman SH, Ginzburg HM, Weiss SH. The AIDS epidemic. N Engl J Med 1985; 312:521-5.
8. Barré-Sinoussi F, Chermann JC, Rey F, et al. Isolation of a T-lymphotropic retrovirus from a patient at risk for acquired immune deficiency syndrome (AIDS). Science 1983; 220:868-70.
9. Gallo, RC, Salahuddin SZ, Popovic M, et al. Frequent detection and isolation of cytopathic retroviruses (HTLV-III) from patients with AIDS and at risk for AIDS. Science 1984; 224:500-3.
10. Levy JA, Hoffman AD, Kramer SM, Landis JA, Shimabukuro JM, Oshiro LS. Isolation of lymphocytopathic retroviruses from San Francisco patients with AIDS. Science 1984; 225:840-2.
11. Council on Scientific Affairs. Status report on the acquired immunodeficiency syndrome: human T-cell lymphotropic virus type III testing. JAMA 1985; 254:1342-5.
12. Heterosexual transmission of human T-lymphotropic virus type III/lymphadenopathy-associated virus. MMWR 1985; 34:561-3.
13. Osterhaus A, Weijer K, Uytedehaag F, Jarrett O, Sundquist B, Morein B. Induction of protective immune response in cats by vaccination with feline leukemia virus iscom. J Immunol 1985; 135:591-6.
14. Wong-Staal F, Shaw GM, Hahn BH, et al. Genomic diversity of human T-lymphotropic virus type III (HTLV-III). Science 1985; 229:759-62.
15. Kalish RS, Schlossman SF. The T4 lymphocyte in AIDS. N Engl J Med 1985; 313:112-3.
16. Levy JA, Holander H, Shimabukuro J, Mills J, Kaminsky L. Isolation of AIDS-associated retroviruses from cerebrospinal fluid and brain of patients with neurological symptoms. Lancet 1985; 2:586-8.

SOUNDING BOARD

THE IMPACT OF THE ACQUIRED IMMUNODEFICIENCY SYNDROME ON MEDICAL RESIDENCY TRAINING

Robert M. Wachter, M.D.

In the past five years, the acquired immunodeficiency syndrome (AIDS) has proved to be a devastating and as yet incurable illness. My own introduction to the syndrome came in 1982, when I was a third-year medical student on my initial rotation in internal medicine. On the previous evening, our team had admitted a young homosexual man with a bizarre history of progressive wasting, fevers, shortness of breath, and new infiltrates on a chest film. My attending physician, having recently read reports of a new (as yet unnamed) syndrome,[1,2] noted that "this *thing* is changing the way we practice medicine."

Now, almost five years later, I am completing my residency in internal medicine in a university setting. Like many of today's interns and residents training in San Francisco, New York, and Los Angeles, I have cared for many more patients with *Pneumocystis carinii* pneumonia than with pneumococcal pneumonia, more patients with Kaposi's sarcoma than with breast cancer, and more patients with cryptococcal meningitis than with meningococcal meningitis. There is a whole generation of residents at certain urban medical centers around the country whose training has been profoundly altered by AIDS. This realization has prompted me to consider the impact of AIDS on medical residency training.

Practical Aspects

Workload

At San Francisco General Hospital, a major center for the care of patients with AIDS, the number of AIDS-related admissions per quarter has increased eightfold over the past two years. In the first quarter of 1985, there were 156 such admissions to the medical service, accounting for about one fourth of all medical admissions. The experience at other teaching hospitals in many of the nation's urban centers has been similar.

Since patients with AIDS come from subgroups that previously had very low rates of hospitalization, the existence of the syndrome has led to an increased workload for the house staff. Because patients with AIDS frequently require expensive care for which hospitals may not be fully reimbursed by a system of payment based on diagnosis-related groups, there is increasing pressure to transfer these patients to municipal, largely teaching, hospitals.[3] The care of these patients is quite labor intensive: as in any immunocompromised host, such common symptoms as fever, shortness of breath, headache, or confusion herald an exhaustive and often invasive workup to exclude a treatable infectious cause. All these factors have contributed to a more difficult house staff experience than occurred in the pre-AIDS era.

Education

As could be anticipated, the educational impact of AIDS at certain teaching hospitals has been tremendous. At San Francisco General Hospital, it is extremely uncommon for an intern not to be caring for at least one or two patients with AIDS at any given time. This means that a large proportion of teaching rounds among residents and attending physicians are devoted to issues involving the care of these patients. In addition, the content of conferences and Grand Rounds is influenced by both the clinical needs of the house staff and attending physicians and the major areas of ongoing research of the faculty. Both these factors have led to the devotion of a substantial amount of conference time to AIDS. Finally, many physicians will never read as much of the general medical literature as they do during their residency. This too has been dominated by AIDS over the past few years. For example, in 1984, 15 percent of the articles and short papers in the *Annals of Internal Medicine* were devoted to AIDS.

House Staff Autonomy

The complexity of AIDS-related illnesses and the unique psychosocial needs of patients with AIDS have resulted in the de facto creation of a new medical subspecialty in AIDS. The same factors have led to the organization of settings for the care of these patients that further serve to define their care as a subspecialty endeavor. At San Francisco General Hospital, all patients with AIDS and related disorders are followed as outpatients in an "AIDS clinic" staffed by physicians, nurses, and other care givers who have chosen to specialize in this area. Similarly, the inpatients are cared for on an "AIDS unit," for purposes of both infection control and provision of quality care. This degree of specialization, which began at San Francisco General in 1983, has since been duplicated elsewhere.[4]

It is undeniable that specialized AIDS units at this hospital have enhanced the care of patients with AIDS by providing comprehensive medical treatment and support services in a single setting. With the data base in AIDS research growing exponentially, it is also clear that the existence of subspecialists in AIDS has been necessary for patient care and for educating other care givers.

The growth of a medical subspecialty in AIDS has had an important influence on the residency experience. The potential for conflict exists between house officers who are seeking some degree of autonomy in caring for their patients and subspecialty attending physicians who have frequently cared for the patients outside the hospital and want to manage their care in the inpatient setting. In addition, the therapy of many of the manifestations of AIDS is under intense investigation. In many of the hospitals staffed by residents, therapy is therefore dictated by research protocol, further diminishing the input of the house staff on patient care. Undoubtedly, the same concerns were raised by house officers with the inception of oncology wards, which share many of the same characteristics. It is likely that, with time, specialized AIDS units will be as acceptable to residents as the more familiar oncology wards.

Emotional Issues

Fear of Transmission

Medical house officers are exposed to blood and body secretions as they care for their patients. This exposure has posed a special concern in the care of patients with AIDS, since recent evidence has shown that a blood-borne virus is responsible for the syndrome.[5,6] In the early days of the AIDS epidemic, fear of transmission caused house officers and other care givers to don masks, gloves, and gowns before even routine contact with patients with AIDS. This inevitably added to the emotional and physical barriers between patients and physicians.

The fear that routine exposure or needle sticks could lead to AIDS has been largely alleviated by recent data,[7,8] but the long latency period of the virus dictates that residents continue to exercise caution. For the most part, however, the days of stringent isolation precautions and failure to visit patients because of fear of transmission have passed. Unfortunately, this may change if evidence of human T-cell lymphotropic virus Type III/lymphadenopathy virus (HTLV-III/LAV) seroconversion or clinical AIDS in health workers not in other risk groups is confirmed.[9]

Frustration with the Limitations of Technology

Many of today's residents spent their formative years in medical training during an era when the ability of the scientific community to solve health care problems seemed limitless. As new diseases such as toxic shock syndrome and legionnaire's disease surfaced, their pathogenesis and treatment were elucidated with dispatch.[10-12] In the case of AIDS, remarkable strides have been achieved in the discovery of an etiologic agent[5,6] and dissemination of a screening assay for blood and plasma.[13] However, as of this writing, a cure remains elusive.

Nowhere are the limitations of technology more evident than in the issue of intensive care for patients with AIDS. In my experience, it is usually a resident who initiates discussion of intubation and mechanical ventilation with a hospitalized patient suffering from *P. carinii* pneumonia. The discussion is emotionally difficult, since the resident often tries to paint a realistic portrait of the probable outcomes of intensive care while trying not to rob the patient of all hope. My colleagues and I have studied this issue at San Francisco General Hospital.[14] Of our first 39 patients with *P. carinii* pneumonia who received mechanical ventilation, 34 (87 percent) died before hospital discharge. During the past year, we have witnessed a considerable increase in the percentage of patients with AIDS who have declined mechanical ventilation and intensive care. Much of the impetus for this change has been generated from within the community of patients with AIDS.[15] Nevertheless, the sentiments of house officers who have cared for patients dying with *P. carinii* pneumonia after protracted and painful stays in the intensive care unit have undoubtedly influenced this trend as well.

The Homosexual Patient

Nationwide, about 70 percent of the patients with AIDS are homosexual or bisexual[16]; in San Francisco the percentage is somewhat higher. In a poll of physicians conducted seven years ago, one third reported discomfort in treating homosexual patients.[17] For the heterosexual resident, the anxiety invoked by dealing with a critically ill patient may be magnified by uneasiness with the patient's sexual orientation.[18] This anxiety may make more traumatic the already difficult tasks of obtaining the sexual history, counseling the patient about the risk of transmitting the infection, and dealing sensitively with the patient's family and lover.

Dealing with the Patient Confronting Death

Interns and residents in internal medicine learn quickly to deal with terminally ill patients. Elaborate defenses are constructed to soften the inevitable blow. It is often not difficult for a resident to accept the death of an elderly patient with widely metastatic cancer as a welcome reprieve from suffering.[19] In other cases intellectualization, peer support, and even gallows humor are used. Dealing with AIDS patients stretches these defenses to their limits. Not in recent memory have so many relatively young, previously healthy people died so quickly, with care givers seemingly powerless to influence the eventual outcome. For house officers already burdened with the traditional stresses of residency,[20,21] involvement in this tragic scenario must extract a substantial psychological toll.

Recommendations

The AIDS epidemic has presented unprecedented challenges to the process of medical training. There are no easy solutions to these challenges, nor are there likely to be any in the near future. With this in mind, the following recommendations regarding medical residency training in the AIDS era are offered.

At certain hospitals, the process of providing labor-intensive care to large numbers of patients with AIDS increases the workload of the house staff to the point at which the care of all patients may be compromised. In these settings, house staff education and morale may also be adversely affected. Each program must assess the number of patients with AIDS per intern and resident and develop ways of reducing the burden. These may include distribution of patients with AIDS to hospitals without house staff, admission of patients treated with an AIDS research protocol to nonteaching services, and redoubled efforts to maximize outpatient and hospice therapy when appropriate. The latter suggestion in particular will have salutary effects for the patients as well. Palliative measures (e.g., control of pain and dyspnea and emotional support) might be more appropriate than invasive therapy for some patients in the terminal stages of AIDS.

In San Francisco, an effective network of outpatient clinics and voluntary support groups for patients with AIDS, coupled with more reliance on oral treatment regimens, has kept the average length of inpatient stay for new patients with AIDS to less than 12 days.[22] Unfortunately, for house staff and patients, this trend toward shorter inpatient stays has not proved universal. In New York, for example, the average length of stay during the initial hospitalization has been 50 days.[22]

Training programs must provide realistic information to prospective applicants about the amount of AIDS at their hospitals. They should also provide the house staff with reasonable guidelines regarding the risk of transmission and methods of minimizing this risk while still providing hands-on care. In addition, each hospital should establish a policy regarding "do not resuscitate" orders for patients with AIDS. At San Francisco General Hospital, physicians are encouraged to discuss this issue with patients within 72 hours of hospitalization. Especially in hospitals where attending physicians are responsible for writing "no code" orders, unambiguously establishing a patient's preference regarding mechanical ventilation decreases the need for haphazard, rushed discussions of this sensitive issue by house officers, patients, and faculty.

All involved parties need to recognize that the AIDS epidemic has added an extraordinary new stress to the already stressful process of medical residency. This should be discussed frankly among house staff, program directors, and other health care providers. Methods of dealing with these stresses, which may include peer or professional counseling or the availability of time on non-AIDS rotations, need to be implemented. Residents must evaluate their own methods of dealing with these stresses to determine whether they add to their ability to cope and to care for their patients.

Conclusions

Nearly five years into the AIDS epidemic, anyone involved in the process of medical education must consider how AIDS is affecting medical residency training. It is true that AIDS has allowed less time for the care and study of patients with more "classic" medical illnesses. It is also true that the emotional and physical toll of medical residency has increased because of AIDS.

On the other hand, the care of patients with AIDS has also provided some rewarding experiences, both personally and professionally. It has yielded new insights into the complexities of the immune system and the devastating manifestations of its breakdown. It has also provided experience in caring for some of the most complex disorders and critically ill patients that one may see during a residency. Although the most profound impact has been felt by residents working in urban centers on the East and West coasts, this may become a more general experience as the epidemic grows. With the possibility of more than 100,000 new cases of AIDS in the next decade,[22] it is becoming increasingly clear that a strong background in the care of these unfortunate patients will prove to be an indispensable attribute of a well-trained internist for the foreseeable future.

References

1. *Pneumocystis* pneumonia — Los Angeles. MMWR 1981; 30:250-2.
2. Kaposi's sarcoma and *Pneumocystis* pneumonia among homosexual men — New York City and California. MMWR 1981; 30:305-8.
3. Nutter DO. Access of care and the evolution of corporate, for-profit medicine. N Engl J Med 1984; 311:917-9.
4. Landesman SH, Ginzburg HM, Weiss SH. The AIDS epidemic. N Engl J Med 1985; 312:521-5.
5. Gallo RC, Salahuddin SZ, Popovic M, et al. Frequent detection and isolation of cytopathic retroviruses (HTLV-III) from patients with AIDS and at risk for AIDS. Science 1984; 224:500-3.
6. Barré-Sinoussi F, Chermann JC, Rey F, et al. Isolation of a T-lymphotropic retrovirus from a patient at risk for acquired immune deficiency syndrome (AIDS). Science 1983; 220:868-71.
7. Hirsch MS, Wormser GP, Schooley RT, et al. Risk of nosocomial infection with human T-cell lymphotropic virus III (HTLV-III). N Engl J Med 1985; 312:1-4.
8. Update: prospective evaluation of health-care workers exposed via the parenteral or mucous-membrane route to blood or body fluids from patients with acquired immunodeficiency syndrome — United States. MMWR 1985; 34:101-3.
9. Update: evaluation of human T-lymphotropic virus Type III/lymphadenopathy-associated virus infection in health-care personnel — United States. MMWR 1985; 34:575-8.
10. Shands KN, Schmid GP, Dan BB, et al. Toxic-shock syndrome in menstruating women: association with tampon use and *Staphylococcus aureus* and clinical features in 52 cases. N Engl J Med 1980; 303:1436-42.
11. McDade JE, Shepard CC, Fraser DW, et al. Legionnaire's disease: isolation of a bacterium and demonstration of its role in other respiratory disease. N Engl J Med 1977; 297:1197-1203.
12. Broomfield B, Dumoff M, Mulkey D, et al. Follow-up on Legionnaires' disease. MMWR 1977; 26:111-2.
13. Provisional Public Health Service inter-agency recommendations for screening donated blood and plasma for antibody to the virus causing acquired immunodeficiency syndrome. MMWR 1985; 34:1-5.
14. Wachter RM, Luce JM, Turner J, Volberding P, Hopewell PC. Intensive care of patients with the acquired immunodeficiency syndrome: outcome and changing patterns of utilization. Am Rev Respir Dis (in press).
15. Steinbrook R, Lo B, Tirpack J, Dilley JW, Volberding PA. Ethical dilemmas in caring for patients with the acquired immunodeficiency syndrome. Ann Intern Med 1985; 103:787-90.
16. Jaffe HW, Bregman DJ, Selik RM. Acquired immune deficiency syndrome in the United States: the first 1,000 cases. J Infect Dis 1983; 148:339-45.
17. Golin CB. MDs assess problems in treating gays. Am Med News, October 27, 1978:21(42):2.
18. Klein M, Pfeffer D. Homosexuality and the physician. New Physician 1985; 34(6):43-8.
19. Wanzer SH, Adelstein SJ, Cranford RE, et al. The physician's responsibility toward hopelessly ill patients. N Engl J Med 1984; 310:955-9.
20. Valko RJ, Clayton PJ. Depression in the internship. Dis Nerv Syst 1975; 36:26-9.
21. Asken MJ, Raham DC. Resident performance and sleep deprivation: a review. J Med Educ 1983; 58:382-8.
22. Ismach JM. AIDS: can the nation cope? Med World News 1985; 26(16): 46-71.

CORRESPONDENCE

CDC'S DEFINITION OF AIDS

To the Editor: The letter from Dr. Klein in the May 22 issue[1] illustrates common points of confusion about the definition of the acquired immunodeficiency syndrome (AIDS) used by the Centers for Disease Control (CDC). As Dr. Klein points out, the definition may lead to the misclassification of some patients as not having AIDS if they have certain other causes of underlying immunodeficiency coexisting with infection with human immunodeficiency virus (HIV, or HTLV-III/LAV).[2] Thus, patients undergoing dialysis who are receiving corticosteroid therapy for autoimmune renal disease and recipients of renal allografts, who are taking drugs to suppress rejection would not be classified as having AIDS under the current definition. Nonetheless, they may have opportunistic diseases secondary to immunodeficiency due to HIV infection. Indeed, renal transplantation itself can be a mode of transmission of HIV infection.[3] The complete list of conditions used to exclude patients with those disorders as representing cases of AIDS in the surveillance definition has been published recently.[4] These exclusionary criteria are limited mainly to immunosuppressive therapy, lymphoid malignant diseases (except those indicative of AIDS), and immunodeficiency syndromes atypical of AIDS (e.g., those occurring with hypogammaglobulinemia).[5]

Other known or possible causes of immunodeficiency,[6,7] such as uremia, diabetes mellitus, alcoholism, sarcoidosis, rheumatic diseases, pregnancy, or nonlymphoid cancers, do not exclude the patients as representing cases of AIDS, according to the CDC's definition. As a result, some patients whose immunodeficiency is not caused by HIV infection may be misclassified as having AIDS. We believe such misclassifications are infrequent because these other causes of immunodeficiency have rarely been associated with the secondary diseases characteristic of AIDS. Therefore, the patient with cryptococcal meningitis described by Dr. Klein could have been reported to the local health department as a case of AIDS, even though he had chronic renal failure.

To monitor epidemic trends, the CDC's surveillance definition of AIDS is restricted to the more severe manifestations that are consistently reported and are relatively specific for HIV infection. As such, the diagnosis of illness due to HIV infection should not depend solely on the surveillance definition; more use should be made of tests for serum antibody to HIV. Regardless of whether they meet the AIDS definition, all patients with HIV infection have a place in a recently published classification system for HIV infections.[8] Patients with secondary infections or cancers (not limited to those in the AIDS definition) may be classified in Group IV, in one or more of the subgroups C, D, and E (Table 1).

Table 1. Summary of Classification System for HIV Infections

Group I.	Acute infection (transient symptoms with seroconversion)
Group II.	Asymptomatic infection
Group III.	Persistent generalized lymphadenopathy
Group IV.	Other manifestations
	A. Chronic constitutional disease
	B. Neurologic disease
	C. Specified secondary infections
	D. Specified secondary cancers
	E. Other conditions

Richard M. Selik, M.D.
Harold W. Jaffe, M.D.
Steven L. Solomon, M.D.
James W. Curran, M.D., M.P.H.
Center for Infectious Diseases
Centers for Disease Control
Atlanta, GA 30333

References

1. Klein RS. More on AIDS in patients on dialysis. N Engl J Med 1986; 314:1386.
2. Coffin J, Haase A, Levy JA, et al. Human immunodeficiency viruses. Science 1986; 232:697.
3. Prompt CA, Reis MM, Grillo FM, et al. Transmission of AIDS virus at renal transplantation. Lancet 1985; 2:672.
4. World Health Organization. Acquired immunodeficiency syndrome (AIDS): WHO/CDC case definition for AIDS. WHO Wkly Epidemiol Rec 1986; 61(10):69-72.
5. Update: acquired immunodeficiency syndrome (AIDS) — United States. MMWR 1984; 32:688-91.
6. Grieco MH, ed. Infections in the abnormal host. New York: Yorke Medical Books, 1980.
7. Weinberg ED. Pregnancy-associated depression of cell-mediated immunity. Rev Infect Dis 1984; 6:814-31.
8. Classification system for human T-lymphotropic virus type III/lymphadenopathy-associated virus infections. MMWR 1986; 35:334-9.

HOW COMMON IS HTLV-III INFECTION IN THE UNITED STATES?

To the Editor: Fairly precise figures for the number of cases of the acquired immunodeficiency syndrome (AIDS) in the United States are based on surveillance data gathered by the Centers for Disease Control. Since the presence of antibodies to human T-cell lymphotrophic virus Type III (HTLV-III) is itself not a reportable condition, and since little information is available on testing for HTLV-III antibody in the general population, the number of residents of this country who have been infected with the virus is unknown. We suggest that the prevalence of this infection in the general U.S. population as well as in identified subgroups may be estimated on the basis of existing data. The critical assumption in our calculations is that the ratio of the number of living patients with AIDS to the number of patients with HTLV-III is constant within different patient groups. To test this assumption we compared the number of living patients with AIDS with the estimated number of patients with HTLV-III in two well-studied populations — intravenous-drug abusers and hemophiliacs.

The total estimate of hemophiliacs in this country[1] is 14,467, of whom at least 62 percent, or 8970, may be

Table 1. Estimated Number of Adults Infected with HTLV-III in the United States.

Group	No. Living with AIDS*	Estimated No. with HTLV-III
Homosexuals or bisexuals	4485	1,345,500
Intravenous-drug abusers	923	270,000
Hemophiliacs	31	8,970
Haitians†	139	41,700
Heterosexual contacts of persons at high risk	48	14,400
Recipients of blood or blood products	69	20,700
Persons at no known risk	214	64,200
	5909	1,765,470

*Centers for Disease Control, surveillance data, July 22, 1985.

†Or persons born in a country where AIDS cases have not been associated with known high risk.

assumed to be infected with HTLV-III according to Western blot electrophoresis.[2] It is known that there are 31 living hemophiliacs with AIDS (Centers for Disease Control, AIDS surveillance, July 22, 1985). Therefore, for every living hemophiliac with AIDS, there are approximately 289 hemophiliacs with HTLV-III. Similarly, the total number of intravenous-drug abusers infected with HTLV-III in this country may be estimated to be 36 percent[3] of 750,000,[1] or 270,000. Since there are 923 living intravenous-drug abusers with AIDS, it follows that for every intravenous-drug abuser with AIDS there are 293 abusers with antibodies to HTLV-III. A recent study revealed that this ratio was smaller in a group of homosexual men — 1:30.[4] However, this group was selected on the basis of attendance at a clinic for sexually transmitted diseases and voluntary participation in the study, and may not be representative of all homosexual men.

If the ratio of living patients with AIDS to those with HTLV-III is approximately 1:300, then the total number of U.S. residents who are infected with HTLV-III can be estimated to be 1,765,470 (Table 1). This figure includes 64,200 persons who do not belong to any identified risk group. Using currently available population data, one can estimate that in the U.S. adult population at no known risk for AIDS, the prevalence of HTLV-III infection is 45 per 100,000.

A recent report from the American Red Cross[5] indicates that the actual prevalence of HTLV-III infection, calculated by screening more than 1 million units of donated blood in the general U.S. population is 38 per 100,000. We believe that the similarity of the calculated and actual prevalence figures supports the accuracy of our assumptions and calculations.

Steven L. Sivak, M.D.,
and Gary P. Wormser, M.D.
New York Medical College
Valhalla, NY 10595

References

1. Hardy AM, Allen JR, Morgan WM, Curran JW. The incidence rate of acquired immunodeficiency syndrome in selected populations. JAMA 1985; 253:215-20.
2. Goedert JJ, Sarngadharan MG, Eyster ME, et al. Antibodies reactive with human T cell leukemia viruses in the serum of hemophiliacs receiving factor VIII concentrate. Blood 1985; 65:492-5.
3. Schupbach J, Haller O, Vogt M, et al. Antibodies to HTLV-III in Swiss patients with AIDS and pre-AIDS and in groups at risk for AIDS. N Engl J Med 1985; 312:265-70.
4. Jaffe HW, Darrow WW, Echenberg DF, et al. The acquired immunodeficiency syndrome in a cohort of homosexual men: a six-year follow-up study. Ann Intern Med 1985; 103:210-4.
5. Schorr JB, Berkowitz A, Cumming PD, Katz AJ, Sandler SG. Prevalence of HTLV-III antibody in American blood donors. N Engl J Med 1985; 313: 384-5.

Clinical Studies

Immune Deficiency Manifestations and Classifications

MEDICAL INTELLIGENCE

T-LYMPHOCYTE SUBPOPULATIONS IN HOMOSEXUAL MEN

Hardy Kornfeld, M.D., Robert A. Vande Stouwe, M.D., Ph.D., Michael Lange, M.D., M. Mohan Reddy, Ph.D., and Michael H. Grieco, M.D.

In the past two years there has been an unprecedented outbreak of Kaposi's sarcoma, *Pneumocystis carinii* pneumonia, and other opportunistic infections in male homosexuals and, to a lesser extent, in drug addicts in the United States.[1,2] These cases have been concentrated in New York City and California, and as of January 13, 1982, 216 cases had been reported to the Centers for Disease Control.[3]

Nineteen cases with immunologic evaluation were reported in December 1981.[4-6] All patients had evidence of cellular immunodeficiency with cutaneous anergy, reduced numbers of T lymphocytes, and impaired lymphocyte transformation. Four patients described by Gottlieb et al.[4] had an altered distribution of T-cell subsets on immunofluorescent staining with monoclonal antibodies. The ratios of Leu-3 positive (helper/inducer) to Leu-2 (suppressor/cytotoxic) lymphocytes were reduced.

It is assumed that the opportunistic infections and Kaposi's sarcoma occurred in these patients as a consequence of acquired immunodeficiency analogous to the complications of treatment with immunosuppressive drugs.[7,8] If this is true then the number of persons at risk for serious illness may be larger than is indicated by the cases of Kaposi's sarcoma and opportunistic infections reported to date.

We have studied 81 male homosexuals in New York City and have found that a large proportion have an altered distribution of T-lymphocyte subpopulations similar to but less pronounced than that found in patients with Kaposi's sarcoma or opportunistic infection. Reduced ratios of OKT4 (helper cells) to OKT8 (suppressor cells)[9,10] were associated with the presence of certain symptoms and with sexual promiscuity but not with the use of inhaled nitrites.

Methods

Eighty-one healthy homosexual volunteers 34.9±8 years of age (mean ±SD) were recruited by advertising in gay newspapers and through a gay health clinic and a university gay student organization. Those with histories of serious systemic illness or immunosuppressive therapy were excluded. Twenty heterosexual men 30.7±5.4 years of age served as controls.

A questionnaire was administered by one of us (H.K.) for information regarding medical history as well as symptoms, drug use, and sexual practices within the previous 12 months. For purposes of standardization, a history of fever was defined as a temperature of 37.8°C or higher for more than one week, weight loss as the unintentional loss of 5 kg or more, and diarrhea as three or more unformed stools per day for more than one week. Lymphadenopathy was defined as persistently enlarged nodes outside the inguinal chains. Recurrent amebiasis was defined as a history of five or more successfully treated discrete episodes in the previous year, and persistent amebiasis as persistently positive stool examinations despite two successive standard treatment regimens.

Mononuclear cells were isolated from heparinized peripheral blood on Ficoll–Hypaque gradients. Monocytes were identified by latex-particle ingestion. After washing, lymphocytes were suspended in Roswell Park Memorial Institute 1640 medium containing 10 percent heat-inactivated fetal calf serum. Lymphocytes positive for OKT4 and OKT8 (Ortho Diagnostic Systems, Raritan, N.J.) were identified by an indirect immunofluorescence assay with fluorescein-conjugated goat antimouse IgG (Meloy, Springfield, Va.) used as the developing antibody. Cells were mounted and slides were examined with a fluorescence microscope. Two hundred latex-negative cells were counted. Simultaneous complete blood counts and differential leukocyte counts were obtained.

Titers of cytomegalovirus antibody were determined by complement fixation.[11]

The means of the percentages and calculated absolute numbers of OKT4-positive and OKT8-positive lymphocytes and the OKT4/OKT8 ratios were compared in different patient groups using Student's t-test. The applicability of the t-test to the data was verified by F tests and graphic inspection of cumulative frequency distributions. Linear regression analysis was used to compare the OKT4/OKT8 ratios with the height of the titers of cytomegalovirus antibody.

Results

Of the 81 homosexual volunteers, 50 were asymptomatic and 31 had a history of one or more symptoms or signs according to the questionnaire. Within the symptomatic group, 2 had weight loss, 2 had thrush, 5 had diarrhea, 7 had fever, 11 had lymphadenopathy, 18 had amebiasis, and 11 had more than one disorder.

The distribution of T-cell subsets was abnormal in both groups of homosexuals as compared with controls, and it differed between the symptomatic and

Table 1. Lymphocyte Subpopulations in Symptomatic and Asymptomatic Male Homosexuals and in Heterosexual Controls.*

Group	%OKT4	Absolute OKT4 Count	%OKT8	Absolute OKT8 Count	OKT4/OKT8 Ratio
		cells/mm³		*cells/mm³*	
Controls (n = 20)	36.6 ±1.0	813.3 ±60.6	20.5 ±0.8	454.0 ±37.3	1.8 ±0.1
Asymptomatic homosexuals (n = 50)	27.4 ±1.4	643.9 ±41.5	28.8 ±1.1	675.1 ±33.3	1.1 ±0.1
Symptomatic homosexuals (n = 31)	22.4 ±1.6	483.5 ±43.0	31.1 ±1.6	651.2 ±42.5	0.8 ±0.1

*Data are reported as means ±SEM. The percentages and absolute counts of OKT4 and the OKT4/OKT8 ratios were significantly different among all three groups (P<0.05 or less). The percentages and absolute counts of OKT8 in symptomatic and asymptomatic homosexuals were higher than in controls (P<0.01 or less) but did not differ from each other.

From the Division of Infectious Diseases and Epidemiology and the Division of Allergy and Clinical Immunology, the Medical Service, St. Luke's–Roosevelt Hospital Center.

asymptomatic homosexuals as well (Table 1). The percentages and absolute counts of OKT4-positive lymphocytes and the OKT4/OKT8 ratios were lower in the homosexuals and were significantly different in all three groups as compared with one another. Of all 81 homosexuals tested, only 14 (17.3 percent) had OKT4/OKT8 ratios within the control range of 1.4 to 2.8. Of these 14 subjects, 12 were in the asymptomatic group and 2 in the symptomatic group. Six asymptomatic and nine symptomatic subjects had OKT4/OKT8 ratios below 0.5. The percentages and absolute counts of OKT8-positive lymphocytes were significantly higher in homosexuals than in controls but did not differ between the two groups of homosexuals.

Tests for cytomegalovirus antibody were positive in 79 of 81 homosexuals, with titers above 1:16 in 63 (77.8 percent). There was no correlation between titers of the antibody and OKT4/OKT8 ratios (r = 0.02). Five of 20 heterosexual controls (25 percent) were positive for cytomegalovirus antibody — all with titers of 1:16 or less.

Sexual promiscuity was associated with reduced OKT4/OKT8 ratios (Fig. 1). Subjects reporting nine or fewer different sexual partners per year tended to have higher ratios than those reporting more sexual partners, although this difference became statistically significant ($P<0.05$) only in comparisons with subjects reporting 50 or more partners.

Long-term use of amyl and butyl nitrite was unrelated to OKT4/OKT8 ratios (Fig. 2). Six of 40 subjects (15 percent) using nitrites at least once a week had normal ratios, whereas 18 of 23 subjects (78.3 percent) who had never used these drugs had low ratios.

Discussion

Reduced OKT4/OKT8 ratios have been reported in a variety of diseases including cytomegalovirus-induced mononucleosis,[12] Epstein–Barr virus infection, influenza, acute and chronic hepatitis B infection, and primary biliary cirrhosis.[13,14] The cause of the reduced ratios in our homosexual subjects is unknown, and their possible relation to the outbreak of Kaposi's sarcoma and opportunistic infections will require longitudinal study. It must be stressed that immunofluorescence staining of lymphocyte subpopulations with monoclonal antibodies reveals only phenotypic cell-surface markers that may not correlate with functional abnormalities.

Prodromal symptoms or signs such as fever, weight loss, diarrhea, and lymphadenopathy for up to 12 months have been reported in many patients with the syndrome of acquired cellular immunodeficiency and Kaposi's sarcoma or opportunistic infection.[3] In this study both symptomatic and asymptomatic homosexuals had reduced OKT4/OKT8 ratios, and there was a significant trend toward lower ratios in the symptomatic subjects. Although the assessment of symptoms was subjective, we believe it is clinically relevant.

Sexual promiscuity as defined by the number of different sexual partners in the previous year was frequently but not invariably associated with low OKT4/OKT8 ratios. The only monogamous volunteer had a ratio of 1.0, whereas another subject, who reported having had more than 400 different partners in the previous year, had a ratio of 1.7. The reduced ratios in the promiscuous subjects may have been due to a higher frequency of sexually transmitted viral infections, particularly cytomegalovirus infection.[15,16] Other factors associated with homosexual practices include mucosal exposure to seminal plasma, which may have immunosuppressive properties,[17] exposure to foreign HLA determinants on spermatozoa, and the use of nitrites.

Goedert et al.[18] recently reported low OKT4/OKT8 ratios in 9 of 15 healthy homosexual men, 8 of whom used nitrites regularly. It was concluded that

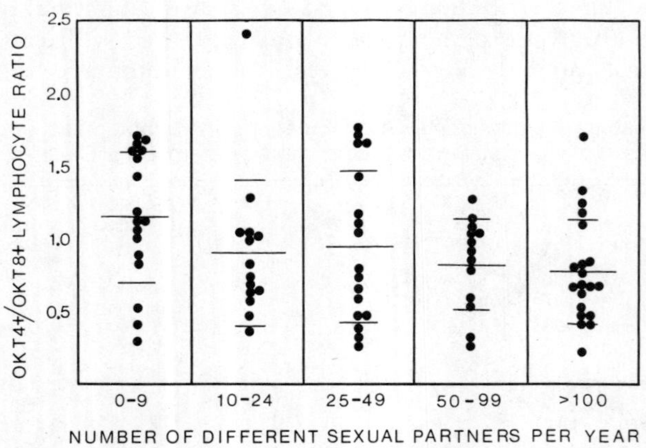

Figure 1. OKT4/OKT8 Ratios and Sexual Promiscuity in Homosexual Men.

The OKT4/OKT8 ratio was higher in subjects reporting nine or fewer different sexual partners per year than in those reporting 50 to 99 partners ($P<0.05$) or 100 or more partners ($P<0.01$) per year. Horizontal lines represent means ±SD.

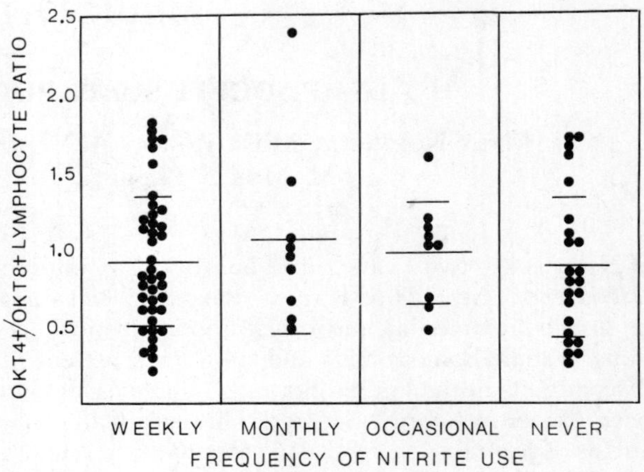

Figure 2. OKT4/OKT8 Ratios and the Use of Inhaled Nitrites in Homosexual Men.

The OKT4/OKT8 ratio was not related to the reported use of nitrites. Horizontal lines represent means ±SD.

nitrites may have had a causative role in altering the T-cell subsets. Although we did not find this association in our subjects, this does not exclude a transient effect, since none of our subjects had taken these drugs within eight hours of testing. Furthermore, the lack of an association between nitrite use and altered T-cell subsets in our study does not exclude the possibility that these drugs have functional immunosuppressive properties.

Whatever the cause and the importance of the altered T-cell subsets in male homosexuals, the finding of a detectable abnormality in over 80 percent of those tested suggests a greater public-health problem than is generally appreciated. Although the volunteers in this study may not be representative of the overall homosexual population in New York City, the strikingly high prevalence of reduced OKT4/OKT8 ratios in our subjects does suggest that this alteration may be present in a large number of homosexual men in the community.

We are indebted to the Columbia University Health Service, the Gay Men's Health Project, and the volunteers from Columbia University for their help; to Dr. Elena Klein for the serologic studies; to Ms. Mary Moriarty for technical assistance; and to Ms. Yolanda Sandoval for preparation of the manuscript.

References

1. *Pneumocystis* pneumonia — Los Angeles. MMWR 1981; 30:250-2.
2. Kaposi's sarcoma and *Pneumocystis* pneumonia among homosexual men — New York City and California. MMWR 1981; 30:305-8.
3. Centers for Disease Control. Epidemiologic aspects of the current outbreak of Kaposi's sarcoma and opportunistic infections. N Engl J Med 1982; 306:248-52.
4. Gottlieb MS, Schroff R, Schanker HM, et al. *Pneumocystis carinii* pneumonia and mucosal candidiasis in previously healthy homosexual men: evidence of a new acquired cellular immunodeficiency. N Engl J Med 1981; 305:1425-31.
5. Masur H, Michelis MA, Greene JB, et al. An outbreak of community-acquired *Pneumocystis carinii* pneumonia. N Engl J Med 1981; 305:1431-8.
6. Siegal FP, Lopez C, Hammer GS, et al. Severe acquired immunodeficiency in male homosexuals, manifested by chronic perianal ulcerative herpes simplex lesions. N Engl J Med 1981; 305:1439-44.
7. Walzer PD, Perl DP, Krogstad DJ, Rawson PG, Schultz MG. *Pneumocystis carinii* pneumonia in the United States: epidemiologic, diagnostic, and clinical features. Ann Intern Med 1974; 80:83-93.
8. Myers BD, Kessler E, Levi J, Pick A, Rosenfeld JB. Kaposi sarcoma in kidney transplant recipients. Arch Intern Med 1974; 133:307-11.
9. Reinherz EL, Kung PC, Goldstein G, Schlossman SF. Separation of functional subsets of human T cells by monoclonal antibody. Proc Natl Acad Sci 1979; 76:4061-5.
10. *Idem.* A monoclonal antibody reactive with the human cytoxic/suppressor T cell subset previously defined by a heteroantiserum termed TH_2^1. J Immunol 1980; 124:1301-7.
11. Cremer NE, Hoffman M, Lennette EH. Analysis of antibody assay methods and classes of viral antibodies in serodiagnosis of cytomegalovirus infection. J Gen Clin Microbiol 1978; 8:153-9.
12. Carney WP, Rubin RH, Hoffman RA, Hansen WP, Healey K, Hirsh MS. Analysis of T lymphocyte subsets in cytomegalovirus mononucleosis. J Immunol 1981; 126:2114-6.
13. Rubin RH, Carney WP, Schooley RT, et al. The effect of infection on T lymphocyte subpopulations: a preliminary report. Int J Immunopharmacol 1981; 3:307-12.
14. Thomas HC. T-cell subsets in patients with acute and chronic HBV infection, primary biliary cirrhosis and alcohol induced liver disease. Int J Immunopharmacol 1981; 3:301-5.
15. Drew WL, Mintz L, Miner RC, Sands M, Ketterer B. Prevalence of cytomegalovirus infection in homosexual men. J Infect Dis 1981; 143:188-92.
16. Lang DJ, Kummer JF. Cytomegalovirus in semen: observations in selected populations. J Infect Dis 1975; 132:472-3.
17. Anderson DJ, Tarter TH. Immunosuppressive effects of mouse seminal plasma components *in vivo* and *in vitro*. J Immunol 1982; 128:535-9.
18. Goedert JJ, Wallen WC, Mann DL, et al. Amyl nitrite may alter T lymphocytes in homosexual men. Lancet 1982; 1:412-6.

MEDICAL INTELLIGENCE

PROGRESSIVE MULTIFOCAL LEUKOENCEPHALOPATHY IN A MALE HOMOSEXUAL WITH T-CELL IMMUNE DEFICIENCY

JAMES R. MILLER, M.D., ROBERT E. BARRETT, M.D., CAROLYN B. BRITTON, M.D., MICHAEL L. TAPPER, M.D., GERALD S. BAHR, M.D., PETER J. BRUNO, M.D., MERLIN D. MARQUARDT, M.D., ARTHUR P. HAYS, M.D., JAMES G. MCMURTRY III, M.D., JACK B. WEISSMAN, M.D., AND MICHAEL S. BRUNO, M.D.

An acquired immune deficiency in male homosexuals that is manifested by infection with one or more opportunistic microorganisms has recently been recognized. These agents have included cytomegalovirus, *Toxoplasma gondii, Pneumocystis carinii, Candida albicans, Mycobacterium avium-intracellulare,* and *Cryptococcus neoformans.*[1-4] A prolonged clinical course with an otherwise self-limited infection, such as herpes simplex infection, has also been described,[3] and a remarkable incidence of Kaposi's sarcoma has been reported.[1-5]

In this milieu, the occurrence of progressive multifocal leukoencephalopathy (PML) might be expected. We present the case of a male homosexual with a T-cell immune deficiency, in whom PML was suspected because of a progressive disorder of the brain stem and cerebellum, as well as a lucent cerebellar lesion demonstrated by computerized tomography (CT). The diagnosis was confirmed by biopsy of the cerebellar lesion.

CASE REPORT

A 39-year-old man was admitted to the hospital on January 4, 1982, because of generalized malaise that had lasted for two months and numbness of the left side of the face and left arm that lasted for two weeks. In December 1981 intestinal amebiasis had been detected and treated, but the patient's symptoms had not been reduced. He began to have "dizziness," with anorexia and weight loss. At admission he also noted blurred vision on lateral gaze and incoordination of the left arm.

Anicteric hepatitis had occurred in 1977. Syphilis, treated with penicillin, had been diagnosed in 1978. Six months before admission an elevated serum antibody titer to cytomegalovirus was recorded.

The patient was a homosexual with frequent sexual contacts. He was also a moderate user of marijuana and a heavy user of amyl nitrite. There was no exposure to other toxins or to animals.

General examination revealed obvious recent weight loss and slight hepatosplenomegaly. Lymphadenopathy was not prominent.

Neurologic examination demonstrated bilateral, horizontal, lateral-gaze nystagmus, diminished pinprick and light-touch sensations on the left face and arm, and incoordination and slightly diminished strength in the left arm.

The white-cell count was 3.3×10^3, with 22 percent polymorphonuclear leukocytes, 13 percent band neutrophils, 51 percent lymphocytes (mostly atypical), 12 percent monocytes, and 2 percent eosinophils. Blood chemistry and electrolyte levels were normal except that the alanine aminotransferase was 57 U (0.645 $\mu mol \cdot sec^{-1} \cdot liter^{-1}$). Serum protein electrophoresis was normal. Immunoglobulins were present at the following levels: IgG, 1450 mg per deciliter (normal, 660 to 1274); IgM, 335 mg per deciliter (normal, 75 to 270); and IgD, 1.7 mg per deciliter (normal, undetectable). Skin tests with purified protein derivative, trichophyton, mumps, and candida antigens did not evoke responses. The proportion of T cells was decreased (57 percent; normal, 60 to 80), and that of B cells was increased (21 percent; normal, 8 to 12) in peripheral-blood leukocytes. The ratio of OKT4 to OKT8 cells was 0.46 (control, 1.95).

Serologic studies demonstrated previous infection but no evidence of active infection from toxoplasma, cytomegalovirus, Epstein–Barr virus, or hepatitis B virus. A serologic test for syphilis was negative. The hemagglutination inhibition titer to JC virus was 1:64, which was consistent with previous infection.

Repeated cultures for infectious agents, including blood and urine studies for cytomegalovirus, were negative.

Cerebrospinal-fluid examination, which included bacterial, fungal, viral, and cytologic studies, gave normal results except for a protein level of 57 mg per deciliter (0.57 g per liter). A repeat examination performed two weeks later showed a negative Venereal Disease Research Laboratory test and Sabin–Feldman dye test, but oligoclonal bands were present that were atypical for demyelinating diseases or acute central-nervous-system infections. IgG made up 11.4 percent of the total cerebrospinal-fluid protein. An electroencephalogram was normal, but a CT scan of the brain showed an area of decreased density in the left cerebellar hemisphere without contrast enhancement or mass effect (Fig. 1).

Left-sided cerebellar and brain-stem signs increased, and the patient became unable to walk. Corticospinal-tract dysfunction was noted in the right limbs. Left carotid and vertebral arteriograms demonstrated no vascular abnormalities or mass effect.

On February 2 the patient was transferred to the New York Neurological Institute, where a cerebellar biopsy was performed a week later. Bacterial, fungal, and viral cultures were negative. There was marked demyelination with relative preservation of axons. A moderate microglial-cell response and occasional giant astrocytes were present, but the few oligodendroglial cells found were not clearly abnormal. Electron microscopy demonstrated intracellular viral particles and filaments typical of PML (Fig. 2). Immunofluorescent-antibody studies demonstrated the presence of papovavirus antigen.

The patient was treated with intravenous vidarabine, 15 mg per kilogram of body weight per day. His condition continued to deteriorate, however, and his respiratory function was compromised. He died on March 1, five days after the initiation of therapy with vidarabine. A buffy-coat culture of blood obtained just before death was positive for cytomegalovirus, but a urine culture was not.

Post-mortem examination of the brain confirmed the biopsy findings. Immunofluorescence studies determined that the papovavirus involved was JC virus.

Examination of other tissues revealed multiple foci of inflammatory cells in the lung, consistent with an ongoing cytomegalovirus infection. Virus was not isolated from the post-mortem cultures. There was no evidence of Kaposi's sarcoma or active infection with other organisms associated with the immunosuppression syndrome described in homosexuals.

DISCUSSION

The acquired immune deficiency observed in homosexuals is now becoming apparent in other groups as well.[6-8] The pathogenesis of this syndrome and the

From the Departments of Neurology, Neuropathology, Neurosurgery, and Medicine, College of Physicians and Surgeons, Columbia University; and the Department of Medicine, Lenox Hill Hospital.

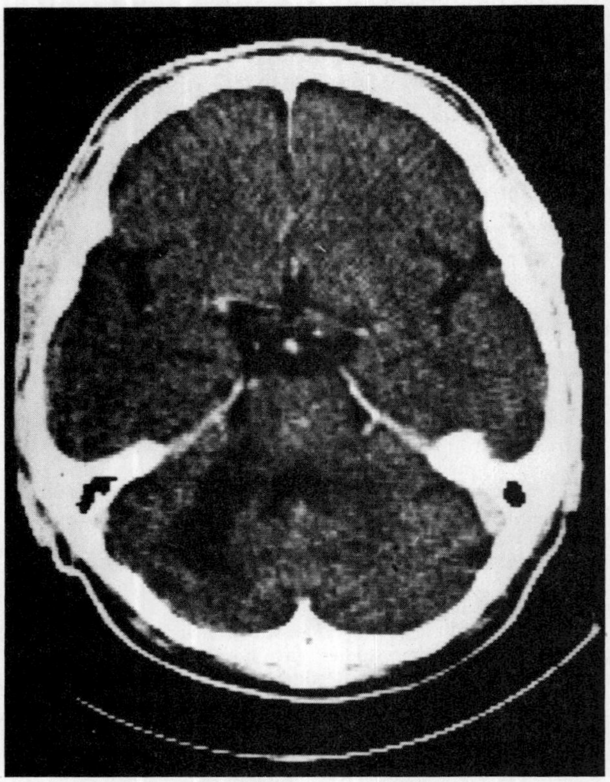

Figure 1. CT Scan with Contrast Enhancement, Demonstrating a Large Lucent Lesion in the Left Cerebellum, without Evidence of Surrounding Edema.

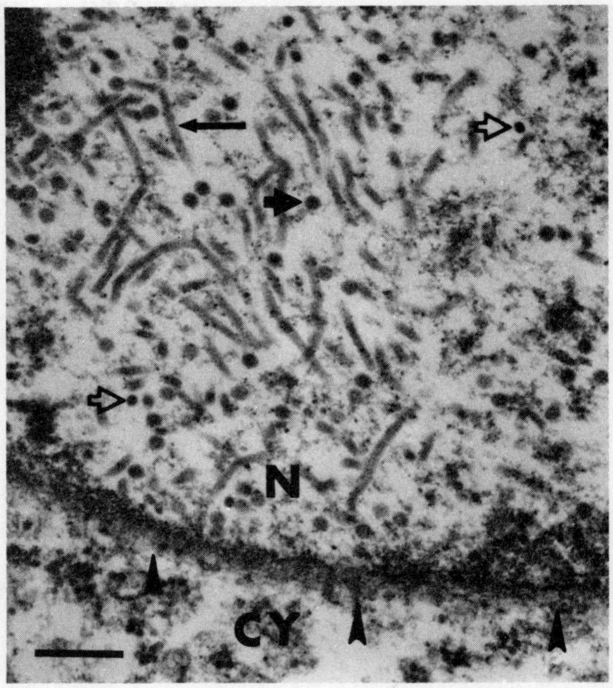

Figure 2. Electron Micrograph of an Oligodendroglial Cell from the Cerebellar Biopsy.

N denotes the nucleus, and CY cytoplasm. The short solid arrow indicates a papovavirus virion (33 to 39 nm), and the long solid arrow indicates filamentous viral forms (18 to 27 nm in width); the open arrows indicate filamentous forms in transverse section, and the arrowheads chromatin clustered at the nuclear margin. (Bar at lower left shows 200 nm.)

reasons for its sudden appearance and spread are unknown. The immune deficiency has been characterized as being predominantly a depression in T-cell function. As in our patient, there is typically a decreased proportion of T helper cells to suppressor cells, as suggested by OKT or other, similar lymphocyte markers.[1-5]

Immunosuppression makes the failure to find serologic evidence of active viral infection in this patient difficult to interpret. Patients with PML usually do not have higher titers of antibody against JC virus than those found in asymptomatie normal persons, probably because of the associated immune disorder.[9] In addition, immunosuppressed patients with symptomatic cytomegalovirus infection do not have the elevated IgM antibody titers against cytomegalovirus that occur during symptomatic infection in immunocompetent persons.[10]

Although serologic studies indicate that about 70 percent of adults worldwide have had at least one infection with JC virus, PML rarely occurs even in the presence of immunosuppression.[9,11,12] In most cases there are multiple central-nervous-system lesions, but approximately 10 percent of cases present as primarily unifocal pontocerebellar disease, as in our patient.[13,14]

The presence of oligoclonal bands in the cerebrospinal fluid has not been a feature of PML. However, these bands have now been recognized in a variety of disorders.[15-19] In these circumstances, the characteristics of the bands may differ from those found in demyelinating or inflammatory disorders, in which they are more often expected.[19] The possibility does exist, however, that the bands may have been related to an unrecognized central-nervous-system infection with another agent.

We are indebted to Dr. Duard L. Walker and his laboratory for the immunofluorescence studies of biopsy and autopsy specimens and for the serologic studies for papovavirus; to Drs. Michael Grieco, Peter Kelsey, and Leonard Chess for characterization of blood lymphocytes; to Dr. Donald Armstrong for the serologic studies for cytomegalovirus; and to Dr. Werner Henle for the serologic tests for Epstein–Barr virus.

References

1. Gottlieb MS, Schroff R, Schanker HM, et al. *Pneumocystis carinii* pneumonia and mucosal candidiasis in previously healthy homosexual men: evidence of a new acquired cellular immunodeficiency. N Engl J Med 1981; 305:1425-31.
2. Masur H, Michelis MA, Greene JB, et al. An outbreak of community-acquired *Pneumocystis carinii* pneumonia: initial manifestation of cellular immune dysfunction. N Engl J Med 1981; 305:1431-8.
3. Siegal FP, Lopez C, Hammer GS, et al. Severe acquired immunodeficiency in male homosexuals, manifested by chronic perianal ulcerative herpes simplex lesions. N Engl J Med 1981; 305:1439-44.
4. Fainstein V, Bolivar R, Mavligit G, Rios A, Luna M. Disseminated infection due to *Mycobacterium avium-intracellulare* in a homosexual man with Kaposi's sarcoma. J Infect Dis 1982; 145:586.

5. Case Records of the Massachusetts General Hospital (Case 11-1982). N Engl J Med 1982; 306:657-68.
6. Update on Kaposi's sarcoma and opportunistic infections in previously healthy persons — United States. MMWR 1982; 31:294, 300-1.
7. Opportunistic infections and Kaposi's sarcoma among Haitians in the United States. MMWR 1982; 31:353-4, 360-1.
8. *Pneumocystis carinii* pneumonia among persons with hemophilia A. MMWR 1982; 31:365-7.
9. Walker DL. Progressive multifocal leukoencephalopathy: an opportunistic viral infection of the central nervous system. In: Vinken PJ, Bruyn GW, eds. Handbook of clinical neurology. Vol. 34. New York: North-Holland Publishing, 1978:307-29.
10. Rasmussen L, Kelsall D, Nelson R, et al. Virus-specific IgG and IgM antibodies in normal and immunocompromised subjects infected with cytomegalovirus. J Infect Dis 1982; 145:191-9.
11. Åström K-E, Mancall EL, Richardson EP Jr. Progressive multifocal leukoencephalopathy: a hitherto unrecognized complication of chronic lymphatic leukaemia and Hodgkin's disease. Brain 1958; 81:93-111.
12. Padgett BL, Walker DL. New human papovaviruses. Prog Med Virol 1976; 22:1-35.
13. Parr J, Horoupian DS, Winkelman AC. Cerebellar form of progressive multifocal leukoencephalopathy (PML). Can J Neurol Sci 1979; 6: 123-8.
14. Jones HR Jr, Hedley-Whyte ET, Freidberg SR, Kelleher JE Jr, Krolikowski J. Primary cerebellopontine progressive multifocal leukoencephalopathy diagnosed premortem by cerebellar biopsy. Ann Neurol 1982; 11:199-202.
15. Laterre EC, Callewaert A, Heremans JF, Sfaello Z. Electrophoretic morphology of gamma globulins in cerebrospinal fluid of multiple sclerosis and other diseases of the nervous system. Neurology (Minneap) 1970; 20:982-90.
16. Link H. Characteristics of the immune response within the CNS in neurological disorders. Acta Neurol Scand [Suppl] 1978; 67:177-90.
17. Roström B, Link H, Norrby E. Antibodies in oligoclonal immunoglobulins in CSF from patients with acute cerebrovascular disease. Acta Neurol Scand 1981; 64:225-40.
18. Roström B, Link H. Oligoclonal immunoglobulins in cerebrospinal fluid in acute cerebrovascular disease. Neurology (NY) 1981; 31:590-6.
19. Miller JR, Burke AM, Bever CT. Occurrence of oligoclonal bands in multiple sclerosis and other CNS diseases. Ann Neurol. (in press).

EDITORIAL

METABOLIC DEFECTS AND IMMUNODEFICIENCY DISORDERS

ROCHELLE HIRSCHHORN, M.D.

IN this issue of the *Journal*, Girot et al. report the occurrence of impaired immune function in two siblings with hereditary orotic aciduria.[1] This observation serves to focus attention on the growing evidence that many of the various abnormalities of immunity may result from inherited metabolic defects in pathways that are not unique to lymphoid cells.

The current classification of primary immunodeficiency disorders rests on the concept that these disorders represent blocks at different steps in the differentiation of immunocompetent cells.[2] Thus, simply stated, there is a common stem cell that is capable of differentiation along either of two pathways. Under the influence of the thymus, it can differentiate to become the T lymphocytes of the cellular immune system, but under the influence of (probably) the bone marrow in human beings, it can differentiate to become the B lymphoid cells of the humoral or antibody-dependent immune system. According to this concept, defects intrinsic to the stem cell would affect both cellular and humoral immunity whereas defects at the level of effector function or at some step in between would affect either B-cell or T-cell function. The subsequent discovery of subsets of lymphocytes, of lymphocyte helper and suppressor functions, and of the complexity of lymphoid-cell interactions added another dimension that is still being explored.[3] An additional dimension was then added by the discovery of unique antigens on the cell surface of T lymphocytes. These antigens appeared to change in an orderly fashion as the cell developed, and more important, differences in these antigens correlated with differences in the functional properties of T lymphocytes. These discoveries and the development of monoclonal antibodies for the easy detection of these antigens[4] led to reexamination of patients with primary (as well as secondary) immunodeficiency disorders for abnormalities in antigen expression. However, despite our increased understanding of the complexity of the steps in differentiation, the conceptual framework for classification of immunodeficiency disorders remains unchanged. The underlying premise still is that immunodeficiency disorders can be classified as reflecting a neat interruption at some specific step in the differentiation of immunocompetent cells. Implicit in this scheme is the assumption that the underlying molecular defects in structural and functional proteins and metabolites are unique to the lymphoid system.

In retrospect, we can see that several empiric observations have suggested that although this conceptual framework was useful at the descriptive level, it may not provide sufficient insight for further definition of primary immunodeficiency disorders at the molecular level. For example, ataxia telangiectasia is an inherited immunodeficiency syndrome in which undifferentiated mesenchymal cells as well as lymphoid cells show increased sensitivity to ionizing radiation. Despite the systemic nature of the defect, the clinically important abnormalities primarily affect immunologic mechanisms and nervous and vascular tissue. Secondly, it has become increasingly apparent that cells differentiate not only with respect to function but also with respect to the relative importance of various biochemical pathways that serve a "housekeeping" role — that is, they allow metabolic steps common to virtually all cells. At the empiric level, it is now appreciated that different types of cells may be susceptible to different "cytotoxic" chemicals; an example is the relative sensitivity of lymphoid cells to purine analogues such as mercaptopurine and azathioprine. Currently, we have insufficient knowledge of or insight into the quantitative or qualitative differences in metabolic pathways of different cell types to predict which organ system will suffer the consequences of the absence of a particular pathway. Fortunately, the combination of serendipity and "experiments of nature" have allowed leaps in our understanding.

Approximately a decade ago, Giblett and co-workers[5] serendipitously discovered that the inherited deficiency of adenosine deaminase, an enzyme of the purine-salvage pathway, results in a severe combined immunodeficiency syndrome with impairment of both cellular and humoral immunity. We now know that this enzyme defect is responsible for an important proportion of the cases of severe combined immunodeficiency syndrome that are inherited in an autosomal recessive fashion. With this clue to guide her, Giblett[6] next found that the genetic deficiency of purine nucleoside phosphorylase, the enzyme distal to adenosine deaminase in the purine-salvage pathway, results in a syndrome of cellular immunodeficiency with essentially normal humoral immunity.[7,8] Investigations in patients who lack the surrounding enzymes of the salvage pathway (hypoxanthine-guanine phosphoribosyltransferase and adenine phosphoribosyltransferase) have not been fruitful, and these patients do not appear to have any immunologic deficit.

The discovery that two defects in the purine-salvage pathway resulted in immunodeficiency disorders suggested that defects in the pyrimidine pathway may also lead to impaired immune function. As Girot and colleagues point out, a reading of the case histories of patients with orotic aciduria suggested that they had a defect in immune function. Until the report by Girot et al., however, there was no documentation of such a defect. The description of the second sibling reported on, whose course was not complicated by therapy with prednisone, provides the strongest evidence for such a conjecture. The attrition of immune function observed in that patient is similar to that observed in some patients with a deficiency of adenosine deaminase and purine nucleoside phosphorylase. It remains to be determined whether the reversal of the immunologic abnormalities will become complete with continued therapy. Studies of additional patients should confirm whether orotic aciduria can be added to the growing list of metabolic defects that have defects in immune function as their primary or secondary manifestations.

Two other disorders have been described in which the major manifestations relate to non-lymphoid systems, but there is also an impairment of immune function. The most striking example is the inherited absence of transcobalamin II, the protein required for the intracellular transport of vitamin B_{12}. In addition to having macrocytic anemia, leukopenia, and thrombocytopenia, patients with this condition have been found to lack immunoglobulins.[7,8] (This finding also raises questions about whether the abnormal autoantibodies seen in pernicious anemia represent a cause or an effect.) Some patients with multiple biotin-dependent carboxylase deficiency have also been reported to have a defect in cell-mediated immunity.[9]

The discovery of specific metabolic defects that give rise to immunodeficiency disorders has allowed the realization that a single molecular defect can give rise to a spectrum of clinical syndromes that, under the current scheme, would be classified separately. Thus, now that the enzyme deficiency can be used to identify patients, it is becoming increasingly apparent that a deficiency of adenosine deaminase or purine nucleoside phosphorylase each gives rise to a spectrum of clinical manifestations. This was initially most obvious in patients with a deficiency of purine nucleoside phosphorylase; the first few cases varied in severity from those with infantile onset and early death to those with much later onset and the occurrence of immunologic attrition during the first decade of life. For adenosine deaminase deficiency, also, the spectrum now extends from severe combined immunodeficiency syndrome with death in early infancy if the condition is untreated, through a slightly milder syndrome with some retention of humoral immunity, to a recently described case of relatively mild, primarily cellular immunodeficiency presenting in childhood (Cowan MJ, Ammann A: personal communication). Indeed, patients have been described who lacked adenosine deaminase in their erythrocytes and were perfectly normal immunologically.[10] Such patients, in contrast to patients with immunodeficiency, have various amounts of adenosine deaminase in their other tissues and, as a result, do not have markedly abnormal concentrations of toxic metabolites. Patients with the milder syndromes appear to have more residual enzyme activity and to accumulate or excrete smaller amounts of abnormal metabolites. (Indeed, our unpublished observations suggest that in vivo concentrations of metabolites more accurately correlate with in vivo enzyme activity and therefore with the presence or absence of immunodeficiency than do in vitro measurements of enzyme activity.) This spectrum of clinical severity reflects a genetic heterogeneity possibly resulting from a series of different mutations at the same genetic locus, similar to those seen with globin-β-chain hemoglobinopathies.

It can be expected that a specific molecular defect will eventually be found for every inherited immunodeficiency disorder. Although such molecular defects would then form the basis for more precise diagnosis, the current conceptual framework can still be expected to remain useful for differential diagnosis. By analogy, one can cite the classification of infections as pneumonia, meningitis, septicemia, and the like, whereas etiologic classification reflects the specific organisms involved — e.g., pneumococcal pneumonia.

The finding of specific molecular defects with toxicity essentially limited to the lymphoid system can also be expected to provide tools for further insight into the normal differentiation and interaction of the components of the lymphoid system and the metabolic pathways involved, and to lead to the development of selective chemotherapeutic and immunomodulatory approaches.

References

1. Girot R, Hamet M, Perignon J-L, et al. Cellular immune deficiency in two siblings with hereditary orotic aciduria. N Engl J Med 1983; 308:700-4.
2. Belohradsky BH, Finstad J, Fudenberg HH, Good RA, Kunkel HG, Rosen F. Meeting report of the Second International Workshop on Primary Immunodeficiency Diseases in Man. Clin Immunol Immunopathol 1974; 2:281-95.
3. Parker CW, ed. Clinical immunology. Vol. 1. Philadelphia: WB Saunders, 1980.
4. Reinherz EL, Schlossman SF. The differentiation and function of human T lymphocytes. Cell 1980; 19:821-7.
5. Giblett ER, Anderson JE, Cohen F, Pollara B, Meuwissen HJ. Adenosine-deaminase deficiency in two patients with severely impaired cellular immunity. Lancet 1972; 2:1067-9.
6. Giblett ER, Ammann AJ, Wara DW, Sandman R, Diamond LK. Nucleoside-phosphorylase deficiency in a child with severely defective T-cell immunity and normal B-cell immunity. Lancet 1975; 1:1010-3.
7. Elliott K, Whelan J, eds. Enzyme defects and immune dysfunction: Ciba Foundation Symposium 68. New York: Excerpta Medica, 1979.
8. Pollara B, Pickering RJ, Meuwissen HJ, Porter IH, eds. Inborn errors of specific immunity. New York: Academic Press, 1979.
9. Cowan MJ, Wara DW, Packman S, et al. Multiple biotin-dependent carboxylase deficiencies associated with defects in T-cell and B-cell immunity. Lancet 1979; 2:115-8.
10. Hirschhorn R, Roegner V, Jenkins T, Seaman C, Piomelli S, Borkowsky W. Erythrocyte adenosine deaminase deficiency without immunodeficiency: evidence for an unstable mutant enzyme. J Clin Invest 1979; 64:1130-9.

ORIGINAL ARTICLE

ABNORMALITIES OF B-CELL ACTIVATION AND IMMUNOREGULATION IN PATIENTS WITH THE ACQUIRED IMMUNODEFICIENCY SYNDROME

H. Clifford Lane, M.D., Henry Masur, M.D., Lynn C. Edgar, M.S., Gail Whalen, B.S., Alain H. Rook, M.D., and Anthony S. Fauci, M.D.

Abstract We studied B-lymphocyte function in 12 homosexual male patients with the acquired immunodeficiency syndrome, 5 healthy homosexual men, and 12 heterosexual controls. In comparison with the heterosexual controls, the patients were found to have elevated numbers of cells spontaneously secreting immunoglobulin, decreased B-cell proliferative responses to T-cell–independent B-cell mitogens, and qualitatively deficient helper T cells. The hyperactive spontaneous B-cell responses as well as the refractoriness to signals for T-cell–independent B-cell activation were highly suggestive of an in vivo polyclonal activation of B cells and may have been responsible for the manifestations of B-cell hyperreactivity, such as hypergammaglobulinemia, seen in these patients. We conclude that the scope of immune dysfunction in the acquired immunodeficiency syndrome involves B cells as well as T cells.

OVER the past two years, a new syndrome has been described that consists of severe opportunistic infections; the development of neoplasms, especially Kaposi's sarcoma; and profound abnormalities of cellular immune function in previously healthy persons.[1-4] The disease was initially described in the male homosexual community, where it has begun to reach epidemic proportions; however, it has also recently been described in Haitian immigrants, hemophiliacs, and users of intravenous drugs. At least 5 percent of the reported cases have had no known predisposing factor.[5] This epidemiology, reminiscent of that of hepatitis B infection, suggests that the disease may be due to an infectious, possibly viral, agent that requires blood-borne transmission. It is as yet uncertain whether the host must have some sort of preexisting immunosuppression such as has been recently demonstrated in the male homosexual community.[6]

Patients with this syndrome have an essentially nonfunctioning cellular immune system because of a selective quantitative defect in the helper/inducer subset of T cells leading to reversal of the normal helper-to-suppressor T-cell ratio among peripheral-blood lymphocytes. This results in suppression of T-cell function both in vivo and in vitro.[1-4,7] In a single case, the ability of a patient's B cells to make immunoglobulin in vitro was found to be normal.[8]

Over the past year, we have had the opportunity to study the mechanisms of antibody production both in vivo and in vitro in patients with the acquired immunodeficiency syndrome (AIDS). In contrast to earlier investigators, we have found marked abnormalities of B-cell activation and immunoregulation directly at the level of the B cell as well as at the level of the T-cell control of B-cell function. These findings are of importance not only in furthering our understanding of the immune mechanisms involved in this syndrome but also in terms of providing insight into its pathophysiology and clinical manifestations.

From the Laboratory of Immunoregulation, National Institute of Allergy and Infectious Diseases; the Critical Care Medicine Department, Clinical Center, National Institutes of Health; and the Division of Virology, Office of Biologics, Food and Drug Administration, Bethesda, Md.

Methods

Patient and Control Groups

Twelve patients with AIDS[5] formed the patient group for the current study. All were homosexual men and ranged in age from 18 to 38 years. No patients were studied during an episode of acute infection. The control groups consisted of five healthy homosexual men, who were matched for age and life style with the majority of the patient group, and 12 healthy heterosexual men, who were studied in parallel with the patient group. The clinical and laboratory features of these three groups are shown in Table 1.

Cell Separations

Peripheral-blood mononuclear cells were separated into T cells and T-cell–depleted cells by means of rosetting with sheep red cells treated with 2-aminoethylisothiuronium bromide hydrobromide (Sigma Chemical, St. Louis). The remaining T cells in the rosette-negative fractions were removed, or T cells were further fractionated into T-cell subsets by monoclonal antibody and complement-mediated lysis. These procedures have been described in detail elsewhere.[9,10]

Culture Conditions

Supernatant immunoglobulin production was determined in cultures performed in 5-ml test tubes containing 5×10^5 peripheral-blood mononuclear cells and 1 ml of RPMI-1640 (Flow Laboratories, McLean, Va.) with 10 percent fetal-calf serum (Dutchland Laboratories, Denver, Pa.). Cultures contained a 1:200 final dilution of pokeweed mitogen (Gibco Laboratories, Grand Island Biological, Grand Island, N.Y.) and were harvested on Day 10.

Proliferative responses were measured in 96-well, round-bottomed microtiter plates (Costar Data Packaging, Cambridge, Mass.). Each well contained 100,000 cells and one of the following: no mitogen at all; 2 μg of phytohemagglutinin A per milliliter (Wellcome Research Laboratories, Beckenham, England); a 1:200 dilution of pokeweed mitogen; or a 1:12,500 dilution of the pure B-cell mitogen formalinized *Staphylococcus aureus* Cowan strain I (SAC) (Bethesda Research Laboratories, Bethesda, Md.). All cultures were performed in a final volume of 200 μl. Cultures containing phytohemagglutinin A or pokeweed mitogen also contained 15 percent human serum from blood group A, whereas cultures containing SAC were performed with 10 percent fetal-calf serum. Proliferative responses to phytohemagglutinin A and SAC were measured on Day 3, and proliferative responses to pokeweed mitogen were measured on Day 5.

Assays

The total numbers of T cells were determined by enumerating the number of cells forming rosettes with sheep red cells; the total numbers of B cells, by staining for surface immunoglobulin. Numbers of T4 and T8 cells were determined by indirect immunofluorescence, with use of a fluorescence-activated cell sorter (Becton-Dickinson, Mountain View, Calif.).[10] Spontaneous secretion of antibody by B cells was measured with a reverse hemolytic plaque-forming cell assay.[11] Supernatant immunoglobulin was measured with enzyme-linked immunosorbent assays, and proliferative responses were measured by the incorporation of [^{3}H]thymidine over a four-hour pulse with 2 μCi of [^{3}H]thymidine (New England Nuclear, Boston, Mass.).

Immunizations

Selected patients and controls received two subcutaneous injections of 5 mg of keyhole-limpet hemocyanin (Calbiochem-Behring, American Hoechst, La Jolla, Calif.), which had been dialyzed against phosphate-buffered saline and passed through a 0.45-μm millipore filter. Injections were spaced two weeks apart. Immunizations were carried out according to peer-reviewed protocols of the National Institutes of Health.

Statistics

Data are expressed as geometric means $\stackrel{\times}{\div}$SEM where appropriate.

Results

The clinical and laboratory features of the patient and control groups are listed in Table 1. Like those described in other studies, our patients with AIDS had a decrease in the number of circulating T lymphocytes and a marked decrease in the ratio of helper/cytotoxic-suppressor, or OKT4/OKT8, T lymphocytes. Worthy of note, however, is the fact that although the mean value for total T cells was lower for the patients than for either control group, the distribution of T-cell values for the patient group was wide and ranged from 138 to 7419 cells per cubic millimeter. Similarly, the range of T4/T8 ratios was from less than 0.1 to 0.7, with patients who had had the most severe opportunistic infections having the lowest ratios. This ratio varied substantially among the five healthy homosexual men studied, ranging from 0.2 to 3.9, with the average for the group significantly lower than that for the heterosexual control group.

Table 1. Clinical and Laboratory Features of Patients with AIDS as Compared with Those of Healthy Homosexual Men and Healthy Heterosexual Men.

Subject No.	Date of Diagnosis	Clinical Features*	Total T Cells	Total B Cells	T4/T8 Ratio	IgG	IgA	IgM
			number per mm^3				*mg/dl*	
Patients with AIDS								
1	1981	Fever, lymphadenopathy, weight loss, CMV viruria	2864	116	0.7	2337	225	249
2	11/81	*Mycobacterium avium-intracellulare* lymphadenitis, MCC, PCP, CMV viremia, retinitis	568	102	0.1	1840	475	86
3	1978	Lymphadenopathy, CMV viruria	1458	19	0.3	3380	142	98
4	2/82	PCP, MCC, CMV viruria, toxoplasmosis retinitis	1279	94	0.1	2440	738	420
5	10/81	Lymphadenopathy, CMV viruria	2329	140	0.5	2030	343	175
6	4/82	PCP, CMV viremia, MCC, perirectal infection	702	80	<0.1	1450	317	148
7	8/82	KS, CMV viremia, recurrent pneumonia, MCC	7419	442	0.2	5570	285	473
8	2/82	PCP, CMV pneumonia, idiopathic hydrocephalus	138	31	<0.1	2210	627	183
9	8/81	Lymphadenopathy, CMV viruria	2011	87	0.4	1690	291	141
10	3/82	Cryptococcal meningitis, disseminated *Mycobacterium avium-intracellulare*, retinitis, CMV viremia	1132	126	<0.1	1610	307	159
11	1/82	KS, MCC, CMV viremia, PCP	676	98	<0.1	2050	703	408
12	4/82	KS, PML, MCC, CMV viremia	1425	78	0.7	2020	694	190
Means $\stackrel{\times}{\div}$SEM			*1253$\stackrel{\times}{\div}$1.3*	*100$\stackrel{\times}{\div}$1.3*	*0.12$\stackrel{\times}{\div}$1.5*	*2222$\stackrel{\times}{\div}$1.1*	*381$\stackrel{\times}{\div}$1.2*	*197$\stackrel{\times}{\div}$1.2*
Healthy homosexual men								
1			2185	232	3.9	1200	85	135
2			1724	159	1.1	1290	151	132
3			1424	17	0.2	1580	226	225
4			2604	156	0.7	1690	308	150
5			1485	147	1.0	1820	220	91
Means $\stackrel{\times}{\div}$SEM			*1833$\stackrel{\times}{\div}$1.1*	*107$\stackrel{\times}{\div}$1.6*	*0.8$\stackrel{\times}{\div}$1.6*	*1497$\stackrel{\times}{\div}$1.1*	*181$\stackrel{\times}{\div}$1.2*	*141$\stackrel{\times}{\div}$1.2*
Healthy heterosexual men (n = 12) (means $\stackrel{\times}{\div}$SEM)			1686$\stackrel{\times}{\div}$1.1	114$\stackrel{\times}{\div}$1.1	2.2$\stackrel{\times}{\div}$1.1	1150$\stackrel{\times}{\div}$1.2	240$\stackrel{\times}{\div}$1.3	185$\stackrel{\times}{\div}$1.3

*CMV denotes cytomegalovirus, MCC mucocutaneous candidiasis, PCP *Pneumocystis carinii* pneumonia, KS Kaposi's sarcoma, and PML progressive multifocal leukoencephalopathy.

The purpose of the present study was to examine the functional capabilities of the circulating B cells in this syndrome. A potential indication of an abnormality in B-cell function was the marked decrease in the proliferative response of the patients' unfractionated peripheral-blood mononuclear cells to a T-cell–dependent B-cell mitogen (pokeweed mitogen) (Figure 1). Because pokeweed mitogen is a T-cell–dependent T-cell and B-cell mitogen and polyclonal activator and because the abnormalities noted could have been merely a manifestation of decreased T-cell function, we also examined the proliferative responses of the patients' unfractionated peripheral-blood lymphocytes to a pure B-cell mitogen — formalinized, intact SAC (Fig. 1). As shown in Figure 1, unfractionated cells from patients demonstrated a profound inability to respond to this T-cell–independent B-cell mitogen.

The B-cell mitogenic capabilities of SAC are not known to be under T-cell influence; however, in order to confirm that the observed decrease in responsiveness to SAC was indeed due to an intrinsic B-cell defect and not simply to the influence of a preponderance of OKT8 suppressor cells, experiments were conducted in which T cells were eliminated before culture. In these experiments, the proliferative response of normal cells to SAC increased from 2000 to 8000 cpm upon removal of T cells, because of a relative increase in the proportion of B cells present in the culture. However, T-cell depletion had no effect on the unresponsiveness to SAC of B lymphocytes from patients with AIDS, with values before and after T-cell depletion of 100 and 100 cpm in Patient 9 and 100 and 300 cpm in Patient 10.

Having established the fact that B cells in AIDS have a decreased proliferative response to B-cell mitogens, we next turned our attention to their ability to secrete antibody either spontaneously (an indicator of activation in vivo) or in response to pokeweed mitogen. In contrast to the earlier indicators of decreased B-cell function in terms of proliferation, the number of circulating B lymphocytes spontaneously secreting antibody in patients with AIDS was found to be approximately 10 times that in the heterosexual control group (Fig. 2). Although the spontaneous secretion of immunoglobulin was elevated in patients with AIDS, their lymphocytes could not be triggered by pokeweed mitogen to produce immunoglobulin (Fig. 3). In fact, for the patients with AIDS, levels of immunoglobulin measured in the cultures triggered by pokeweed mitogen were not sub-

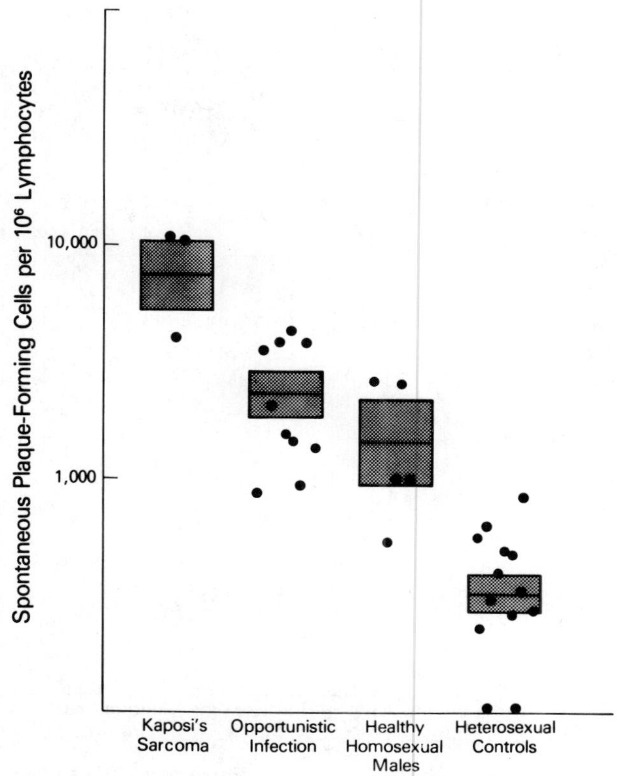

Figure 2. Enumeration of Spontaneous Plaque-Forming Cells in Patients with Kaposi's Sarcoma, Patients with Opportunistic Infections Only, Healthy Homosexual Men, and Healthy Heterosexual Men.

Patients with AIDS have evidence of substantial polyclonal B-cell activation in vivo.

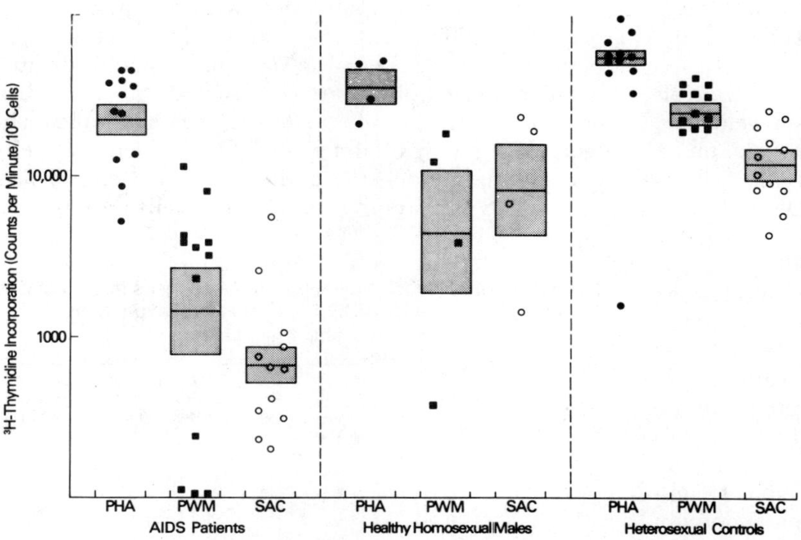

Figure 1. Proliferative Responses of Unfractionated Peripheral-Blood Mononuclear Cells from Patients with AIDS, Healthy Homosexual Men, and Healthy Heterosexual Men to the T-Cell Mitogen Phytohemagglutinin A (PHA), the T-Cell and B-Cell Mitogen Pokeweed (PWM), and the T-Cell–Independent B-Cell Mitogen Staphylococcus aureus Cowan Strain I (SAC).

Responses to the B-cell mitogen are the most severely reduced.

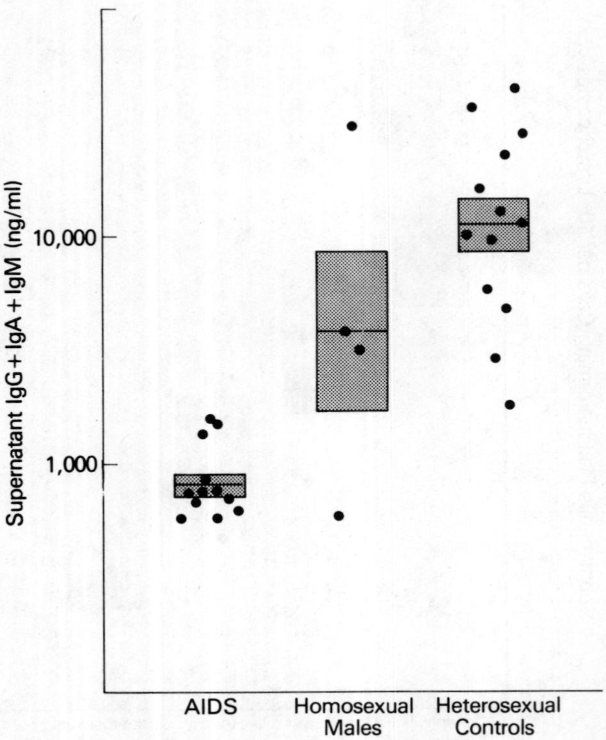

Figure 3. Pokeweed-Mitogen–Induced Production of Supernatant Immunoglobulin.

This T-cell–dependent B-cell function is essentially absent in patients with AIDS.

stantially different from those measured in the unstimulated cultures (data not shown).

A defect in immunoglobulin production induced by pokeweed mitogen can be due to a defect in T cells, B cells, or both. In order to localize the site of such a defect, allogeneic cocultures were performed. In experiments in which B cells from patients or controls were cultured with normal T cells, control B cells (two allogeneic donors) produced a geometric mean (×÷SEM) of 20,335×÷1.1 ng of immunoglobulin, whereas B cells from four patients with AIDS produced 3831×÷2.0 ng of immunoglobulin. As reflected in the large SEM for the patient group, the B cells from some but not all patients with AIDS could be induced to secrete immunoglobulin when cocultured with normal allogeneic T cells. Thus, on the whole, B cells from patients with AIDS were intrinsically defective in their ability to be induced to secrete immunoglobulin. Next, the ability of T4 cells from two patients and a normal donor to provide help and the ability of T8 cells from these same persons to suppress were assayed in a system of immunoglobulin production driven by pokeweed mitogen (Fig. 4). In order to control for allogeneic effects, cells from a second normal subject were used as the indicator population. As shown in Figure 4, the T4 cells from the patients with AIDS exhibited a qualitative defect in their ability to provide help, whereas the T8 cells functioned normally in this system.

Having thus established in a variety of mitogen-driven systems that B cells from patients with AIDS exhibit marked abnormalities of immunoregulation, we next sought to determine whether these same phenomena applied to an antigen-specific response. We have previously shown that two weeks after immunization with keyhole-limpet hemocyanin, the peripheral blood of normal volunteers contained a population of lymphocytes that could be triggered in vitro with antigen or pokeweed mitogen to produce specific antibody or to undergo substantial blast transformation. At the same time, the serologic response in vivo to keyhole-limpet hemocyanin was at its peak.[9] As shown in Table 2, patients with AIDS did not respond either in vivo or in vitro to immunization with this potent primary antigen, with healthy homosexual men again having a response between that of the patients and that of the homosexual controls.

Discussion

The present study has demonstrated marked abnormalities of B-cell activation and immunoregulation in patients with AIDS. These abnormalities include an inability to develop a proliferative response to the pure B-cell mitogen SAC and an increase in the number of cells spontaneously secreting immunoglobulin. These findings are consistent with a marked degree of polyclonal activation in vivo, such as is seen after certain viral infections and in some connective-tissue diseases.[12]

In normal persons, the circulating B-cell pool contains B cells at various stages of activation. The resting B cells can be induced to undergo proliferation by a variety of stimuli, including SAC; the partially activated B cells, when provided with adequate T-cell help, can differentiate into antibody-secreting cells under the influence of pokeweed mitogen; and the fully differentiated B cells are represented by the number of cells in the peripheral blood that spontaneously secrete immunoglobulin.[11,13,14] Thus, given this well-documented model, the peripheral blood of patients with AIDS appears to lack resting B cells and to have

Table 2. Antigen-Specific Lymphocyte Responses in Vivo and in Vitro in Patients with AIDS, Healthy Homosexual Men, and Healthy Heterosexual Men.

	Patients with AIDS (N = 5)	Healthy Homosexual Men (N = 3)	Healthy Heterosexual Men (N = 6)
	means ×÷ SEM		
Serologic response of anti-KLH antibody*	1789×÷1.6	5309×÷1.2	17,900×÷1.2
In vitro proliferative response (cpm/10^5 cells)	190×÷1.2	3906×÷4.8	10,543×÷1.3
In vitro specific antibody production*	<1	4.2×÷1.7	39×÷1.7

*DT_M units per milliliter (1 unit is the amount of anti-KLH IgM present in 1 ml of a 1:10,000 dilution of a hyperimmune reference serum and is approximately 1 ng).[9]

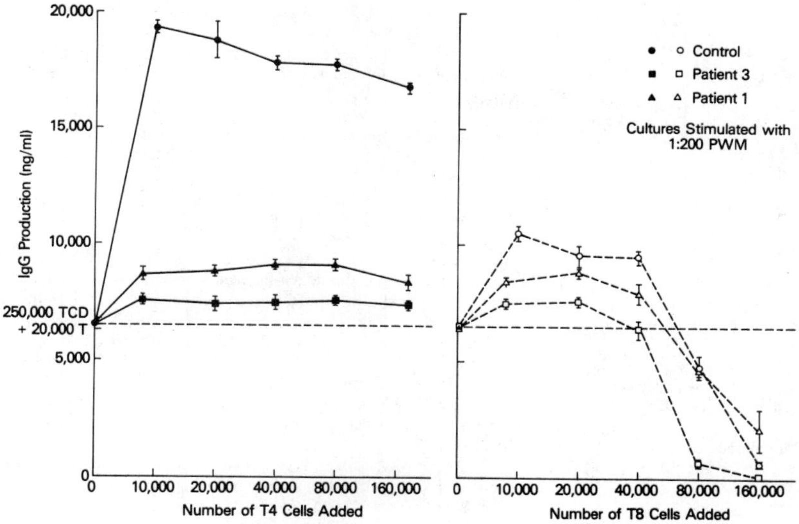

Figure 4. Functional Capabilities of T4+ and T8+ Lymphocytes from Two Patients with AIDS and One Control in a System of Pokeweed-Mitogen (PWM)–Driven Immunoglobulin Production.

T4+ and T8+ populations are assayed in cultures containing 250,000 T-cell–depleted lymphocytes plus 20,000 T cells from a healthy allogeneic donor. The T4+ lymphocytes from patients are qualitatively defective, whereas the T8+ lymphocytes function normally.

decreased numbers of partially activated cells and increased numbers of fully differentiated B cells.

These findings of polyclonal B-cell activation in vivo are very suggestive of viral stimulation or transformation. Polyclonal activation in vivo has been noted during acute infection with members of the herpesvirus family, most notably Epstein–Barr virus.[15] In this regard, as noted in Table 1, all our patients were culture-positive for cytomegalovirus from at least one site, and in the 11 patients tested, all were culture-positive for Epstein–Barr virus. Thus, the extreme polyclonal activation reported here may represent a viral B-cell activation or transformation either by a known agent occurring in the absence of the normal regulatory T-cell influences or by an as yet unknown agent that could be related to the cause of the syndrome.

Our patient group had elevated levels of serum IgG and IgA. This finding has been reported by others and has been interpreted as evidence of intact humoral immune responses.[2-4,7] In the light of the current data, this conclusion must be reexamined. It is quite possible that the elevated levels of serum immunoglobulin in such patients are due to intense polyclonal B-cell activation in vivo and that although the immunoglobulin levels are quantitatively normal or high, they are qualitatively defective. This is demonstrated in this study by the fact that patients with this syndrome do not make serum antibody in response to the potent immunogen keyhole-limpet hemocyanin. The failure to diagnose many of the infections seen in this group of patients serologically may also be related to this B-cell abnormality. In addition, the occurrence of B-cell polyclonal activation may be responsible for the autoimmune thrombocytopenia that has recently been reported in homosexual men[16] and for the elevated levels of circulating immune complexes reported in those men and in patients with AIDS.[1]

The polyclonal B-cell activation reported here is almost surely due to a primary B-cell defect. In diseases that are also associated with polyclonal activation, such as systemic lupus erythematosus, it has been debated for years whether or not the observed phenomena are due to excess T-cell help, decreased T-cell suppression, or direct B-cell activation.[17] In AIDS, the lack of functional helper T cells together with the increased proportion of suppressor T cells places the origin of polyclonal B-cell activation in vivo directly at the level of the B cell.

Whether the decreased level of T-cell function observed in patients with AIDS is explicable solely on the basis of decreased numbers of T4 cells is unknown. Our data (Fig. 4) indicate that with respect to immunoglobulin production, the T4 cells in two patients with AIDS were qualitatively as well as quantitatively abnormal. In addition, in the milieu of normal allogeneic T4 cells, the T8 cells appeared to function normally. Previous investigators reporting abnormally activated suppressor cells in patients with AIDS have used unfractionated T-cell populations; thus, quantitative differences may have been misinterpreted as qualitative differences.

The findings in healthy homosexual men are particularly noteworthy. In each instance in which it was studied, this control group had altered immune function in comparison to that of the heterosexual control group. The variation in the group was substantial, however, with one member of the group having a high T4/T8 ratio of 3.9 and entirely normal proliferative responses to mitogens. The relation of these immunologic abnormalities in healthy homosexual men to AIDS as defined by the Centers for Disease Control is unknown. The factors underlying these observations on abnormal immune responses in healthy homosexual men reported here and by others[6,7] are currently under investigation.

The cause of AIDS remains a mystery. Our data suggest that at the level of the B cell, there is uniform evidence of polyclonal B-cell activation that is highly suggestive of viral stimulation. The nature of the T-cell dysfunction is more difficult to ascertain. It is possible that a lymphocytotropic virus specifically destructive of T4 cells is involved; however, few data have been published to support this possibility. Whatever its cause, AIDS has become a substantial public-health problem that is clearly not limited to one or two segments of society. Further studies more precisely delineating the immunopathophysiology of AIDS may shed important light on the cause of this disorder and ultimately on its treatment.

We are indebted to Dr. Gerald V. Quinnan and Ms. Jody Manischewitz for performing the cytomegalovirus cultures and to Ms. Ann London for editorial assistance.

References

1. Gottleib MS, Schroff R, Schanker HM, et al. *Pneumocystis carinii* pneumonia and mucosal candidiasis in previously healthy homosexual men: evidence of a new acquired cellular immunodeficiency. N Engl J Med 1981; 305:1425-31.
2. Masur H, Michelis MA, Greene JB, et al. An outbreak of community-acquired *Pneumocystis carinii* pneumonia: initial manifestation of cellular immune dysfunction. N Engl J Med 1981; 305:1431-8.
3. Siegal FP, Lopez C, Hammer GS, et al. Severe acquired immunodeficiency in male homosexuals, manifested by chronic perianal ulcerative herpes simplex lesions. N Engl J Med 1981; 305:1439-44.
4. Friedman-Kien AE, Laubenstein LJ, Rubinstein P, et al. Disseminated Kaposi's sarcoma in homosexual men. Ann Intern Med 1982; 96:693-700.
5. Update on acquired immune deficiency syndrome (AIDS) — United States. MMWR 1982; 31:507-14.
6. Kornfeld H, Vande Stouwe RA, Lange M, Reddy MM, Grieco MH. T-lymphocyte subpopulations in homosexual men. N Engl J Med 1982; 307:729-31.
7. Stahl RE, Friedman-Kien A, Dubin R, Marmor M, Zolla-Pazner S. Immunologic abnormalities in homosexual men: relationship to Kaposi's sarcoma. Am J Med 1982; 73:171-8.
8. Mildvan D, Mathur U, Enlow RW, et al. Opportunistic infections and immune deficiency in homosexual men. Ann Intern Med 1982; 96:700-4.
9. Lane HC, Volkman DJ, Whalen G, Fauci AS. In vitro antigen-induced, antigen-specific antibody production in man: specific and polyclonal components, kinetics, and cellular requirements. J Exp Med 1981; 154: 1043-57.
10. Reinherz EL, Kung PC, Goldstein G, Schlossman SF. Further characterization of human inducer T cell subsets defined by monoclonal antibody. J Immunol 1979; 123:2894-6.
11. Fauci AS, Whalen G, Burch C. Activation of human B lymphocytes. XV. Spontaneously occurring and mitogen-induced indirect anti-sheep red blood cell plaque-forming cells in normal human peripheral blood. J Immunol 1980; 124:2410-3.
12. Budman DR, Merchant EB, Steinberg AD, et al. Increased spontaneous activity of antibody forming cells in the peripheral blood of patients with active SLE. Arthritis Rheum 1977; 20:829-33.
13. Fauci AS, Lane HC, Volkman DJ. Activation and regulation of human immune responses: implications in normal and disease states. Ann Intern Med 1983; 99:61-75.
14. Kuritani T, Cooper MD. Human B cell differentiation. II. Pokeweed mitogen-responsive B cells belong to a surface immunoglobulin D-negative subpopulation. J Exp Med 1982; 155:1561-6.
15. van Furth R, Schuit HRE, Hijmans W. The formation of immunoglobulins by human tissues *in vitro*. IV. Circulating lymphocytes in normal and pathological conditions. Immunology 1966; 11:29-40.
16. Morris L, Distenfeld A, Amorosi E, Karpatkin S. Autoimmune thrombocytopenic purpura in homosexual men. Ann Intern Med 1982; 96:714-7.
17. Fauci AS. Immunoregulation in autoimmunity. J Allergy Clin Immunol 1980; 66:5-17.

ORIGINAL ARTICLE

ACID-LABILE ALPHA INTERFERON

A Possible Preclinical Marker for the Acquired Immunodeficiency Syndrome in Hemophilia

M. Elaine Eyster, M.D., James J. Goedert, M.D., Man-Chiu Poon, M.D., and Olivia T. Preble, Ph.D.

Abstract Many homosexual men with the acquired immunodeficiency syndrome (AIDS) have an unusual acid-labile form of human leukocyte, or alpha, interferon in their serum. Male patients with classic hemophilia treated with lyophilized clotting-factor concentrates are also at high risk for the development of AIDS. To determine whether the level of alpha interferon may be a preclinical marker of early subclinical disease, we examined stored plasma and serum from three hemophilic patients with AIDS. Persistently elevated levels of the acid-labile form of alpha interferon were found in all three patients. In two patients the appearance of circulating alpha interferon preceded the onset of clinical disease by 3 to 10 months. In contrast, alpha-interferon levels were not elevated in 43 of 46 unselected patients with hemophilia; three of these patients had transient elevations. These results suggest that acid-labile alpha interferon may be a marker that can be used to identify affected asymptomatic members of high-risk groups before the onset of clinical disease.

THE acquired immunodeficiency syndrome (AIDS) is defined as biopsy-confirmed Kaposi's sarcoma or life-threatening opportunistic infections in previously healthy persons who are under 60 years of age and who have no underlying immunosuppressive condition.[1] The clinical manifestations may be the result of a severe, selective depletion of helper or inducer T lymphocytes and a consequent reversal of the ratio of helper to suppressor T lymphocytes.[2]

Homosexual men are at high risk for AIDS[1,3-6]; many homosexuals who have AIDS have an unusual acid-labile form of human leukocyte, or alpha, interferon in their serum.[7] Male patients with classic hemophilia (hemophilia A) treated with lyophilized clotting-factor concentrate are also at high risk for AIDS.[8-12] The status of alpha interferon in their serum has not been reported.

To determine whether the presence of alpha interferon may allow early recognition of patients with subclinical AIDS, we examined stored plasma and serum from three hemophilic patients with AIDS. When samples were evaluated after the development of AIDS, persistently elevated levels of the acid-labile form of alpha interferon were found in all three patients. In two of them the appearance of circulating alpha interferon preceded the onset of clinical disease by 3 to 10 months. In contrast, alpha-interferon levels were normal in 46 unselected patients with asymptomatic hemophilia, except for transient elevations in three patients. These results suggest that acid-labile alpha interferon may be a marker that can be used to identify affected but asymptomatic persons in high-risk groups before the onset of clinical disease.

From the Division of Hematology, Department of Medicine, Milton S. Hershey Medical Center, Pennsylvania State University, Hershey, Pa.; the Environmental Epidemiology Branch, National Cancer Institute, Bethesda, Md.; the Division of Hematology/Oncology, Department of Medicine, University of Alabama in Birmingham, and Birmingham Veterans Administration Medical Center, Birmingham, Ala.; and the Department of Pathology, Uniformed Services University of Health Sciences, Bethesda, Md.

Supported in part by grants (R07426 and R07439) from the Uniformed Services University of the Health Sciences, under a contract (Y01 CP 00502) with the National Cancer Institute, and under contracts (ME82051 and ME82130) from the Pennsylvania Department of Health.

Case Histories

Case 1

A 36-year-old white man from Pennsylvania who had had mild hemophilia A and common variable hypogammaglobulinemia for 16 years received monthly infusions of fresh-frozen plasma and occasional infusions of antihemophilic factor (factor VIII concentrate).[11] During 1981 he was admitted to the hospital five times for recurrent pansinusitis. On February 17, 1982, radical maxillary and sphenoid-sinus surgery was performed. Profuse postoperative bleeding necessitated treatment with large doses of antihemophilic factor. Bloody diarrhea, with cultures that were positive for *Clostridium difficile,* was resolved with oral vancomycin in late March; non-bloody diarrhea containing no identifiable microorganism developed in late April and persisted for the next few months. A rectal biopsy performed in July, by which time the patient had lost 18 kg in weight, disclosed small eosin-staining particles, and electron microscopy revealed the typical cysts of cryptosporidiosis.

A laboratory evaluation in September showed profound lymphopenia with marked depletion of helper T cells (the total lymphocyte count was 300, with 17 percent helper cells and 64 percent suppressor cells; the helper/suppressor ratio was 0.26). Low titers of antibodies against hepatitis B surface antigen (31 sample ratio units) were detected by radioimmunoassay, and antibodies against cytomegalovirus (1:8) and herpes Type 1 (1:64) by indirect hemagglutination. Diarrhea and weight loss continued despite furazolidone therapy, and the patient died in October 1982. A postmortem examination (performed at Geisinger Medical Center in Danville, Pa.) revealed micronodular cirrhosis, disseminated candidiasis, cytomegalovirus pneumonia, and cryptosporidiosis. The multiple opportunistic infections in this patient are typical of AIDS and unprecedented in common variable hypogammaglobulinemia.

Case 2

A 10-year-old white boy from Pennsylvania with severe hemophilia A treated at home with factor VIII concentrate was otherwise well until October 1982, when he was admitted to the hospital with fever, cough, and dyspnea of three weeks' duration.[8] At physical examination the temperature was 38.4°C and the respiratory rate was 60 per minute. Chest x-ray films showed a bilateral interstitial pneumonitis. The absolute number of circulating lymphocytes was depressed (580 cells per cubic millimeter), and the helper/suppressor ratio was markedly reduced (0.1), with 5 percent helper cells and 46 percent suppressor cells. Serum immunoglobulin levels were elevated. An open-lung biopsy demonstrated extensive infiltration with *Pneumocystis carinii* and *Cryptococcus neoformans*. Intravenous therapy with sulfamethoxazole–trimethoprin and amphotericin B led to complete resolution of the pneumonitis. However, the T-cell abnormalities persisted with an absolute deficiency of helper cells and a helper/suppressor ratio of 0.2 (as of January 12, 1983).

Case 3

A 55-year-old white man from Alabama with severe hemophilia A treated at home with factor VIII concentrate had anorexia and progressive weight loss beginning in September 1981.[8,12] In March 1982 herpes zoster developed but resolved after five days of treatment with vidarabine. In June the patient was hospitalized for fever and respiratory symptoms associated with bibasilar infiltrates; he improved with the administration of broad-spectrum antibiotics. Laboratory studies performed in August revealed persistent lymphopenia (1050 cells per cubic millimeter) with 6 percent helper cells and 30 percent suppressor cells (helper/suppressor ratio, 0.2). In September the patient was hospitalized again, with fever, cough, and a cumulative weight loss of 47 kg. Chest x-ray films revealed bilateral infiltrates, and an open-lung biopsy showed *P. carinii.* The patient responded to treatment with sulfamethoxazole–trimethoprim, but eight weeks later *Mycobacterium avium-intracellulare* was cultured from a lung-biopsy specimen and subsequent sputum specimens. In addition to prophylactic sulfamethoxazole–trimethoprim with folinic acid, isoniazid with pyridoxine, rifampin, clofazimine, and ansamycin was started in December. The lymphopenia and inverted helper/suppressor ratio (0.1 to 0.3) persisted (as of January 1983).

Methods

Interferon was quantitated in 96-well microtiter plates, with the use of human GM 2504 fibroblasts; a challenge was performed with encephalomyocarditis virus, as previously described.[7,13] The interferon titer was defined as the reciprocal of the highest twofold dilution of the serum or plasma sample that would protect 50 percent of the cells from virus-induced cytopathology. For determination of antiviral activity on nonhuman cells, interferon was assayed in duplicate on GM 2504 cells and on bovine (MDBK) cells; the challenge was performed with vesicular stomatitis virus. Antiviral activity on bovine cells is a characteristic of human alpha interferon; human beta and gamma interferons are inactive on these cells. To confirm the identity of interferons from hemophilic patients with AIDS, each interferon was incubated with highly specific rabbit antibodies against purified human alpha, beta, and gamma interferons, as previously described,[13] and residual interferon was assayed on GM 2504 cells. The stability of alpha interferon at pH 2 was determined as described elsewhere.[7,13] Each sample was tested in duplicate. When the above methods were used in studies in approximately 80 laboratory workers and healthy blood donors of both sexes between the ages of 18 and 60 years, all serum samples but one were negative for alpha interferon[7,13] (and Preble OT: unpublished data).

Thirty-seven unselected male patients with hemophilia A and nine with hemophilia B, who served as controls, gave informed consent for a clinical evaluation, interview, and phlebotomy during routine clinic visits for comprehensive care at the Hershey Medical Center from September through December 1982. They included 45 whites and 1 black and ranged in age from 6 to 61 years (median, 24.5 years). One man was homosexual; the other 45 patients or their parents denied homosexual activity.

Interferon levels in the controls were determined in coded samples of serum that had been separated from clotted blood in serum-separation tubes and frozen at −70°C until use. Coded samples from the three patients with AIDS were either serum or citrated platelet-poor plasma that had been stored at −70°C. The validity of using stored samples for this assay has been verified by finding acid-labile alpha interferon in the expected proportion of serum samples from patients with systemic lupus erythematosus, even though the samples had been stored for as long as 10 years (Preble OT: unpublished data). Repeated freezing and thawing had no effect on either the titer or properties of the acid-labile alpha interferon in the serum from the patients with systemic lupus or those with AIDS (Preble OT: unpublished data). Additional controls included coded specimens of serum from 40 healthy laboratory workers of both sexes, citrated plasma from 20 healthy Hershey Medical Center employees of both sexes between the ages of 18 and 45 years, plasma from 17 patients (including 7 children between 6 and 14 years of age) with coagulation disorders treated at the Center, and serum from three adults with various disorders (aplastic anemia, dysmyelopoiesis, and myelofibrosis) who received multiple transfusions. Preservative-free heparin (100 U per milliliter) was routinely added to all plasma samples before quantitation of interferon, to prevent clotting.

Phenotypic helper/suppressor ratios were determined in peripheral-blood lymphocytes by means of commercially available reagents, as previously described.[12,14,15]

Results

The circulating alpha-interferon levels and concurrent clinical status of the three hemophiliacs with AIDS are shown in Table 1. In all three cases, no interferon was detected in samples obtained 16 to 53 months before the onset of AIDS. In Cases 1 and 2, however, alpha interferon was clearly elevated 3 to 10 months before an opportunistic infection. Case 2, in particular, was apparently healthy when alpha interferon was first detected. The alpha interferon in each of 12 serum and plasma samples from these three patients was partially inactivated by acid pH, with a fourfold to eightfold reduction in titer at pH 2, as previously reported in homosexuals with AIDS[7] and patients with systemic lupus erythematosus.[13] In con-

Table 1. Serial Alpha-Interferon Levels in Three Hemophilic Patients with AIDS.

Case No.	Date	Alpha-Interferon Level (IU/ml)*	Clinical Status
1	01/09/80	Negative	Well, receiving intermittent ampicillin and fresh-frozen plasma
	10/08/80	Negative	Well, receiving intermittent antibiotics for chronic sinusitis
	06/17/81	12†	Recurrent sinusitis with purulent drainage, receiving penicillin
	02/19/82	25†	Postoperative bleeding
	04/30/82	Not done	Diarrhea
	07/26/82	25†	Cryptosporidiosis with diarrhea and weight loss
	09/15/82	25 †	Pneumonia
	10/12/82	25†	Antemortem (see text)
2	09/19/79	Negative	Well
	06/19/80	Negative	Well
	12/10/80	Negative	Well
	06/10/81	Negative	Well
	07/14/82	20–25	Well
	10/25/82	12†	Pneumocystis and cryptococcal pneumonia
	11/17/82	25†	Recovering, receiving sulfamethoxazole–trimethoprim and amphotericin B
	01/12/83	10–12†	Well; helper/suppressor ratio of 0.2
3	10/20/76	Negative	Well
	05/11/78	Negative	Diabetes mellitus, otherwise well
	10/26/82	8–10†	Recovering from *Pneumocystis carinii* pneumonia, receiving sulfamethoxazole–trimethoprim
	12/13/82	100†	Pulmonary *Mycobacterium avium-intracellulare;* throat culture positive for cytomegalovirus
	01/05/83	8–10	Intermittent nausea, ascites, otherwise well; helper/suppressor ratio of 0.3

*Negative denotes ≤4 IU per milliliter. Levels determined in citrated plasma samples, unless otherwise indicated.

†Level in serum.

trast, reference human alpha interferon was completely stable under the same conditions.

Borderline levels of alpha interferon (6 IU per milliliter) were detected in serum obtained from 2 of the 37 controls with hemophilia A and from 1 of the 9 controls with hemophilia B. One control, a self-reported homosexual who had a helper/suppressor ratio of 1.49 (normal mean ±SD, 1.9±0.7), was asymptomatic and had no detectable interferon four months later. Another control, whose helper/suppressor ratio was slightly low (1.09), had an interferon level of 12 IU per milliliter three months later. After nine months, no serum interferon was detected and he was healthy. A third control, an ethanol abuser with chronic hepatitis, thrombocytopenia, and a normal helper/suppressor ratio (1.74), had no detectable interferon at three or six months. Follow-up of these control patients is continuing. No interferon was found in the three adults given multiple transfusions for various disorders. Likewise, none was found in any of the 60 healthy adults or in any of the 17 children or adults with coagulation disorders who served as additional controls.

Discussion

In a recent study of homosexual men in New York City high serum levels of alpha interferon were present in 63 percent of the men with AIDS and in 29 percent of those with enlarged lymph nodes.[7] Only 2 of 25 clinically healthy homosexual men had circulating alpha interferon[7]; both these men had inverted helper/suppressor ratios.[16] Only 1 of approximately 80 healthy laboratory workers and normal blood donors had detectable serum interferon[7,13] (and Preble OT: unpublished data). Other investigators have also found that the prevalence of detectable serum interferon is very low (1 to 3 percent) in normal subjects,[17,18] possibly reflecting transient viral infections.

All three of our hemophilic patients with AIDS had persistently elevated levels of alpha interferon during and after opportunistic infections. In two patients, circulating alpha interferon appeared 3 to 10 months before clinical disease and in the absence of known inducers of interferon, such as acute viral infections. Very low levels of alpha interferon were occasionally detected in 3 of 46 controls with hemophilia, one of whom was homosexual and therefore had at least two risk factors. On repeat examination after three months, only a heterosexual patient with hemophilia and a low helper/suppressor ratio had elevated levels, and interferon was no longer detected in his serum after nine months. No interferon was detected in the serum or plasma of 80 controls without hemophilia. None of the subjects had clinical evidence of autoimmune diseases.

Although the exact cause of interferon induction in these patients is uncertain, alpha interferon may have biologic relevance to the immune defects and cause of AIDS. All classes of human interferon have potent effects on antibody production, cell-mediated immunity, and natural-killer-cell activity.[19] Natural alpha interferon comprises at least 15 proteins that differ from one another in molecular weight and biologic activities in vitro.[20] Why so many forms of human alpha interferon exist and whether they perform different functions in vivo are not yet known. Viruses and other microorganisms that proliferate within cells are potent inducers of alpha interferon in cultures of mononuclear cells, such as monocytes, natural killer cells, and B lymphocytes.[21] Lymphocytes or other cells from persons with certain genotypes may respond to viral infection or other inducers by producing disproportionately large quantities of a normally minor component of human alpha interferon. Such a mechanism could account for endogenous production of acid-labile alpha interferon in patients with autoimmune disease, as well as in those with AIDS. Alternatively, epidemiologic evidence suggests that AIDS may be caused by a transmissible agent[22-25] and production of acid-labile alpha interferon may be a specific response to this agent. No information is yet available to distinguish between these two possibilities, since the latter hypothesis can be tested only if an "AIDS agent" is isolated.

The alpha interferon found in homosexual men and hemophiliacs with AIDS is an unusual, acid-labile form previously reported in patients with autoimmune disease.[13] Since it is seldom detected in the serum of healthy people, it has the potential for use as a specific marker for the early detection of AIDS. However, further research will be necessary before assay of circulating acid-labile alpha interferon can be used as a screening procedure. In particular, the accuracy of elevated levels of alpha interferon in identifying patients in whom AIDS will subsequently develop will have to be compared with the accuracy of other currently available indicators, including thymosin α_1 levels,[26] helper/suppressor ratios, and other T-cell phenotypes. Laboratory testing should be used only as an adjunct to a careful clinical evaluation with special attention to lymphadenopathy and early symptoms, such as intermittent diarrhea and weight loss. Large, carefully controlled studies of transfusion recipients will also be required to determine whether alpha interferon or other surrogate markers of AIDS can be used to screen blood products for a putative transmissible agent.

We are indebted to Drs. T.V. Shankey, D.L. Mann, D.M. Strong, and A. Landay for determining the helper/suppressorratios; Dr. H. Masur for providing a serum sample from Case 3; to Drs. D. Francis and L. Nerurkar for viral-antibody testing; to Dr.C.J. Favino for the postmortem examination of Case 1; to Elizabeth White for expert technical assistance; and to Dianna Jessee for help in the preparation of the manuscript.

References

1. Update on acquired immune deficiency syndrome (AIDS) — United States. MMWR 1982; 31:507-14.
2. Fauci AS. The syndrome of Kaposi's sarcoma and opportunistic infections: an epidemiologically restricted disorders of immunoregulation. Ann Intern Med 1982; 96:777-9.

3. Gottlieb MS, Schroff R, Schanker HM, et al. *Pneumocystis carinii* pneumonia and mucosal candidiasis in previously healthy homosexual men: evidence of a new acquired cellular immunodeficiency. N Engl J Med 1981; 305:1425-31.
4. Masur H, Michelis MA, Greene JB, et al. An outbreak of community-acquired *Pneumocystis carinii* pneumonia: initial manifestation of cellular immune dysfunction. N Engl J Med 1981; 305:1431-8.
5. Siegal FP, Lopez C, Hammer GS, et al. Severe acquired immunodeficiency in male homosexuals, manifested by chronic perianal ulcerative herpes simplex lesions. N Engl J Med 1981; 305:1439-44.
6. Friedman-Kien AE, Laubenstein LJ, Rubinstein P, et al. Disseminated Kaposi's sarcoma in homosexual men. Ann Intern Med 1982; 96:693-700.
7. DeStefano E, Friedman RM, Friedman-Kien AE, et al. Acid-labile human leukocyte interferon in homosexual men with Kaposi's sarcoma and lymphadenopathy. J Infect Dis 1982; 146:451-5.
8. Update on acquired immune deficiency syndrome (AIDS) among patients with hemophilia A. MMWR 1982; 31:644-6, 652.
9. Lederman MM, Ratnoff OD, Scillian JJ, Jones PK, Schacter B. Impaired cell-mediated immunity in patients with classic hemophilia. N Engl J Med 1983; 308:79-83.
10. Menitove JE, Aster RH, Casper JT, et al. T-lymphocyte subpopulations in patients with classic hemophilia treated with cryoprecipitate and lyophilized concentrates. N Engl J Med 1983; 308:83-6.
11. Eyster ME, Koch KL, Abt AB, Shankey TV. Cryptosporidiosis in a hemophiliac with acquired immunodeficiency. Blood 1982; 60:Suppl 1:211a. abstract.
12. Poon M-C, Landay A, Prasthofer EF, Stagno S. Acquired immunodeficiency syndrome with *Pneumocystis carinii* pneumonia and *Mycobacterium avium-intracellulare* in a previously healthy patient with classic hemophilia: clinical, immunologic and virologic findings. Ann Intern Med (in press).
13. Preble OT, Black RJ, Friedman RM, Klippel JH, Vilcek J. Systemic lupus erythematosus: presence in human serum of an unusual acid-labile leukocyte interferon. Science 1982; 216:429-31.
14. Slease RB, Wistar R Jr, Scher I. Surface immunoglobulin density on human peripheral blood mononuclear cells. Blood 1979; 54:72-87.
15. Slease RB, Strong DM, Wistar R Jr, Budd RE, Scher I. Determination of surface immunoglobulin density on frozen-thawed mononuclear cells analyzed by fluorescence-activated cell sorter. Cryobiology 1980; 17:523-9.
16. Goedert JJ, Neuland CY, Wallen WC, et al. Amyl nitrite may alter T lymphocytes in homosexual men. Lancet 1982; 1:412-6.
17. Levin S, Hahn T. Evaluation of the human interferon system in viral disease. Clin Exp Immunol 1981; 46:475-83.
18. Hooks JJ, Jordan GW, Cupps T, Moutsopoulos HM, Fauci AS, Notkins AL. Multiple interferons in the circulation of patients with systemic lupus erythematosus and vasculitis. Arthritis Rheum 1982; 25:396-400.
19. Friedman RM, Vogel SM. Interferon with special emphasis on the immune system. Adv Immunol (in press).
20. Nagata S, Mantei N, Weissmann C. The structure of one of the eight or more distinct chromosomal genes for human interferon — α. Nature 1980; 287:401-8.
21. Epstein LB. The comparative biology of immune and classical interferons. In: Cohen S, Pick E, Oppenheim JJ, eds. Biology of the lymphokines. New York: Academic Press, 1979:443-514.
22. Possible transfusion-associated acquired immune deficiency syndrome (AIDS) — California. MMWR 1982; 31:652-4.
23. A cluster of Kaposi's sarcoma and *Pneumocystis carinii* among homosexual male residents of Los Angeles and Orange Counties, California. MMWR 1982; 31:305-7.
24. Gerstoft J, Malchow-Møller A, Bygbjerg I, et al. Severe acquired immunodeficiency in European homosexual men. Br Med J 1982; 285:17-9.
25. Marmor M, Friedman-Kien AE, Laubenstein L, et al. Risk factors for Kaposi's sarcoma in homosexual men. Lancet 1982; 1:1083-6.
26. Hersh EM, Reuben JM, Rios A, et al. Elevated serum thymosin α_1 levels associated with evidence of immune dysregulation in male homosexuals with a history of infectious diseases or Kaposi's sarcoma. N Engl J Med 1983; 308:45-6.

SPECIAL ARTICLE

A PATHOGENIC RETROVIRUS (HTLV-III) LINKED TO AIDS

SAMUEL BRODER, M.D., AND ROBERT C. GALLO, M.D.

APPROXIMATELY three years ago an apparently new and unexplained disorder called the acquired immunodeficiency syndrome (AIDS) was recognized. Prompt worldwide recognition of this syndrome was brought about by a truly remarkable collaboration between practicing physicians in several parts of the United States and epidemiologists at the Centers for Disease Control. AIDS immediately became the subject of a number of reports, many of which have appeared in the *Journal*.[1-9] The disorder is an epidemic immunosuppressive disease that predisposes to life-threatening infections with opportunistic organisms, Kaposi's sarcoma, and less commonly, other neoplasms such as non-Hodgkin's lymphomas. Characteristically, AIDS is associated with a depletion of T cells, especially the helper/inducer subset bearing the OKT4 surface marker.

One of the major frustrations for practicing physicians and the public alike has been the inability of the scientific community to define the origin of this disease. Perhaps John Donne, in 1624, in reference to his own life-threatening illness, was able to capture some of the frustrating emotions felt by patients with AIDS, persons thought to be at risk of AIDS, and their physicians:

> I observe the Phisician, with the same diligence, as hee the disease; I see hee feares, and I feare with him: I overtake him, I overrun him in his feare, and I go the faster, because he makes his pace slow; I feare the more, because he disguises his fear, and see it with more sharpnesse, because hee would not have me see it.[10]

But recently, several converging lines of research have linked a human T-cell lymphotropic retrovirus (HTLV-III) to the pathogenesis of AIDS,[11-14] and this knowledge has brought us closer to understanding the disease. We would like to highlight some of the recent developments that are likely to have immediate clinical relevance and briefly review some of the ideas and basic research that led to the current understanding of retroviruses in AIDS.

Current discoveries can perhaps best be understood in the larger context of research on human retroviruses.[15-20] A retrovirus encodes its genetic information in RNA and uses a unique viral enzyme called reverse transcriptase to copy its genome into DNA. Usually, retroviruses contain three genes, including a gene for the viral internal core proteins, called *gag*, the polymerase or reverse transcriptase gene, called *pol*, and the gene for the envelope glycoprotein, called *env*. The transcription-initiation signals for a retrovirus lie within the long terminal repeat sequences that flank the virus as it exists within the host-cell genome in a DNA form (called a provirus). Certain viral genes are sometimes replaced by a cell-derived DNA sequence known as an *onc* gene, which allows some animal retroviruses to transform appropriate target cells acutely. However, members of the HTLV family of human retroviruses as well as the vast majority of naturally occurring animal retroviruses do not carry known *onc* genes as they are conventionally defined. Retroviruses have been unequivocally linked to certain cancers and immunodeficiency states in animals, but evidence for human counterparts of the animal retroviruses was slow to develop. Indeed, at one time most investigators questioned the existence of human retroviruses and their relevance to human diseases. Beginning in 1970, after the discovery of reverse transcriptase by Baltimore[21] and Temin and Mizutani,[22] molecular and biologic approaches adapted to detect low-level expression of retroviruses in human tissues,[23] as well as techniques for the routine long-term culture of various hematopoietic cells, were developed in the Laboratory of Tumor Cell Biology at the National Cancer Institute. Both strategies proved useful in isolating and identifying human retroviruses in the United States and soon thereafter in several other parts of the world.

The long-term growth of mature human T cells was made possible in 1976, when a protein called T-cell growth factor (TCGF) was identified.[24] This protein, later called interleukin-2, has been purified, its gene cloned, and its membrane receptor characterized.[25-27] With TCGF the routine establishment of T-cell lines from normal persons and patients with various diseases, including certain T-cell neoplasms, became possible. Cultured cells derived from American patients with TCGF-receptor–positive T-cell lymphoproliferative disease were the source of the first isolates of human retroviruses, obtained in 1978 and 1980. Large-scale virus production was possible at the outset. These viruses were given the name "human T-cell leukemia/lymphoma virus" (HTLV) when the work was published in 1980[16] and 1981,[17] after immunologic, biochemical, and genetic analyses had proved that the agent was not an animal-virus contaminant,[15] and that it could be detected repeatedly in the same patient. In culture this unique virus could infect and transform human T cells.[15,19,28] In certain settings, infected cells acquired new functional properties, including the capacity to respond to soluble antigen in the absence of accessory cells.[29] In other settings, however, transformation of an immune T cell was associated with a cytopathic effect occurring upon further contact with the virus.[30]

The virus was then found to be endemic in southern

From the Clinical Oncology Program and the Laboratory of Tumor Cell Biology, National Cancer Institute, Bethesda, Md.

Japan[15,31] and later in Africa and certain parts of the Western hemisphere, including the southeastern portion of the United States, and it was linked to the origin of adult T-cell leukemia.[15]

Later it became apparent that HTLV should be viewed as a family of related T-cell lymphotropic retroviruses and not as a single virus. The prototypical member of the family (first isolated from American, Japanese, and Caribbean patients with adult T-cell leukemia) is referred to as HTLV-I. The second member of the family is designated HTLV-II.[20] The genes of HTLV-I and HTLV-II have been cloned and analyzed in detail.[32-34] We shall summarize the established molecular and biologic features of the HTLV family and discuss some of the more promising developments for future research.

These viruses do not possess known *onc* genes, and yet (in the case of HTLV-I and HTLV-II) they can acutely transform cells in vitro. Since the first isolation of HTLV-I, more than 100 isolates of this virus have been obtained. HTLV-I is the only member of this family that has been identified in Japan thus far; the virus in Japan is identical to the HTLV-I found in the United States and the Caribbean, implying relatively recent divergence, prevention of divergence by biologic imperatives, or both. Unlike HTLV-I, the latest addition to the HTLV family — HTLV-III — is characterized by substantial genetic polymorphism — a point that we will consider in more detail later.

Several features related to the genetic organization of the HTLV-I provirus and its pattern of insertion into the host genome are worth noting. Usually, only one provirus is integrated into the DNA of a given host cell.[35,36] Although HTLV-I can integrate into many different chromosomal loci, analysis of HTLV-bearing leukemias and lymphomas has shown that the viral integration is monoclonal — i.e., in each tumor cell in a given patient the viral sequence is integrated in the same place.[15,35-37] Since HTLV-I (as either a complete or defective virus) can integrate into many different chromosomal loci,[37,38] these findings demonstrate that HTLV-I infects the host before neoplastic transformation of the first T cell. In other words, the process does not reflect a late passenger-virus effect, thus supporting a direct role for HTLV-I in the process of leukemogenesis.

The knowledge that HTLV-I has no common pattern of chromosomal integration, yet can transform normal T cells in vitro under certain circumstances, suggests that there is a *trans* mechanism for the leukemogenic effect of this virus — i.e., a diffusible viral-protein product mediates at least one step in the transformation. In this regard, it is necessary to discuss a special segment of the virus, called the pX region.[32] To date, all viruses of the HTLV family have been shown to have a unique pX sequence at the 3′ end of the viral genome. In an analysis of one molecular clone of HTLV-I, the pX region had genetic information for four polypeptides.[32] However, more recent work with other variants of HTLV-I and comparisons of HTLV-I and HTLV-II[34,39] (and Ratner L: unpublished data) indicate that there is a 3′, 1011-nucleotide-long region that is highly conserved and has but one open reading frame, with a coding capacity for a protein with a molecular weight of about 40,000. Indeed, a discrete messenger RNA transcribed from the pX region has been defined by Franchini et al.,[40] and more recently the protein product has been identified (Lee T, Sodroski J, Haseltine W, et al.: unpublished data).

Recently, Sodroski et al. have proposed a process of *trans*-acting transcriptional activation in the leukemogenesis induced by this virus.[41] (Such *trans*-acting viral gene products are known to exist in certain DNA tumor-virus systems.[42,43]) From these investigators' data, the hypothesis can be drawn that the pX region encodes a substance capable of activating transcription in regulatory sequences of distantly situated long terminal repeats of the virus. This would explain how the virus itself could play a part in amplifying viral replication through what is, in effect, a positive-feedback loop. By direct extension, one can propose a model in which such a factor coincidentally interacts with similar regulatory sequences of cellular genes, such as those that participate in cell division, and thereby serves as one element in initiating the uncontrolled growth of transformed cells. Mutations in the pX region might profoundly affect a range of biologic activities, including virus-mediated transformation or cytopathic effect.

It is worth recapitulating certain very recent data regarding the HTLV family. Although HTLV-I and HTLV-II are quite distinct viruses, their genomes have some homologous sequences, especially in the pX region.[34] Also, Hahn et al. have recently found a variant of HTLV-I in Africa,[44] and perhaps future research will reveal clinical manifestations that can be linked to subtle molecular changes in this virus. Moreover, viruses very similar to HTLV-I are present in many Old World monkeys,[45-48] but they can be distinguished from human retroviruses by molecular analyses.[47] The wide distribution of HTLV-I in Africa[15,48] and the presence of a closely related virus in troops of Old World monkeys support the hypothesis that the HTLV family originated in Africa and that at least one member arrived in the Americas by way of the slave trade.[49] Moreover, the presence of HTLV-I in Japan and the identity of this virus with the HTLV-I in Africa, the United States, and the Caribbean is consistent with the speculation that HTLV-I arrived in Japan relatively recently, perhaps brought there by the 16th-century Portuguese mariners who had contacts with Africa and Japan during the same period.[49]

In contrast to HTLV-I, isolated from numerous patients with adult T-cell leukemia and linked to this neoplasm by consistent epidemiologic and molecular biologic results, HTLV-II has been isolated only in a patient with leukemia[20] and in an intravenous-drug abuser[50] and has not been conclusively linked to human disease by seroepidemiologic results to date.

One can summarize the salient features of HTLVs by noting that all members of the family (including the agent believed to cause AIDS) have at least eight features in common: (1) they are exogenous viruses isolated from mature T cells, especially OKT4+ T cells; (2) they infect mature T cells in vitro, although other kinds of cells can serve as targets for infection under certain circumstances[51]; (3) they have a reverse transcriptase with similar biochemical features (e.g., similar size and preference for magnesium); (4) they possess some cross-reacting antigens; (5) they have major core proteins of similar size; (6) they exhibit some homology in nucleotide sequence; (7) they have a pX sequence at the 3′ end of the genome; and (8) upon in vitro infection of some T cells, they induce formation of multinucleated giant cells.

The hypothesis that a T-cell tropic retrovirus might cause AIDS was developed in 1982 and was stimulated by a number of considerations, including the knowledge that another retrovirus — feline leukemia virus — causes immunodeficiencies in cats.[52] Moreover, well-characterized retroviruses in the HTLV family were known to have tropism for T cells, to exert cytopathic effects on target cells, to alter T-cell functions, to kill immune T cells in certain situations, to exhibit transmissibility by intimate contact or blood products, and probably to have originated in Africa.[15] Obviously, these are features that would be expected of a putative AIDS-causing virus. Nonetheless, at the beginning of these studies (and even more recently) several other factors attracted considerable attention as primary causes of AIDS,[53] including self-administration of amyl nitrate, antigen overload, immunosuppressive properties of sperm, the Epstein–Barr virus, cytomegalovirus, and a fungus.

The hypothesis that AIDS is caused by one or more immunosuppressive T-cell tropic retroviruses received direct empirical support in 1983.[54-57] Key seroepidemiologic data were provided by Essex and Lee and their colleagues,[54] who discovered the presence of antibodies to cell-membrane antigen of HTLV-I–infected T cells in a substantial number of patients with AIDS. This antigen is now known to be part of the envelope of HTLV-I. At the same time, an observation made by Barré-Sinoussi et al. in France reinforced the possibility that a then-uncharacterized member of the HTLV family might have a role in the pathogenesis of AIDS: the detection of a retrovirus, initially termed lymphadenopathy-associated virus, in a homosexual man who was thought to have a possible prodrome of AIDS.[57] These workers concluded that the new retrovirus belonged in the HTLV family but was distinct from the other members then defined.[57] Two parallel findings supported these ideas: the frequent detection of antibodies to a membrane (HTLV-I or HTLV-II envelope) protein in serum from patients with AIDS,[54] who usually lack antibodies to internal core structural proteins of HTLV-I and HTLV-II[58]; and the infrequent isolation of HTLV-I and HTLV-II virions from patients with AIDS, even in the presence of antibodies to HTLV-I envelope determinants.

As these studies were intensified by workers at the National Cancer Institute and at the Pasteur Institute, it became clear that cytopathic retroviruses resembling, but not identical to, the known members of the HTLV family could be detected in a large number of patients with AIDS. In fact, such viruses were detected as early as November 1982 but not reported until 1984 because of the original inability to propagate these cytopathic retroviruses reliably on a wide scale.[12] HTLV-I and HTLV-II can be grown reproducibly in T cells, either by supporting the primary cells with TCGF or by establishing replication in newly infected T cells, which eventually become immortal. T cells infected by HTLV-III, on the other hand, quickly degenerate, and the virus can be lost. As a consequence, the inability to document unambiguously the relation between individual isolates impeded research within any given laboratory and collaboration among laboratories.[59]

Accumulating case reports provided potentially important clinical and epidemiologic data relating to T-cell tropic retroviruses in AIDS,[60,61] but there still was no certainty that each isolate represented the same retrovirus. A variety of designations for retroviruses detected in patients with AIDS appeared in the literature[61] (e.g., LAV, IDAV1, and IDAV2). In theory, each isolate might have been a different, newly discovered human retrovirus presenting as an opportunistic infection, with no bearing on the pathogenesis of AIDS.

One major hurdle was overcome by identifying a neoplastic T-cell target population that was susceptible to infection by the new AIDS-related member of the HTLV family (as free virus) but capable of maintaining high rates of growth and virus production despite the cytopathic effect in other T-cell systems.[11] This made it possible to harvest large amounts of virus continuously and offered new research opportunities. First of all, it permitted the development of both immunologic and nucleic acid probes of a retrovirus linked to AIDS. This development in turn permitted a precise definition of the latest addition to the HTLV family — HTLV-III — as a specific retrovirus but one that differed from HTLV-I and HTLV-II on morphologic, immunologic, and genetic grounds. Secondly, it made it possible to determine that each of 48 new viral isolates obtained from patients with AIDS or at risk for AIDS represented the same agent; this has now been done for over 90 isolates in the Laboratory of Tumor Cell Biology. Thirdly, it made it feasible to begin distributing specimens of virus to interested researchers on a regular basis. Finally, and most important from a practical viewpoint, it provided the opportunity to produce sufficient antigen for nationwide seroepidemiologic studies, especially blood-bank screening.

As noted above, HTLV-III shares many properties with HTLV-I and HTLV-II, including T-cell tropism and a propensity to infect T cells with the OKT4+ (helper/inducer) phenotype. All three viruses also have similar reverse transcriptases, at least some cross-reactive antigens, major structural proteins of similar size, and the capacity to induce multinucleated giant cells. Moreover, recent nucleic acid hybridization studies have revealed some homologies among all three members of the HTLV family and the presence of a pX region[62] (and Ratner L, Wong-Staal F, Gallo RC: unpublished data). It is of interest that pX is highly conserved in HTLV-I and HTLV-II and that both these viruses can transform T cells in vitro. By contrast, although a pX region is found in HTLV-III, it is much less conserved in this virus, and perhaps this is related to the cytopathic effect of HTLV-III, as well as our inability thus far to demonstrate a transforming capacity in this agent.

HTLV-III is a highly replicating virus in vivo. This feature represents another departure from what has previously been observed in members of the HTLV family, which are capable of existing for long periods in an unexpressed proviral form. Perhaps because of the rapid replication (coupled with the lack of fidelity in retroviral replication), there is a noteworthy diversity in the restriction-endonuclease cleavage patterns seen among HTLV-III isolates from different patients to date, indicating a genetic polymorphism not found in other viruses within the HTLV family (Shaw G, Hahn B, Wong-Staal F, Gallo RC: unpublished data). Therefore, we believe that HTLV-III really represents a set of closely related but varying genetic forms, and that lymphadenopathy-associated virus is one of these forms.

At this point HTLV-III has been isolated from the blood or lymph nodes of over 95 persons. The virus can now be recovered from over 90 percent of patients with early-stage AIDS (Markham P, Salahuddin SZ, Gallo RC: unpublished data). However, it is worth noting that with the technologies currently available, the virus cannot always be recovered intact from patients who have late-stage, fulminant AIDS, perhaps because the OKT4+ subset of T cells thought to harbor the virus is so profoundly diminished. In the future, the availability of sensitive tests for HTLV-III antigenemia or circulating antigen–antibody complexes may obviate some of the difficulties inherent in relying on intact isolation of the virus as an index of viral replication in vivo.

It has recently been possible to recover the virus from the seminal fluid (Zagury D, Salahuddin SZ, Markham P, Sarngadharan MG, Gallo RC: unpublished data) and saliva (Groopman J, Salahuddin SZ, Markham P, Sarngadharan MG, Gallo RC: unpublished data) of patients with AIDS. These observations may provide additional insights on the transmission and pathogenesis of this disease.

HTLV-III has never been isolated from healthy heterosexual donors (115 unsuccessful attempts), and it was isolated from only 1 of 22 nonpromiscuous homosexual men (from a region of the United States without a high risk of AIDS) who appeared to be healthy. AIDS developed in this man six months later.[12]

In nearly 90 percent of patients with AIDS it was possible to detect circulating antibodies reactive against HTLV-III.[14] In more recent testing, using a combination of enzyme-linked immunosorbent and electroblot (Western) assays for detecting antibodies, all patients with AIDS were positive,[63] but only 1 of 286 controls was positive. Moreover, seropositivity for HTLV-III can identify blood donors who have been suspected (on clinical and epidemiologic grounds) of transmitting AIDS through transfused blood products (Groopman J, Sarngadharan MG, Gallo RC: unpublished data).

Knowledge of HTLV-III may affect many phases of basic research with clinical implications. First of all, there are new possibilities for identifying early cases of AIDS and assessing the risks of the disease. One practical application is a kit for rapid antibody screening to prevent donation of blood products by persons infected by HTLV-III. The Department of Health and Human Services has taken steps to make a nationwide system for serum screening available by transferring the virus and other reagents to the private sector. This will be done under a licensing arrangement, to facilitate large-scale studies. (The current licensees include Abbott Laboratories, E.I. du Pont de Nemours/Biotech and Co., Electro-Nucleonics, Litton Industries, and Travenol–Genentech Diagnostics.) The availability of such tests is likely to pose a number of difficult questions — at least in the short term. For example, what does one tell a seropositive health-care provider or pregnant woman?

Secondly, the discovery of an immunosuppressive retrovirus in AIDS could serve as a stimulus to reexamine endemic forms of cancer that pose special public-health problems for some nations in the Third World. Could some of the cases of Kaposi's sarcoma and Burkitt's lymphoma in equatorial Africa be at least partly explained by a subtle, retrovirus-associated immune abnormality? Is there a reservoir for HTLV-III in an exceedingly remote portion of central Africa, from which the virus was only recently introduced into urban centers in that region of the world? If so, is it possible that population shifts in the mid-1970s (e.g., see discussion of travel patterns involving Haiti and Zaire by Piot et al.[64]) conveyed the virus to North America? These latter issues are, of course, speculative because of insufficient information at this time.

Thirdly, the identification of HTLV-III makes it possible to study the effect of more than one retrovirus infecting a given patient. Approximately 10 percent of patients with AIDS have serologic evidence of infection involving another virus in the HTLV family (usually HTLV-I but sometimes HTLV-II). Does infection with a combination of these viruses affect the clinical presentation or course of AIDS? Do clusters of HTLVs play a part in other diseases?

Fourthly, current technology may make it possible to begin formulating rational interventions directed against a cause rather than the manifestations of AIDS. In the future, it may be possible to develop a vaccine for persons who belong to certain risk groups and thereby prevent the disease. Moreover, strategies for restoring immune function by interrupting viral replication in AIDS or pre-AIDS (perhaps by inhibiting reverse transcriptase) or eliminating virus-bearing cells, coupled with bone-marrow transplantation, may be developed when the biology of this new agent is understood. Indeed, the availability of HTLV-III has permitted relatively rapid screening systems for biologic and pharmaceutical agents that can block replication of the virus. Approximately 12 years ago, it was demonstrated that certain rifamycins can inhibit the reverse transcriptase of animal retroviruses,[65,66] and these findings were extended to other compounds.[67] Suramin (a drug widely used in the treatment of African trypanosomiasis and onchocerciasis, but not traditionally considered an antiviral agent) was shown to inhibit the reverse transcriptases of animal retroviruses.[68] This observation received very little attention at the time, but we have recently learned that suramin protects normal OKT4+ (helper/inducer) T cells against the cytopathic effect of HTLV-III in vitro (Mitsuya H, Broder S: unpublished data) and also blocks the infectivity and replication of the virus (Popovic M, Broder S, Gallo RC: unpublished data) in a special neoplastic T-cell clone that is permissive for replication of HTLV-III and partially resistant to its cytopathic effect.[11] The drug has recently been shown to be an inhibitor of the reverse transcriptase of HTLV-III (Fischinger P, Arthur L, Gilden R, Sarin P, Broder S, Gallo RC: unpublished data), making inhibition of the transcriptase the likely cause of these effects. A pilot trial of suramin, testing whether in vivo replication of HTLV-III can be blocked in patients with AIDS — and if so, whether an improvement of the immunodeficiency state can be detected — is now under way at the Clinical Center of the National Institutes of Health. (We wish to stress that the purpose of the first phase of the trial is to learn whether the drug can be safely administered to patients with AIDS.)

Finally, the simultaneous availability of a virus that routinely transforms T cells (HTLV-I) and of a related virus that kills T cells (HTLV-III) might offer a unique opportunity to analyze the mechanisms critical to human cell growth and destruction.

We are indebted to Dr. Flossie Wong-Staal for a critical reading of the manuscript and for many helpful suggestions.

References

1. *Pneumocystis* pneumonia — Los Angeles. MMWR 1981; 30:250-2.
2. Kaposi's sarcoma and *Pneumocystis* pneumonia among homosexual men — New York City and California. MMWR 1981; 30:305-8.
3. Gottlieb MS, Schroff R, Schanker HM, et al. *Pneumocystis carinii* pneumonia and mucosal candidiasis in previously healthy homosexual men: evidence of a new acquired cellular immunodeficiency. N Engl J Med 1981; 305:1425-31.
4. Masur H, Michelis MA, Greene JB, et al. An outbreak of community-acquired *Pneumocystis carinii* pneumonia: initial manifestation of cellular immune dysfunction. N Engl J Med 1981; 305:1431-8.
5. Siegal FP, Lopez C, Hammer GS, et al. Severe acquired immunodeficiency in male homosexuals, manifested by chronic perianal ulcerative herpes simplex lesions. N Engl J Med 1981; 305:1439-44.
6. Centers for Disease Control Task Force on Kaposi's Sarcoma and Opportunistic Infections. Epidemiologic aspects of the current outbreak of Kaposi's sarcoma and opportunistic infections. N Engl J Med 1982; 306: 248-52.
7. Curran JW, Lawrence DN, Jaffe H, et al. Acquired immunodeficiency syndrome (AIDS) associated with transfusions. N Engl J Med 1984; 310:69-75.
8. Harris C, Small CB, Klein RS, et al. Immunodeficiency in female sexual partners of men with the acquired immunodeficiency syndrome. N Engl J Med 1983; 308:1181-4.
9. Clumeck N, Sonnet J, Taelman H, et al. Acquired immunodeficiency syndrome in African patients. N Engl J Med 1984; 310:492-7.
10. Donne J. Devotions upon emergent occasions. VI. Meditation. In: Coffin CM, ed. The complete poetry and selected prose of John Donne. New York: Modern Library, 1952:421-2.
11. Popovic M, Sarngadharan MG, Read E, Gallo RC. Detection, isolation, and continuous production of cytopathic retroviruses (HTLV-III) from patients with AIDS and pre-AIDS. Science 1984; 224:497-500.
12. Gallo RC, Salahuddin SZ, Popovic M, et al. Frequent detection and isolation of cytopathic retroviruses (HTLV-III) from patients with AIDS and at risk for AIDS. Science 1984; 224:500-2.
13. Schüpbach J, Popovic M, Gilden RV, Gonda MA, Sarngadharan MG, Gallo RC. Serological analysis of a subgroup of human T-lymphotropic retroviruses (HTLV-III) associated with AIDS. Science 1984; 224: 503-5.
14. Sarngadharan MG, Popovic M, Bruch L, Schüpbach J, Gallo RC. Antibodies reactive with human T-lymphotropic retroviruses (HTLV-III) in the serum of patients with AIDS. Science 1984; 224:506-8.
15. Gallo RC. Human T-cell leukaemia-lymphoma virus and T-cell malignancies in adults. Cancer Surv 1984; 3:113-59.
16. Poiesz BJ, Ruscetti FW, Gazdar AF, Bunn PA, Minna JD, Gallo RC. Detection and isolation of type C retrovirus particles from fresh and cultured lymphocytes of a patient with cutaneous T-cell lymphoma. Proc Natl Acad Sci USA 1980; 77:7415-9.
17. Poiesz BJ, Ruscetti FW, Reitz MS, Kalyanaraman VS, Gallo RC. Isolation of a new type C retrovirus (HTLV) in primary uncultured cells of a patient with Sézary T-cell leukemia. Nature 1981; 294:268-71.
18. Hinuma Y, Nagata K, Hanaoka M, et al. Adult T-cell leukemia: antigen in an ATL cell line and detection of antibodies to the antigen in human sera. Proc Natl Acad Sci USA 1981; 78:6476-80.
19. Miyoshi I, Kubonishi I, Yoshimoto S, et al. Type C virus particles in a cord T-cell line derived by co-cultivating normal human cord leukocytes and human leukaemic T cells. Nature 1981; 294:770-1.
20. Kalyanaraman VS, Sarngadharan MG, Robert-Guroff M, et al. A new subtype of human T-cell leukemia virus (HTLV-II) associated with a T-cell variant of hairy cell leukemia. Science 1982; 218:571-3.
21. Baltimore D. RNA-dependent DNA polymerase in virions of RNA tumour viruses. Nature 1970; 226:1209-11.
22. Temin HM, Mizutani S. RNA-directed DNA polymerse in virions in Rous sarcoma virus. Nature 1970; 226:1211-3.
23. Sarngadharan MG, Allaudeen HS, Gallo RC. Reverse transcriptase of RNA tumor viruses and animal cells. Methods Cancer Res 1976; 12:3-47.
24. Morgan DA, Ruscetti FW, Gallo R. Selective *in vitro* growth of T lymphocytes from normal human bone marrows. Science 1976; 193:1007-8.
25. Taniguchi T, Matsui H, Fujita T, et al. Structure and expression of a cloned cDNA for human interleukin-2. Nature 1983; 302:305-10.
26. Clark SC, Arya SK, Wong-Staal F, et al. Human T-cell growth factor: Partial amino acid sequence, cDNA cloning, and organization and expression in normal and leukemic cells. Proc Natl Acad Sci USA 1984; 81:2543-7.
27. Leonard WJ, Depper JM, Uchiyama T, Smith KA, Waldmann TA, Greene WC. A monoclonal antibody that appears to recognize the receptor for human T-cell growth factor: partial characterization of the receptor. Nature 1982; 300:267-9.
28. Popovic M, Sarin PS, Robert-Guroff M, et al. Isolation and transmission of human retrovirus (human T-cell leukemia virus). Science 1983; 219:856-9.
29. Mitsuya H, Guo H-G, Cossman J, Megson M, Reitz MS, Broder S. Functional properties of antigen-specific T cells infected by human T-cell leukemia/lymphoma virus (HTLV-I). Science 1984; 225:1484-6.
30. Mitsuya H, Guo H-G, Megson M, Trainor C, Reitz MS Jr, Broder S. Transformation and cytopathogenic effect in an immune human T-cell clone infected by HTLV-I. Science 1984; 223:1293-6.
31. Hinuma Y. Adult T cell leukemia (ATL) virus. (in Japanese). J Clin Sci 1983; 19:291-8.
32. Seiki M, Hattori S, Hirayama Y, Yoshida M. Human adult T-cell leukemia virus: complete nucleotide sequence of the provirus genome integrated in leukemia cell DNA. Proc Natl Acad Sci USA 1983; 80:3618-22.

33. Chen ISY, McLaughlin J, Golde DW. Long terminal repeats of human T-cell leukaemia virus II genome determine target cell specificity. Nature 1984; 309:276-9.
34. Shaw GM, Gonda MA, Flickinger BH, Hahn B, Gallo RC, Wong-Staal F. Genomes of evolutionarily divergent members of the human T-cell leukemia virus family (HTLV-I and HTLV-II) are highly conserved, especially in pX. Proc Natl Acad Sci USA 1984; 81:4544-8.
35. Wong-Staal F, Hahn B, Manzari V, et al. A survey of human leukaemias for sequences of human retrovirus. Nature 1983; 302:626-8.
36. Yoshida M, Seiki M, Yamaguchi K, Takatsuki K. Monoclonal integration of human T-cell leukemia provirus in all primary tumors of adult T-cell leukemia suggests causative role of human T-cell leukemia virus in the disease. Proc Natl Acad Sci USA 1984; 81:2534-7.
37. Wong-Staal F. Possible molecular mechanisms of virus transformation. In: Broder S, moderator. T-Cell lymphoproliferative syndrome associated with human T-cell leukemia/lymphoma virus. Ann Intern Med 1984; 100:543-57.
38. Seiki M, Eddy R, Shows TB, Yoshida M. Nonspecific integration of the HTLV provirus genome into adult T-cell leukaemia cells. Nature 1984; 309:640-2.
39. Haseltine WA, Sodroski J, Patarca R, Briggs D, Perkins D, Wong-Staal F. Structure of 3′ terminal region of type II human T lymphotropic virus: evidence for new coding region. Science 1984; 225:419-21.
40. Franchini G, Wong-Staal F, and Gallo RC. Human T-cell leukemia virus (HTLV-I) transcripts in fresh and cultured cells of patients with adult T-cell leukemia. Proc Natl Acad Sci USA (in press).
41. Sodroski JG, Rosen CA, Haseltine WA. *Trans*-acting transcriptional activation of the long terminal repeat of human T lymphotropic viruses in infected cells. Science 1984; 225:381-5.
42. Nevins JR. Mechanism of activation of early viral transcription by the adenovirus EIA gene product. Cell 1981; 26:213-20.
43. Brady J, Bolen JB, Radonovich M, Salzman N, Khoury G. Stimulation of simian virus 40 late gene expression by simian virus 40 tumor antigen. Proc Natl Acad Sci USA 1984; 81:2040-4.
44. Hahn BH, Shaw GM, Popovic M, Lo Monico A, Gallo RC, Wong-Staal F. Molecular cloning and analysis of a new variant of human T-cell leukemia virus (HTLV-Ib) from an African patient with adult T-cell leukemia-lymphoma. Int J Cancer (in press).
45. Miyoshi I, Taguchi H, Yoshimoto S, Fujishita M, Ohtsuki Y. Natural infection in monkeys with adult T-cell leukemia virus or a closely related agent. In: Gallo RC, Essex M, Gross L, eds. Human T-cell leukemia/lymphoma viruses. New York: Cold Spring Harbor Laboratories, 1984:313-21.
46. Guo H-G, Wong-Staal F, Gallo RC. Novel viral sequences related to human T-cell leukemia virus in T cells of a seropositive baboon. Science 1984; 223:1195-7.
47. Saxinger WC, Lange-Wantzin G, Thomsen K, et al. Human T cell leukemia virus: A diverse family of related exogenous retroviruses of humans and Old World primates. In: Gallo RC, Essex M, Gross L, eds. Human T-cell leukemia/lymphoma viruses. New York: Cold Spring Harbor Laboratories, 1984:323-30.
48. Fleming AF, Yamamoto N, Bhusnurmath SR, Maharajan R, Schneider J, Hunsmann G. Antibodies to ATLV (HTLV) in Nigerian blood donors and patients with chronic lymphocytic leukaemia or lymphoma. Lancet 1983; 2:334-5.
49. Gallo RC, Sliski A, Wong-Staal F. Origin of human T-cell leukaemia/lymphoma virus. Lancet 1983; 2:962-3.
50. Hahn BH, Popovic M, Kalyanaraman VS, et al. Detection and characterization of an HTLV II provirus in a patient with AIDS. In: Gottlieb MS, Groopman JE, eds. UCLA Symposia in Molecular and Cellular Biology, New Series. New York: Alan R Liss, 1984:73-81.
51. Clapham P, Nagy K, Cheingsong-Popov R, Exley M, Weiss RA. Productive infection and cell-free transmission of human T-cell leukemia virus in a nonlymphoid cell line. Science 1983; 222:1125-7.
52. Hardy WD Jr, Hess PW, MacEwen EG, et al. Biology of feline leukemia virus in the natural environment. Cancer Res 1976; 36:582-8.
53. Haverkos HW, Curran JW. The current outbreak of Kaposi's sarcoma and opportunistic infections. CA 1982; 32:330-9.
54. Essex M, McLane MF, Lee TH, Falk L, Howe CWS, Mullins JI. Antibodies to cell membrane antigens associated with human T-cell leukemia virus in patients with AIDS. Science 1983; 220:859-62.
55. Gelmann EP, Popovic M, Blayney D, et al. Proviral DNA of a retrovirus, human T-cell leukemia virus, in two patients with AIDS. Science 1983; 220:862-5.
56. Gallo RC, Sarin PS, Gelmann EP, et al. Isolation of human T-cell leukemia virus in acquired immune deficiency syndrome (AIDS). Science 1983; 220:865-8.
57. Barré-Sinoussi F, Chermann C, Rey F, et al. Isolation of a T-lymphotropic retrovirus from a patient at risk for acquired immune deficiency syndrome (AIDS). Science 1983; 220:868-71.
58. Robert-Guroff M, Blayney DW, Safai B, et al. HTLV-I-specific antibody in AIDS patients and others at risk. Lancet 1984; 2:128-31.
59. Weiss R. Acquired immune deficiency syndrome: retroviruses linked with AIDS. Nature 1984; 309:12-3.
60. Vilmer E, Barré-Sinoussi F, Rouzioux C, et al. Isolation of new lymphotropic retrovirus from two siblings with haemophilia B, one with AIDS. Lancet 1984; 1:753-7.
61. Montagnier L, Chermann JC, Barré-Sinoussi F, et al. A new human T-lymphotropic retrovirus; characterization and possible role in lymphadenopathy and acquired immune deficiency syndromes. In: Gallo RC, Essex M, Gross L, eds. Human T-cell leukemia/lymphoma viruses. New York: Cold Spring Harbor Laboratories, 1984:363-79.
62. Arya SK, Gallo RC, Hahn BH, et al. Homology of genome of AIDS-associated virus with genomes of human T-cell leukemia viruses. Science 1984; 225:927-30.
63. Safai B, Sarngadharan MG, Groopman JE, et al. Seroepidemiological studies of human T-lymphotropic retroviruses type III in acquired immunodeficiency syndrome. Lancet 1984; 1:1438-40.
64. Piot P, Quinn TC, Taelman H, et al. Acquired immunodeficiency syndrome in a heterosexual population in Zaire. Lancet 1984; 2:65-9.
65. Ting RC, Yang SS, Gallo RC. Reverse transcriptase, RNA tumour virus transformation, and derivatives of rifamycin SV. Nature [New Biol] 1972; 236:163-6.
66. Gurgo C, Bridges S, Green M. Rifamycins. In: Came PE, Caliguiri LA, eds. Handbook of experimental pharmacology. Vol. 61. Berlin: Springer-Verlag, 1982:519-55.
67. Chandra P, Steel LK, Ebener U, et al. Chemical inhibitors of oncornaviral DNA polymerases: biological implications and their mode of action. Pharmacol Ther 1977; 1:231-87.
68. De Clercq. Suramin: a potent inhibitor of the reverse transcriptase of RNA tumor viruses. Cancer Lett 1979; 8:9-22.

SPECIAL ARTICLE

AIDS — AN IMMUNOLOGIC REEVALUATION

MAXIME SELIGMANN, M.D., LEONARD CHESS, M.D., JOHN L. FAHEY, M.D., ANTHONY S. FAUCI, M.D., PETER J. LACHMANN, M.D., JOHANNA L'AGE-STEHR, M.D., JACOB NGU, M.D., ANTHONY J. PINCHING, M.D., FRED S. ROSEN, M.D., THOMAS J. SPIRA, M.D., AND JOSEPH WYBRAN, M.D.

THE acquired immunodeficiency syndrome (AIDS) is a novel, epidemic form of immunodeficiency that has been widely recognized within the past three years.[1-3] Full-blown AIDS, as defined clinically by the Centers for Disease Control surveillance definition, is characterized by opportunistic infections and malignant diseases in patients without a known cause for immunodeficiency.[4] This clinical pattern has been associated with certain epidemiologic features and immunologic abnormalities. We take the view that AIDS represents a broad spectrum of conditions, including the full-blown syndrome, persistent lymphadenopathy with other clinical manifestations, and a disorder not associated with symptoms — all in persons having similar characteristic immunologic abnormalities. However, there are as yet no known pathognomonic immunologic features that precisely delineate this syndrome. There is strong evidence that the etiologic agent in this group of conditions is a lymphocytotropic retrovirus or a closely related group of such retroviruses, designated LAV/IDAV (lymphadenopathy-associated virus/immunodeficiency-associated virus) by the Pasteur Institute (Paris)[5] and HTLV-III (human T-cell lymphocytotropic virus III) by the National Cancer Institute (Bethesda).[6]

AIDS has been recognized almost exclusively in certain "at-risk" groups. Most of the patients in the developed countries are homosexually active men.[1-3] Intravenous-drug abusers are another group at risk,[7,8] as are recipients of blood products,[9,10] particularly patients with hemophilia who are receiving factor VIII concentrates.[11-13] The disease has also occurred in both males and females in Central Africa and in the Caribbean.[14-16] It has occurred in heterosexual partners of all the aforementioned groups[17,18] and also in infants of women in at-risk groups.[19,20] The epidemiologic pattern has a striking resemblance to the spread of hepatitis B and strongly suggests that a transmissible agent is present in the blood and other body fluids of affected persons.

A number of opportunistic infections have been observed in patients with AIDS. They are caused most prominently by *Pneumocystis carinii*, cytomegalovirus, atypical mycobacteria, *Toxoplasma gondii*, candida, herpes simplex virus, *Cryptococcus neoformans*, and cryptosporidium.[1-3,21-23] The frequent occurrence of Kaposi's sarcoma is another highly distinctive feature of AIDS.[24] This disease is otherwise extremely rare in patients under 60 years of age, except in Central Africa.[25]

The characteristics of AIDS illustrate the complexity of the interactions occurring between the environment and the immunologic system of the host. AIDS is the latest of a large number of examples of defects in immunity that may result from or may be associated with transmissible agents. The purpose of this report is to describe the distinctive immunologic features of AIDS, to evaluate their importance, and to explore their relations to the features of other primary and secondary immunodeficiency diseases.

IMMUNOLOGIC ABNORMALITIES

Description

AIDS is a distinctive disease of the immune system, and a number of immunologic abnormalities have been described thus far (Table 1). The diagnosis of AIDS cannot be made solely on the basis of any one of these immunologic abnormalities; however, a characteristic pattern has emerged. In the full-blown syndrome, there is an acquired, persistent quantitative and functional depression within the T4-lymphocyte subset, associated with hyperactivity of B cells.[26,27]

Because of the reliance on the phenotypic designation of T-cell subsets in evaluating patients with AIDS, it is essential to understand the normal differentiation and functions of these cells. During early T-cell development, both the T4 (or Leu-3) and T8 (or Leu-2) surface molecules are expressed simultaneously on the same cell. With further maturation, T cells express either the T4 or the T8 antigen. As a consequence, the T4 and T8 antigens identify mutually exclusive subsets that are phenotypically stable.[28]

The association of a particular T-cell subset with a given function has caused some confusion in the analysis of immunologic data in AIDS. For example, T4 cells have commonly been associated with helper functions, and T8 cells with cytotoxic or suppressor functions (or both).[29] This dichotomy is an oversimplification. The T4 population has been shown to contain not only helper cells but also cytotoxic cells as well as suppressor inducer and effector cells.[30] In addition, the T8 population contains cells capable of augmenting and amplifying the interaction of T4 cells with B cells.[31] Thus, describing T4 cells as helper cells and T8 cells as suppressor/cytotoxic cells is not justified. More important, it has recently become clear that T4 cells and T8 cells recognize foreign antigens in the context of distinct major histocompatibility antigens (cognitive functions). Thus, T4 cells recognize antigen

From the Working Group on AIDS of the Clinical Immunology Committee of the International Union of Immunologic Societies/World Health Organization.

in association with the Class II major histocompatibility complex (HLA-D), and T8 cells recognize those in association with Class I (HLA-A, HLA-B, and HLA-C).[32] Abnormalities in the number of T4 or T8 cells can be associated with abnormalities in cognitive functions of T cells and may lead to immunoincompetence.

Functional studies with purified populations of T cells, including subgroups within the T4 and T8 subsets, will be important in defining the immunologic alterations in AIDS. Patients with the lymphadenopathy syndrome have a selective decrease in a specific subgroup of T4 cells (Leu-8+ or TQ-1+ cells) not responsible for the induction of B-cell responses.[33] In addition, reported functional abnormalities such as decreased proliferative responses to certain mitogens and antigens may merely reflect a decreased proportion of a given subset within the unfractionated mononuclear-cell suspension. In contrast, one may also see qualitative defects within a particular subset, with or without a quantitative diminution in numbers of the subset in question.

The activation and growth of T cells are regulated by a number of antigen-nonspecific peptides. For example, antigen-activated monocytes release a molecule termed interleukin-1, which triggers proliferation of thymocytes and antigen-stimulated peripheral T cells.[34] After antigen and interleukin-1 triggering, T cells synthesize and secrete another peptide (interleukin-2), which is essential for clonal expansion of the antigen-triggered T cell.[35] It has been proposed that a defect in the synthesis or secretion (or both) of interleukin-2 is associated with AIDS.[36,37] In fact, it has been shown that the addition of interleukin-2 to cell cultures can restore some immune functions in vitro. On the basis of these studies, interleukin-2 is currently being administered to patients with AIDS in Phase-I trials. It is clear that more detailed studies of the production, regulation, and responsiveness of interleukin-2, as well as studies of interleukin-2 receptors on cells from patients with AIDS, should be carried out. The evaluation of other lymphokines is also important. For instance, it has been shown that γ-interferon is a product of triggered T4 cells that has a major role in the activation of macrophages.[38] Its production is defective in AIDS, and exogenous γ-interferon has been shown to restore macrophage activation in vitro.[39]

Clinical Spectrum

Patients who present with Kaposi's sarcoma alone generally have a less severe immune defect than patients with opportunistic infections. This difference may be manifested by the presence of skin-test reactivity to some antigens and a less profound defect in the T4 subset.[40]

A number of unanticipated immunologic complications have been observed with high frequency in patients with AIDS. Among these are an extreme hypersensitivity to trimethoprim–sulfamethoxazole and recrudescence of atopy. Although these manifestations have been observed in other immunodeficiency diseases, the mechanism of these phenomena is poorly understood.

In addition to patients with full-blown AIDS, there are patients in all the risk groups for AIDS who have chronic generalized lymphadenopathy or constitutional signs and symptoms, including fever, fatigue, malaise, night sweats, weight loss, anorexia, oral candidiasis, and diarrhea.[41] Some patients also have thrombocytopenia.[42] These features in various combinations appear to be parts of the full clinical spectrum of AIDS on the basis of epidemiologic association. In some patients such features may represent a true prodrome of AIDS, whereas in others they may represent an end point or forme fruste. However, similar features may also be seen in unrelated conditions. A feature is considered prodromal when it has been consistently seen in patients whose illness has subsequently progressed to full-blown AIDS. However, not all patients with full-blown AIDS have passed through an identifiable prodromal stage. Currently, there is no specific test to predict which are likely to have the full-blown disease.

On immunologic testing, these patients are heterogeneous. Some have low T4-cell numbers, and some have high T8-cell numbers; consequently, a majority have a low T4:T8 ratio.[40] Some patients have cutaneous anergy, polyclonal hypergamma-globulinemia, and diminished in vitro proliferative responses.

Table 1. Immunologic Abnormalities in AIDS.

I. Abnormalities that characterize the syndrome
   1. Lymphopenia
   2. Selective T-cell deficiency based on a quantitative reduction within the antigenic subset designated by T4 or Leu-3 monoclonal antibodies
   3. Decreased or absent delayed cutaneous hypersensitivity to both recall and new antigens
   4. Elevated serum immunoglobulins, predominantly IgG and IgA in adults and including IgM in children
   5. Increased spontaneous immunoglobulin secretion by individual B lymphocytes

II. Consistently observed abnormalities
   1. Decreased in vitro lymphocyte proliferative responses
      a. Mitogens
      b. Antigens
      c. Alloantigens ; autoantigens
   2. Decreased cytotoxic responses
      a. Natural killer cells
      b. Cell-mediated cytotoxicity (T-cell)
   3. Decreased ability to mount a de novo antibody response to a new antigen
   4. Altered monocyte function
   5. Elevated serum levels of immune complexes

III. Other reported abnormalities
   1. Increased levels of acid-labile α-interferon
   2. Antilymphocyte antibodies
   3. Suppressor factors
   4. Increased levels of β-2 microglobulin and α-1 thymosin; decreased serum thymulin levels

Histologically, the lymph nodes of the majority of these patients show follicular hyperplasia with or without parafollicular hyperplasia; some show follicular involution or a mixed pattern.[41] Immunohistologic studies have demonstrated infiltration of germinal centers by T8 cells, disruption of the germinal center's follicular dendritic reticulum-cell structure, depletion of T4 cells with a predominance of T8 cells in T-cell areas, and plasma-cell infiltration.[43,44] Patients whose disease has subsequently progressed to full-blown AIDS have tended to have depletion of circulating T4 cells, cutaneous anergy, follicular involution, or germinal-center disruption.

Some persons at risk, such as healthy homosexually active men, have a high incidence of viral infections such as cytomegalovirus and Epstein–Barr virus infections that, in the acute stage, can result in the transient appearance of several of the immunologic abnormalities listed in Table 1. Both infections can cause increased spontaneous polyclonal B-cell activation and a reversal of the normal T4:T8 ratio. However, it is critical to appreciate that the reversal of the T4:T8 ratio is due for the most part to an elevated level of T8 cells and not to a depletion of T4 cells.[45,46] In marked contrast, the reversal of the T4:T8 ratio characteristic of full-blown AIDS is due almost invariably to a selective profound diminution in the T4 subset.

Longitudinal cohort studies of populations at risk for AIDS will establish the natural history and implications of the various immunologic abnormalities involved, which may include those related to AIDS and those related to intercurrent events.[47] It will be important to correlate these immunologic abnormalities with evidence of prior infection with HTLV-III or LAV, whether by virus isolation or seroconversion.

Cause and Pathogenesis

The present evidence indicates that the etiologic agent of AIDS is either a single or a closely related group of lymphocytotropic retroviruses designated LAV/IDAV or HTLV-III[5,6] and known to be distinct from HTLV-I and HTLV-II.[48] Such a virus (or viruses), with characteristic morphologic features, has been isolated from the blood or node lymphocytes of a substantial number of patients from all risk groups, including children, who have had full-blown AIDS or lymphadenopathy.[49] In addition, antibodies to viral constituents have been detected in serum from the vast majority of such patients. A substantial proportion of asymptomatic members of high-risk groups are also seropositive.[50,51] It seems likely that cross-reactivity of some of these antibodies with HTLV-I envelope proteins explains the prior finding, in the serum of some patients with AIDS, of positive membrane immunofluorescence against HTLV-I-infected cells.

The lymphocytotropic viruses have cytopathic effects on lymphocytes but fail to transform them. These viruses appear to have a positive tropism for activated T4 lymphocytes, and HTLV-III has been successfully propagated in a human neoplastic T-cell line.[6,52] It is not yet known whether these viral agents have a selective tropism for the Leu-8+ or TQ-1+ subset of T4+ cells or for other cells of the immune system, such as earlier cells in the T-cell lineage, B cells, or antigen-presenting cells. In theory, the virus could destroy its target cell or its precursor or both, interfere with the growth or cognitive function of its target cell, or interfere with the biosynthesis of molecules involved in its function. The etiologic virus could interact directly with B lymphocytes and cause polyclonal activation, or this may be the consequence of a primary effect of the virus on T4 cells. In addition to affecting T4 cells, the virus may also interfere with the functions of antigen-presenting cells. Alternatively, impaired antigen-presenting-cell function due to down regulation of Ia expression may be secondary to the T4-cell defect.[53] Many of the immunologic abnormalities observed in AIDS may be secondary to the host response, although some could be direct effects of the retrovirus infection. These abnormalities include the presence of immune complexes, antilymphocyte antibodies, suppressor factors, and acid-labile interferon.[54-57]

Regardless of immunologic state, is everyone equally susceptible to infection with the retrovirus and its consequences? If this is not the case, predisposing or contributing factors must apply. These could include immunogenetic variation, intercurrent infections, alloantigenic stimulation, or drugs.[58] Any of these potentiating factors could act either to predispose the host to infection or to determine the expression and clinical outcome of the infection. Enhanced susceptibility to the retrovirus may result from a relative immunodeficiency or from prolonged or repeated activation of target cells, which could facilitate penetration or spread of the retrovirus in the immune system.

Relevant Data from Other Human Diseases and Animal Models

In looking for the pathogenetic mechanisms that underlie the immune defect in AIDS, it may be helpful to consider the mechanisms of immune defects in other conditions.

Primary Immunodeficiency States

Among the primary immunodeficiency diseases, AIDS most closely resembles the immunologic alterations observed in children with a defect in purine nucleoside phosphorylase.[59] Children with this abnormality have a marked diminution in T cells but normal or elevated levels of immunoglobulins. They are unduly susceptible to opportunistic infections. It has been proposed that accumulation of the metabolites deoxyguanosine and deoxyguanosine triphosphate is cytotoxic to dividing lymphocytes in this deficiency.[60] Because of these observations, it appears worthwhile to look for abnormal accumulations of purine metabolites in patients with AIDS.

In some immunodeficiencies, a primary immunologic defect appears to lead to secondary immunologic defects. Boys with X-linked agammaglobulinemia and many adults with common varied immunodeficiency have primary defects in B-cell development.[59] Nonetheless, impaired cellular immunity may occur in some of these patients. T-cell dysregulatory phenomena are noted in the majority in whom the T-cell abnormality is clearly secondary to the B-cell defect.[61] An elevation of T8 cells in the blood is accompanied by suppression of immunoglobulin synthesis by normal B cells. An animal model of this phenomenon has been observed in bursectomized chickens.[62]

Immunodeficiency Associated with Other Environmental Factors

Nutritional Status

The commonest cause of T-cell immunodeficiency worldwide is protein-calorie malnutrition. Malnourished children have defects in macrophage and T-cell function accompanied by hypergammaglobulinemia and increased susceptibility to infections.[63] These effects are particularly marked in malnourished children with measles, an infection that itself causes T-cell anergy (see below). Bacterial superinfection in these children is a major cause of serious disease and death.

Antigen Overload

It has been proposed that if the immune system is chronically overstimulated by a high antigenic load in association with various chronic infections, this overstimulation may interfere with the host's capacity to eliminate infectious agents.[64,65] This is one explanation advanced for the abnormal response to Epstein–Barr virus infection in children with malaria, which may (rarely) lead to the development of Burkitt's lymphoma,[66] and it may be one explanation for the low clinical resistance to *Mycobacterium leprae* in the lepromatous form of leprosy in which a poor T-cell response is accompanied by hypergammaglobulinemia, autoantibody formation, and immune-complex disease.[67]

Failure of the Effector Mechanisms of the Immune Response

Very rarely, unremarkable measles-virus infection is followed by the development after some years of a fatal progressive neurologic disease, subacute sclerosing panencephalitis. It is currently believed that the pathogenesis of this condition involves a sequestered intracellular infection that, once established, cannot be eliminated; progressive viral destruction of neurons and progressive hyperimmunization continue relentlessly.[68] In AIDS as well as in AIDS-related lymphadenopathy, retrovirus production continues despite the presence of detectable titers of antibodies to LAV/IDAV or HTLV-III.[6,49]

Infections That Primarily Affect Components of the Immune System

There are other examples of viruses that infect cellular components of the immune system and thereby evade normal immune responses. Acute measles-virus infection is accompanied by clinically important T-cell immunodeficiency and anergy, but destruction of T cells is not an adequate explanation for the observed anergy.

Infectious mononucleosis involves an Epstein–Barr virus infection of B cells that stimulates a T-cell response to the virus-infected cell. These T cells give rise to a temporary and self-limited immunosuppression by activating the suppressor network.[69] Certain pedigrees are genetically predisposed to have an unfavorable outcome after Epstein–Barr virus infections, such as fatal mononucleosis, B-cell lymphoma, agammaglobulinemia, or aplastic anemia.[70] Before the infection develops, no phenotypic abnormality in T-cell distribution or function is apparent. However, once the infection occurs, these patients become profoundly lymphopenic.[71] This disease illustrates importantly how a relatively innocuous pathogen may have far-reaching and devastating immunologic consequences in a geneticallly susceptible host.

Congenital virus infections with either rubella or cytomegalovirus can produce a marked immunosuppression associated with a heavy virus burden and opportunistic infections.[72]

Animal Models

One of the most relevant models for AIDS is infection with the feline leukemia virus.[73] This lymphocytotropic retrovirus more commonly gives rise to profound immunosuppression with lymphopenia and opportunistic infections than to leukemia.

A retrovirus-induced form of transmissible immunodeficiency (which has been called "simian AIDS") has been observed in macaques.[74] The type D retrovirus is lymphocytotropic. However, the syndrome observed in affected monkeys differs in important ways from AIDS, in that the monkeys usually have hypogammaglobulinemia and neutropenia with a profound depletion of all lymphocyte populations.

Therapy of AIDS

Since the pathogenesis of AIDS has not been fully delineated, all therapeutic approaches have been empirical. These have included identical-twin and allogeneic bone-marrow transplantation, lymphocyte plasmapheresis, and administration of recombinant α-interferon, natural-product γ-interferon, natural-product and recombinant interleukin-2, thymic factors, and isoprinosine. Recombinant α-interferon has been reported to induce remissions of cutaneous Kaposi's sarcoma in some patients.[75] Bone-marrow transplantations and lymphocyte transfusions have resulted in some cases in partial immunologic reconstitution with no detectable clinical improvement. All other approaches are still being tested and no final results are available.

Special Problems in Developing Countries

It seems doubtful that the surveillance criteria adopted in the industrialized countries for the identification of AIDS are necessarily valid in developing countries. The wide distribution of parasitic infections with known immunosuppressive activity leading to opportunistic infections, and the coexistence of multiple parasites in the same subject, make it difficult to identify patients with AIDS on the basis of the current epidemiologic criteria and immunologic aberrations. Future studies on AIDS in developing countries are of utmost importance and should take these difficulties into account. The varying incidence of Kaposi's sarcoma among different ethnic groups demands further investigation.

Useful data might be obtained from an epidemiologic survey to determine whether there has been an increase in the prevalence of Kaposi's sarcoma in the young in endemic areas, or an immunologic study of relevant populations with special attention paid to such variables as parasitic infection.

Future Goals

Although the recent identification of the likely etiologic agent (or agents) in AIDS will greatly facilitate research in this area, it nonetheless does not diminish the importance of delineating the immunopathogenesis of the disease. A natural consequence of this identification is the development of reliable serologic tests that will allow specific detection of the infection, screening programs, and epidemiologic studies.

The following broad objectives remain to be achieved: (1) establishment of the clinical implications of positive serology and of virus detection (this would include the whole spectrum of asymptomatic subjects who may have protective immunity, carriers, and patients with mild or progressive disease); (2) characterization of predisposing or potentiating factors, such as immunogenetic variants, local and systemic immunosuppressive effects, or factors that could activate target cells; (3) characterization of factors that confer resistance to the retrovirus (or viruses) or its effects; (4) identification of features that can predict clinical progression; (5) elucidation of the basic immunobiologic defect (or defects) underlying the disease; this can be furthered by the development of more informative functional tests and cell markers (this goal should be more readily achieved by the study of patients in the early stages of AIDS); (6) development of rational therapy based on more precise immunologic understanding of the disease; and (7) development of a safe, protective vaccine against the retrovirus; the potential utility of such a vaccine will depend on an understanding of how the immune system might cope with the virus and how the virus might evade immune elimination.

As was the case with primary immunodeficiencies, an understanding of the immunopathogenesis of AIDS will provide insights into the normal physiology of the immune system.

References

1. Gottlieb MS, Schroff R, Schanker HM, et al. *Pneumocystis carinii* pneumonia and mucosal candidiasis in previously healthy homosexual men: evidence of a new acquired cellular immunodeficiency. N Engl J Med 1981; 305:1425-31.
2. Masur H, Michelis MA, Greene JB, et al. An outbreak of community-acquired *Pneumocystis carinii* pneumonia: initial manifestation of cellular immune dysfunction. N Engl J Med 1981; 305:1431-8.
3. Siegel FP, Lopez C. Hammer GS, et al. Severe acquired immunodeficiency in male homosexuals, manifested by chronic perianal ulcerative herpes simplex lesions. N Engl J Med 1981; 305:1439-44.
4. Update on acquired immunodeficiency syndrome (AIDS) — United States. MMWR 1982; 31:507-14.
5. Barré-Sinoussi F, Chermann JC, Rey F, et al. Isolation of a T lymphotropic retrovirus from a patient at risk for acquired immune deficiency syndrome (AIDS). Science 1983; 220:868-71.
6. Popovic M, Sarngadharan MG, Read E, Gallo RC. Detection, isolation, and continuous production of cytopathic retroviruses (HTLV-III) from patients with AIDS and pre-AIDS. Science 1984; 224:497-500.
7. Wormser GP, Krupp LB, Hanrahan JP, Gavis G, Spira TJ, Cunningham-Rundles S. Acquired immunodeficiency syndrome in male prisoners: new insights into an emerging syndrome. Ann Intern Med 1983; 98:297-303.
8. Masur H, Michelis MA, Wormser GP, et al. Opportunistic infection in previously healthy women: initial manifestations of a community-acquired cellular immunodeficiency. Ann Intern Med 1982; 97:533-9.
9. Ammann AJ, Cowan MJ, Wara D, et al. Acquired immunodeficiency syndrome in an infant: possible transmission by means of blood products. Lancet 1983; 1:956-8.
10. Jett JR, Kuritsky JN, Katzmann JA, Homburger HA. Acquired immunodeficiency syndrome associated with blood-product transfusions. Ann Intern Med 1983; 99:621-4.
11. Davis KC, Horsburgh CR, Hasiba U, Schocket AL, Kirkpatrick CH. Acquired immunodeficiency syndrome in a patient with hemophilia. Ann Intern Med 1983; 98:284-6.
12. Poon M-C, Landay A, Prasthofer EF, Stagno S. Acquired immunodeficiency syndrome with *Pneumocystis carinii* pneumonia and *Mycobacterium avium-intracelllulare* infection in a previously healthy patient with classic hemophilia. Ann Intern Med 1983; 98:287-90.
13. Elliott JL, Hoppes WL, Platt MS, Thomas JG, Patel IP, Gansar A. The acquired immunodeficiency syndrome and *Mycobacterium avium-intracellulare* bacteremia in a patient with hemophilia. Ann Intern Med 1983; 98:290-3.
14. Brunet JB, Bouvet E, Chaperon J, et al. Acquired immunodeficiency syndrome in France. Lancet 1983; 1:700-1.
15. Vieira J, Frank E, Spira TJ, Landesman SH. Acquired immune deficiency in Haitians: opportunistic infections in previously healthy Haitian immigrants. N Engl J Med 1983; 308:125-9.
16. Clumeck N, Sonnet J, Taelman H, et al. Acquired immunodeficiency syndrome in African patients. N Engl J Med 1984; 310:492-7.
17. Pitchenik AE, Shafron RD, Glasser RM, Spira TJ. The acquired immunodeficiency syndrome in the wife of a hemophiliac. Ann Intern Med 1984; 100:62-5.
18. Harris C, Small CB, Klein RS, et al. Immunodeficiency in female sexual partners of men with the acquired immunodeficiency syndrome. N Engl J Med 1983; 308:1181-4.
19. Oleske J, Minnefor A, Cooper R Jr, et al. Immune deficiency syndrome in children. JAMA 1983; 249:2345-9.
20. Rubinstein A, Sicklick M, Gupta A, et al. Acquired immunodeficiency with reversed T_4/T_8 ratios in infants born to promiscuous and drug-addicted mothers. JAMA 1983; 249:2350-6.
21. Greene JB, Sidhu GS, Lewin S, et al. *Mycobacterium avium-intracellulare:* a cause of disseminated life-threatening infection in homosexuals and drug abusers. Ann Intern Med 1982; 97:539-46.
22. Lerner CW, Tapper ML. Opportunistic infection complicating acquired immune deficiency syndrome: clinical features of 25 cases. Medicine 1984; 63:155-64.
23. Mildvan D, Mathur U, Enlow RW, et al. Opportunistic infections and immune deficiency in homosexual men. Ann Intern Med 1982; 96: 700-4.
24. Friedman-Kien AE, Laubenstein LJ, Rubenstein P, et al. Disseminated Kaposi's sarcoma in homosexual men. Ann Intern Med 1982; 96:693-700.
25. Downing RG, Eglin RP, Bayley AC. African Kaposi's sarcoma and AIDS. Lancet 1984; 1:478-80.
26. Schroff RW, Gottlieb MS, Prince HE, Chai LL, Fahey JL. Immunological studies of homosexual men with immunodeficiency and Kaposi's sarcoma. Clin Immunol Immunopathol 1983; 27:300-14.
27. Lane HC, Masur H, Edgar LC, Whalen G, Rook AH, Fauci AS. Abnormalities of B-cell activation and immunoregulation in patients with the acquired immunodeficiency syndrome. N Engl J Med 1983; 309:453-8.
28. Reinherz EL, Schlossman SF. The differentiation and function of human T lymphocytes. Cell 1980; 19:821-7.
29. Reinherz EL, Kung PC, Goldstein G, Schlossman SF. Separation of functional subsets of human T cells by a monoclonal antibody. Proc Natl Acad Sci USA 1979; 76:4061-5.
30. Thomas Y, Rogozinski L, Irigoyen OH, et al. Functional analysis of human T cell subsets defined by monoclonal antibodies. IV. Induction of suppressor cells within the $OKT4^+$ population. J Exp Med 1981; 154:459-67.

31. Friedman SM. Hunter SB, Irigoyen OH, Kung PC, Goldstein G, Chess L. Functional analysis of human T cell subsets defined by monoclonal antibodies. II. Collaborative T–T interactions in the generation of TNP-altered-self–reactive cytotoxic T lymphocytes. J Immunol 1981; 126: 1702-5.
32. Krensky AM, Reiss CS, Mier JW, Strominger JL, Burakoff SJ. Long-term human cytolytic T-cell lines allospecific for HLA-DR6 antigens are OKT4^{+}. Proc Natl Acad Sci USA 1982; 79:2365-9.
33. Nicholson JKA, McDougal JS, Spira TJ, Cross GD, Jones BM, Reinherz EL. Immunoregulatory subsets of the T helper and T suppressor cell populations in homosexual men with chronic unexplained lymphadenopathy. J Clin Invest 1984; 73:191-201.
34. Mizel SB, Mizel D. Purification to apparent homogeneity of murine interleukin 1. J Immunol 1981; 126:834-7.
35. Smith KA, Lachman LB, Oppenheim JJ, Favata MF. The functional relationship of the interleukins. J Exp Med 1980; 151:1551-6.
36. Rook AH, Masur H, Lane HC, et al. Interleukin-2 enhances the depressed natural killer and cytomegalovirus-specific cytotoxic activities of lymphocytes from patients with the acquired immune deficiency syndrome. J Clin Invest 1983; 72:398-403.
37. Hauser GJ, Bino F, Rosenberg H, Zakuth V, Geller E, Spirer Z. Interleukin-2 production and response to exogenous interleukin-2 in a patient with acquired immune deficiency syndrome (AIDS). Clin Exp Immunol 1984; 56:l4-7.
38. Kasahara T, Hooks JJ, Dougherty SF, Oppenheim JJ. Interleukin-2-mediated immune interferon (IFN-γ) production by human T cells and T cell subsets. J Immunol 1983; 130:1784-9.
39. Murray HW, Rubin BY, Masur H, Roberts RB. Impaired production of lymphokines and immune (gamma) interferon in the acquired immunodeficiency syndrome. N Engl J Med 1984; 310:883-9.
40. Fahey JL, Prince H, Weaver M, et al. Quantitative changes in T helper and T suppressor/cytotoxic lymphocyte subsets that distinguish acquired immune deficiency syndrome from other immune subset disorders. Am J Med 1984; 76:95-100.
41. Metroka CE, Cunningham-Rundles S, Pollack MS, et al. Generalized lymphadenopathy in homosexual men. Ann Intern Med 1983; 99:585-91.
42. Morris L, Distenfeld A, Amorosi E, Karpatkin S. Autoimmune thrombocytopenic purpura in homosexual men. Ann Intern Med 1982; 96:714-7.
43. Modlin RL, Meyer PR, Hofman FM, et al. T-lymphocyte subsets in lymph nodes from homosexual men. JAMA 1983; 250:1302-5.
44. Janossy G, Pinching AJ, Basill M, et al. An immunohistological approach to persistent lymphadenopathy and its relationship to the acquired immunodeficiency syndrome. Clin Exp Immunol (in press).
45. Carney WP, Iacoviello V, Hirsch MS. Functional properties of T lymphocytes and their subsets in cytomegalovirus mononucleosis. J Immunol 1983; 130:390-3.
46. Reinherz EL, O'Brien C, Rosenthal P, Schlossman SF. The cellular basis for viral-induced immunodeficiency: analysis by monoclonal antibodies. J Immunol 1980; 125:1269-74.
47. Pinching AJ, McManus TJ, Jeffries RJ, et al. Studies of cellular immunity in male homosexuals in London. Lancet 1983; 2:126-30.
48. Schüpbach J, Popovic M, Gilden RV, Gonda MA, Sarngadharan MG, Gallo RC. Serologic analysis of a subgroup of human T-lymphotropic retroviruses (HTLV-III) associated with AIDS. Science 1984; 224:503-5.
49. Vilmer E, Barre-Sinoussi F, Rouzioux C, et al. Isolation of new lymphotropic retrovirus from two siblings with haemophilia B, one with AIDS. Lancet 1984; 1:753-7.
50. Sarngadharan MG, Popovic M, Bruch L, Schüpbach J, Gallo RC. Antibodies reactive with human T-lymphotropic retroviruses (HTLV-III) in the serum of patients with AIDS. Science 1984; 224:506-8.
51. Brun-Vezinet F, Rouzioux C, Barré-Sinoussi F, et al. Detection of IgG antibodies to lymphadenopathy-associated virus in patients with AIDS or lymphadenopathy syndrome. Lancet 1984; 1:1253-6.
52. Klatzmann D, Barré-Sinoussi F, Nugeyre MT, et al. Selective tropism of lymphadenopathy associated virus (LAV) for helper-inducer T lymphocytes. Science 1984; 225:59-63.
53. Belsito DV, Sanchez MR, Baer RL, Valentine F, Thorbecke GJ. Reduced Langerhans' cell Ia antigen and ATPase activity in patients with the acquired immunodeficiency syndrome. N Engl J Med 1984; 310:1279-82.
54. DeStefano E, Freidman RM, Friedman-Kien AE, et al. Acid-labile human leukocyte interferon in homosexual men with Kaposi's sarcoma and lymphadenopathy. J Infect Dis 1981; 146:451-5.
55. Laurence J, Gottlieb AB, Kunkel HG. Soluble suppressor factors in patients with acquired immune deficiency syndrome and its prodrome: elaboration in vitro by T lymphocyte-adherent cell interactions. J Clin Invest 1983; 72:2072-81.
56. Williams RC Jr, Masur H, Spira TJ. Lymphocyte-reactive antibodies in acquired immune deficiency syndrome. J Clin Immunol 1984; 4:118-23.
57. Kloster BE, Tomar RH, Spira TJ. Lymphocytotoxic antibodies in the acquired immune deficiency syndrome (AIDS). Clin Immunol Immunopathol 1984; 30:330-5.
58. Hurtenbach U, Shearer GM. Germ cell-induced immune suppression mice: effect of inoculation of syngeneic spermatozoa on cell-mediated immune responses. J Exp Med 1982; 155:1719-29.
59. Rosen FS, Cooper MD, Wedgwood RJP. The primary immunodeficiencies. N Engl J Med 1984; 311:235-42, 300-10.
60. Ullman B, Gudas LJ, Clift SM, Martin DW Jr. Isolation and characterization of purine-nucleoside phosphorylase-deficient T-lymphoma cells and secondary mutants with altered ribonucleotide reductase: genetic model for immunodeficiency disease. Proc Natl Acad Sci USA 1979; 76:1074-8.
61. Waldmann TA, Durm M, Broder S, Blackman M, Blaese RM, Strober W. Role of suppressor T cells in pathogenesis of common variable hypogammaglobulinaemia. Lancet 1974; 2:609-11.
62. Blaese RM, Weiden PR, Koski I, Dooley N. Infectious agammaglobulinemia: transmission of immunodeficiency with grafts of agammaglobulinemic cells. J Exp Med 1974; 140:1097-101.
63. Smythe PM, Schonland M, Brereton-Stiles GG, et al. Thymolymphatic deficiency and depression of cell-mediated immunity in protein-calorie malnutrition. Lancet 1971; 2:939-44.
64. Williamson WA, Greenwood BM. Impairment of the immune response to vaccination after acute malaria. Lancet 1978; 1:1328-9.
65. Virgin HWIV, Unanue ER. Suppression of the immune response to Listeria monocytogenes. I. Immune complexes inhibit resistance. J Immunol 1984; 133:104-9.
66. Dalldorf G. Lymphomas of African children: with different forms or environmental influences. JAMA 1962; 181:1026-8.
67. Nath I, van Rood JJ, Mehra NK, Vaidya MC. Natural suppressor cells in human leprosy: the role of HLA-D-identical peripheral lymphocytes and macrophages in the *in vitro* modulation of lymphoproliferative responses. Clin Exp Immunol 1980; 42:203-10.
68. Joseph BS, Oldstone MBA. Immunologic injury in measles versus infection. II. Suppression of immune injury through antigenic modulation. J Exp Med 1975; 142:864-76.
69. Haynes BF, Schooley RT, Payling-Wright CR, Grouse JE, Dolin R, Fauci AS. Emergence of suppressor cells of immunoglobulin synthesis during acute Epstein–Barr virus-induced infectious mononucleosis. J Immunol 1979; 123:2095-101.
70. Purtilo DT, Yang JPS, Cassel CK, et al. X-linked recessive progressive combined variable immunodeficiency (Duncan's disease). Lancet 1975; 1:935-41.
71. Sullivan JL, Byron KS, Brewster FE, Baker SM, Ochs HD. X-linked lymphoproliferative syndrome: natural history of the immunodeficiency. J Clin Invest 1983; 71:1765-78.
72. Schimke RN, Bolano C, Kirkpatrick CH. Immunologic deficiency in the congenital rubella syndrome. Am J Dis Child 1969; 118:626-33.
73. Essex M, Hardy WD Jr, Cotter SM, Jakowski RM, Sliski A. Naturally occurring persistent feline oncornavirus infections in the absence of disease. Infect Immun 1975; 11:470-5.
74. Gravell M, London WT, Houff SA, et al. Transmission of simian acquired immunodeficiency syndrome (SAIDS) with blood or filtered plasma. Science 1984; 223:74-6.
75. Krown SE, Real FX, Cunningham–Rundles S, et al. Preliminary observations on the effect of recombinant leukocyte A interferon in homosexual men with Kaposi's sarcoma. N Engl J Med 1983; 308:1071-6.

CASE RECORD OF THE MASSACHUSETTS GENERAL HOSPITAL

CASE 11-1982

Presentation of Case

A 29-year-old man was admitted to the hospital because of chronic uticaria, proteinuria, and cryoglobulinemia.

He was well until five years earlier, when episodes of diffuse urticaria developed, sometimes accompanied by edema of the tongue, lips, periorbital areas, and extremities. Most of the episodes were spontaneous, although some were precipitated by the ingestion of aspirin. Some of them were accompanied by dyspnea, without wheezing. An antihistamine provided relief of symptoms. During the year before admission he experienced increased fatigue, and for several months he observed Raynaud's phenomenon. Three months before entry he felt a firm nodule in the right testis. One month before admission general malaise occurred. Examination at this hospital showed small lymph nodes in the left cervical, right supraclavicular, and both axillary and inguinal regions. The liver and spleen were not felt. A firm, tender nodule, 0.5 cm in diameter, was palpated at the inferior pole of the right testis.

The urine gave a ++ test for protein; the sediment contained 10 white cells, more than 100 red cells, and moderate numbers of granular and red-cell casts per high-power field. The hematocrit was 30.4 percent; the white-cell count was 4900, and the total eosinophil count 106 per cubic millimeter (normal, 150 to 350). The erythrocyte sedimentation rate was 70 mm per hour. The urea nitrogen was 10 mg per 100 ml (4 mmol per liter), the glucose 89 mg per 100 ml (4.9 mmol per liter), and the protein 6.5 g (the albumin 3.3 g, and the globulin 3.2 g) per 100 ml. The serum aspartate aminotransferase (SGOT) was 34 U per milliliter (0.27 μmol · sec^{-1} per liter), the lactic dehydrogenase (LDH) 122 U per milliliter (2.03 μmol · sec^{-1} per liter), and the alkaline phosphatase 30 IU (0.5 μmol · sec^{-1}) per liter. The thyroxine was 6.9 μg per 100 ml (89 nmol per liter), and the triiodothyronine-resin uptake 25 percent; the thyroid-stimulating hormone was 2.4 μU per milliliter. A test for antinuclear antibodies was positive in a titer of 1:256, with homogeneous and speckled patterns; a test for rheumatoid factor was positive in a titer of 1:64. The total hemolytic complement was 60 U; C3 was 42 mg, and C4 12 mg per 100 ml. A test for hepatitis B surface antigen was positive, and a test for hepatitis B surface antibodies was negative. A serologic test for syphilis and an LE-cell test were negative. Immunoelectrophoresis revealed that IgG, IgA, and IgM precipitin arcs were normal; agarose-gel electrophoresis gave a normal pattern. A test for serum cryoprecipitate gave a ++++ reaction; the precipitate consisted of homogeneous IgM kappa and heterogeneous IgG and IgA proteins. In a 24-hour specimen of urine the protein was 5 g; the creatinine clearance was 158 liters (0.03 ml per second). X-ray films of the chest were normal; no hilar lymphadenopathy was visible. He was admitted to the hospital.

The patient had a homosexual life style and had been treated for gonococcal urethritis in the past. He had observed variable cervical lymphadenopathy over a period of several years. There was no history of fever, jaundice, overt hepatitis, blood transfusion, gross hematuria, arthralgia, or use of illicit drugs.

The temperature was 37.2°C, the pulse 80, and the respirations 16. The blood pressure was 130/80 mm Hg.

On examination he appeared well. No jaundice was observed. Urticarial lesions were present on all the extremities and the abdomen; no other cutaneous lesions were seen. Shotty lymphadenopathy was found in both cervical, axillary, and inguinal regions. The head, neck, lungs, and heart were normal. The liver and spleen were not felt. There was no peripheral edema, clubbing, or cyanosis. Neurologic examination was negative. The genitalia were normal except for slight tenderness of the right epididymis.

The urine gave a + test for protein; the sediment contained 5 white cells, innumerable red cells, moderate bacteria, and occasional granular and red-cell casts per high-power field. The hematocrit was 34.2 percent; the white-cell count was 4100, with 75 percent neutrophils, 24 percent lymphocytes, and 1 percent monocytes. The platelet count was 177,000, and the reticulocyte count 2.9 percent; the erythrocyte sedimentation rate was 78 mm per hour. The prothrombin time and the partial thromboplastin time were normal. The bleeding time was eight minutes and 30 seconds. The haptoglobin was 12 mg per 100 ml. The creatinine was 1.1 mg per 100 ml (97 μmol per liter), the conjugated bilirubin 0.2 mg per 100 ml (3 μmol per liter), the total bilirubin 0.5 mg per 100 ml (9 μmol per liter), the iron 75 μg per 100 ml (13 μmol per liter), the iron-binding capacity 296 μg per 100 ml (53.0 μmol per liter), and the protein 6.5 g (the albumin 3.2 g, and the globulin 3.3 g) per 100 ml. In a 24-hour specimen of urine the creatinine was 1730 mg per 100 ml (13.9 mmol · kg^{-1}), and the protein 5.2 g. The folic acid was 8.8 ng per 100 ml (20 nmol per liter), and the ferritin 288 ng per milliliter. An LE-cell test was negative on two occasions. A test for hepatitis B surface antigen was positive, and a test for hepatitis B surface antibodies was negative; tests for hepatitis B e antigen and antibody were positive. Direct and indirect Coombs tests were negative. Tests for antimitochondrial antibodies, anti-smooth-muscle antibodies, and anti-native DNA antibodies were negative. A skin test with mumps antigen was negative, and a test with candida antigen was positive. A serologic test for syphilis was negative. The cryoprecipitate contained hepatitis B surface antigen in a titer considerably lower than that detected in serum. Micropscopical examination of a stained smear and a fixed specimen of bone marrow showed normal cellularity, normal numbers of megakaryocytes, and normal red-cell and white-cell maturation, with an increase in eosinophils; there was no evidence of myeloma or lymphoma.

A urologic consultant made a diagnosis of epididymitis and prescribed cephalexin. On the third hospital day multiple biopsies were performed. Microscopical examination of a specimen of skin of the flank showed a slight mixed perivascular infiltrate with mild dermal edema; several small dermal vessels contained sludged erythrocytes and platelets; there were no findings suggestive of cryoglobulinemia. Immunofluorescence examination of the specimen showed focal deposition of IgM and IgA within vessel walls, consistent with urticaria. Microscopical examination of a small cervical lymph node (Fig. 1 and 2) revealed partial replacement by a vascular proliferation that appeared to originate in the lymph-node sinuses and encroached on the paracortex; there were rare spindle-cell foci and occasional slit-like spaces that encompassed red cells; occasional mitoses were observed, but no nuclear atypicality was present; follicular hyperplasia was noted in the residual nodal tissue, with increased plasma cells in the paracortex and medulla. Special stains for intracellular immunoglobulins revealed both light-chain types within the plasma cells. The nature of the vascular lesion was unclear. Microscopical examination of a specimen of the liver disclosed mild chronic persistent hepatitis, with evidence of hepatitis B surface antigen in rare hepatocytes. Microscopical examination of a renal-biopsy specimen revealed immune-complex glomerulonephritis, with granular deposition of immunoglobulin and complement components along the glomerular basement membranes and in the mesangium. The patient was discharged on the seventh hospital day.

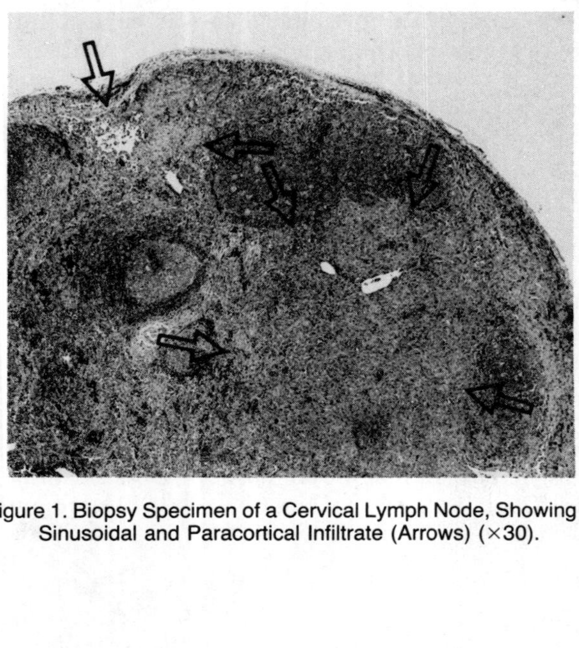

Figure 1. Biopsy Specimen of a Cervical Lymph Node, Showing a Sinusoidal and Paracortical Infiltrate (Arrows) (×30).

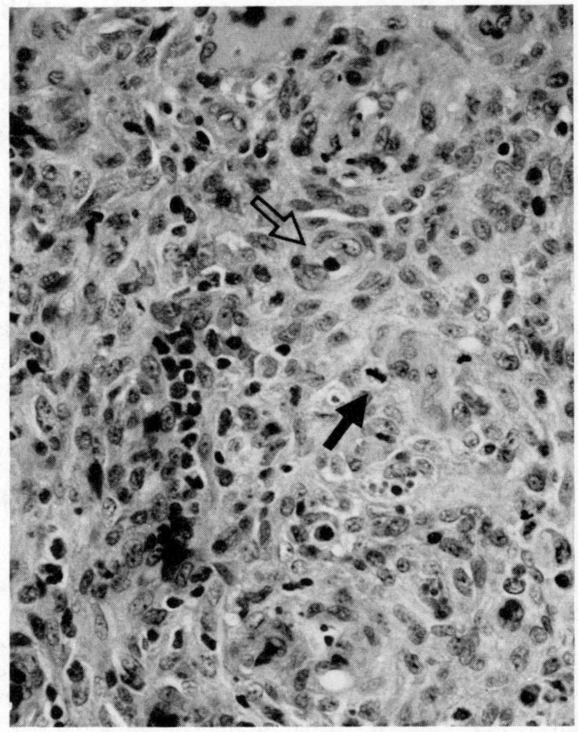

Figure 2. Biopsy Specimen of a Cervical Lymph Node, Showing Small Capillary-like Blood Vessels (Open Arrow) and Spindle Cells (×400).
Note the mitotic figure (solid arrow).

At a follow-up visit in the clinic three days after discharge examination again disclosed shotty cervical, axillary, and epitrochlear lymphadenopathy and bilateral slightly tender inguinal lymph nodes, 3 cm in diameter.

A diagnostic procedure was performed.

Differential Diagnosis

Dr. Raphael Dolin*: This young man, who had apparently been in good health except for a five-year history of chronic urticaria, had a subacute illness manifested principally by increasing fatigue, Raynaud's phenomenon, and general malaise. Examination at this hospital revealed generalized lymphadenopathy and a tender nodule in the right testis. Initially, a number of laboratory abnormalities indicated the presence of multisystem involvement. They included mild anemia, an elevated erythrocyte sedimentation rate, hematuria, proteinuria, cryoglobulinemia, low complement levels, and positive tests for rheumatoid factor and antinuclear antibodies.

*Director, Infectious Disease Unit and professor of medicine, University of Vermont College of Medicine, Burlington, Vt.

The patient also had circulating hepatitis B surface antigen.

Thus, there was evidence of disease involving the liver, kidneys, skin, testis, hematopoietic system, and lymph nodes, along with the presence of cryoglobulins and other immunoglobulins of unusual reactivity. As part of the diagnostic workup the attending physicians biopsied virtually all the involved organs, and although the histopathologic studies provided additional information the nature of much of the underlying process remained unclear. I shall approach this problem by considering each organ system separately, beginning with those in which the histopathologic diagnosis appears most clear and then attempting to correlate the findings with a unifying diagnosis.

With respect to the hepatic involvement, the patient had chronic infection with hepatitis B virus (HBV), with histologic evidence of chronic persistent hepatitis and hepatitis B surface antigen in the blood and hepatocytes. The absence of hepatosplenomegaly and other signs of liver disease is typical of this entity, and the results of liver-function tests were normal. Of interest is the information that the patient was a homosexual. The rate of infection with hepatitis B[1] and several sexually transmitted agents is extremely high in homosexuals.[2] We learn subsequently that the patient's serum gave positive tests for both e antigen and anti-e antibody. The precise nature of e antigen is not clear, but recent studies suggest that it is a subunit of the nucleocapsid of the virus, antigenically distinct from hepatitis B surface antigen.[3] E antigen appears to circulate in two forms, one with a small molecular size and a larger one with molecular size of approximately 300,000 daltons, which is associated with IgG. E antigen is associated with infectivity and active liver disease, whereas the development of anti-e antibody is reported to be a favorable prognostic sign since it is generally, although not invariably, associated with resolution of chronic hepatitis B infection and liver disease.[4] The simultaneous presence of both e antigen and anti-e antibody, as described in this case, is distinctly unusual; it was reported to occur in only 4 percent of chronic carriers of hepatitis B in a recent large study.[5]

I shall turn now to the interpretation of the immunoglobulin abnormalities. There was a ++++ test for serum cryoprecipitate, which consisted of a homogeneous IgM kappa component and heterogeneous IgG and IgA immunoglobulins. This cryoprecipitate represents a mixed cryoglobulin of the Type II category in the classification of Brouet et al.[6] In that classification Type I cryoglobulin consists of a monoclonal immunoglobulin or Bence Jones protein, Type II consists of a monoclonal component with component activity against polyclonal immunoglobulins of one or more classes, and Type III consists of mixtures of polyclonal immunoglobulins, occasionally including nonimmunoglobulin proteins. In the Type II cryoglobulin the monoclonal component has rheumatoid factor activity directed against the Fc portion of the other immunoglobulins and probably accounts for the rheumatoid factor found in this case. The antinuclear-antibody activity reflected generation of other autoantibodies. It is of interest that in the majority of the reported cases of Type II cryoglobulinemia the monoclonal IgM component has contained kappa light chains,[7] as was also observed in this case.

Mixed cryoblobulinemia, Types II and III, has been described in association with a number of diseases, including lymphoproliferative disorders, collagen vascular diseases, autoimmune disorders, vasculitis, and various acute and chronic infections. When mixed cryoglobulinemia is observed without an underlying illness the disorder is referred to as "essential" (EMC) and is characterized clinically by arthralgia or arthritis, purpura, weakness, vasculitis, and glomerulonephritis. It has been said that Type II cryoglobulinemia is more frequently associated with lymphoproliferative disease, whereas Type III is more commonly accompanied by collagen vascular diseases, autoimmune disorders, infection, or no underlying disease.[6] However, there is sufficient overlap among the diseases associated with each type of mixed cryoglobulinemia that classification into Type II versus Type III is of limited diagnostic value in the individual patient.

The infectious diseases associated with mixed cryoglobulins include syphilis,[8] subacute bacterial endocarditis,[9] lymphogranuloma venereum,[10] toxoplasmosis,[11] lepromatous leprosy,[12] and malaria,[13] none of which, except perhaps for lymphogranuloma venereum, are suggested by the data provided. In these settings the cryoglobulins represent circulating immune complexes that contain immunoglobulins with antibody activity against the infectious agent, often along with antigens of the infectious agent or the agent itself in certain viral infections. The most notable example of this circumstance is the association of mixed cryoglobulinemia with hepatitis B infection,[13] but it has also been described in association with infectious mononucleosis induced by both the Epstein–Barr virus (EBV)[14] and cytomegalovirus (CMV).[15] The association with hepatitis B infection has been particularly striking, and one group of investigators reported that 74 percent of patients with the diagnosis of essential mixed cryoglobulinemia have proved to have hepatitis B virus surface antigen in cryoprecipitates.[16] These investigators postulated that in many cases essential mixed cryoglobulinemia reflects the presence of occult hepatitis B infection. In a recent report from this institution, however, investigators did not find a similarly high rate of HBV infection in patients with essential mixed cryoglobulinemia.[17] In this case we are told that hepatitis B surface antigen (HBsAg) was present "in a titer considerably lower than that detected in serum," which suggests that the cryoprecipitate did not contain circulating immune complexes involving HBsAg, since one would expect an increased concentration of HBsAg or anti-HBsAg if that were the situation. One could raise the question whether the immune complexes contained other hepatitis B antigens and antibodies, such as e antigen and anti-e antibodies, and I wonder whether the cryoprecipitate was examined for their presence. Another useful approach would have been electron microscopical examination of the cryoprecipitate, which has been used for direct visualization of virus particles in immune complexes, including HBV[16] and herpesviruses such as EBV and CMV.[18] E antigen, however, is a soluble, nonparticulate antigen and would be unlikely to be seen on routine electron microscopical study. It should be noted that in the application of these techniques either antigen or antibody activity may be lost when cryoprecipitates are purified and that immune complexes themselves may interfere with the measurement of either antigen or antibody. Finally, it is clear that in some patients with hepatitis B infection immune complexes that are entirely unrelated to recognized HBV antigens may be detected. Nonetheless, elucidation of the nature of the immune complexes in this patient might provide useful information concerning the underlying disease.

Immune complexes, regardless of their source, have been implicated in the pathogenesis of disease involving virtually all organs, including those involved in this case. What determines the site of tissue injury induced by immune complexes or whether any injury occurs at all is not entirely understood. The pathogenesis probably involves a complex interplay of multiple factors, among the most important being the composition of the immune complexes in terms of size, antibody class and subclass, the state of antigen or antibody excess, and the presence of anti-immunoglobulin activity. Clearly, the immune status of the host and the functional capacity of the host's reticuloendothelial system also play a part. A feature of this patient's illness that can be linked to immune complexes is the Raynaud's phenomenon, which has been described with all three types of cryoglobulinemia. Although we are not given a history of cold-induced or cold-aggravated symptoms they are often not present.[6,7]

This patient's renal disease also appears to have been immune-complex mediated, and a biopsy is described as revealing "immune-complex glomerulonephritis." The original presentation with hematuria, red-cell casts, and proteinuria, subsequently documented at an excretion of more than 5 g per day, indicates active glomerulonephritis, probably with both membranous and proliferative components. A number of renal lesions have been associated with immune-complex injury and with cryoglobulinemia, including diffuse and focal proliferative glomerulonephritis, membranoproliferative glomerulonephritis, and membranous glomerulonephritis.[19] Characteristic crystalline inclusions have been demonstrated by electron microscopical examination in kidneys with cryoglobulinemia-associated disease.[20] The renal lesion most frequently associated with chronic HBV infection, particularly in children, has been the membranous type of glomerulonephritis.[21] In patients with this lesion immune complexes containing HBsAg have been implicated by detection of HBsAg, immunoglobulins, and complement in the affected glomeruli, by elution of a high titer of anti-HBsAg from glomeruli, and by visualization of HBV-like particles within the glomeruli. Despite this evidence, questions have been raised regarding the pathogenesis of HBV-associated glomerulonephritis because of the large size of HBsAg-containing immune complexes, which would have a minimum size of 3,000,000 daltons if the entire antigen were present in the complexes. In experimental studies in which bovine serum albumin-antibody immune complexes were administered to rabbits only complexes of a size less than 1,000,000 daltons were found in the glomerular basement membrane and subepithelial regions, inducing membranous glomerulonephritis.[22] Takekoshi and his colleagues[23] pointed out that e antigen, with a molecular size of 300,000 daltons even when associated with IgG, is more likely to induce membranous glomerulonephritis in association with HBV, and they subsequently demonstrated e antigen in the kidneys of two children with chronic HBsAg infection and membranous glomerulonephritis. It would be of interest to know if the renal tissue in this case was examined for the presence of HBsAg or e antigen.

The most common cutaneous lesion associated with mixed cryoglobulinemia is purpura, most frequently involving the lower extremities, as a result of small-vessel vasculitis in the dermis.[6,7] A variety of other skin manifestations have been attributed to immune-complex injury, including those associated with circulating immune complexes containing HBsAg. Urticaria with lymphocytic venulitis and focal necrosis has been most often associated with acute hepatitis B infection. Chronic hepatitis (B or non-B related) has been accompanied more often by palpable purpura, reflected histopathologically in a neutrophilic vasculitis of small dermal vessels.[24] In this case the skin biopsy showed a slight mixed perivascular infiltrate with mild dermal edema. I assume that the lack of findings suggestive of cryoglobulinemia refers to the absence of small-vessel vasculitis. Focal disposition of IgM and IgA within vessel walls was demonstrated by immunofluorescence. These findings are consistent with urticaria but tell us little about its pathogenesis. The patient had a five-year history of urticaria. Some episodes were precipitated by the ingestion of aspirin, so that, at least in part, the urticaria may not have been immunologically mediated. Attempts to define the cause of chronic urticaria have been frustrating in many cases, and authors of several large series have reported that specific precipitating factors are identified in less than 20 percent of the cases.[25] The histopathologic pattern of skin lesions in cases of chronic idiopathic urticaria is very similar to that described in this patient.[25] There is, however, a group of patients with chronic urticaria in whom circulating immune complexes are present as well as immunoglobulins in vessel walls, and no dermal vasculitis can be demonstrated. Whether these cases reflect a coincidence of chronic urticaria and circulating immune complexes or whether the two are pathogenetically related by as yet undefined mechanisms remains unresolved.

The results of the bone-marrow examination in this case are similarly not very revealing except for the absence of abnormal findings. The patient had mild anemia when first seen, and the hematocrit had risen slightly by the time of admission. The cause of the anemia is not clear except that it does not appear to have been related to iron or folic acid deficiency. The reticulocyte count was slightly elevated, and the haptoglobin level was markedly decreased, suggesting the possibility of a hemolytic component. Both direct and indirect Coombs tests were negative, but it is conceivable that the patient had Coombs-negative autoimmune anemia. The anemia could also have been related to any of the chronic illnesses under consideration.

The central question in this case concerns the cause of the diffuse lymphadenopathy. On the initial presentation small lymph nodes were palpable in the left cervical, right supraclavicular, and both axillary and inguinal regions. The nodes were described as shotty on admission and again on a follow-up visit three days after discharge. However, at that time the inguinal lymph nodes were slightly tender and 3 cm in diameter suggesting some progression of the process. In a patient of any age, but particularly a young adult, who presents with these findings one needs to consider the possibility of infectious mononucleosis. The most common cause of this syndrome is, of course, Epstein–Barr virus (EBV) infection, which is characterized by the typical triad of fever, sore throat, and lymphadenopathy.[26] The lymphadenopathy is generally confined to the posterior cervical nodes, but generalized involvement of lymph nodes occurs rarely and can include those in the inguinal area. The hematologic hallmark of this syndrome is a relative and absolute mononuclear leukocytosis with atypical lymphocytes. This finding is present in 70 percent of the cases, peaking during the second and third weeks of the illness. Since we are given only a total white-cell count (4900) on the initial presentation, a low total eosinophil count, and no differential count or mention of atypical lymphocytes, we have insufficient information to determine whether the patient had hematologic findings suggestive of infectious mononucleosis. On admission the white-cell count had fallen further to 4100, with 75 percent neutrophils, 24 percent lymphocytes, and 1 percent monocytes. Again, there is no mention of atypical lymphocytes. EBV-induced infectious mononucleosis is associated with the development of heterophil antibodies, but we are not told that tests for heterophil agglutinins were performed. Because of the presence of multiple circulating immunoglobulins of unusual reactivity the interpretation of the presence of heterophil agglutinins would have required differential absorption with guinea-pig kidney and beef red cells. The identification of EBV as the causative agent of heterophil-positive infectious mononucleosis has led to the recognition of a broad spectrum of clinical manifestations associated with infection due to this virus. These include asymptomatic infection, heterophil-negative mononucleosis syndromes,[27] particularly in children, and an isolated hepatic or neurologic illness, with or without a positive heterophil-agglutination test.[28] The most important tests to identify EBV infection are EBV-specific antibody determinations. A fourfold or greater rise in IgG titers to EBV-viral capsid antigen (VCA) establishes the diagnosis of acute EBV infection, but often, as is probably in this case, the patient presents late in the course of the illness at a time when a high stable titer is already present. Examination of the serum for IgM-VCA antibodies may help to establish the diagnosis. However, the recent demonstration of IgM-VCA antibodies in an asymptomatic older population unlikely to have a primary EBV infection[29] as well as the finding of IgM antibodies in patients with several types of recurrent herpesvirus infection indicate that the presence of IgM antibodies does not document recent primary infection. The pattern of development of antibodies to Epstein–Barr nuclear antigen and to early antigen, particularly anti-D, may also be useful in the diagnosis of recent infection.[30]

EBV-induced mononucleosis is usually a self-limited lymphoproliferative illness, although fatal X-linked syndromes in which agammaglobulinemia or lymphoma developed have been reported.[31] Primary EBV infection accompanied by a diffuse polyclonal B-cell lymphoma has also been recognized,[32] but neither the histopathologic examination of the lymph node nor the clinical findings support the diagnosis of lymphoma in this case.

The major cause of heterophil-negative infectious mononucleosis is cytomegalovirus infection.[33] CMV mononucleosis is most often manifested as an acute or subacute febrile illness in which a sore throat is usually absent. Lymphadenopathy is less prominent than in EBV-induced mononucleosis and is frequently absent. However, there is a spectrum of CMV-induced disease and an overlap with EBV-induced infectious mononucleosis, and thus the cause in an individual case cannot be determined with certainty on clinical grounds. The distinction between EBV-associated and CMV-associated illness can be complicated further by simultaneous infection with both viruses, as has been reported recently in four cases of heterophil-negative infectious mononucleosis.[34] Because of the propensity of herpesviruses to cause latent infection such episodes of dual infection may well represent reactivation of latent infection with one virus at the time when a primary infection with a different virus is occurring.

The question of cytomegalovirus infection is particularly relevant in this setting because of the extraordinarily high prevalence of CMV infection in homosexual men, probably as a result of sexual transmission. In one recent study the authors reported that 95 percent of homosexual men attending a clinic for sexually transmitted diseases had antibody to CMV, as compared with 54 percent of heterosexual men.[35] At the same clinic 14 percent of homosexual men between 18 and 29 years of age were found to be excreting CMV in the urine, although they were reported to be asymptomatic.[35] Retrospective analysis by the same group of investigators detected 15 cases of CMV mononucleosis over a nine-year period, including four in homosexual men. It would have been important to obtain viral cultures for CMV from urine and a buffy coat in the patient under discussion as well as to obtain acute and convalescent serum specimens for anti-CMV antibodies. An IgM anti-CMV determination might also have been helpful, despite the previously discussed problems in the interpretation of IgM titers.

Hematologic abnormalities identical to those in EBV-induced mononucleosis may be seen in CMV-induced mononucleosis, although the atypical lymphocytosis generally is less pronounced than in EBV-induced mononucleosis. Except for heterophil antibodies all the immunoglobulin abnormalities associated with EBV-induced mononucleosis can be seen in CMV-induced disease. Many of the immunopathologic features of this case have been reported in cases of infectious mononucleosis. Cryoglobulins have been found in 70 to 90 percent of the cases of infectious mononucleosis, although they are ordinarily present only transiently during the acute illness, are in a low concentration, and are rarely associated with lesions. Cryoglobulins have also been implicated in the pathogenesis of the urticaria that is occasionally seen in patients with acute mononucleosis. Immune complexes from one such patient were demonstrated to contain IgG, IgM, IgA, C3, C4, C5, and EBV-VCA antibodies, along with viral particles resembling EBV.[18] Immune-complex glomerulonephritis, although uncommon, has also been reported in patients with EBV[36] and CMV infections.[37] CMV antigens and antibodies and EBV antibodies have been detected in the kidneys of such patients, and the findings from one study suggested that mild glomerulonephritis may be relatively common in patients with infectious mononucleosis, although it is rarely associated with appreciable symptoms of proteinuria.[38] Autoimmune hemolytic anemia and thrombocytopenia have also been reported with both EBV-induced and CMV-induced disease.[39]

For the sake of completeness I should mention that toxoplasmosis can cause an infectious-mononucleosis syndrome, but the absence of characteristic lymph-node histopathologic changes argues against that diagnosis. Serologic tests for toxoplasmosis ordinarily show a high level of antibodies at the time of the acute illness.

An additional diagnosis that merits serious consideration in this case is the lymphoproliferative syndrome known as immunoblastic lymphadenopathy or angioimmunoblastic lymphadenopathy.[40,41] This disease is seen most frequently in older patients (fifth and sixth decades), although patients as young as this one have been reported. Most of the patients present with fever, sweats, and weight loss, accompanied by generalized lymphadenopathy, hepatosplenomegaly, and a rash. The rash is commonly maculopapular or morbilliform, although urticaria has also been described. The lymph nodes are often 2 to 3 cm in diameter, are generally firm and mobile, and may or may not be tender. Regional as opposed to generalized lymphadenopathy has also been reported. The laboratory findings include anemia, which is frequently hemolytic and Coombs-positive. Various white-cell findings have been described, the most common being lymphopenia, and eosinophilia has also been observed variably. The patients generally manifest a polyclonal hypergammaglobulinemia, and cryoglobulins have been reported as well.[42] Loss of delayed skin-test reactivity and depression in a variety of in vitro tests of T-cell function have been noted. The disease is of unknown cause but is generally regarded as a polyclonal lymphoproliferative response to antigenic stimulation. Specific precipitating agents, most commonly drugs, are implicated in only about a third of the cases. The patient under discussion was afebrile and lacked many of the constitutional symptoms associated with immunoblastic lymphadenopathy. Generalized lymphadenopathy was present, but there was no hepatosplenomegaly. A number of laboratory abnormalities that have been described in cases of immunoblastic lymphadenopathy, including anemia nad cryoglobulinemia, were seen in this case, but hypergammaglobulinemia was not present since both agarose-gel electrophoresis and immunoelectrophoresis were normal. In addition, this patient reacted to a candida skin test. Although he lacked many of the typical features of immunoblastic lymphadenopathy, sufficient variants of the syndrome have been reported so that it is risky to exclude this diagnosis on clinical grounds alone.

The histopathologic findings in the lymph node, however, provided much stronger evidence against immunoblastic lymphadenopathy, which is characterized by a diffuse process obliterating the normal architecture and consisting of marked proliferation and arborization of small vessels, a mixed cellular proliferation with prominent immunoblasts, a few small lymphocytes and variable numbers of plasma cells, eosinophils, and histiocytes, and an accumulation of an amorphous acidophilic interstitial material. These features are in contrast to the focal findings described in this case, which are more consistent with an alternative diagnosis. It should also be noted that the pathological findings described in lymph nodes in cases of immunoblastic lymphadenopathy have been reported in skin-biopsy specimens and occasionally in bone-marrow specimens from patients with this disorder, and their absence in this patient is further evidence against the diagnosis. A word of caution is in order, however. It is fairly common for the diagnosis to be obscure on examination of initial biopsy specimens, and serial biopsies have been required on occasion to establish this diagnosis.

The final diagnosis that I shall consider is the lymphadenopathic form of Kaposi's sarcoma. Consideration of this entity should be placed in the context of the emergence of a series of remarkable observations concerning diseases among homosexual men. First of all, it is apparent that the frequency of sexually transmitted diseases among certain groups of homosexual men is extraordinarily high.[1,2] In addition to hepatitis B and CMV infection, alluded to earlier, many of these men have a history of gonorrhea, syphilis, lymphogranuloma venereum, herpes genitalis, amebiasis, and giardiasis. We are told that the patient under discussion had been treated for gonococcal urethritis in the past, and he presented with a tender testicular nodule, which resolved partially during the course in the hospital. From the information provided it is difficult to say whether the diagnosis of epididymitis was correct, but tetracycline might have been a better choice of therapy, since chlamydia as well as gonococci are important causes of epididymitis in this setting. However, the location of the nodule and the clinical course are consistent with the diagnosis that was made. The extraordinary observation has also been made that in addition to sexually transmitted diseases we are now witnessing in previously healthy homosexual men the emergence of infections that had formerly been restricted to severely immunocompromised patients. Currently, 60 cases of pneumocystis infection in homosexual men have been reported to the Centers for Disease Control (CDC).[43,44] The disease in these cases has been associated with a high fatality rate, reaching nearly 60 percent. Other infections generally associated with severe immunosuppression that have been observed in previously healthy homosexual men include disseminated cryptococcosis, central nervous system toxoplasmosis, severe perianal herpes simplex infection, and disseminated atypical mycobacteriosis. Many of these patients also have had serologic evidence of CMV infection, and in patients in whom appropriate viral cultures were obtained CMV was often cultured from blood, urine, or lungs.

Even more extraordinary is the recognition of at least 54 cases of Kaposi's sarcoma among homosexual men as reported to the CDC through August 1981.[44,45] Kaposi's sarcoma is an uncommon malignant neoplasm with an estimated annual frequency in the United States of 0.02 to 0.06 per 100,000.[46] Earlier it had been observed principally in three settings: among elderly men in North America and Europe[47]; in equatorial Africa in an endemic belt similar to that observed for Burkitt's lymphoma, where it frequently affects children and young adults[48]; and in renal-transplant recipients and other patients receiving intensive immunosuppressive therapy.[49]

Clinically, Kaposi's sarcoma is manifested by the presence of skin lesions, which consist of macules, plaques, or nodules, reddish-purple to dark-blue, that may appear anywhere on the skin or mucous membranes but are most commonly found in the lower extremities. These lesions may form large plaques and even fungating masses, which can become ulcerated and eroded. Involvement of lymph nodes, bones, and viscera can occur before, simultaneously with, or after the appearance of the skin lesions. Metastatic spread and direct extension of the lesions have been described.

Taylor et al.[50] classified Kaposi's sarcoma into four clinical types based largely on the appearance of the skin lesions in cases in Africa — nodular, florid, infiltrative, and lymphadenopathic forms. The first three forms are seen largely in patients over the age of 25 years and rarely involve lymph nodes. The nodular form is indolent, whereas the florid and infiltrative forms are locally aggressive. In contrast, the lymphadenopathic form is seen in patients below the age of 25 years, often children, in whom skin lesions are few or absent. In the last group an aggressive course with visceral involvement may be seen. Cases in the United States have not fit as neatly within this classification, but the majority of the elderly men with this disease have had a chronic course, with a mean survival of 8 to 13 years.[51]

The histopathologic features of Kaposi's sarcoma consist of proliferation of small vessels lined by endothelial cells with large nuclei, spindle-cell foci with some nuclear pleomorphism, and slit-like spaces containing red cells. In lymph nodes the same histopathologic pattern is observed but in nodular foci, which may partially replace lymph-node tissue. Depending on the relative proportion of these findings, three histopathologic types have been proposed[50,52] — the mixed-cell pattern, the mononuclear (spindle-cell) pattern, and the anaplastic pattern. The lymphadenopathic form most frequently has a mixed-cell pattern.

The cause of Kaposi's sarcoma is unknown. Several investigators have suggested the possibility of a causal relation with CMV, perhaps similar to that suggested for EBV and Burkitt's lymphoma. The evidence presented thus far consists of a serologic association between CMV and Kaposi's sarcoma,[53,54] the demonstration of herpes-like virus particles in tissue cultures prepared from Kaposi's sarcoma tissue,[55] and the detection of CMV-DNA in cells from Kaposi's sarcoma tissue.[56] This evidence, of course, does not distinguish between a causative relation and persistent infection in such cases. Similarly, the cell of origin of Kaposi's sarcoma has not been defined. Many investigators have suggested that this tumor is a malignant neoplasm of reticuloendothelial cells. It is of interest that it is associated with a markedly increased frequency of second primary cancers, largely reticuloendothelial malignant tumors.[57] Transitional stages between Kaposi's sarcoma and reticuloendothelial malignant tumors have also been reported, leading Safai and Good[51] and others to suggest that the increased frequency of reticuloendothelial malignant tumors in patients with Kaposi's sarcoma may not reflect the occurrence of multiple primary tumors but may be different manifestations of a single malignant process.

In the case under discussion we are told specifically that the patient had urticaria but no other rash or skin lesions, and thus we would have to postulate the lymphadenopathic form of Kaposi's sarcoma, in which skin lesions are rare or absent. It should be pointed out, however, that in cases reported to the CDC skin lesions had often been overlooked initially, particularly if present in small numbers or in unusual locations. Patients with the lymphadenopathic form come to medical attention principally because of constitutional symptoms such as malaise and often with fever and weight loss. The histopathologic findings in the lymph node described in this case are consistent with the diagnosis of Kaposi's sarcoma. In addition, the biopsy showed follicular hyperplasia in the residual nodal tissue with evidence of polyclonal stimulation of plasma cells, suggesting that polyclonal proliferation was occurring as well. Lymphoid hyperplasia and plasma-cell infiltration have on occasion been reported in lymph nodes in which Kaposi's sarcoma was present, so that confusion with the histologic appearance of lymphoma or a plasmacytoma may occur.[58]

Can the hematologic and immunologic features of this case be attributed to Kaposi's sarcoma as well? Unfortunately, we are at a disadvantage in this regard since no detailed report of the laboratory findings in Kaposi's sarcoma in homosexual patients has been published at this time. Hypergammaglobulinemia was described earlier in patients with Kaposi's sarcoma, and several patients with Kaposi's sarcoma, and plasma-cell dyscrasia accompanied by paraproteinemia have also been described.[59] Interestingly enough, three cases of autoimmune hemolytic anemia associated with Kaposi's sarcoma have been reported, including two in which the anemia preceded the recognition of Kaposi's sarcoma by one to eight years.[60]

In discussing the question of unusual immunoglobulins with Dr. Alvin Friedman-Kein of New York University, who has seen many of the New York patients with Kaposi's sarcoma, and Dr. Mary Guinan of the CDC I was informed that cryoglobulinemia and rheumatoid factor have not been observed in the reported cases, although immune complexes have been detected frequently. Therefore, one cannot exlude the possiblity of a relation between the cryoglobulinemia and Kaposi's sarcoma in this case. As stated previously, high titers of anti-CMV antibody are present in these patients, but in addition in many of the recent cases there have been extraordinarily high titers of anti-EBV antibodies as well, raising further interesting questions regarding the potential role of EBV.

The majority of the recent homosexual patients with Kaposi's sarcoma and many earlier patients with that tumor are severely immunosuppressed, particularly with respect to cell-mediated immunity. Many of the latter patients have lymphocyte counts below 1000 per cubic millimeter, as in this case, but, unlike this patient, they are generally skin-test negative. It is of interest that only patients with Kaposi's sarcoma who have been reported to be consistently skin-test negative. It is of interest that only patients with Kapsosi's sarcoma who have been reported to be consistently skin-test positive are those described as having the benign, localized form of the disease.[61]

The major unanswered question, which looms over this entire discussion, is what accounts for this extraordinary cluster of cases of Kaposi's sarcoma and opportunistic pathogens in this population. Most of the cases have been reported from two locations, New York and California, but cases in other areas are also being recognized, and it is unlikely that it is a localized phenomenon. Is there an outbreak of immunosuppression related to environmental factors, to an infectious agent, or perhaps to a summation of infections in such patients? Are we dealing with activation of a latent agent that induces immunosuppression or that itself has pluripotential expressions of disease? Are we then observing the sequelae of immunosuppression, such as pneumocytstis infection or Kaposi's sarcoma? The role of cytomegalovirus, which can cause immunosuppression and has been implicated in Kaposi's sarcoma, clearly needs to be examined further, and perhaps the role of EBV as well. The CDC has begun an intensive case-control study, which should help to identify some of the risk factors.

In summary, I believe that this patient had Kaposi's sarcoma. He had many of the features of immunoblastic lymphadenopathy, but the histopathologic pattern does not support that diagnosis. In addition, he had chronic hepatitis B infection with chronic persistent hepatitis, mixed cryoglobulinemia, and immune-complex glomerulonephritis. Although we are not given specific information with which to make the diagnosis, I suspect that evidence of CMV or EBV infection was found. Biopsy of an additional lymph node was probably the procedure selected to yield a definitive diagnosis.

Dr. Robert E. Scully: I shall call on Dr. Haupert, who took care of this patient, to make some comments.

Dr. Garner T. Haupert, Jr.: Although the glomerulonephritis, hepatitis, and cryoimmunoglobulinemia seemed compatible with chronic hepatitis B virus infection and antigenemia, in our view that diagnosis did not adequately explain the substantial anemia and diffuse peripheral lymphadenopathy. Since our concern about an underlying lymphoproliferative disorder had not been allayed by the findings on the initial lymph-node biopsy we asked Dr. Stephen P. Dretler to excise a second lymph node.

Dr. Jules L. Dienstag: At the time of admission, because of the circulating hepatitis B surface antigen, glomerulonephritis, and urticaria, we attributed the clinical findings to hepatitis B-associated immune-complex disease with cryoglobulinemia. However, we were very puzzled by the anemia of relatively recent onset and the diffuse lymphadenopathy, which are not characteristic of this syndrome.

Dr. Scully: Dr. Calderwood, will you give us the medical students' diagnosis?

Dr. Stephen B. Calderwood: They focused their attention on the chronic urticarial skin lesions, the immune-complex glomerulonephritis, the circulating Type II cryoglobulin, and the presence of hepatitis B surface antigen in the serum. They discussed a variety of diagnoses, including viral infections, such as those due to hepatitis B virus and Epstein–Barr virus, lymphoproliferative disease, and angioimmunoblastic lymphadenopathy. They thought that the findings in the original lymph-node-biopsy specimen were suggestive of angioimmunoblastic lymphadenopathy but that the clinical course was atypical. They chose angioimmunoblastic lymphadenopathy as their first diagnosis and favored a repeated lymph-node biopsy as the diagnostic procedure.

Clinical Diagnoses

Hepatitis B virus infection, chronic, with chronic persistent hepatitis and immune-complex glomerulonephritis.
Type II mixed cryoglobulinemia.
? Underlying lymphoproliferative disease.

Dr. Raphael Dolin's Diagnoses

Kaposi's sarcoma.
Chronic hepatitis B infection, with chronic persistent hepatitis.
Mixed cryoglobulinemia.
Immune-complex glomerulonephritis.
? Crytomegalovirus or Epstein–Barr virus infection.

Pathological Discussion

Dr. Nancy L. Harris: The cervical-lymph-node biopsy mentioned in the case record was performed six months before the first report of the epidemic of Kaposi's sarcoma in young homosexual men.[45] The interpretation of the specimen was a matter of considerable debate among staff members of the Department of Pathology. Some observers thought that the findings were suggestive or even diagnostic of Kaposi's sarcoma, but the majority concluded that a definite diagnosis of neoplasia was unwarranted. Primary lymphadenopathic Kaposi's sarcoma was at that time believed to be very unusual in Caucasian adults, and even those who thought that Kaposi's sarcoma was the probable diagnosis were reluctant to believe that it could be other than a local, even possibly incidental finding. As Dr. Haupert mentioned, the predominant impression of the clinicians was that the patient had an underlying lymphoproliferative disorder accounting for the cryoglobulinemia and for the systemic symptoms. Consequently, the procedure described at the end of the case record was a biopsy of an enlarged inguinal lymph node.

The specimen, 3.5 cm in diameter, was almost completely replaced by hemorrhagic spindle-cell sarcoma. Its appearance removed any doubt about whether the previously observed vascular proliferation was neoplastic. The histologic features were typical of the mixed pattern of Kaposi's sarcoma, in which islands of well-formed capillaries alternate with areas of pure spindle-cell proliferation. Even in the spindle-cell areas slit-like spaces containing red cells were usually seen (Fig. 3). Electron microscopical examination showed small blood vessels lined by typical endothelial cells, with Weibel–Palade bodies, undifferentiated or fibroblast-like spindle cells, and histiocytic cells with phagocytosed erythrocytes. Red cells were present within capillary lumens and free in tissue spaces.

A diagnosis of primary lymphadenopathic Kaposi's sarcoma was made on the basis of the findings in the second lymph-node-biopsy specimen. As observed by Dr. Dolin, the lymphadenopathic form of Kaposi's sarcoma has previously been rare outside Africa. However, according to the recent reports of Kaposi's sarcoma in homosexual men lymph-node involvement, with or without skin lesions, is seen frequently.[45,62-64] In addition, these homosexual patients have had a high mortality rate, similar to that in African children and in contrast to that in most Western adults with the disease.

The cell of origin of Kaposi's sarcoma is still controversial. Morphologic observations clearly indicate that the neoplastic cell has the capacity to form vascular channels. The tumor cells have been shown to contain factor VIII antigen, which is present only in vascular endothelial cells and megakaryocytes.[65] The finding of endothelial cells, phagocytic histiocytes, and fibroblasts or myofibroblasts on electron micro-

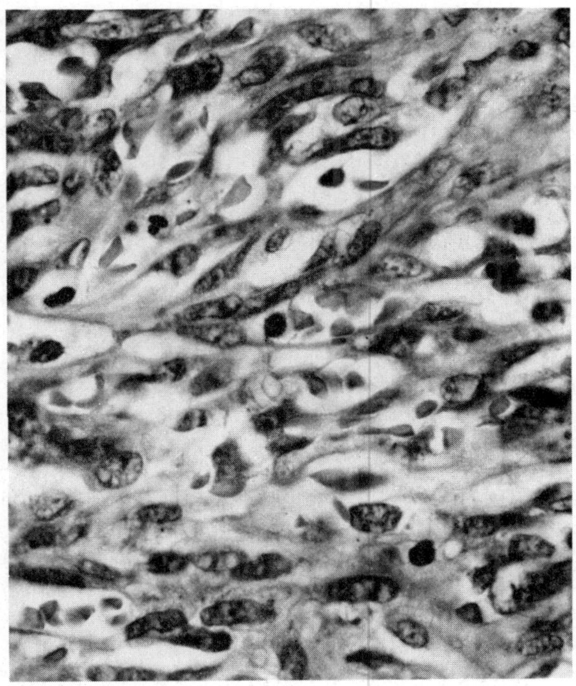

Figure 3. Biopsy Specimen of an Inguinal Lymph Node, Showing the Sarcomatous Pattern of Spindle Cells and Numerous Small Capillary-like Spaces Containing Red Cells (×640).

scopical examination suggests that the neoplastic cell may be a multipotential mesenchymal cell.[66] On the basis of histochemical studies and the observation that the lesions tend to follow the lymphatic system it has been suggested that Kaposi's sarcoma is a tumor of lymphatic-vascular rather than blood-vascular origin.[67] This hypothesis is also favored by the preferential occurrence of tumors in areas of lymphatic stasis, such as the lower extremities. Because of the high rate of association of Kaposi's sarcoma with lymphoid neoplasia and abnormal immune states a reticuloendothelial origin has also been proposed.[51,52,57]

The reticuloendothelial system, as defined in the broadest sense, is now known to be composed of a number of distinct cell lines. Although it was earlier thought that reticulum cells gave rise to lymphocytes, we now know that small lymphocytes proliferate by way of blast transformation and are not derived from the fixed reticulum cells of the lymph node. It has also been shown that the Kupffer cells of the liver and sinus histiocytes of the spleen and lymph nodes as well as pulmonary alveolar macrophages are derived from circulating blood monocytes. This group of cells has been called the mononuclear phagocyte system.[68] The remaining fixed elements of the lymph node are fibroblasts, fixed reticulum cells, and blood vessels, all of which are thought to be distinct from lymphocytes. Most tumors of the reticuloendothelial system are malignant lymphomas — tumors of lymphocytes, not of reticulum cells, macrophages, or endothelial cells. If blood vessels are considered part of the reticuloendothelial system Kaposi's sarcoma may be a reticuloendothelial neoplasm; there is no evidence that it is a form of malignant lymphoma.

The coincidence of Kaposi's sarcoma and malignant lymphoma probably reflects the tendency of both diseases to occur with increased frequency in immunosuppressed patients, such as renal-transplant recipients. The observation that the lesions of Kaposi's sarcoma in transplant recipients may wax and wane with increasing and decreasing immunosuppressive therapy[49] suggests that Kaposi's sarcoma, in particular, is an opportunistic neoplasm in immunologically compromised hosts.

Dr. Scully: Dr. McCluskey, do you want to comment about the renal findings?

Dr. Robert T. McCluskey: Examination of the renal-biopsy specimen showed some glomerular mesangial hypercellularity and thickening of the capillary walls, with prominent granular deposits of IgG, C3, and C1q along the peripheral capillary loops. There were conspicuous IgM-containing deposits in mesangial regions. Staining for HBsAg was positive in mesangial regions, and e antigen was found in deposits along the glomerular basement membranes.

Dr. Dienstag: We detected hepatitis B surface antigen, hepatitis B e antigen, and antibody to hepatitis B core antigen in the cryoprecipitate but not in concentrations greater than those in the serum. In previous studies of patients with cryglobulinemia and extrahepatic disease associated with hepatitis B infection we found the concentration of HBsAg in cryoprecipitates higher than that in serum.[69-71] Therefore, we were left with a dilemma. The patient had two different diseases — Kaposi's sarcoma and hepatitis B infection. Did the glomerulonephritis result from glomerular deposition of HBsAg–anti-HBs or HBeAg–anti-HBe antigen-antibody complexes, or both? Alternatively, despite the immunopathologic evidence of hepatitis B antigen deposition in the kidney, could deposition of a tumor antigen[72,73] have been responsible for the glomerulonephritis?

Dr. Kurt J. Bloch: In view of the apparent discrepancy between the findings on the serologic and immunofluorescence studies additional antigen (such as cytomegalovirus[74])-antibody systems should be sought in the renal-biopsy material.

Dr. McCluskey: I favor the idea that the glomerulonephritis was related to immune complexes containing hepatitis antigens. The demonstration of HBsAg and e antigen in glomeruli was convincing. Attempts to demonstrate CMV antigen in glomeruli were unsuccessful. The most direct way of implicating a given system of immune complexes in the pathogenesis of glomerular lesions is to demonstrate their presence in glomeruli; complexes that are found in the circulation are sometimes irrelevant. Furthermore, I am skeptical of reports in which it has been stated that antigens related to a malignant tumor have been demonstrated in glomerular deposits.

Dr. Bloch: With respect to the emergence of Kaposi's sarcoma in homosexual men it is possible that simultaneous or sequential infection with several viruses that can cause immunosuppression is responsible for the emergence of this tumor. Whether cytomegalovirus has a more specific causative role in Kaposi's sarcoma is still uncertain.[75]

Dr. Richard A. Moscicki: I examined the lymphocytes from a sample of this patient's blood for the presence of T-cell subsets. The distribution of T-cell subset markers was as follows: 54 percent of the lymphocytes bore the T3 marker; 16 percent bore T4; and 33 percent bore T8. The ratio of T4-bearing to T8-bearing cells was 0.5 (normal, 1.7). A similar alteration has been observed in viral disease, including that caused by Epstein–Barr virus[76] and cytomegalovirus.[77]

Dr. Harris: After the diagnosis of Kaposi's sarcoma was made the patient's serum was tested for antibodies to cytomegalovirus and was positive in a titer of 1:2048. There was no evidence of excretion of a virus in the urine. The patient was referred to Dr. Sheldon Kaufman, who began treatment with weekly vinblastine (700 mg) administered intravenously for six months. All the lymphadenopathy resolved. There has never been any evidence of the skin lesions of Kaposi's sarcoma.

Dr. Haupert: Nephrotic-range proteinuria has continued, and there has been a gradual but definite decrease in the glomerular filtration rate. Because the renal pathological findings resembled in some ways those seen in membranous nephropathy we treated the patient with alternate-day high-dose prednisone for two months, since this therapy has been found to benefit some patients with idiopathic membranous glomerulonephritis.[78] There was, however, no diminution in the proteinuria, and the prednisone was stopped.

Since patients of this type manifest some signs of immunocompetence and since we have no proved efficacious therapy for this type of nephropathy, we have been particularly hesitant to institute cytotoxic or immunosuppressive therapy in addition to or in lieu of vinblastine treatment. This man is currently on monthly vinblastine maintenance therapy and feeling well, with resolution of the lymphadenopathy.

Anatomical Diagnoses

Kaposi's sarcoma, involving cervical and inguinal lymph nodes, lymphadenopathic type.

(Type II cryglobulinemia.)

Immune-complex glomerulonephritis.

Chronic persistent hepatitis with hepatitis B surface antigen.

Addendum

Dr. Dolin: This interesting case is an example of a previously recognized disease, Kaposi's sarcoma, emerging in new setting. Physicians need to be aware of this possibility and to be alert for the presence of unusual opportunistic infections in homosexual male patients as well. Unraveling the reasons for the emergence of these disorders in this group of patients should provide important insights into the pathogenesis of these diseases.

Dr. Harris: Since this conference three publications describing unusual opportunistic infections and Kaposi's sarcoma in previously healthy persons, principally homosexual men, have appeared in this journal.[79-81] Just as described by Dr. Moscicki in the patient under discussion, Gottlieb et al.[79] found decreased helper/suppressor ratios in four patients with *Pneumocystis carinii* pneumonia, one of whom had Kaposi's sarcoma, and in two additional patients with Kaposi's sarcoma without infection. Evidence of depressed cellular immunity was found by Masur et al.[80] and Siegal et al.[81] using other techniques in 15 additional patients.

References

1. Szmuness W, Much MI, Prince AM, et al. On the role of sexual behavior in the spread of hepatitis B infection. Ann Intern Med 1975; 83:489-95.
2. Phillips SC, Mildvan D, William DC, Gelb AM, White MC. Sexual transmission of enteric protozoa and helminths in a venereal-disease-clinic population. N Engl J Med 1981; 305:603-6.
3. Takahashi K, Imai M, Miyakawa Y, Iwakiri S, Mayumi M. Duality of hepatitis B e antigen in serum of persons infected with hepatitis B virus: evidence for the nonidentity of e antigen with immunoglobulins. Proc Natl Acad Sci USA 1978; 75:1952-6.
4. Hoofnagle JH, Dusheiko GM, Seeff LB, Jones EA, Waggoner JG, Bales ZB. Seroconversion from hepatitis B e antigen to antibody in chronic type B hepatitis. Ann Intern Med 1981; 94:744-8.
5. Villarejos VM, Andersen-Visoná K, Serra JC, Frösner GG, Deinhardt F. Anti-DNA, anti-HBc correlations with RIA-detected HBeAg and anti-HBe in chronic H BsAg carriers. J Med Virol 1980; 5:265-71.
6. Brouet C, Clauvel J-P, Danon F, Klein M, Seligman M. Biologic and clinical significance of cryoglobulins: a report of 86 cases. Am J Med 1974; 57:775-88.
7. Gorevic PD, Kassab HJ, Levo Y, et al. Mixed cryoglobulinemia: clinical aspects and long-term follow-up of 40 patients. Am J Med 1980; 69: 287-308.
8. Lassus A. Development of rheumatoid factor activity and cryoglobulins in primary and secondary syphilis. Int Arch Allergy Appl Immunol 1969; 36:515-22.
9. Hurwitz D, Quismorio FP, Friou GJ. Cryoglobulinaemia in patients with infectious endocarditis. Clin Exp Immunol 1975; 19:131-41.
10. Lassus A, Mustakallio KK, Wager O. Autoimmune serum factors and IgA elevation in lymphogranuloma venereum. Ann Clin Res 1970; 2:51-6.
11. Wager O, Mustakallio KK, Räsänen JA. Mixed IgA-IgG cryoglobulinemia: immunological studies and case reports of three patients. Am J Med 1968; 44:179-87.
12. Bonomo L, Dammacco F. Immune complex cryoglobulinemia in lepromatous leprosy: a pathogenetic approach to some clinical features of leprosy. Clin Exp Immunol 1971; 9:175-81.
13. Houba V, Lambert PH, Voller A, Soyanwo MAO. Clinical and experimental investigation of immune complexes in malaria. Clin Immunol Immunopathol 1976; 6:1-12.
14. Capra JD, Winchester RJ, Kunkel HG. Cold-reactive rheumatoid factors in infectious mononucleosis and other diseases. Arthritis Rheum 1969; 12: 67-73.
15. Wager O, Räsänen JA, Hagman A, Klemola E. Mixed cryoimmunoglobulinemia in infectious mononucleosis and cytomegalovirus mononucleosis. Int Arch Allergy Appl Immunol 1968; 34:345-61.
16. Levo Y, Gorevic PD, Kassab HJ, Zucker-Franklin D, Franklin EC. Association between hepatitis B virus and essential mixed cryoglobulinemia. N Engl J Med. 1977; 296:1501-4.
17. Popp JW Jr, Dienstag JL, Wands JR, Bloch KJ. Essential mixed cryoglobulinemia without evidence for hepatitis B virus infection. Ann Intern Med 1980; 92:379-83.
18. Wands JR, Perrotto JL, Isselbacher KJ. Circulating immune complexes and complement sequence activation in infectious monnucleosis. Am J Med 1976; 60:269-72.
19. Raij L, Michael AF. Immunologic aspects of kidney disease. In: Parker CW, ed. Clinical immunology. Philadelphia: WB Saunders, 1980:1051-87.
20. Feiner H, Gallo G. Ultrastructure in glomerulonephritis associated with cryoglobulinemia: a report of six cases and review of the literature. Am J Pathol 1977; 88:145-62.
21. Dienstag JL. Hepatitis B as an immune complex disease. Semin Liver Dis 1981; 1:45-55.
22. Germuth FG, Rodriguez E. Immunopathology of the renal glomerulus: immune complex deposit and antibasement membrane disease. Boston: Little, Brown, 1973.
23. Takekoshi Y, Tanaka M, Miyakawa Y, Yoshizawa H, Takahashi K, Mayumi M. Free "small" and IgG-associated "large" hepatitis B e antigen in the serum and glomerular capillary walls of two patients with membranous glomerulonephritis. N Engl J Med 1979; 300:814-9.
24. Popp JW Jr, Harrist TJ, Dienstag JL, et al. Cutaneous vasculitis associated with acute and chronic hepatitis. Arch Intern Med 1981; 141:623-9.
25. Yecies LD, Kaplan AP. Urticaria. In: Parker CW, ed. Clinical immunology. Philadelphia: WB Saunders, 1980:1306-15.
26. Schooley RT, Dolin R. Epstein–Barr virus (infectious mononucleosis). In: Mandell GL, Douglas RG, Bennett JE, eds. Principles and practice of infectious diseases. New York: John Wiley, 1979:1324-41.
27. Schmitz H, Volz D, Krainick-Riechert C, Scherer M. Acute Epstein–Barr virus infections in children. Med Microbiol Immunol 1972; 158:58-63.
28. Grose C, Henle W, Henle G, Feorino PM. Primary Epstein–Barr virus infections in acute neurologic diseases. N Engl J Med 1975; 292:392-5.
29. Sumaya CV. Endogenous reactivation of Epstein–Barr virus inections. J Infect Dis 1977; 135:374-9.
30. Henle W, Henle GE, Horwitz CA. Epstein–Barr virus specific diagnostic tests in infectious mononucleosis. Hum Pathol 1974; 5:551-65.
31. Purtilo DT, Paquin L, DeFlorio D, Virzi F, Sakhuja R. Immunodiagnosis and immunopathogenesis of the X-linked recessive lymphoproliferative syndrome. Semin Hematol 1979; 16:309-43.
32. Robinson JE, Brown N, Andiman W, et al. Diffuse polyclonal B-cell lymphoma during primary infection with Epstein–Barr virus. N Engl J Med. 1980; 302:1293-7.
33. Horwitz CA, Henle W, Henle G, et al. Heterophil-negative infectious mononucleosis and mononucleosis-like illness: laboratory confirmation of 43 cases. Am J Med 1977; 63:947-57.
34. Lemon SM, Hutt LM, Huang Y-T, Blum J, Pagano JS. Simultaneous infection with multiple herpesviruses. Am J Med 1979; 66:270-6.
35. Drew WL, Mintz L, Miner RC, Sands M, Ketterer B. Prevalence of cytomegalovirus infection in homosexual men. J Infect Dis 1981; 143:188-92.

36. Oldstone MBA, Theofilopoulos AN, Gunvén P, Klein G. Immune complexes associated with neoplasia: presence of Epstein–Barr virus antigen-antibody complexes in Burkitt's lymphoma. Intervirology 1974; 4:292-302.
37. Ozawa T, Stewart JA. Immune-complex glomerulonephritis associated with cytomegalovirus infection. Am Soc Clin Pathol 1979; 1:103-7.
38. Woodroffe AJ, Row PG, Meadows R, Lawrence JR. Nephritis in infectious mononucleosis. Q J Med 1974; 43:451-60.
39. Worlledge SM, Dacie JV. Haemolytic and other anaemias in infectious mononucleosis. In: Carter RL, Penman HG, eds. Infectious mononucleosis. Oxford: Blackwell, 1969:82-98.
40. Lukes RJ, Tindle BH. Immunoblastic lymphadenopathy: a hyperimmune entity resembling Hodgkin's disease. N Engl J Med 1975; 292:1-8.
41. Frizzera G, Moran EM, Rappaport H. Angio-immunoblastic lymphadenopathy with dysproteinaemia. Lancet 1974; 1:1070-3.
42. Schultz DR, Yunis AA. Immunoblastic lymphadenopathy with mixed cryoglobulinemia: a detailed case study. N Engl J Med 1975; 292:8-12.
43. *Pneumocystis* pneumonia — Los Angeles. MMWR 1981; 30:250-2.
44. Follow-up on Kaposi's sarcoma and *Pneumocystis* pneumonia. MMWR 1981; 30:409-10.
45. Kaposi's sarcoma and *Pneumocystis* pneumonia among homosexual men — New York City and California. MMWR 1981; 30:305-8.
46. Oettle AG. Geographical and racial differences in the frequency of Kaposi's sarcoma as evidence of environmental or genetic causes. Acta Unio Int Contra Cancrum 1962; 18:330-63.
47. Davis J. Kaposi's sarcoma: present concept of clinical course and treatment. NY State J Med 1968; 68:2067-73.
48. Dutz W, Stout AP. Kaposi's sarcoma in infants and children. Cancer 1960; 13:684-94.
49. Myers BD, Kessler E, Levi J, Pick A, Rosenfeld JB, Tikvah P. Kaposi's sarcoma in kidney transplant recipients. Arch Intern Med 1974; 133:307-11.
50. Taylor JF, Templeton AC, Vogel CL, Ziegler JL, Kyalwazl SK. Kaposi's sarcoma in Uganda: a clinico-pathological study. Int J Cancer 1971; 8: 122-35.
51. Safai B, Good RA. Kaposi's sarcoma: a review and recent developments. CA 1981; 31:2-12.
52. Reynolds WA, Winkelmann RK, Soule EH. Kaposi's sarcoma: a clinicopathologic study with particular reference to its relationship to the reticuloendothelial system. Medicine (Baltimore) 1965; 44:419-43.
53. Giraldo G, Beth E, Kourilsky FM, et al. Antibody patterns to herpes-viruses in Kaposi's sarcoma: serological association of European Kaposi's sarcoma with cytomegalovirus. Int J Cancer 1975; 15:839-48.
54. Giraldo G, Beth E, Henle W, et al. Antibody patterns to herpesviruses in Kaposi's sarcoma. II. Serological association of American Kaposi's sarcoma with cytomegalovirus. Int J Cancer 1978; 22:126-31.
55. Giraldo G, Beth E, Haguenau F. Herpes-type virus particles in tissue culture of Kaposi's sarcoma from different geographic regions. J Natl Cancer Inst. 1972; 49:1509-26.
56. Giraldo G, Beth E, Huang E-S. Kaposi's sarcoma and its relationship to cytomegalovirus (CMV). III. CMV DNA and CMV early antigens in Kaposi's sarcoma. Int J Cancer 1980; 26:23-9.
57. Safai B, Miké V, Giraldo G, Beth E, Good RA. Association of Kaposi's sarcoma with second primary malignancies: possible etiopathogenic implications. Cancer 1980; 45:1472-9.
58. Lubin J, Rywlin AM. Lymphoma-like lymph node changes in Kaposi's sarcoma: two additional cases. Arch Pathol 1971; 92:338-41.
59. Law IP. Kaposi sarcoma and plasma cell dyscrasia. JAMA 1974; 229: 1329-31.
60. Schreiber ZA, Haim S, Gellei B, Tatarsky I. Autoimmune hemolytic anemia in the course of Kaposi's sarcoma — report of a case. Cancer 1973; 32:922-5.
61. Master SP, Taylor JF, Kyalwazi SK, Ziegler JL. Immunological studies in Kaposi's sarcoma in Uganda. Br Med J 1970; 1:600-2.
62. Gottlieb GJ, Ragaz A, Vogel JV, et al. A preliminary communication on extensively disseminated Kaposi's sarcoma in young homosexual men. Am J Dermatopathol 1981; 3:111-4.
63. Hymes KB, Cheung T, Greene JB, et al. Kaposi's sarcoma in homosexual men — a report of eight cases. Lancet 1981; 2:598-600.
64. Thomsen HK, Jacobsen M, Malchon-Møller A. Kaposi's sarcoma among homosexual men in Europe. Lancet 1981; 2:688.
65. Nadji M, Morales AR, Ziegles-Weissman J, Penneys NS. Kaposi's sarcoma: immunohistologic evidence for an endothelial origin. Arch Pathol Lab Med 1981; 105:274-5.
66. Templeton AC. Kaposi's sarcoma. Pathol Annu 1981; 16:315-36.
67. Dorfman RF. Kaposi's sarcoma. The contribution of enzyme histochemistry to the identification of cell types. In: Ackerman LV, Murray JF, eds. Symposium on Kaposi's sarcoma. Basel: S Karger, 1963:151.
68. van Furth R, Langevoort HL, Schaberg A. Mononuclear phagocytes in human pathology — proposal for an approach to improved classification. In: van Furth R, ed. Mononuclear phagocytes in immunity, infection, and pathology. Oxford: Blackwell, 1975:1-15.
69. Wands JR, Mann E, Alpert E, Isselbacher KJ. The pathogenesis of arthritis associated with acute hepatitis-B surface antigen-positive hepatitis: complement activation and characterization of circulating immune complexes. J Clin Invest 1975; 55:930-6.
70. Farivar M, Wands JR, Benson GD, Dienstag JL, Isselbacher KJ. Cryoprotein complexes and peripheral neuropathy in a patient with chronic active hepatitis. Gastroenterology 1976; 71:490-3.
71. Dienstag JL, Rhodes AR, Bhan AK, Dvorak AM, Mihm MC Jr, Wands JR. Urticaria associated with acute viral hepatitis type B: studies of pathogenesis. Ann Intern Med 1978; 89:34-40.
72. Costanza ME, Pinn V, Schwartz RS, Nathanson L. Carcinoembryonic antigen-antibody complexes in a patient with colonic carcinoma and nephrotic syndrome. N Engl J Med 1973; 289:520-2.
73. Couser WG, Wagonfeld JB, Spargo BH, Lewis EJ. Glomerular deposition of tumor antigen in membranous nephropathy associated with colonic carcinoma. Am J Med 1974; 57:962-70.
74. Richardson WP, Colvin RB, Cheeseman SH, et al. Glomerulopathy associated with cytomegalovirus viremia in renal allografts. N Engl J Med 1981; 305:57-63.
75. Giraldo G, Beth E, eds. The role of viruses in human cancer. Vol. 1. New York: Elsevier/North Holland, 1980:57-73.
76. Reinherz EL, O'Brien C, Rosenthal P, Schlossman SF. The cellular basis for viral-induced immunodeficiency: analysis by monoclonal antibodies. J Immunol 1980; 125:1269-74.
77. Carney WP, Rubin RH, Hoffman RA, Hansen WP, Healey K, Hirsch MS. Analysis of T lymphocyte subsets in cytomegalovirus mononucleosis. J Immunol 1981; 126:2114-6.
78. Collaborative study of the adult idiopathic nephrotic syndrome. A controlled study of short-term prednisone treatment in adults with membranous nephropathy. N Engl J Med 1979; 301:1301-6.
79. Gottlieb MS, Schroff R, Schanker HM, et al. *Pneumocystis carinii* pneumonia and mucosal candidiasis in previously healthy homosexual men: evidence of a new acquired cellular immunodeficiency. N Engl J Med 1981; 305:1425-30.
80. Masur H, Michelis MA, Greene JB, et al. An outbreak of community-acquired *Pneumocystis carinii* pneumonia: initial manifestation of cellular immune dysfunction. N Engl J Med 1981; 305:1432-8.
81. Siegal FP, Lopez C, Hammer GS, et al. Severe acquired immunodeficiency in male homosexuals, manifested by chronic perianal ulcerative herpes simplex lesions. N Engl J Med 1981; 305:1439-44.

CASE RECORD OF THE MASSACHUSETTS GENERAL HOSPITAL

CASE 2-1986

Presentation of Case

A 58-year-old woman was admitted to the hospital because of fever and pulmonary infiltrates.

Approximately 10 years before admission a murmur was noted. Seven years before entry a stroke occurred, with a left-visual-field defect; atrial fibrillation was discovered, with evidence of mitral stenosis. Warfarin and digoxin were administered. One year later exertional dyspnea developed and gradually worsened, with the subsequent appearance of orthopnea and paroxysmal nocturnal dyspnea. Ten months before entry she was admitted to another hospital with pulmonary edema. She was transferred to this hospital, where cardiac catheterization confirmed the presence of mitral stenosis, with a calculated mitral-valve area of 1.1 cm^2, and mild aortic regurgitation. A mitral-valve replacement was performed after resection of a calcified mitral valve with rheumatic deformity. The intraoperative course was complicated by mitral regurgitation secondary to inadequate function of the prosthetic valve, and the prosthesis was repositioned, with the assistance of an intraaortic balloon pump. In the postoperative period the temperature rose to 40°C; all cultures were negative, and a cephalosporin was administered, with gradual defervescence during the next three weeks. Numerous transfusions were administered. Leukopenia was noted. Evidence of hyperthyroidism was found, and a radioiodine scan of the thyroid gland disclosed a nodule in the right lobe with increased uptake of radionuclide; methimazole was administered. The white-cell count fell to as low as 800, with 50 percent neutrophils. Methimazole and many other medications were discontinued, and the white-cell count rose to 4000, with a normal differential count. Microscopical examination of an aspirated specimen of bone marrow disclosed no abnormality. The patient was discharged on the 41st hospital day, on methimazole, warfarin, digoxin, ethacrynic acid, and potassium chloride.

The patient later received radioiodine treatment at another facility, and methimazole was discontinued. She was then well until three months before admission, when her family began to notice intermittent mild confusion, diminished alertness, and progressive fatigue. A gingivectomy was performed, and it was not clear whether she received appropriate antibiotic prophylaxis. Six weeks before admission fever developed, with rise of the temperature to 39.4°C associated with sweats, and the patient was readmitted to the first hospital, where physical examination yielded no diagnostic findings. Laboratory studies showed mild anemia; the white-cell count was 2100, with 20 percent band forms. X-ray films of the chest revealed evidence of a median sternotomy and mitral-valve replacement. Multiple blood cultures were negative. An echocardiogram disclosed no abnormality of the prosthetic heart valve. Cephalothin and gentamicin were given but were discontinued because of a rash; cefoperazone was substituted, but fever persisted. The erythrocyte sedimentation rate was 74 mm per hour. A diagnosis of polymyalgia rheumatica was considered, and prednisone, 30 mg daily, was begun, with prompt defervescence. The patient was discharged on prednisone, 30 mg daily, digoxin, and warfarin.

During the next few days she felt well, but fever soon recurred, with increasing weakness. Her family observed that she had doubled the prednisone dose to 60 mg daily and that she was uncertain as to her use of digoxin. Nine days before admission she returned to the same hospital. Her temperature was 39.9°C; physical examination disclosed no new findings. The hemoglobin was 10.9 g per 100 ml; the white-cell count was 14,600, with 14 percent band forms. X-ray films of the chest showed clear lungs. A computed tomographic (CT) scan of the abdomen revealed no abnormality. A CT scan of the thorax showed a mass to the right of the trachea, believed consistent with a thyroid nodule; an anterior mediastinal mass was seen, with lymphadenopathy in the region of the aortopulmonary window. Bradycardia developed; the digoxin level was 5.5 ng per milliliter, and digoxin was withheld. Repeated bacteriologic cultures remained negative. On the fifth hospital day another x-ray film of the chest was reported to show a prominent reticulonodular pattern throughout both lungs. A diuretic was administered, but the radiographic pattern did not change. She was transferred to this hospital.

The patient had lost 9.1 kg in weight during the preceding year. There was a history of exposure to pulmonary tuberculosis in the past. She had worked in remote years as a fabric cutter and occasionally used hair spray. A nonproductive cough had developed recently. There was no history of chest pain, recent dyspnea, rheumatic fever, diabetes mellitus, hypertension, use of tobacco, alcohol, or illicit drugs, or travel to the Midwest or California; the patient had not left eastern Massachusetts during the past three years.

The temperature was 40.1°C, the pulse was 84, and the respirations were 24. The blood pressure was 140/80 mm Hg.

On examination the patient appeared chronically and acutely ill. No rash or splinter hemorrhages were found. Shotty axillary lymphadenopathy was noted. The head was normal except that two microhemorrhages were seen in the left retina; no Roth spots were observed. The oropharynx was dry, with evidence of moniliasis. The neck was supple; a soft nodule, 1 by 1 cm, was palpated in the right thyroid lobe. The carotid pulses were ++, without a bruit. Diffuse crackles and scattered rhonchi were heard in both lungs, with a few expiratory wheezes bilaterally. The heart was slightly enlarged, and the rhythm was irregular; the prosthetic-valve sounds were crisp; no murmur or S3 sound was heard. The breasts and abdomen were normal. No peripheral edema, clubbing, or cyanosis was found. Pelvic and rectal examinations were negative. A stool specimen gave a negative test for occult blood. Neurologic examination disclosed slight disorientation as to the day and date; there was a questionable left homonymous visual-field defect. The tendon reflexes were ++ and equal, and a left Babinski sign was present.

The urine gave a trace-positive test for protein; the sediment contained 2 white cells, 3 granular casts, and numerous bacteria per high-power field. The hematocrit was 28.3 percent; the white-cell count was 3700, with 73 percent neutrophils, 17 percent band forms, 7 percent lymphocytes, 1 percent monocytes, and 2 percent eosinophils. The platelet count was 199,000, and the reticulocyte count 1 percent; the erythrocyte sedimentation rate was 139 mm per hour. The prothrombin time was 11.4 seconds, with a control of 11 seconds; the partial thromboplastin time was 41.9 seconds. The urea nitrogen was 66 mg per 100 ml (24 mmol per liter), the creatinine 1.9 mg per 100 ml (170 μmol per liter), the glucose 110 mg per 100 ml (6.1 mmol per liter), the calcium 7.7 mg per 100 ml (1.9 mmol per liter), the phosphorus 5.7 mg per 100 ml (1.8 mmol per liter), the uric acid 9.2 mg per 100 ml (0.55 mmol per liter), the conjugated bilirubin 0.9 mg per 100 ml (2 μmol per liter), the total bilirubin 1.3 mg per 100 ml (2.2 μmol per liter), the cholesterol 120 mg per 100 ml (3.1 mmol per liter), the triglyceride 356 mg, and the protein 6.0 g (the albumin 2.6 g and the globulin 3.4 g) per 100 ml. The sodium was 130 mmol, the potassium 3.6 mmol, the chloride 87 mmol, the carbon dioxide 26 mmol, and the osmolality 278 mOsm per liter. The serum aspartate aminotransferase (SGOT) was 32 U, the lactic dehydrogenase (LDH) 291 U, the creatine kinase (CK) 24 U, the amylase 3 U, and the alkaline phosphatase 38 U per liter. An electrocardiogram demonstrated atrial fibrillation at a ventricular rate of 80 and a mean QRS axis of +75°; the T waves were flattened, with slight inversion in Leads V_2 through V_6. X-ray films of the chest (Fig. 1 and 2) revealed slight cardiac enlargement; multiple confluent nodules, 5 to 7 mm, were scattered diffusely throughout both lungs. A specimen of arterial blood, drawn while the patient was breathing oxygen at 2 liters per minute, revealed that the partial pressure of oxygen (PaO_2) was 65 mm Hg, the partial pressure of carbon dioxide ($PaCO_2$) 37 mm Hg, and the pH 7.50. A lumbar puncture yielded clear, colorless cerebrospinal fluid that contained 710 red cells and no white cells per cubic millimeter; the glucose was 64 mg per 100 ml (3.6 mmol per liter), and the protein 18 mg per 100 ml; microscopical examination of specimens of the fluid after Gram and Ziehl–Neelsen stains disclosed no microorganisms. Microscopical examination of a Gram-stained specimen of urine showed a moderate number of neutrophils and mixed bacterial flora.

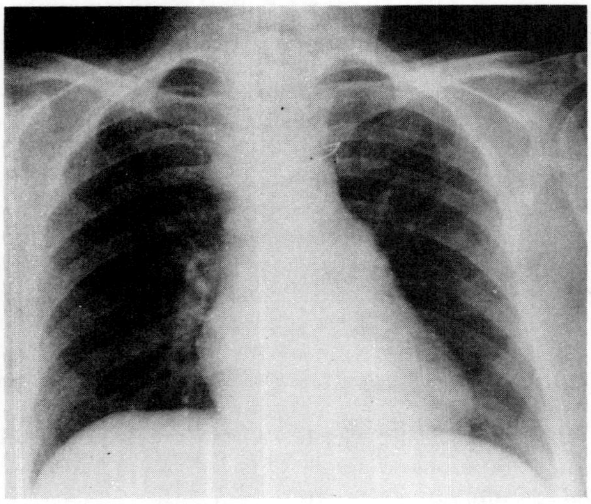

Figure 1. Radiograph of the Chest Taken on Admission, Demonstrating Diffuse Ill-Defined 5-mm to 7-mm Nodular Opacities.

A right paratracheal opacity suggests lymphadenopathy.

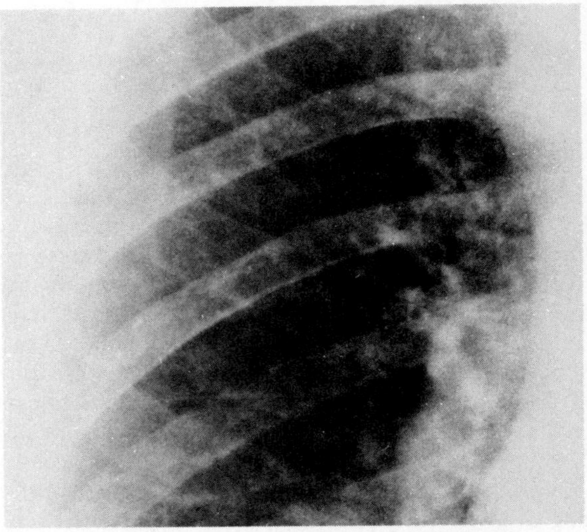

Figure 2. Detailed View of the Right Upper Lobe.

A diagnostic procedure was performed.

Differential Diagnosis

Dr. Barry W. Levine*: May we begin with a review of the x-ray films?

*Assistant physician, Massachusetts General Hospital; assistant clinical professor of medicine, Harvard Medical School.

Dr. David L. Spizarny: An anteroposterior film obtained nine days before admission demonstrates clear lungs. The heart is slightly enlarged, and the main pulmonary artery is prominent. There is a right paratracheal opacity consistent with lymphadenopathy, which was not present on a postoperative film taken 10 months previously. A very slight impression on the trachea above the thoracic inlet is compatible with the known goiter. Films of the chest obtained on the day of admission (Fig. 1 and 2) demonstrate no change in the cardiomediastinal silhouette or in the right paratracheal opacity. Multiple ill-defined nodular opacities, 5 to 7 mm in diameter, are visible throughout the lungs. No pleural effusions are seen. A prosthetic mitral valve and median sternotomy wires are present.

Dr. Levine: Several features of the case record are relevant to the differential diagnosis. The first is the administration of numerous transfusions after the repositioning of the prosthetic mitral valve. Secondly, at some time during the 10 months before the admission under discussion the patient had undergone a gingivectomy, followed by the development of a low-grade fever, an elevated sedimentation rate, increasing weakness, weight loss, and the administration of high-dose steroid therapy. She was also noted to be confused. A history of previous exposure to tuberculosis was obtained. The pertinent findings included multiple negative blood cultures, an echocardiogram showing no vegetations on the heart valves, unilateral hilar lymphadenopathy, and an anterior mediastinal mass. Physical examination revealed oral moniliasis and shotty lymphadenopathy. The laboratory evaluation disclosed a sedimentation rate elevated to a level that in my experience is seen only in association with tuberculosis, tumors, and autoimmune diseases. The x-ray films of the chest taken nine days before transfer to this hospital were reported to show clear lungs, but by the time of admission films of the chest demonstrated a diffuse pattern of confluent nodules 5 to 7 mm in diameter. The tempo of the clinical course was consistent with a smoldering, indolent process that suddenly became rapidly progressive, with the appearance of pulmonary infiltrates. At the time of the detection of the infiltrates the patient was ill enough to prompt an invasive procedure, even before sputum smears for either ordinary bacteria or tubercle bacilli were obtained.

In a 2½-year period 201 examples of the acquired immunodeficiency syndrome (AIDS) were reported in persons who could not be placed in a high-risk group for this disease.[1] Thirty-five of these patients had received transfusions of single-donor blood components within five years of the diagnosis of the syndrome. As in cases of typical disease, these persons were susceptible to the development of various opportunistic infections and malignant tumors. They differed in that 25 percent were 50 years of age or older, and most of them were female. The most frequent opportunistic infection was due to *Pneumocystis carinii*, which was found in 34 percent of the patients. Esophageal moniliasis occurred in six patients, and nontuberculous mycobacterial infection occurred in three patients. The median time between transfusion and the diagnosis was 28 months, with a range of 5 to 65 months. This diagnostic possibility is suggested in this case.

All cases of the acquired immunodeficiency syndrome and tuberculosis reported in Dade County, Florida, between January 1980 and June 1983 have been reviewed.[2] Tuberculosis was diagnosed in 25 of 45 Haitians with the syndrome. The higher prevalence among Haitian patients is probably related to the general increased frequency of tuberculosis in Haiti. In the 28 patients with tuberculosis and the acquired immunodeficiency syndrome the tuberculosis preceded the development of Kaposi's sarcoma or other opportunistic infections by 1 to 17 months. According to the investigators in this study the early emergence of *Mycobacterium tuberculosis* probably reflected the virulence of the organism, which was able to cause disease at an earlier stage of immunosuppression. The frequency of atypical mycobacterial infection was also high — 11.3 percent in Haitian and 8.3 percent in non-Haitian patients with the syndrome. Disease with atypical mycobacteria occurred during a later stage of the immunodeficiency syndrome. In the case under discussion the weight loss, persistent fever, negative blood cultures, and mental confusion suggest a process other than cardiac in origin, perhaps compatible with AIDS. The findings on the x-ray films of the chest are suggestive of a rapidly progressive acinar process, such as a virulent opportunistic infection.

In 1979, 27,699 cases of tuberculosis were reported to the Centers for Disease Control.[3] The distribution of the disease was uneven. In the city of Boston, for example, there were 26.7 cases per 100,000 persons, whereas in the suburb of Newton there were only 5.6 cases per 100,000. Many factors, including age, race, socioeconomic status, and geographic location, seem to account for this heterogeneous distribution. In most circumstances tuberculosis is spread by airborne particles 1 to 5 μm in diameter. On the average 30 percent of close contacts are found to be infected. However, only 5 percent of newly infected persons are unable to limit replication of the tubercle bacilli, and infection progresses to disease within a year or two. Age and sex affect resistance. Morbidity is greater in young women and older persons of both sexes. Diabetes, postgastrectomy states, and therapy with drugs such as steroids or other immunosuppressants also decrease resistance. Among persons in whom the disease does not develop soon after an initial exposure to tuberculosis approximately 5 percent will have the disease later in life if they have a dormant focus of tubercle bacilli. Disease results from regrowth of bacilli within an old infected focus.[4] The most important test for establishing the diagnosis of tuberculosis is the demonstration of acid-fast bacilli in expectorated sputum. However, the sputum smear may be unreliable. Between 22 and 66 percent of patients with tuberculosis have negative smears and positive cultures. In a recent study 26 percent of the patients with proved mycobacterial disease had persistently negative examinations of sputum.[5] To identify tubercle bacilli on microscopical examination of a smear 10^4 organisms must be present. In patients with closed tuberculous lesions it is not unusual for sputum studies to be negative. Examination of sputum is negative in 60 to 80 percent of patients with minimal to moderately advanced noncavitary tuberculosis and in 30 to 40 percent of patients with more advanced disease.[5]

Miliary tuberculosis is the result of hematogenous dissemination of tubercle bacilli caused by the erosion of an active tuberculous process into a blood vessel. Within the lung the blood-borne bacilli cause lesions 0.5 to 2 mm in diameter. Any process that decreases cellular immunity can predispose to the development of miliary tuberculosis — for example, starvation, immunosuppression, and viral illnesses such as measles. The process may be massive and sudden, leading to overwhelming systemic infection.[6] More extensive pulmonary opacifications can result when large quantities of caseous and liquefied material containing tubercle bacilli enter a bronchus from an adjacent infected area. This form of tuberculosis has a much more confluent acinar pattern, with lesions demonstrable on radiologic examination that are similar to those found in the case under discussion, and can be associated with a much more acute course.

M. avium intracellulare belongs in the category of the Runyon Group 3 nonchromogenic mycobacteria. Unlike tuberculosis, *M. avium intracellulare* infection is not transmitted from person to person. There is an increased frequency of this syndrome in victims with the acquired immunodeficiency syndrome (AIDS). Clinical descriptions of infection due to *M. avium intracellulare* began appearing approximately 30 years ago. Patients with this disease were usually older, white, and male, as compared with those with tuberculosis. A large number had underlying chronic lung disease, such as chronic obstructive lung disease, bronchiectasis, previous tuberculosis with scarring, or silicosis.[7] The symptoms of this infection include fever, weight loss, night sweats, and a productive cough. X-ray films of the chest usually show underlying chronic lung disease. The infection progresses slowly, and often a period of observation is necessary to determine its activity. Unlike tuberculosis, the process is indolent and not virulent and therefore would not present in the form of overwhelming sepsis.

Another possible source of infection to be considered in this case is subacute or acute bacterial endocarditis, which develops in approximately 2 percent of patients who receive a prosthetic valve.[8] Dental procedures, especially those associated with gingival bleeding, have long been known to be associated with endocarditis.[9] The patient under discussion, who had a prolonged, indolent course with recurrent fever and malaise, also had undergone such a dental procedure. The laboratory data included an elevated sedimentation rate, anemia, and a leftward shift in the white-cell count, all of which are consistent with bacterial endocarditis. However, all the blood cultures were negative. Since the mid-1950s it has been stated that no more than six blood cultures are needed to establish confirmation of the diagnosis of bacterial endocarditis.[10] In approximately 80 percent of the patients the first blood culture is positive.[11] In only 33 percent of patients with endocarditis is echocardiographic examination useful in demonstrating vegetations on an aortic, mitral, or tricuspid valve.[12] The negative blood cultures and normal echocardiogram prompt me to exclude the diagnosis of endocarditis in this patient.

Up to December 1984, 9608 cases of AIDS were reported in the United States, and increasing numbers are being identified in other Western countries. Its occurrence is no longer confined to the major high-risk groups — Haitians, homosexuals, hemophiliacs, and drug addicts. The investigators at the Centers for Disease Control estimate that up to a million Americans have been exposed to the AIDS virus, and the prevalence of exposure is increasing. In 1982 54 percent of a group of 85 New York male homosexuals had evidence of exposure.[13] In 1983 AIDS could be attributed to transfusions in only 31 cases. However, the latency period of the development of the disease was long, up to five years. As the viral pool increases and three million Americans receive blood transfusions every year there may be a marked increase in the number of cases over the next few years.[14] This patient therefore was at a relatively high risk for the development of AIDS at the time that she received the transfusions. Fortunately, screening for the AIDS virus has become an easy test, and transfusion-related AIDS should no longer be a problem.

The results of recent studies suggest that susceptibility to tuberculosis is related to genetic factors, in particular the presence of HLA-DR3 antigens.[15] Alteration in host-resistance factors through genetic restructuring could make a virulent disease, such as tuberculosis, much more common.

On the basis of this patient's previous exposure to tuberculosis, the history of multiple transfusions, the use of prednisone, and the indolent course marked by fever, weight loss, and mental confusion I conclude that she had post-transfusion AIDS. I believe that this state led to acute tuberculosis as a result of bronchial spread of the bacilli. I also suspect that an examination of lung tissue showed very limited granulomatous inflammation, with a great many organisms because the patient's immunosuppression allowed her to shed numerous tubercle bacilli. A sputum smear for acid-fast bacilli would have been helpful. I suspect that the diagnostic procedure was a closed-lung biopsy.

My final diagnoses are acute tuberculous pneumonia and the acquired immunodeficiency syndrome.

A Physician: Does the possibility of a fungal pneumonia enter into the differential diagnosis?

Dr. Levine: Yes. I was influenced by the exposure to tuberculosis and recent literature that has pointed out an increased frequency of tuberculosis, even preceding other opportunistic infections, in persons with AIDS. However, any virulent opportunistic infection, including fungal diseases, must be considered.

A Physician: Will you comment on your choice of a closed-lung biopsy as opposed to an open biopsy?

Dr. Levine: In a patient with overwhelming sepsis, such as tuberculosis, presenting with a diffuse homogeneous lung process a transbronchial biopsy via the bronchoscope is an appropriate procedure and has a relatively high yield.

A Physician: Would septic pulmonary emboli ever present in this fashion?

Dr. Levine: Septic pulmonary emboli could have this presentation. However, as in cases of subacute bacterial endocarditis or other forms of endocarditis, the blood cultures should be positive, and all the cultures in this case were negative.

A Physician: In patients with AIDS there is usually a combination of infections. Why did you choose the diagnosis of tuberculosis rather than tuberculosis in combination with pneumocystis infection or other combinations of infections?

Dr. Levine: Tuberculosis was my preference in view of the features in the case record. Any number of combined infections could have given a similar pattern on the x-ray films. Dr. Spizarny, is the radiologic pattern specific for any type of infection?

Dr. Spizarny: The radiographic differential diagnosis of ill-defined, 5-mm to 7-mm nodules includes infections such as bronchogenic tuberculosis, viral pneumonias such as varicella pneumonia, and fungal pneumonias as well as neoplasms such as alveolar-cell carcinoma and metastatic carcinoma. This nodular pattern would not be the typical appearance of pneumocystis pneumonia.

A Physician: How do you interpret the presence of the anterior mediastinal mass? Could it have been due to cytomegalovirus infection?

Dr. Levine: I suspect that it was produced by tuberculous lymphadenopathy and that erosion of the lymph-node infection into a bronchus caused the pulmonary infection.

A Physician: Why is it necessary to make a diagnosis of AIDS in this patient? Couldn't the whole illness be explained by tuberculosis exacerbated by prednisone therapy?

Dr. Levine: The patient was given prednisone therapy late in the course because of a diagnosis of polymyalgia rheumatica. She had previously experienced confusion, weight loss, and a low-grade fever.

A Physician: Will you comment on the use of the tuberculin skin test in such a setting?

Dr. Levine: It was not performed in this case. In general, skin tests are very important. There is a reaction called tuberculin shock, in which patients become anergic when they have overwhelming tuberculous infections. Although a skin test might have been helpful in this case, I would not have been surprised if it was negative.

A Physician: How do you explain the appearance of confusion and microhemorrhages in the patient's left eye?

Dr. Levine: The appearance of confusion is compatible with the acquired immunodeficiency syndrome. Patients can have microhemorrhages in the eyes without any underlying disease. We do not have the pathognomonic findings for subacute bacterial endocarditis, such as Roth spots, which are due to septic emboli. I considered the hemorrhages nonspecific.

A Physician: Could the fulminant course of the disease as well as the diffuse nodules throughout the lung fields be consistent with Wegener's or lymphomatoid granulomatosis?

Dr. Levine: The tempo of the illness, with clear lungs on x-ray films of the chest obtained nine days before admission, is much more consistent with an infectious process than with either of those diseases.

Clinical Diagnosis

Pneumonia, ? tuberculous.

Dr. Barry W. Levine's Diagnoses

Acute tuberculous pneumonia.
Acquired immunodeficiency syndrome.

Pathological Discussion

Dr. Eugene J. Mark: Flexible fiberoptic bronchoscopic examination was performed, and three biopsy specimens were obtained (Fig. 3). One specimen consisted of a small pulmonary artery, a second consisted of approximately 20 alveoli with interstitial thickening, and a third consisted of approximately 30 alveoli with alveolar consolidation.

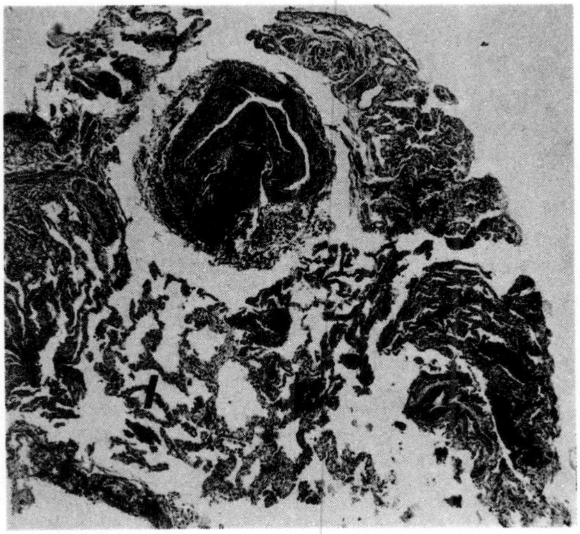

Figure 3. Transbronchial-Lung-Biopsy Specimens, Which Include a Small Pulmonary Artery (A), Lung Tissue with Interstitial Thickening (I), and Tissue with Alveolar Consolidation (C) (×36).

The interstitial fibrosis in one of the biopsy specimens was associated with hemosiderin in alveolar macrophages and in the interalveolar septa (Fig. 4). Among the causes of interstitial fibrosis and hemosiderin deposition in the lung is mitral-valve disease.[16] Other histopathologic changes in the lung in patients with chronic mitral stenosis include medial and intimal hypertrophy of pulmonary arterioles, intimal hyperplasia and adventitial fibrosis of pulmonary veins, interstitial and intraalveolar edema, and distention of lymphatics.[17-20] The presence of fibrosis and hemosiderin may have been the result of the patient's prior mitral-valve disease but is probably an incidental finding because there is no clinical or radiologic evidence of "mitral lung disease."

The alveolar consolidation in one of the specimens was characterized by filling of the alveoli with histiocytes, neutrophils, and fibrin (Fig. 5), indicating infection, but no granulomas were present. The differential diagnosis of a histiocytic pneumonia includes mycobacterial and fungal disease. For this reason an acid-fast stain was performed, and examination revealed numerous long, beaded acid-fast mycobacteria within the exudate (Fig. 6).

Tuberculous pneumonia with extensive air-space inflammation in the absence of granulomas or palisading histiocytes indicates rapidly spreading pulmonary disease related either to a large inoculum of organisms or to poor immunologic response, or both. In this case it is probable that an infected bronchial lymph node ruptured into a bronchus, spilling large numbers of organisms into the airways.

The patient was begun on isoniazid, streptomycin, and rifampin. Clinical improvement was slow. A suspicion of the acquired immunodeficiency syndrome arose. Serum was obtained to test for HTLV-III antibodies, and the result was positive. It was supposed, but never proved, that blood transfusions at the time of the mitral-valve replacement were the source of the HTLV-III virus. The patient gradually felt better, the fever disappeared, the abnormalities shown on the radiographs of the chest improved, and she was discharged home two weeks after the biopsy. Culture of a biopsy specimen grew *M. tuberculosis hominis*. Culture of the spinal fluid obtained at lumbar puncture was negative.

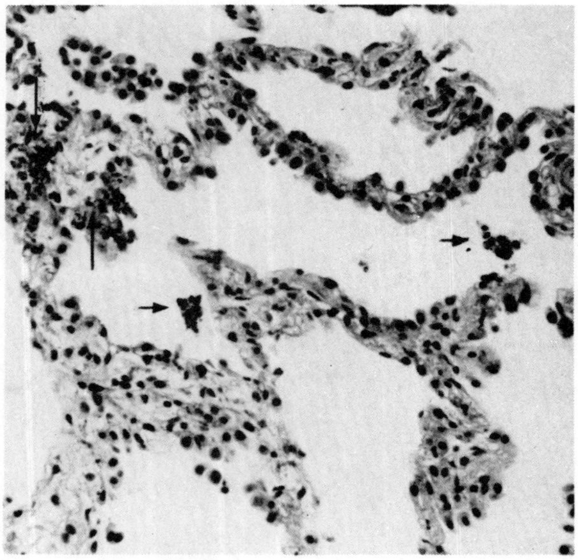

Figure 4. Interstitial Fibrosis and Hemosiderin Deposition in Alveolar Macrophages (Short Arrows) and in the Interstitium (Long Arrows) (×200).

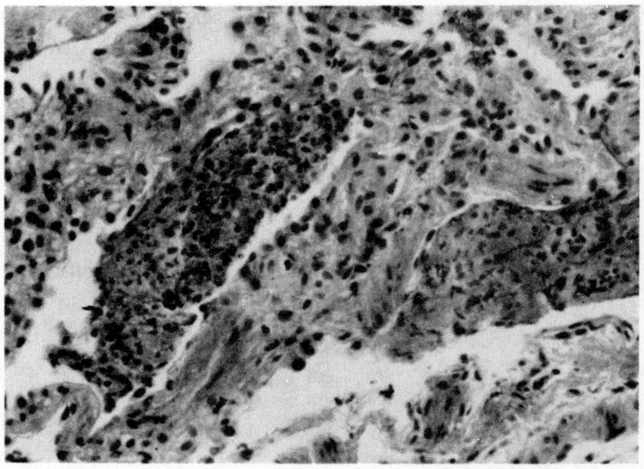

Figure 5. Filling of an Alveolus (Left) and an Alveolar Duct (Right) with Histiocytes and Neutrophils (×200).

We selected this case for discussion when the only diagnosis was tuberculous pneumonia and pulmonary hemosiderosis. The subsequent finding of HTLV-III antibodies has complicated the case. Two months after discharge from this hospital the patient was admitted to her local hospital because of fever with a temperature of 40.6°C and a clinical and radiologic diagnosis of severe congestive heart failure with acute pulmonary edema. The attending physicians were aware that she had HTLV-III antibodies. Bronchial secretions obtained by bronchoscopic examination showed no mycobacteria or pneumocystis. An open-lung biopsy was contemplated, but the patient was believed to be too ill to tolerate it. She was treated empirically with gentamicin, clindamycin, cefotaxime sodium, trimethoprim–sulfamethoxazole, and pentamidine. She continued to receive antituberculous medications and warfarin. After one week she became afebrile and was discharged. After stabilization of her cardiac condition she was started on various antibiotics on the assumption that she had an opportunistic infection.

One week later she became confused and jaundiced, according to her family. Her attending physician asked her to come to his office. On the day of the scheduled appointment she ran out of her house in a confused state, fell on the street, and hit her head. She was brought to the emergency room in a coma. An emergency CT scan of the brain revealed, in addition to two old infarcts, two densities suggestive of recent contusions, one in the right frontal region and one

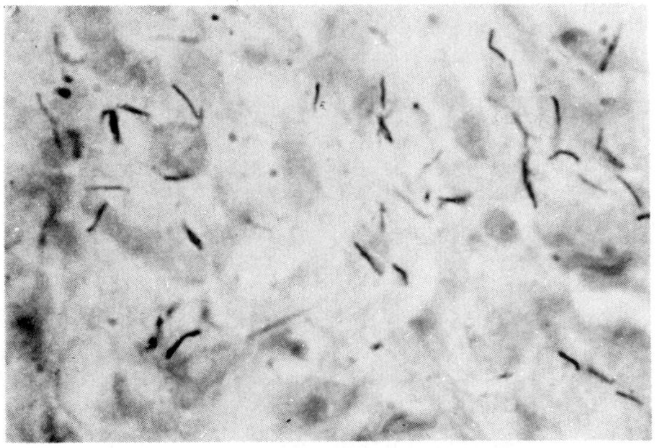

Figure 6. Numerous Mycobacteria (Acid-Fast Stain, ×1250).

lateral to the anterior horn of the right ventricle. She was jaundiced; the serum SGOT was 520 U, the LDH 800 U, the alkaline phosphatase 245 U per liter, and the prothrombin time 46 seconds. A clinical diagnosis of acute hepatitis was made. The patient died a few hours later in the hospital. An autopsy was not done.

Although the patient had antibodies to the HTLV-III virus, this case does not fulfill the criteria for the acquired immunodeficiency syndrome because she was never proved to have an opportunistic infection or a malignant tumor related to this disorder. We can only speculate that an immunosuppressed state may have been responsible for her poor response to treatment for tuberculosis and for the terminal episode of acute, fulminant hepatitis.

A Physician: Since only one of the three biopsy specimens was positive for acid-fast organisms and the diagnosis would have been missed if that specimen had not been obtained, bronchial washings might have been a helpful additional diagnostic procedure.

Dr. Mark: Yes. Prebronchoscopic sputum specimens, bronchoscopic washings, and postbronchoscopic sputum specimens all yield a higher number of positive cultures of *M. tuberculosis* than the corresponding transbronchial biopsy in the same patient.[21,22] A recent study of 179 patients with mycobacterial disease of the lung was concerned with the recovery of organisms by culture of bronchial brushings and bronchial secretions obtained during fiberoptic bronchoscopic examination. Of these patients 48 underwent fiberoptic bronchoscopic study during the course of their illness. Of the 48 patients 25 had positive smears or cultures of expectorated sputum. Twenty-three of the 25 patients had positive cultures of bronchoscopic specimens obtained after examination of three or more expectorated sputum specimens was negative for acid-fast bacilli. In 3 of the 23 patients nodular lesions were demonstrated on the radiographs of the chest, and mycobacterial disease was confirmed by thoracotomy and resection of the nodules. The remaining 20 patients did not undergo thoracotomy. Eleven of these 20 patients had a positive examination of bronchial brushings, only 8 had both a positive examination of sputum and positive bronchial brushings, and 1 had a positive examination of bronchial brushings only. In 19 patients the species of mycobacterium was identified; in 11 it was *M. tuberculosis*, in 2 it was *M. kansasii*, and in 6 it was *M. intracellulare*.[21] Needle-aspiration biopsy has also been used in the diagnosis of pulmonary tuberculosis.[22,23]

A Physician: How often does one miss pneumocystis infection if one does only a bronchoscopic study and not an open-lung biopsy?

Dr. Mark: *P. carinii* can be identified by bronchopulmonary lavage,[24,25] bronchial brushing,[26] bronchoscopic biopsy,[27,28] needle-aspiration biopsy,[29] and open biopsy.[30-33] The accuracy of the diagnosis in patients who are immunosuppressed because of drugs or cancer, with the use of a positive autopsy finding as the criterion for the diagnosis, increases directly with the volume of tissue available for examination. In one study, in which 17 consecutive patients who were immunosuppressed had synchronous percutaneous aspiration-needle biopsy, cutting-needle biopsy, transbronchial biopsy, and open biopsy of the lung, the yield of specific diagnoses from these techniques was 12, 24, 29,and 59 percent, respectively.[34] Our experience has been similar. Most patients at this hospital have either a transbronchial biopsy or an open-lung biopsy.

The frequency of identification of pneumocystis in patients with AIDS is higher than in patients immunosuppressed because of drugs or cancer, probably because the number of organisms is greater in patients with AIDS. In a study of 60 transbronchial-lung biopsies and 1 open-lung biopsy in 40 homosexual male patients with AIDS the frequency of a positive diagnosis of pneumocystis infection on biopsy, bronchoalveolar lavage, and bronchial brushing was remarkably similar. The bronchial-lung biopsy was positive for pneumocystis in 66 percent of the cases, the bronchoalveolar-lavage specimen was positive in 69 percent, and the bronchial-brushing specimen was positive in 64 percent.[25] There was an 84 percent correlation between the findings on transbronchial brushing and those on biopsy. The correlation of positive brushings and biopsy was highest in specimens obtained before treatment, in which the organisms were most abundant. Bronchoscopic brushing and bronchoalveolar lavage increased the frequency of positive diagnoses over that of biopsy alone in patients after treatment, when organisms were less abundant.[25]

Dr. Charles R. Felton: It is worth emphasizing that although the frequency of bacteremia associated with bronchoscopic examination is relatively low and the need for antimicrobial prophylaxis with bronchoscopic study has not been established,[35] the American Heart Association has suggested that antimicrobial prophylaxis be used when bronchoscopic examination is performed on patients with valvular heart disease,[36] and this suggestion has been supported by others.[37]

A Physician: Were T-lymphocyte subsets determined on admission in this case?

Dr. Mark: The ratio of OKT4 to OKT8 lymphocytes was 0.38, which is a reversal of the normal ratio. This finding is consistent with AIDS but not diagnostic. Reversal of the normal ratio of helper lymphocytes to suppressor lymphocytes is seen in other diseases, particularly in infections with Epstein–Barr virus, herpesvirus, and cytomegalovirus.[38]

Anatomical Diagnoses

Tuberculous pneumonia.

HTLV-III antibody positivity.

References

1. Chamberland ME, Castro KG, Haverkos HW, et al. Acquired immunodeficiency syndrome in the United States: an analysis of cases outside high-incidence groups. Ann Intern Med 1984; 101:617-23.
2. Pitchenik AE, Cole C, Russell BW, et al. Tuberculosis, atypical mycobacteriosis, and the acquired immunodeficiency syndrome among Haitian and non-Haitian patients in south Florida. Ann Intern Med 1984; 101:641-5.
3. Glassroth J, Robins AG, Snider DE Jr. Tuberculosis in the 1980's. N Engl J Med 1980; 302:1441-50.
4. Stead WW. Pathogenesis of a first episode of chronic pulmonary tuberculosis in man: recrudescence of residuals of the primary infection or exogenous reinfection? Am Rev Respir Dis 1967; 95:729-45.
5. Kim TC, Blackman RS, Heatwole KM, Kim T, Rochester DF. Acid-fast bacilli in sputum smears of patients with pulmonary tuberculosis: prevalence and significance of negative smears pretreatment and positive smears post-treatment. Am Rev Respir Dis 1984; 129:264-8.
6. Reichman L, ed. International conference on tuberculosis. Chest 1979; 76: Suppl:737-817.
7. Yeager H Jr, Raleigh JW. Pulmonary disease due to *Mycobacterium intracellulare*. Am Rev Respir Dis 1973; 108:547-52.
8. Watanakunakorn C. Infective endocarditis as a result of medical progress. Am J Med 1978; 64:917-9.
9. Drapkin MS. Endocarditis after use of an oral irrigation device. Ann Intern Med 1977; 87:455.
10. Belli J, Waisbren BA. The number of blood cultures necessary to diagnose most cases of bacterial endocarditis. Am J Med Sci 1956; 232:284-8.
11. Walker SR, Shumway NE, Merigan TC. Management of infected cardiac valve prostheses. JAMA 1969; 208:531-3.
12. Wann LS, Dillon JC, Weyman AE, Feigenbaum H. Echocardiography in bacterial endocarditis. N Engl J Med 1976; 295:135-9.
13. Clark M, Cappola V. AIDS: a growing 'pandemic'? Newsweek. April 29, 1985:71.
14. Curran JW, Barker LF. The acquired immunodeficiency syndrome associated with transfusion: the evolving perspective. Ann Intern Med 1984; 100:298-300.
15. van Eden W, De Vries RRP, Stanford JL, Rook GAW. HLA-DR3 associated genetic control of responses to multiple skin tests with new tuberculins. Clin Exp Immunol 1983; 52:287-92.
16. Goyette EM, Farinacci CJ, Forsee JH, Blake HA. The clinicopathologic correlation of lung biopsies in mitral stenosis. Am Heart J 1954; 47:645-52.
17. Heath D, Whitaker W. The pulmonary vessels in mitral stenosis. J Pathol Bacteriol 1955; 70:291-8.
18. Goodale F Jr, Sanchez G, Friedlich AL, Scannell JG, Myers GS. Correlation of pulmonary arteriolar resistance with pulmonary vascular changes in patients with mitral stenosis before and after valvulotomy. N Engl J Med 1955; 252:979-83.
19. Heath D, Hicken P. The relation between left atrial hypertension and lymphatic distension in lung biopsies. Thorax 1960;15:54-8.
20. Vogt T, Fauser A, Schlosser V, Mittermayer C. Patho-histologische befunde an probeexcisionen der lunge bei patienten nach mitralkommisurotomie und morphometrische untersuchungen des oberen und unteren lungenlappens. Bull Soc Int Chir 1975; 34:145-51.
21. Funahashi A, Lohaus GH, Politis J, Hranicka LJ. Role of fiberoptic bronchoscopy in the diagnosis of mycobacterial diseases. Thorax 1983; 38:267-70.
22. Robicheaux G, Moinuddin SM, Lee LH. The role of aspiration biopsy cytology in the diagnosis of pulmonary tuberculosis. Am J Clin Pathol 1985; 83:719-22.
23. Dahlgren SE, Ekström P. Aspiration cytology in the diagnosis of pulmonary tuberculosis. Scand J Respir Dis 1972; 53:196-201.
24. Drew WL, Finley RN, Mintz L, Klein HZ. Diagnosis of *Pneumocystis carinii* pneumonia by bronchopulmonary lavage. JAMA 1974; 230: 713-5.
25. Hartman B, Koss M, Hui A, Baumann W, Athos L, Boylen T. *Pneumocystis carinii* pneumonia in the acquired immunodeficiency syndrome (AIDS): diagnosis with bronchial brushings, biopsy, and bronchoalveolar lavage. Chest 1985; 87:603-7.
26. Repsher LH, Schröter G, Hammond WS. Diagnosis of *Pneumocystis carinii* pneumonitis by means of endobronchial brush biopsy. N Engl J Med 1972; 287:340-2.
27. Jaffe JP, Maki DG. Lung biopsy in immunocompromised patients: one institution's experience and an approach to management of pulmonary disease in the compromised host. Cancer 1981; 48:1144-53.
28. Puksa S, Hutcheon MA, Hyland RH. Usefulness of transbronchial biopsy in immunosuppressed patients with pulmonary infiltrates. Thorax 1983; 38: 146-50.
29. Gibney RTN, Man GCW, King EG, leRiche J. Aspiration biopsy in the diagnosis of pulmonary disease. Chest 1981; 80:300-3.
30. Singer C, Armstrong D, Rosen PP, Walzer PD, Yu B. Diffuse pulmonary infiltrates in immunosuppressed patients: prospective study of 80 cases. Am J Med 1979; 66:110-20.
31. Canham EM, Kennedy TC, Merrick TA. Unexplained pulmonary infiltrates in the compromised patient: an invasive investigation in a consecutive series. Cancer 1983; 52:325-9.
32. Haverkos HW, Dowling JN, Pasculle AW, Myerowitz RL, Lerberg DB, Hakala TR. Diagnosis of pneumonitis in immunocompromised patients by open lung biopsy. Cancer 1983; 52:1093-7.
33. McKenna RJ Jr, Mountain CF, McMurtrey MJ. Open lung biopsy in immunocompromised patients. Chest 1984; 86:671-4.
34. Burt ME, Flye MW, Webber BL, Wesley RA. Prospective evaluation of aspiration needle, cutting needle, transbronchial, and open lung biopsy in patients with pulmonary infiltrates. Ann Thorac Surg 1981; 32:146-53.
35. Durack DT. Prophylaxis of infective endocarditis. In: Mandell GL, Douglas RG, Bennett JE, eds. Principles and practice of infectious diseases. 2nd ed. New York: John Wiley, 1984:539-44.
36. Kaplan EL, Anthony BF, Bisno A, et al. Prevention of bacterial endocarditis. Circulation 1977; 56:139A-43A.
37. Keys TF. Antimicrobial prophylaxis for patients with congenital or valvular heart disease. Mayo Clin Proc 1982; 57:171-5.
38. Carney WP, Rubin RH, Hoffman RA, Hansen WP, Healey K, Hirsch MS. Analysis of T lymphocyte subsets in cytomegalovirus mononucleosis. J Immunol 1981; 126:2114-6.

CASE RECORD OF THE MASSACHUSETTS GENERAL HOSPITAL

CASE 9-1986

Presentation of Case

A 40-month-old girl was admitted to the hospital because of respiratory distress.

The child was born of a full-term normal delivery, one year after her mother's tuberculin test had converted to a positive reaction, without known contact with tuberculosis, and isoniazid was administered to the mother. At the age of 12 months the child was well and thriving, with a weight of 10.4 kg (75th percentile). She was taken by her parents to visit Haiti for one month. The child experienced diarrhea and conjunctivitis during the trip but had no major illness. At 13 months a hypochromic, microcytic anemia was found; the hemoglobin was 9.1 g per 100 ml, and the reticulocyte count was 2.4 percent; the serum iron, iron-binding capacity, and a hemoglobin electrophoresis were normal. Iron was administered by mouth, without improvement. At the age of 20 months she was treated for pneumonia with erythromycin and sulfisoxazole and appeared to improve. Several weeks later a tuberculin skin test was negative. At about the same time her mother noticed that the child had progressive cervical lymphadenopathy and was weaker and more clumsy than others of her age. She had several bouts of nocturnal fever and sweats and repeated episodes of otitis media. At the age of 24 months oral thrush appeared and was treated with nystatin. During the next few weeks the lymphadenopathy became generalized. A productive cough developed, her nocturnal temperature rose to 39.4°C, and the left upper eyelid became swollen. She was admitted to the hospital.

The child was black. Her mother was born in Haiti and later immigrated to the United States; her father was a native of this country. Her maternal grandmother died of carcinoma of an unknown primary site. The child had received no transfusions. There were no cats at home, and there was no family history of sickle-cell or other anemia, leukemia, lymphoma, or acquired immunodeficiency syndrome (AIDS). No household contacts had recognized AIDS, lymphadenopathy, homosexual activities, or history of drug abuse. There was no family history of autoimmune or endocrine disease.

The temperature was 37.6°C, the height 84 cm (25th percentile), and the weight 10.8 kg (25th percentile). The child appeared chronically ill. Cervical lymph nodes, 1 to 2 cm, were palpable, and smaller nodes were felt in the occipital, postauricular, axillary, and inguinal regions. White patches were seen on the oral mucous membrane. The lungs and heart were normal. The liver descended 6 cm below the right costal margin, with a span of 11 cm; the spleen was felt 4 cm below the left costal margin. Neurologic examination was negative.

The urine gave a ++ test for protein; the sediment contained 10 white cells per high-power field. The hematocrit was 27.2 percent; the white-cell count was 19,600, with 13 percent neutrophils, 78 percent lymphocytes, 3 percent atypical lymphocytes, and 6 percent monocytes. The platelet count was 355,000, and the reticulocyte count 2 percent. The erythrocyte sedimentation rate was 135 mm per hour. The ferritin was 49 ng per milliliter. The iron was 34 μg per 100 ml (6.1 μmol per liter), the iron-binding capacity 315 μg per 100 ml (56.4 μmol per liter), the uric acid 4.3 mg per 100 ml (0.26 mmol per liter), and the protein 11.4 g per 100 ml. Serum electrophoresis revealed that the albumin was 28 percent, the $alpha_1$ globulin 2 percent, the $alpha_2$ globulin 9 percent, the beta globulin 6 percent, and the gamma globulin 55 percent. The serum aspartate aminotransferase (SGOT) was 76 U, the lactic dehydrogenase (LDH) 279 U, and the alkaline phosphatase 27 U per liter. X-ray films of the chest (Fig. 1) showed homogeneous involvement of both lungs by miliary nodules, 1 to 2 mm, with a suggestion of hilar lymphadenopathy; no pleural effusion was noted; the cardiomediastinal silhouette was normal. Films of the paranasal sinuses were normal. Ultrasonographic examination of the upper portion of the abdomen disclosed enlargement of the liver and spleen; both kidneys appeared normal; the gallbladder was not seen, and there was no evidence of ascites. A

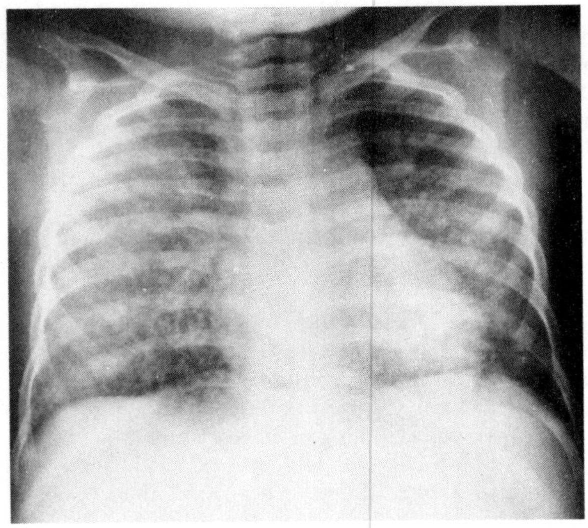

Figure 1. Radiograph of the Chest Obtained When the Patient Was 24 Months Old, Demonstrating a Diffuse Miliary Nodular Interstitial Infiltrate with Slightly Enlarged Hilar Lymph Nodes.

culture of the oral lesions yielded *Candida albicans.* A serologic test for cytomegalovirus antibody was positive; tests for hepatitis B surface antigen and antibody, a serologic test for syphilis, a heterophil antibody test, and a test for toxoplasma antibody were negative. The IgG was 6970 mg (normal for the patient's age, 492 to 1224), the IgA 300 mg (normal, 23 to 124), and the IgM 466 mg per 100 ml (normal, 49 to 190). The C3 was 138 mg (normal, 83 to 177), the C4 13 mg (normal, 15 to 45), and the Factor B 44 mg per 100 ml (normal, 17 to 42). Skin tests with tuberculin, mumps, and candida antigens were negative. A test for T-cell subsets in the peripheral blood showed that the ratio of OKT4 to OKT8 reactive cells was 1:6 instead of the usual ratio of approximately 2:1. Microscopical examination of a biopsy specimen of a supraclavicular lymph node showed atypical follicular and diffuse hyperplasia believed most suggestive of viral lymphadenitis. Microscopical examination of an aspirated specimen of bone marrow was negative except for an increase in mature lymphocytes and mature plasma cells. Microscopical examination of an open-biopsy specimen of the lung disclosed polymorphous hyperplasia of the bronchial and pleural lymphoid tissue. There were atypical small lymphocytes and plasma cells similar to those seen in the interfollicular region of the previous lymph-node-biopsy specimen, but no germinal centers were observed. No viral inclusions were seen, and microscopical examination of specimens stained for acid-fast bacilli, *Pneumocystis carinii*, and other microorganisms was negative. Cultures of the pulmonary-biopsy specimen, urine, and a buccal swab yielded cytomegalovirus (CMV); a culture of the buffy coat for CMV was negative. A test on the peripheral blood for human T-cell lymphotropic virus Type III (HTLV-III) antibody was positive. A test on the child's mother for HTLV-III antibody was positive, and a test on her father was negative; both parents gave negative tests for cytomegalovirus antibody. Microscopical examination of stained smears of sputum, bone marrow, and lymph node was negative for acid-fast bacilli, and cultures of these specimens and of gastric aspirates yielded no tubercle bacilli. The child was given a course of human interferon-alpha, without improvement in the lymphadenopathy or in the changes shown on x-ray films of the chest. Her course was complicated by left otitis media. She was discharged home on the 79th hospital day with a queried diagnosis of AIDS.

Three months later the child was returned to the hospital because of respiratory distress and a temperature of 40°C. X-ray films of the chest disclosed worsening of the diffuse bilateral pulmonary nodules in the interval; evidence of hepatosplenomegaly was noted. A blood culture yielded *Streptococcus pneumoniae*, and penicillin was given, with rapid defervescence. The child was discharged on the ninth hospital day. At the age of 32 months she was readmitted because of progressive dyspnea and cyanosis, and evidence of a respiratory-syncytial-virus infection was found. X-ray films of the chest were unchanged. The patient improved on supportive treatment and was discharged on the 20th hospital day on trimethoprim–sulfamethoxazole. Thirty-four days later she was readmitted because of fever, and pneumococcal bacteremia was again found and treated with penicillin. She complained of abdominal pain. An upper gastrointestinal series revealed irregularity of the midportion of the esophagus and thickening of the gastric, duodenal, and small-intestine folds, with flocculation of barium. An ultrasonographic examination of the abdomen disclosed bilateral renal enlargement, with increased echogenicity of the renal cortexes in comparison with the liver. The child was discharged on penicillin on the 15th hospital day. Twenty-four days later she was returned to the hospital because of rise of the temperature to 38.7°C and an extensive vesicular eruption of the tongue. A diagnosis of herpetic stomatitis was made, and acyclovir was administered by vein, with improvement. The patient's mother required treatment for active pulmonary tuberculosis; the patient received a brief course of isoniazid and rifampin; culture was negative, and she was continued on isoniazid. She was discharged on the 12th hospital day.

At the age of 39 months the child was again admitted to the hospital because of severe anorexia, fever, and increasing dyspnea. X-ray films of the chest revealed diffuse miliary infiltrates and confluent bibasilar densities; the thoracic spine appeared normal. A feeding gastrostomy was performed. During her convalescence a blood culture yielded *C. albicans.* Amphotericin was begun, and she was discharged home on the 31st hospital day, to receive amphotericin on an outpatient basis, along with isoniazid and pyridoxine. Seven days later, during a visit to the hospital to receive amphotericin, examination disclosed that the temperature was 37.7°C, the pulse was 140, and the respirations were 56. The blood pressure was 105/60 mm Hg. Diffuse rales were heard throughout both lungs. X-ray films of the chest showed that the bibasilar infiltrates were more extensive (Fig. 2). Trimethoprim–sulfamethoxazole was again prescribed. Her sister, one year of age, was reported to be febrile, with poor oral intake and weight loss. Two days later the child returned to the hospital and received another injection of amphotericin. Increased respiratory distress was noted, and she was readmitted.

The temperature was 37.7°C, the pulse was 140, and the respirations were 56. The blood pressure was 80/50 mm Hg.

On examination the child was a dyspneic, cachectic girl with small extremities. The left tympanic membrane was perforated, with exudation of white, purulent material; the right tympanic membrane appeared scarred and dull. Prominent cervical, axillary, and inguinal lymphadenopathy was found. White lesions were observed over the tongue and oral mucosa. The lungs were clear, although flaring and intercostal retraction were noted. The heart was normal. The abdomen was distended, with diminished bowel sounds;

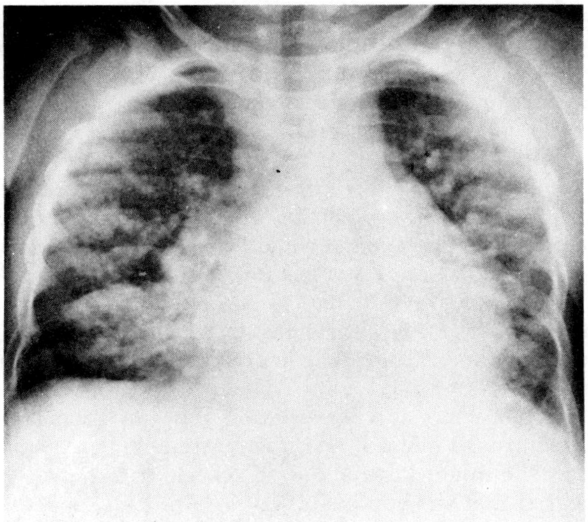

Figure 2. Radiograph of the Chest Taken at 40 Months of Age, Showing Extension of the Miliary Nodular Interstitial Infiltrates and Confluent Bibasilar Infiltrates with Air Bronchograms.

the edge of the liver was palpated 6 cm below the right costal margin, and the spleen was felt 4 cm below the left costal margin. Diffuse tenderness was noted over the spine. There was ++ digital clubbing. Neurologic examination was negative except for diffuse weakness of all extremities; the tendon reflexes were + and equal, and the plantar responses were flexor.

The urine gave a ++ test for protein; the sediment contained 10 white cells and 2 red cells per high-power field. The hematocrit was 19.8 percent; the white-cell count was 12,000, with 40 percent neutrophils, 2 percent band forms, 40 percent lymphocytes, and 18 percent monocytes. The platelet count was 316,000, and the erythrocyte sedimentation rate was more than 145 mm per hour. The urea nitrogen was 10 mg per 100 ml (4 mmol per liter), the glucose 96 mg per 100 ml (5.3 mmol per liter), and the calcium 8.3 mg per 100 ml (2.1 mmol per liter). The sodium was 130 mmol, the potassium 2.8 mmol, and the carbon dioxide 22 mmol per liter. X-ray films of the chest were little changed. A film of the abdomen revealed a gastrostomy tube; there was an intravenous line in the vicinity of the midportion of the inferior vena cava; the liver and spleen appeared enlarged, and confluent consolidations were observed in both lung bases, with a diffuse miliary infiltrate; there was destruction of the right side of the 11th thoracic vertebral body and its pedicle. Films of the thoracic spine confirmed the presence of destruction of the right side of the 11th dorsal vertebra and pedicle, with a lateral compression fracture of the vertebral body; the adjacent vertebral bodies and ribs appeared intact.

Isoniazid, pyridoxine, and trimethoprim–sulfamethoxazole were continued, and the patient was given intravenously administered fluids and sodium chloride. Periodic injections of amphotericin were administered. The child's tachypnea diminished, but she complained of abdominal and back pain, with relief after paregoric. Blood clots were observed in her stools. She vomited intermittently and passed diarrheal stools that gave positive tests for occult blood. Fever was present on most days. A test for *Clostridium difficile* toxin was positive in a titer of 1:6250. Repeated blood cultures were negative. Vancomycin was administered by mouth, and other oral intake was restricted; hyperalimentation was begun. The child complained of frequent anterior chest pains, which were relieved by sitting forward. An electrocardiogram showed sinus tachycardia at a rate of 127, with a mean QRS axis of +150°. An echocardiogram revealed dilatation of the pulmonary artery and the right-ventricular-outflow tract and a small pericardial effusion; no other abnormality was detected. Additional x-ray films of the chest disclosed improvement in the diffuse nodular pulmonary infiltrate; there was a suggestion of periosteal reaction along several ribs. The child began to complain of pain in both legs and was observed to grasp her leg with her hand and to move it in response to painful stimuli. A neurologic consultant found that the cranial nerves were normal. The upper extremities were normal except for a slight decrease in motor power consistent with her cachexia. The lower extremities were functionless; the knee jerks were absent, and the ankle reflexes were ++++ bilaterally, with sustained clonus. On repeated examination one hour later the ankle jerks were absent, and clonus could not be elicited. There were bilateral Babinski signs. A lumbar myelographic examination showed complete block of flow of contrast material at the superior aspect of the 12th dorsal vertebra; the destructive process that involved the right side of the 11th thoracic vertebra was again noted (Fig. 3).

A diagnostic procedure was performed.

Differential Diagnosis

Dr. Sarah H. Cheeseman*: In summary, this child enjoyed good health for her first year of life, but then a chronic illness developed, characterized by a failure to thrive, generalized lymphadenopathy, hepatosplenomegaly, reticulonodular pulmonary infiltrates, and multiple intercurrent infections. Finally, at three years and four months of age, she was admitted to the hospital with new bilateral lower-lobe consolidation, distention of the abdomen, and a destructive process in a lower thoracic vertebra and its pedicle. In the course of this hospital admission pericarditis and a spinal-cord compression syndrome developed. This unfortunate series of events followed a visit to Haiti, her mother's country of origin, and occurred in the setting of the development of active tuberculosis in the mother despite isoniazid prophylaxis at the time of her tuberculin conversion. In addition, we are given serologic data indicating that both the mother and the child had been infected with HTLV-III.

*Associate professor of medicine, pediatrics, and molecular genetics and microbiology, University of Massachusetts Medical School, Worcester, Massachusetts.

Dr. Herman, may we review the x-ray films now?

Dr. Thomas E. Herman: The first radiograph of the chest, obtained when the child was 24 months of age, demonstrates a diffuse miliary interstitial pattern with nodules about 1 mm in diameter throughout the lungs (Fig. 1). A radiograph of the chest taken at 40 months of age (Fig. 2) shows more extensive infiltrates, which are confluent at the bases with air bronchograms. The final film (Fig. 3), obtained with the patient's head down after placement of Pantopaque in the lumbar subarachnoid space, demonstrates complete block at the T12 level. The T11 vertebral body and right-sided pedicle are partially destroyed.

Dr. Cheeseman: I shall divide my discussion of this child's illness into three phases — the time up to and including the first hospital admission, the next five admissions, and the final admission described in the case record.

The features that evolved between her return from Haiti and the first admission were an anemia not responsive to iron, pneumonia, several episodes of otitis media, cervical lymphadenopathy, and thrush. At this point her pediatrician had to try to distinguish between multiple unrelated episodes and underlying disease or immunodeficiency. The pneumonia, which responded to erythromycin and sulfisoxazole, and repeated episodes of otitis media could well have occurred in any child. Oral thrush is hardly surprising after what must have been nearly continuous antibiotic therapy for four months, and the cervical lymphadenopathy might have reflected only her frequent otitis. The anemia could have been the result of frequent infections. By the time of admission to the hospital, however, she had gained only 0.4 kg, or 1 lb, in a little over a year, suggesting a chronic systemic disease or an immunodeficiency syndrome, congenital or acquired.

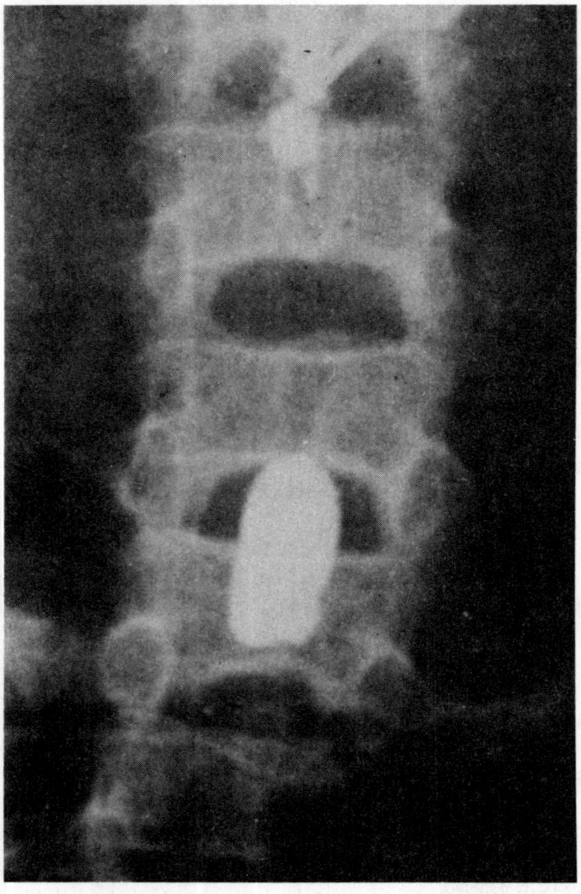

Figure 3. Pantopaque Myelogram, Taken with the Patient's Head Down, Revealing Destruction of the Right Side of the T11 Vertebral Body and Pedicle.

Complete block to the flow of Pantopaque is evident at the superior end plate of the T12 vertebral body.

The patient's illness apparently began soon after her return from Haiti, and it is reasonable to consider what she might have acquired on her trip there. We are told that she had conjunctivitis and can speculate that it may have been the hemorrhagic form associated with enterovirus 70, which is currently widespread in the Caribbean,[1] but that possibility has no relevance to anything that followed. Malnutrition, malaria, tuberculosis, and infantile diarrhea are major public health problems in Haiti.[2,3] Of these possibilities, it is unlikely that malnutrition developed while she was traveling, and she should certainly have recovered on her return. The diarrhea seems to have been transient and would not explain her persistent problems. She could have contracted malaria as a cause of the anemia, recurrent fever, and hepatosplenomegaly, but it would not account for the lymphadenopathy or pulmonary infiltrates. She might have been exposed to active tuberculosis while visiting Haiti or, in fact, here in the United States, since her mother's tuberculin reaction had converted, meaning that she had acquired primary tuberculosis shortly before the child's conception. Even though the mother received prophylactic therapy, presumably preventing active and infective disease, the conversion indicates infectious tuberculous contacts who may still have been in the child's environment.

Tuberculosis could explain nearly every feature of this patient's illness to date. The pneumonia could have been a presentation of primary pulmonary tuberculosis, the symptoms of which may clear in several weeks, although the radiologic abnormalities persist much longer.[4] Recurrent otitis may also be tuberculous. The weakness and clumsiness might have represented the typical fatigue of the tuberculous child, and the cutaneous delayed hypersensitivity develops late on rare occasions. Even unilateral eyelid edema has been described in patients with tuberculosis, but in association with a primary lesion of the conjunctiva and an enlarged preauricular node. I think that the interval in this case was too long after the travel to link the illness to the conjunctivitis in Haiti, and Lincoln and Sewell[4] tell us that primary tuberculosis of the skin and mucous membranes is rarely associated with hematogenous dissemination. We would have to invoke hematogenous spread to explain the generalized superficial lymphadenopathy, hepatosplenomegaly, urine-sediment abnormality, and reticulonodular pulmonary infiltrates by tuberculosis. In fact, the picture is strongly suggestive of acute miliary tuberculosis and a vigorous work-up aimed at this possibility was undertaken, but the results did not support a diagnosis of tuberculosis.

Instead, the studies raised the question of the acquired immunodeficiency syndrome (AIDS). The patient was anergic, with inversion of the usual helper–suppressor ratio of T lymphocytes and strikingly elevated levels of IgG, IgA, and IgM. The lymph-node biopsy showed follicular hyperplasia, the usual finding in the lymphadenopathy syndrome in homosexual men,[5-7] which is often a precursor of AIDS and, like AIDS, is associated with the presence of antibody to HTLV-III. I shall not dwell on the issue of whether being Haitian is a risk factor for AIDS, since this child and her mother had antibody to HTLV-III and must be considered infected, whether by virtue of the mother's coming from Haiti or other aspects of her life experience. It is probable that the child did acquire the virus from her mother, probably transplacentally,[8] although in one case transmission has been attributed to breast milk.[9]

On the assumption that the child had HTLV-III infection, can I say that she had AIDS? The case definition used by the Centers for Disease Control for surveillance is the occurrence of disease at least moderately predictive of underlying cellular immune deficiency in the absence of prior disease or therapy known to be associated with defective cellular immunity.[10] In children infections that may be congenital and not indicative of immunodeficiency (specifically, toxoplasmosis and herpes simplex infection in the first month of life and cytomegalovirus infection in the first six months) must be excluded, as must primary immunodeficiency states.[11] This patient's healthy first year and higher than normal immunoglobulin levels exclude many of the congenital immunodeficiencies, including severe combined immunodeficiency and DiGeorge's syndromes. The Wiskott–Aldrich syndrome is unusual in girls, being X-linked, and this patient did not have the eczema and thrombocytopenia that characterize this disease. We must think twice about ataxia telangiectasia, since conjunctival telangiectases may be mistaken initially for conjunctivitis and her weakness and clumsiness could have been evidence of ataxia, but I shall assume that the absence of these findings on repeated physical examination is genuine and therefore dismiss this possibility. A review of her diagnoses to date in the light of the list of infections accepted by the Centers for Disease Control as criteria for AIDS shows that oral candidiasis does not qualify; only candidal esophagitis does. Cytomegalovirus must be demonstrated by histopathological examination, not merely culture, because Craighead[12] obtained positive lung cultures in 8 of 69 unselected autopsies on patients who died on a medical–surgical ward. This virus may be either a commensal or a pathogen in the same location.

Despite this failure to fit within the surveillance definition there is much to suggest that the child did have AIDS. At the recent AIDS Conference in Atlanta, Georgia, Dr. James M. Oleske stated that non-iron-deficiency anemia and elevated immunoglobulin levels strongly suggest the presence of AIDS rather than primary immunodeficiency,[13] and Dr. Arthur J. Ammann presented data to show that HTLV-III antibodies were also a valid discriminator, not being present in any of 61 children who met the World Health Organization diagnostic criteria for the diagnosis of the primary immunodeficiency diseases.[14] The purpose of the surveillance definition is not diagnosis in an individual patient but virtual certainty that all the patients being included in the study of a new entity have the disease, and thus very stringent criteria are chosen.

On the other hand, our clinical appreciation of the spectrum of AIDS is growing. In children with AIDS a prominent feature has been lymphoid interstitial pneumonitis, an otherwise rare disease predominantly affecting middle-aged women, often in association with Sjögren's syndrome and dysgammaglobulinemia.[15] The presence of a reticulonodular pattern on radiographs of the chest is even said to be pathognomonic by radiologists at a center experienced in pediatric AIDS, eliminating the need for a lung biopsy.[16] Histologic examination reveals that small lymphocytes and plasma cells infiltrate the pulmonary interstitium and sometimes the visceral pleura. Involvement of the hilar or mediastinal lymph nodes or parietal pleura, as well as cellular atypia, signals lymphomatous transformation. The pulmonary architecture is not destroyed, but the patients have a restrictive defect and impaired carbon monoxide diffusing capacity. The clinical manifestations are cough and dyspnea, with or without fever. The patients have usually been treated with steroids, although with uncertain justification and no controlled trials. Some of the patients improve remarkably even after years of symptoms; others, especially those over 50 years of age, may die from pulmonary complications or malignant lymphoma.[15,17] The groups from Miami and New Jersey who have seen large numbers of cases of childhood AIDS think that lymphoid interstitial pneumonitis should be considered part of the disease,[18,19] and there is a similar suggestion with regard to adults, particularly Haitians.[20]* I believe that lymphoid interstitial pneumonitis was the pulmonary lesion described in this child. I would ascribe the protein and cells in the urine to the glomerulopathy also reported in association with AIDS in both children[21] and adults.[22]

The events of the five subsequent admissions conform to the diagnostic impression and pattern of childhood AIDS. There were two episodes of *Streptococcus*

*The CDC diagnostic criteria for pediatric AIDS were revised after this discussion was presented and now include histologically verified lymphoid interstitial pneumonitis in a child under 13 years of age with antibody to HTLV-III. (MMWR 1985; 34:373-5.)

pneumoniae bacteremia; a review of AIDS in children recorded pneumococcal bacteremia in 38 percent of the patients.[23] A bout of respiratory-syncytial-virus infection required admission to the hospital at the age of two years and eight months, and the patient was discharged on trimethoprim–sulfamethoxazole, presumably either as empiric therapy or prophylaxis against *Pneumocystis carinii* infection. Herpetic stomatitis occurred, probably representing the child's primary infection. Since it was treated with acyclovir we do not know whether it would have lasted the month required of mucocutaneous herpes simplex infections to become a criterion for AIDS. An additional pulmonary process characterized by bibasilar consolidation developed, but I suspect that the isoniazid and pyridoxine were instituted as prophylaxis when the mother's tuberculosis became active. If the intent had been therapeutic two antituberculous drugs would have been used. Candidemia occurred and in this setting apparently was not even thought worthy of detailed description.

The final admission outlined in the case record was precipitated by respiratory distress, which seemed to improve without the addition of new therapeutic agents. However, the patient then had clubbing, right-axis deviation demonstrable on the electrocardiogram, and dilatation of the right-ventricular-outflow tract shown on the echocardiogram, indicative of advanced chronic lung disease and perhaps cor pulmonale. It may be that very small perturbations were enough to produce respiratory decompensation and simply being on bed rest in the hospital was enough to produce a transient improvement. She also had abdominal distention, which may have resulted from air swallowing associated with tachypnea, may have been a manifestation of malnutrition, or may have been an early stage of the colitis induced by the toxin of *Clostridium difficile*. The presence of colitis was documented later in the hospital course and was probably related to the administration of multiple antibiotics or peritoneal seeding by tumor or infection. She had symptoms of pericarditis, and a small pericardial effusion was demonstrated on the echocardiogram. Of greatest importance, half of the T11 vertebral body, including the pedicle, had been destroyed over a period of four to six weeks, and paraplegia due to spinal-cord compression developed.

The major causes to be considered for the spinal lesion are infection and tumor. Each of these categories includes a number of possibilities. To begin with infection, the patient had already had signs of bloodstream invasion and thus the potential for hematogenous seeding by *Strep. pneumoniae* and *Candida albicans*. The possibility of yet another agent, a new infection, cannot be overlooked. She had a Broviac catheter in the inferior vena cava, used for amphotericin therapy and hyperalimentation, as a potential portal of entry for *Staphylococcus epidermidis, Staph. aureus,* other skin flora, and gram-negative rods. All these organisms can cause osteomyelitis; vertebral osteomyelitis can give rise to an epidural abscess and spinal-cord compression. These infections usually involve the anterior portion of the vertebral body rather than the pedicle and usually affect the disk space and adjacent vertebral body as well. Furthermore, bacterial vertebral osteomyelitis is rare in children; it occurred in only 1 of 26 patients with osteomyelitis in a series from this hospital[24] and in only 2 of 163 patients from the University of Texas Southwestern.[25] Pericarditis may be an associated finding.[24]

Fungal osteomyelitis due to candida and aspergillus may occur in immunosuppressed hosts. The common locations seem to be the same as for hematogenous bacterial osteomyelitis.[26] The deep mycoses also reach bone by the hematogenous route and preferentially affect the anterior portion of the vertebral body. African histoplasmosis due to *Histoplasma duboisii* has a predilection for pedicles, but *H. capsulatum,* the form found in the United States, very rarely produces bone lesions.[27-29] Coccidioides may spare the disk space, and blastomyces may involve the pedicles.[27] We can exclude coccidioidomycosis on the basis of the lack of a history of appropriate travel; however, blastomycosis may be acquired in Massachusetts.

Actinomycosis can produce vertebral disease by direct extension from a pulmonary focus through multiple tissue planes. A hallmark of actinomycotic lung disease is said to be a wavy periosteal reaction in the overlying ribs,[30] but in this case we do not know the relation of the periosteal change mentioned in the case record to the parenchymal disease. However, the characteristic "soap-bubble" appearance of the vertebral body and involvement of the posterior ends of the ribs seen in actinomycosis[27,30] were absent.

Tuberculous spondylitis does favor the lower thoracic vertebras, which may be seeded from the bloodstream or from infected lymph nodes. This lesion occurred frequently in children in the days when tuberculosis was common. The usual site is the vertebral body, but an onset of involvement in the pedicle has been described in some patients,[29] all of whom were more than 10 years old and had paraspinal abscesses, as did this child. Despite the previous negative investigations for tuberculosis the question of this diagnosis must be reopened at this juncture. Her mother's need for therapy suggests that the patient had been newly exposed to active disease, and the efficacy of isoniazid prophylaxis in the setting of profound immunocompromise is uncertain at best.

When we speak of tumors associated with AIDS we always think of Kaposi's sarcoma, although it has been more frequent in homosexual men than any other risk group and is particularly uncommon in children. In the two published cases of its occurrence in infants[31] it assumed a so-called lymphadenopathic form, with abnormally small nodes infiltrated by the tumor. Bony involvement in adults with Kaposi's sarcoma is described in association with overlying florid exophytic nodules or woody fibrosis and brawny edema,[32] which were not observed in this patient.

We must also consider other tumors, although both primary bone tumors and metastases involving the vertebras are rare in childhood.[33,34] The tumors mentioned as capable of producing vertebral lesions and paraplegia in children are neuroblastoma, Ewing's sarcoma, embryonal rhabdomyosarcoma, leukemia, and non-Hodgkin lymphoma, particularly Burkitt's lymphoma. In one textbook of pediatric oncology[34] it is stated that "the rapid development of paraplegia in a child less than five years of age should be assumed on statistical grounds to be due to a neuroblastoma until proven otherwise." Since neuroblastomas are derived from neural-crest tissue one almost invariably finds a paraspinal mass and often destruction of a pedicle, although sometimes the tumor is entirely within the epidural space. Neuroblastoma is often widely metastatic and can produce a picture of systemic illness like that seen in this patient.[35] If neuroblastoma proved to be the explanation for the entire illness, however, it should have been found on one of the many biopsies performed earlier.

When Ewing's sarcoma involves a vertebra, it usually arises from a process rather than the body and extends into the canal to produce spinal-cord compression. The amount of vertebral bony change in this case seems out of proportion to that described for Ewing's sarcoma, which is also predominantly a disease of slightly older children, 5 to 10 years of age.[36] Embryonal rhabdomyosarcoma occurs in this patient's age group and may metastasize to the spine and be associated with a paravertebral mass. Primary sites include the cavities of the head and neck, the pelvic organs, including the genital organs, and the skin or muscles of the trunk and extremities.[37] The orbit is a particularly common site,[38] but if the swelling of the eyelid that occurred before the first admission was caused by a rhabdomyosarcoma it should not have subsided and should have been noted on one of the physical examinations.

In areas of Africa where Burkitt's lymphoma is endemic paraplegia is a frequent manifestation of this disease. It may be associated with a block demonstrable on myelographic examination or may occur in its absence.[39,40] Paravertebral masses are frequently present, but bone changes are not marked.[39] The authors of a recent report of a series of cases[41] described epidural spinal compression as a presenting manifestation, albeit a rare one, of non-Hodgkin lymphoma or leukemia in children in this country. The tumors were Burkitt's lymphoma or B-cell leukemia, with one exception, and bony destruction was seen in only one child, in whom the disease did involve the pedicles.

Non-Hodgkin lymphoma has been occurring with unusual frequency in homosexual men in the United States, many of whom had the lymphadenopathy syndrome and some of whom had frank AIDS before the appearance of lymphoma.[42,43] Lymphoma in this setting may be of the Burkitt or another histologic type, is usually high-grade, and almost always involves extranodal sites, frequently the brain. In all but 1 of the 90 cases in a recent reported series[43] the tumor was of B-cell origin, and Epstein–Barr-virus DNA has been found in such tumors.[44] In the setting of immunosuppression for organ transplantation primary B-cell lymphoma of the brain has been related to Epstein–Barr virus,[45] and polyclonal lymphocytic proliferation as well as monoclonal tumors have occurred. The pathogenesis of this process has been explored with great care in the recently published description of a child with a severe combined immunodeficiency syndrome who was maintained in a gnotobiotic environment until he became seriously ill after bone marrow was transplanted from a sibling. This child was the famous "bubble boy" from Houston, Texas. He was found to have acquired Epstein–Barr-virus infection from the donor, without engraftment, and his viscera were studded with nodular lymphoid tumors; some of them were polyclonal, but others were monoclonal and clearly lymphomatous.[46] Similar lymphomatous transformation has been described in association with lymphocytic interstitial pneumonitis.[47] Also, the Epstein–Barr-virus genome has apparently been detected in lung tissue from children with lymphoid interstitial pneumonitis and AIDS, in one of whom a central nervous system lymphoma eventually developed.[48] We may have to apply the same caution to the detection of Epstein–Barr virus in the lung as we do to cytomegalovirus, since Epstein–Barr-virus genomes have been found in a variety of types of exfoliated respiratory tract cells in patients in whom cytologic studies were performed for the question of lung cancer and in whom levels of Epstein–Barr-virus antibodies were not suggestive of active disease.[49]

I believe that either tuberculosis or non-Hodgkin lymphoma could explain the new pulmonary infiltrates, the pericardial effusion, the vertebral changes, and the cord compression. Either might also account for the abdominal distention. North American blastomycosis can mimic tuberculosis but would have to be considered less likely than tuberculosis, a more common infection to which the child had known exposure. I reject the diagnosis of conventional bacterial osteomyelitis with an epidural abscess on the grounds that the asymmetry of the involvement and sparing of the disk would be extremely unusual in that disease. It is generally said that involvement of the vertebral pedicle suggests a metastatic tumor, but that statement applies to adult patients.[28,50] Preservation of the disk space also favors a malignant tumor[28,50] but has occurred in patients with tuberculosis affecting only one vertebral body,[51] as in this case. The type of malignant tumor that I am considering, however, is characteristically associated with little bone change, and this child had lost a substantial amount of bone in a very short time. I think that this lysis was too rapid to be attributed to tuberculosis. In short, the bone destruction was atypical in pattern for tuberculosis and atypical in quantity for lymphoma. The choice between these two diagnoses is very difficult, but I lean toward non-Hodgkin lymphoma. I suspect that the bibasilar pulmonary consolidation proved to be lymphomatous transformation of a preexisting lymphocytic interstitial pneumonitis.

I believe that the diagnostic procedure was performed with therapeutic intent as well and was a biopsy with decompression of the spinal cord. I would be interested to know if there are any data on the child's state of infection with Epstein–Barr virus.

Dr. David L. Gang: We have some data. IgG antibody to viral capsid antigen (VCA) was positive at a dilution of 1:10,240, and IgA antibody to VCA was positive at 1:80. IgG antibody to early antigen (EA) was positive at 1:1280 in a diffuse pattern, and the IgA titer was less than 1:10. Titers against Epstein–Barr-virus nuclear antigen (EBNA) were less than 1:2. These titers are very high. Do you want to comment in that regard?

Dr. Cheeseman: Such very high titers are known to occur in patients with AIDS. It is very interesting that she had not mounted a response to EBNA. Anti-EBNA is a late-occurring antibody that tends to signal convalescence and control of the disease, and its absence would fit with my supposition that this child's system had not controlled the primary Epstein–Barr-virus infection.

Dr. Gang: I shall ask Dr. Pasternack, of the Pediatric Infectious Disease Service, to comment on the treatment of this patient.

Dr. Mark S. Pasternack: I should like to underscore a few of the points that Dr. Cheeseman has made in trying to highlight some of the differences between AIDS as it is seen in children and adults.

First of all, the report that this child's HTLV-III antibody was positive came late in her illness. For some time we wondered whether the entire illness was a severe secondary immunodeficiency syndrome due to congenital or acquired cytomegalovirus infection, because cytomegalovirus was grown from her lung and other tissues. The other possibility was that the cytomegalovirus infection was a harbinger of another disorder such as AIDS. The positive antibody titer against HTLV-III resolved that differential diagnosis.

Dr. Cheeseman has emphasized the importance of serious bacterial infection in children with this syndrome, an aspect that is not stressed in consideration of infection in adult patients with AIDS. Indeed, this patient's course, with serious bacterial disease and recurrent bacteremia, is typical of children with AIDS, in whom the usual bacterial pathogens may cause serious illness and even death. In fact, this child's sibling also had HTLV-III antibody and died of fulminant pneumococcal sepsis.

The progressive pulmonary disease was a problem in management because open-lung biopsy could not be undertaken repetitively, and in young children it is difficult to perform more limited biopsies, such as transbronchial biopsy. The decision whether the progressive pulmonary disease was atypical lymphoid proliferation or persistent or newly acquired pneumocystis infection was very difficult, and the multiple courses of trimethoprim–sulfamethoxazole that were administered reflected our frustration in trying to manage progressive pulmonary disease in a child in whom we did not have the luxury of repetitive open-lung biopsies.

Dr. Gang: Dr. Cohn, you were the patient's private physician. Will you comment on her course outside the hospital?

Dr. Herbert E. Cohn: In the early stage of her illness, when anemia and recurrent infections were the paramount features, we began to suspect the presence of an underlying disorder after otitis media recurred and periorbital cellulitis developed. These episodes did respond effectively to antibiotic therapy. When cytomegalovirus was grown from three different sites we thought that the patient had systemic cytomegalovirus infection even though the organism was not demonstrated histologically, and we began to be concerned about her immune capabilities.

In regard to the second phase of her illness as defined by Dr. Cheeseman, we attempted continuously to maintain adequate nutrition since it was the only treatment that we had to offer. The course was one of progressive pulmonary involvement and debility, and we believed that she would soon succumb to respiratory failure due to cytomegalovirus infection. She had severe anorexia at about 39 months of age, and I believe that she would have died at that time if she had not been brought into the hospital for the surgical placement of a feeding gastrostomy tube.

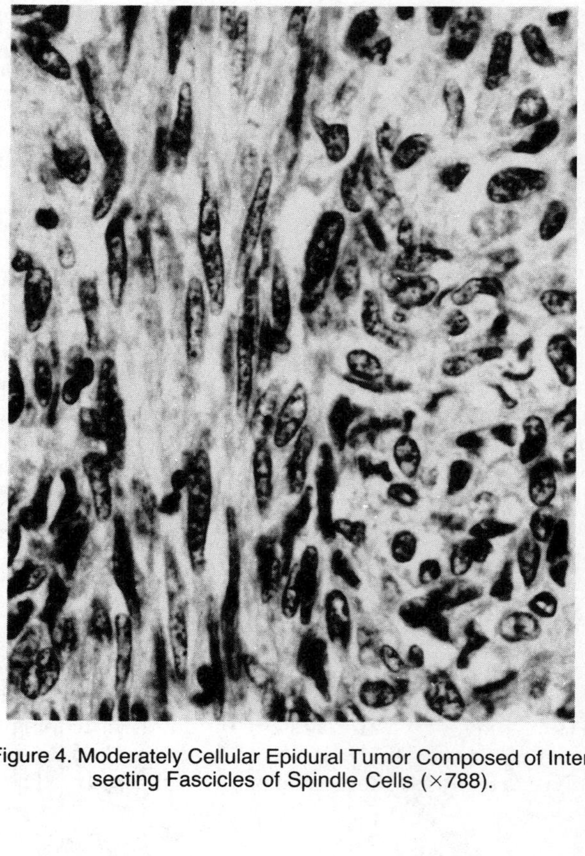

Figure 4. Moderately Cellular Epidural Tumor Composed of Intersecting Fascicles of Spindle Cells (×788).

A Physician: Was the infection acquired transplacentally?

Dr. Cheeseman: In view of the additional information about the sibling who had a positive serologic test for HTLV-III and died of overwhelming pneumococcal disease and in the setting of the development of active tuberculosis in the mother despite isoniazid prophylaxis, one has to be very suspicious that the mother transmitted the infection transplacentally to both children. Convincing data favor transplacental transmission in some cases — for example, the onset of illness within the first three months of life in infants of HTLV-III–positive mothers and the demonstration of HTLV-III genomes in thymic cells in a premature infant. I believe that the latter finding has been reported only in abstract form. However, if a child with the disease is seen long after the time of birth it is very difficult to prove transplacental rather than horizontal transmission during the perinatal period. At that time there is very close contact between the mother and baby, including exposure to blood and secretions.

A Physician: Did the possibility of Kawasaki's disease enter your differential diagnosis?

Dr. Cheeseman: Although we say that Kawasaki's disease is a diagnosis that one makes as the illness evolves over time, we are not talking about the duration of time in the case under discussion. In Kawasaki's disease the presence of only a few enlarged cervical lymph nodes and not generalized lymphadenopathy is characteristic, and there is a rash, which this child never had. The distinctive rash, conjunctivitis, red tongue, fissured lips, and fever are followed by desquamation usually within 10 days to two weeks, and the total illness lasts two to four weeks. Coronary-artery aneurysms, which develop during the acute phase, may give rise to sequelae, but this child's pericardial involvement was not suggestive of the cardiac tamponade that may occur when an aneurysm ruptures. Kawasaki's disease would have been a consideration at the time that lymphadenopathy first developed in this child, however.

Clinical Diagnoses

Acquired immunodeficiency syndrome, with cytomegalovirus infection and ? *Pneumocystis carinii* pneumonia.

Malignant tumor, with metastasis to thoracic vertebra and epidural space.

Dr. Sarah H. Cheeseman's Diagnoses

Acquired immunodeficiency syndrome.

Lymphoid interstitial pneumonitis, ? with lymphomatous transformation.

Non-Hodgkin lymphoma of vertebra, with spinal-cord compression.

Pathological Discussion

Dr. Gang: The diagnostic procedure, performed by Dr. Paul H. Chapman, was a decompressive laminectomy at levels T10 through T12, with subtotal resection of a friable, vascular, pink-gray epidural mass.

Light-microscopical examination of the specimen revealed a moderately cellular tumor composed of interwoven bands of slightly pleomorphic spindle cells suggestive of a schwannian origin (Fig. 4). Immunoperoxidase studies for S-100 protein were negative. Since only half of malignant nerve-sheath tumors contain this protein on immunohistochemical examination, the diagnosis of a schwannian origin was not excluded by the negative result.[52] However, electron-microscopical examination of the tumor revealed thick and thin filaments in parallel array in virtually all the cells as well as scattered condensations of electron-dense Z-band material characteristic of rhabdomyosarcoma (Fig. 5).

The patient had a difficult postoperative course characterized by increasingly severe respiratory distress and died 18 days after the operation. At postmortem examination an atypical lymphoplasmacytic infiltrate was found to involve massively the lungs, lymph nodes, spleen, accessory spleens, bone marrow, salivary glands, kidneys, liver, stomach, thymus, and intestine. The lungs appeared diffusely consolidated and

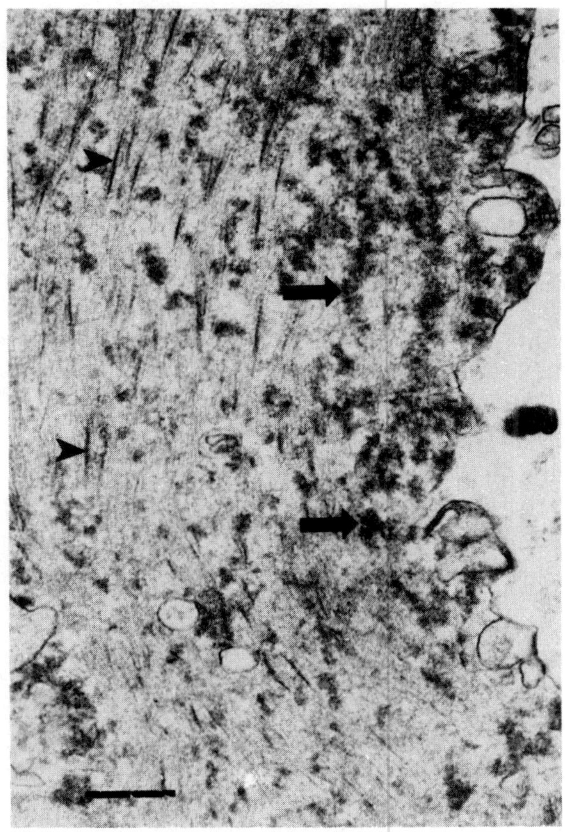

Figure 5. Electron Micrograph (×38,000; Bar = 0.395 μm).
A portion of one of the neoplastic spindle cells shows innumerable thin and thick filaments (arrowheads) and "puffs" of early Z-bands (arrows).

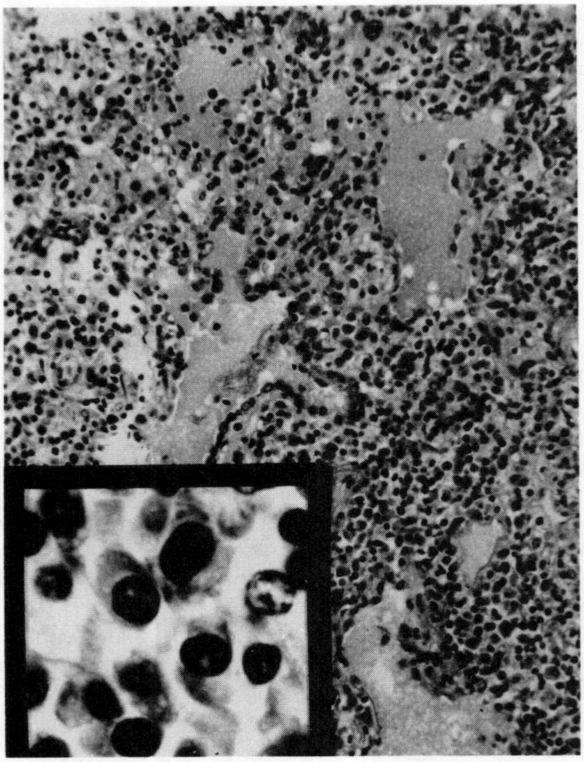

Figure 6. Septal Widening in the Lung by a Dense Lymphoplasmacytic Infiltrate (×200; Inset, ×1250).

edematous, and examination showed extensive interstitial, subpleural, and peribronchial infiltration by a polymorphous population of lymphoplasmacytic cells (Fig. 6). Immunoperoxidase staining revealed an equal distribution of kappa and lambda light chains among the infiltrating cells consistent with a polyclonal proliferation. A polyclonal light-chain distribution was also found in infiltrates in the liver and bone marrow. The immediate cause of death was respiratory failure as a result of the tumor-like infiltrate and acute pulmonary edema.

The pulmonary infiltrates in this case were similar in pattern to those of lymphoid interstitial pneumonitis (LIP) described in 4 of 10 children with AIDS from New Jersey, in 6 of 14 infants with AIDS and LIP from Miami, and 8 of 14 children with AIDS, nodular pulmonary densities, and LIP followed at the Albert Einstein Medical School, in New York.[18,53] Goldman et al.[54] stated that biopsy-proved LIP is now accepted as consistent with AIDS in children.

The other major finding at autopsy was the presence of widely disseminated spindle-cell tumor in the spleen, large and small bowel, abdominal lymph nodes, vertebral bodies, cervical epidural space, and gallbladder morphologically similar to the recently biopsied paraspinal mass. No tumor was identified at the biopsy site. The primary tumor appeared to have arisen in the gallbladder, where the lower portion of the lumen was completely occluded and scattered nodules were present above the obstruction (Fig. 7). Microscopical examination (Fig. 8) showed a large, bulging tumor stretching the overlying attenuated epithelium.

Malignant tumors associated with AIDS in children appear to be rare. Two of the 14 infants described by Scott et al.[53] had disseminated lymphadenopathic Kaposi's sarcoma, but at autopsy there was no evidence of Kaposi's sarcoma or other tumors in the eight cases reported by Joshi et al.[55]

Examination of the brain revealed an encephalomyelitis typical of that seen in patients with AIDS. In multiple areas we found a perivascular cellular infiltrate containing atypical mononuclear cells and activated glial cells without neutrophils. Occasional plasmacytoid cells were seen.

Autopsy tissue from a salivary gland, lymph node, and lung were sent to Dr. Warren A. Andiman, at Yale University. He analyzed the tissues, extracting whole cellular DNA from these organs. All three specimens contained small amounts of Epstein–Barr-virus DNA (one to two genome copies per cell).

The finding of high antibody titers to Epstein–Barr-virus antigens, the presence of Epstein–Barr-virus genomes in several body tissues, and the associated lymphoproliferative disorder suggests that this patient had an Epstein–Barr-virus–associated lymphoproliferative disorder similar to that of the famous 12-year-old "bubble boy" with combined immunodeficiency who died with multiple tumor-like B-cell proliferations containing Epstein–Barr-virus genomes.[56] The Epstein–Barr virus is a well-known inducer of polyclonal and monoclonal B-cell lymphoproliferative disease after organ transplantation.[57,58] It is possible that the polymorphous and seemingly polyclonal proliferation of plasmacytoid lymphocytes in this case represented an oligoclonal lymphoma in which more than one cell line had become neoplastic. We hope to be able to look for rearrangement of immunoglobulin-gene DNA within the proliferating lymphoid cells in the near future.

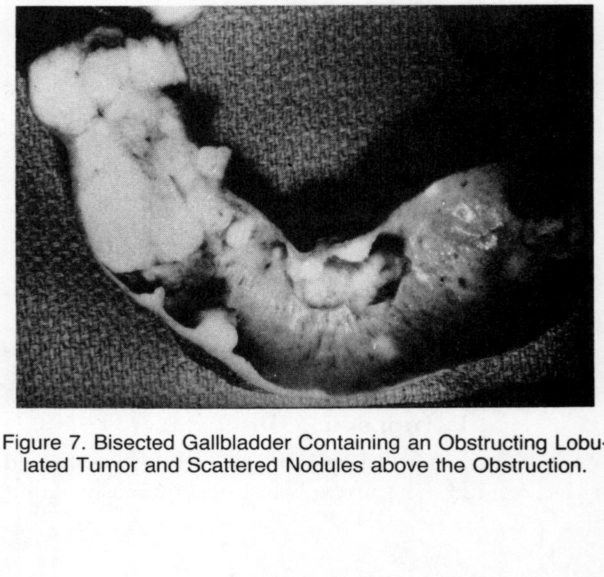

Figure 7. Bisected Gallbladder Containing an Obstructing Lobulated Tumor and Scattered Nodules above the Obstruction.

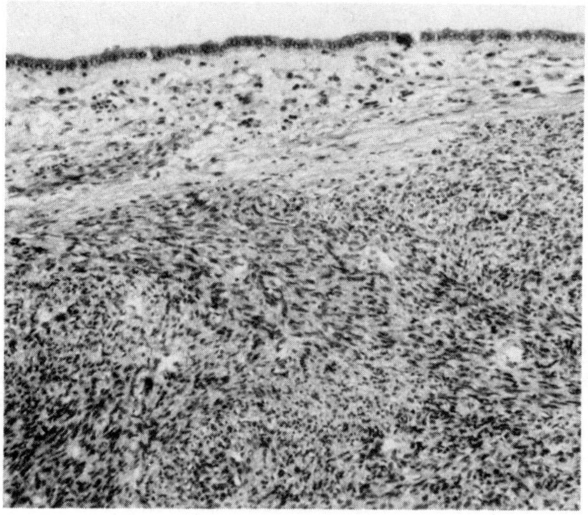

Figure 8. Gallbladder Tumor (×125).
An attenuated mucosa is stretched over a cellular spindle-cell tumor morphologically similar to the epidural mass.

A Physician: Dr. Cohn, what will you tell the mother regarding her positive HTLV-III titer?

Dr. Cohn: I am uncertain. When she told me that she was pregnant again, I informed her that there was little hope that she would have a viable baby. She is aware that she has a positive HTLV-III test. If she were to ask me if she should become pregnant again I would advise her against it. I would suggest waiting for five years to evaluate her state of health and find out what might be known at that time about this very devastating condition.

Anatomical Diagnoses

Acquired immunodeficiency syndrome.

Rhabdomyosarcoma of probable gallbladder origin, with extensive metastases.

Lymphoproliferative disorder associated with Epstein–Barr-virus infection.

Encephalomyelitis.

References

1. Acute hemorrhagic conjunctivitis — Latin America. MMWR 1981; 30:450-1.
2. Berggren WL, Ewbank DC, Berggren GG. Reduction of mortality in rural Haiti through a primary-health-care program. N Engl J Med 1981; 304: 1324-30.
3. Barry M, Stansfield SK, Bia FJ. Haiti and the Hôpital Albert Schweitzer. Ann Intern Med 1983; 98:1018-20.
4. Lincoln EM, Sewell EM. Tuberculosis in children. New York: McGraw-Hill, 1963.
5. Guarda LA, Butler JJ, Mansell P, Hersh EP, Reuben J, Newell GR. Lymphadenopathy in homosexual men: morbid anatomy with clinical and immunologic correlations. Am J Clin Pathol 1983; 79:559-68.
6. Ioachim HL, Lerner CW, Tapper ML. Lymphadenopathies in homosexual men: relationships with the acquired immune deficiency syndrome. JAMA 1983; 250:1306-9.
7. Brynes RK, Chan WC, Spira TJ, Ewing EP Jr, Chandler FW. Value of lymph node biopsy in unexplained lymphadenopathy in homosexual men. JAMA 1983; 250:1313-7.
8. Rogers MF. AIDS in children: a review of the clinical, epidemiologic and public health aspects. Pediatr Infect Dis 1985; 4:230-6.
9. Ziegler JB, Johnson RO, Cooper DA, Gold J. Postnatal transmission of AIDS-associated retrovirus from mother to infant. Lancet 1985; 1:896-7.
10. Jaffe HW, Bregman DJ, Selik RM. Acquired immune deficiency syndrome in the United States: the first 1,000 cases. J Infect Dis 1983; 148:339-45.
11. Update: Acquired immunodeficiency syndrome (AIDS) — United States. MMWR 1984; 32:688-91.
12. Craighead JE. Pulmonary cytomegalovirus infection in the adult. Am J Pathol 1971; 63:487-504.
13. Minnefor A, Oleske J, Zabala M, et al. Clinical findings in pediatric acquired immune deficiency syndrome. Presented at the International Conference on Acquired Immunodeficiency Syndrome (AIDS). Atlanta, April 14-17, 1985.
14. Ammann AJ, Kaminsky L, Cowan M, Levy JA. Antibodies to AIDS-associated retrovirus distinguish between pediatric primary and acquired immunodeficiency diseases. JAMA 1985; 253:3116-8.
15. Strimlan CV, Rosenow EC III, Weiland LH, et al. Lymphocytic interstitial pneumonitis: review of 13 cases. Ann Intern Med 1978; 88:616-21.
16. Goldman HS, Zipkowski MN, Charytan M, Rubinstein A, Morecki R. Lymphocytic interstitial pneumonitis in children with AIDS: a perfect radiographic-pathologic correlation. Presented at the 28th Annual Meeting, Society for Pediatric Radiology, Boston, April 18-21, 1985.
17. Vath RR, Alexander CB, Fulmer JD. The lymphocytic infiltrative lung diseases. Clin Chest Med 1982; 3:619-34.
18. Joshi VV, Oleske JM, Minnefor AB, et al. Pathologic pulmonary findings in children with the acquired immunodeficiency syndrome: a study of ten cases. Hum Pathol 1985; 16:241-6.
19. Saldana MJ, Mones JM, Scott GB, Fischl MA. Lymphoid interstitial pneumonia in the acquired immunodeficiency syndrome. Presented at the International Conference on Acquired Immunodeficiency Syndrome (AIDS), Atlanta, April 14-17, 1985.
20. Couderc LJ, Matheron S, Solol-Celigny PH, et al. Lymphoid interstitial pneumonitis (LIP) in Haitians and Africans: an AIDS-linked entity? Presented at the International Conference on Acquired Immunodeficiency Syndrome (AIDS), Atlanta, April 14-17, 1985.
21. Montane B, Scott G, Ziueruelo G, Freundlich M, Abitbol C, Strauss J. Urinary and renal histological changes in children with acquired immunodeficiency syndrome (AIDS). Presented at the International Conference on Acquired Immunodeficiency Syndrome (AIDS). Atlanta, April 14-17, 1985.
22. Pardo V, Aldana M, Colton RM, et al. Glomerular lesions in the acquired immunodeficiency syndrome. Ann Intern Med 1984; 101:429-34.
23. Shannon KM, Ammann AJ. Acquired immune deficiency syndrome in childhood. J Pediatr 1985; 106:332-42.
24. Waldvogel FA, Medoff G, Swartz MN. Osteomyelitis: a review of clinical features, therapeutic considerations and unusual aspects. N Engl J Med 1970; 282:198-206, 260-6, 316-22.
25. Dich VQ, Nelson JD, Haltalin KC. Osteomyelitis in infants and children. Am J Dis Child 1975; 129:1273-8.
26. Simpson MB, Merz WG, Kurlinski JP, Solomon MH. Opportunistic mycotic osteomyelitis: bone infections due to *Aspergillus* and *Candida* species. Medicine (Baltimore) 1977; 56:475-82.
27. Rhangos WC, Chick EW. Mycotic infections of bone. South Med J 1964; 57:664-74.
28. Gorse GJ, Pais MJ, Kusske JA, Cesario TC. Tuberculous spondylitis: a report of six cases and a review of the literature. Medicine (Baltimore) 1983; 62:178-93.
29. Bell D, Cockshott WP. Tuberculosis of the vertebral pedicles. Radiology 1971; 99:43-8.
30. Flynn MW, Felson B. The roentgen manifestations of thoracic actinomycosis. Am J Roentgenol Radium Ther Nucl Med 1970; 110:707-16.
31. Buck BE, Scott GB, Valdes-Dapena M, Parks WP. Kaposi sarcoma in two infants with acquired immune deficiency syndrome. J Pediatr 1983; 103:911-3.
32. Ziegler JL, Templeton AC, Vogel CL. Kaposi's sarcoma: a comparison of classical, endemic, and epidemic forms. Semin Oncol 1984; 11:47-52.
33. Silverman FN. The neck, spine, and pelvis. In: Silverman FN, ed. Caffey's pediatric x-ray diagnosis: an integrated imaging approach. 8th ed. Chicago: Year Book, 1985:267-358.
34. Hooper R. Intracranial and spinal tumors. In: Jones PG, Campbell PE, eds. Tumours of infancy and childhood. Oxford: Blackwell, 1976:231-94.
35. Jones PG. Tumours of the adrenal gland and retroperitoneum. In: Jones PG, Campbell PE, eds. Tumours of infancy and childhood. Oxford: Blackwell, 1976:537-95.
36. *Idem.* Bone tumours. In: Jones PG, Campbell PE, eds. Tumours of infancy and childhood. Oxford: Blackwell, 1976:723-75.
37. *Idem.* Sarcomas of soft tissues. In: Jones PG, Campbell PE, eds. Tumours of infancy and childhood. Oxford: Blackwell 1976:777-836.
38. Billson FA. Tumours of the eye and orbit. In: Jones PG, Campbell PE, eds. Tumours of infancy and childhood. Oxford: Blackwell, 1976:397-440.
39. Cockshott WP, Evans KT. Childhood paraplegia in lymphosarcoma (Burkitt's tumour). Br J Radiol 1963; 36:914-20.

40. Ziegler JK, Bluming AZ, Morrow RH, Fass L, Carbone PP. Central nervous system involvement in Burkitt's lymphoma. Blood 1970; 36:718-28.
41. Pui C-H, Dahl GV, Hustu HO, Murphy SB. Epidural spinal cord compression as the initial finding in childhood acute leukemia and non-Hodgkin lymphoma. J Pediatr 1985; 106:788-92.
42. Levine AM, Meyer PR, Begandy MK, et al. Development of B-cell lymphoma in homosexual men: clinical and immunologic findings. Ann Intern Med 1984; 100:7-13.
43. Ziegler JL, Beckstead JA, Volberding PA, et al. Non-Hodgkin's lymphoma in 90 homosexual men: relation to generalized lymphadenopathy and the acquired immunodeficiency syndrome. N Engl J Med 1984; 311:565-70.
44. Lind SE, Gross PL, Andiman WA, Stone GC, Schooley RT, Harris NL. Malignant lymphoma presenting as Kaposi's sarcoma in a homosexual man with the acquired immunodeficiency syndrome. Ann Intern Med 1985; 102:338-40.
45. Hochberg FH, Miller G, Schooley RT, Hirsch MS, Feorino P, Henle W. Central-nervous-system lymphoma related to Epstein–Barr virus. N Engl J Med 1983; 309:745-8.
46. Shearer WT, Ritz J, Fiengold MJ, et al. Epstein–Barr virus-associated B-cell proliferations of diverse clonal origins after bone marrow transplantation in a 12-year-old patient with severe combined immunodeficiency. N Engl J Med 1985; 312:1151-9.
47. Kradin RL, Young RH, Kradin LA, Mark EJ. Immunoblastic lymphoma arising in chronic lymphoid hyperplasia of the pulmonary interstitium. Cancer 1982; 50:1339-43.
48. Markowitz RI. Epstein–Barr virus related illness in two infants with AIDS (abstract). Presented at the 28th Annual Meeting of the Society for Pediatric Radiology, Boston. April 15-18, 1985.
49. Lung ML, So SY, Chan KH, Lam WK, Lam WP, Ng MH. Evidence that respiratory tract is a major reservoir for Epstein–Barr virus. Lancet 1985; 1:899-92.
50. Paus B. Tumour, tuberculosis and osteomyelitis of the spine: differential diagnostic aspects. Acta Orthop Scand 1973; 44:372-82.
51. Rahman NU. Atypical forms of spinal tuberculosis. J Bone Joint Surg (Br) 1980; 62:162-5.
52. Weiss SW, Langloss JM, Enzinger FM. Value of S-100 protein in the diagnosis of soft tissue tumors with particular reference to benign and malignant Schwann cell tumors. Lab Invest 1983; 49:299-308.
53. Scott GB, Buck BE, Leterman JG, Bloom FL, Parks WP. Acquired immunodeficiency syndrome in infants. N Engl J Med 1984; 310:76-81.
54. Goldman HS, Ziprkowski MN, Charytan M, Rubinstein A, Morecki R.. Lymphocytic interstitial pneumonitis in children with AIDS: a perfect radiographic-pathologic correlation. AJR 1985; 145:868a.
55. Joshi VV, Oleske JM, Minnefor AB, Singh R, Bokhari T, Rapkin RH. Pathology of suspected acquired immune deficiency syndrome in children: a study of eight cases. Pediatr Pathol 1984; 2:71-87.
56. Shearer WT, Ritz J, Finegold MJ, et al. Epstein-Barr virus-associated B-cell proliferations of diverse clonal origins after bone marrow transplantation in a 12-year-old patient with severe combined immunodeficiency. N Engl J Med 1985; 312:1151-9.
57. Hanto DW, Gajl-Peczalska KJ, Frizzera G, et al. Epstein-Barr virus (EBV) induced polyclonal and monoclonal B-cell lymphoproliferative diseases occurring after renal transplantation. Ann Surg 1983; 198:356-69.
58. Cleary ML, Warnke R, Sklar J. Monoclonality of lymphoproliferative lesions in cardiac-transplant recipients: clonal analysis based on immunoglobulin-gene rearrangements. N Engl J Med 1984; 310:477-82.

ORIGINAL ARTICLE

RISK OF NOSOCOMIAL INFECTION WITH HUMAN T-CELL LYMPHOTROPIC VIRUS III (HTLV-III)

MARTIN S. HIRSCH M.D., GARY P. WORMSER, M.D., ROBERT T. SCHOOLEY, M.D., DAVID D. HO, M.D., DONNA FELSENSTEIN, M.D., CYRUS C. HOPKINS, M.D., CAROL JOLINE, R.N., FREDERICK DUNCANSON, M.D., M.G. SARNGADHARAN, PH.D., CARL SAXINGER, PH.D., AND ROBERT C. GALLO, M.D.

Abstract Infection with human T-cell lymphotropic virus III (HTLV-III) is closely linked to the acquired immunodeficiency syndrome (AIDS). We evaluated the risk of nosocomial infection with HTLV-III by testing for antibodies to HTLV-III among hospital employees, including victims of needle-stick exposure, endoscopists, pathologists, and laboratory workers. Assays for antibody against the virus were performed by enzyme-linked immunosorbent assay and electrophoretic (Western blot) techniques.

Although all 22 of our patients with AIDS and 6 of 7 with AIDS-related complex were found to have antibodies to HTLV-III when both assays were employed, none of the 85 employees with nosocomial exposure to specimens from patients with AIDS were positive for HTLV-III antibody. These studies must be regarded as preliminary, but they suggest that when current hospital isolation procedures are employed, the risk of nosocomial transmission of HTLV-III is low.

RECENT studies indicate a close association between newly discovered human retroviruses and the acquired immunodeficiency syndrome (AIDS).[1-9] The vast majority of patients with AIDS have antibodies to human T-cell lymphotropic virus III (HTLV-III), whereas the frequency of antibodies to this virus among low-risk control populations — e.g., blood donors — is less than 1 percent.[4,6] In addition, over 95 isolates of HTLV-III have been obtained from persons who have AIDS or are at risk for it.[3,7-9]

Of great concern is the risk of contracting HTLV-III for persons caring for patients with AIDS, as well as for laboratory workers performing clinical and research studies on specimens derived from this population. Several hundred needle-stick exposures to blood or tissue from patients with AIDS have been reported to a registry established by the Centers for Disease Control.[10]

We have studied the HTLV-III serologic status of hospital employees considered at high risk after accidental inoculation or repeated exposure to specimens from patients with AIDS over a three-year period. Specimens were collected at two medical centers, in Massachusetts and New York. The employees studied included 33 victims of needle-stick or blood exposure, 8 endoscopists, 8 pathologists, and 20 laboratory workers handling AIDS specimens.

METHODS

Populations Studied

Between February 1981 and April 1, 1984, 32 patients meeting the criteria of the Centers for Disease Control for the diagnosis of AIDS[11] were treated at the Massachusetts General Hospital; at the same time, 57 patients with AIDS were seen at the Westchester County Medical Center. Of these, 22 were evaluated for HTLV-III antibodies in this study. In addition, seven men with the syndrome known as AIDS-related complex were evaluated. AIDS-related complex is defined as a constellation of signs, symptoms, and laboratory abnormalities that may possibly predict the subsequent development of AIDS.[12] Although definitions of criteria for the diagnosis of the complex vary, we used Krause's criteria,[12] which include two clinical findings among the following: fever for longer than three months, weight loss of more than 10 percent of the baseline body weight, lymphadenopathy for longer than three months, chronic diarrhea, fatigue, and night sweats; plus two laboratory abnormalities among the following: reduced numbers of helper T cells, a diminished helper/suppressor T-cell ratio, decreased lymphoproliferative responses, and increased serum globulins.

Hospital employees enrolled in this serologic study included persons who reported they had experienced accidental inoculations with needles used in patients with AIDS as well as others who were repeatedly exposed to specimens from such patients. Included in the latter group were gastroenterologist endoscopists, bronchoscopists, surgeons, and research scientists and technicians. Most had repeated exposures over a period of one to three years. Serum samples from hospital employees were obtained between September 1983 and June 1984.

Measurement of Antibodies to HTLV-III

Enzyme-Linked Immunosorbent Assay (ELISA)

The wells of 96-well Immulon plates were coated overnight with a lysate of density-banded HTLV-III at 0.5 μg of protein per well in 100 μl of 50 mM sodium bicarbonate buffer, pH 9.6. The wells were washed with water and incubated for 20 minutes with 100 μl of 5 percent bovine serum albumin in phosphate-buffered saline. The wells were washed again in water, and then 100 μl of 20 percent normal goat serum in phosphate-buffered saline were added to each well, followed by 5 or 10 μl of the test serum samples. These were allowed to react for two hours at room temperature. The wells were washed three times with 0.05 percent Tween-20 in phosphate-buffered saline and incubated for one hour at room temperature with peroxidase-labeled goat antiserum to human immunoglobulin G at a dilution of 1:2000 in 1 percent normal goat serum in phosphate-buffered saline. The wells were washed four times successively with 0.05 percent Tween-20 in phosphate-buffered saline and four times with phosphate-buffered saline, and reacted with 100 μl of the substrate mixture containing 0.05 percent orthophenylene diamine and 0.005 percent hydrogen peroxide in phosphate–citrate buffer, pH 5.0. The reactions were stopped by the addition of 50 μl of 4N sulfuric acid, and the color yield was measured with a Dynatech

From the Infectious Disease Unit, Massachusetts General Hospital, Harvard Medical School, Boston; the Division of Infectious Diseases, Department of Medicine, Westchester County Medical Center and New York Medical College, Valhalla, N.Y.; the Department of Cell Biology, Litton Bionetics, Inc., Kensington, Md.; and the Laboratory of Tumor Cell Biology, National Cancer Institute, Bethesda, Md.

Supported in part by grants (CA 12464, CA 35020, and CA 37461) from the National Institutes of Health and by the Mashud A. Mezerhane B Fund. Drs. Ho and Felsenstein are Fellows of the American Cancer Society.

ELISA reader. Assays were done in duplicate, and an absorbance reading that was more than three times the average of four normal negative-control readings was taken to be positive.

Electrophoretic (Western Blot) Technique

HTLV-III was lysed and fractionated by electrophoresis on a 12 percent polyacrylamide slab gel in the presence of sodium dodecyl sulfate. The protein bands on the gel were electrophoretically transferred to a nitrocellulose sheet according to the procedure of Towbin et al.[13] Strip solid-phase radioimmunoassays were then performed. The sheet was incubated at 37°C for two hours with 5 percent bovine serum albumin in 10 mM TRIS–hydrochloric acid, pH 7.5, containing 0.9 percent sodium chloride, and cut into 0.5-cm strips. Each strip was incubated for two hours at 37°C and for two hours at room temperature in a screw-cap tube containing 2.5 ml of buffer 1 (20 mM TRIS–hydrochloric acid, pH 7.5; 1 mM EDTA; 0.2 M sodium chloride; 0.3 percent Triton X-100; and 2 mg of bovine serum albumin and 0.2 mg of human Fab per milliliter). Test serum samples (25 μl) were then added to individual tubes containing the strips, and incubation was continued for one hour at room temperature and overnight in the cold. The strips were washed three times with a solution containing 0.5 percent sodium deoxycholate, 0.1 M sodium choloride, 0.5 percent Triton X-100, 1 mM phenylmethylsulfonyl fluoride, and 10 mM sodium phosphate, pH 7.5. The strips were incubated for one hour at room temperature with 2.4 ml of buffer 1 and 0.1 ml of normal goat serum. Affinity-purified and ^{125}I-labeled goat antiserum to human immunoglobulin (μ chain and Fc fragment) (1.25×10^6 cpm) was added to the reaction mixture, and the incubation was continued for 30 minutes at room temperature. The strips were washed as described, dried, mounted, and exposed to x-ray film.

Results

All serum samples were obtained in Boston, Mass., or Valhalla, N.Y., and sent under code for serologic analysis at the National Cancer Institute. Serum samples were screened by ELISA, and if they were negative, by the more sensitive Western blot technique.

Patients with AIDS and AIDS-Related Complex

The serum samples from all 22 patients confirmed as having AIDS by the Centers for Disease Control were found to be positive for HTLV-III antibodies when both serologic techniques were employed. ELISA alone identified 12 of these patients (55 percent; Table 1). The patients with AIDS consisted of 20 homosexual men, 1 two-year-old Haitian child, and 1 woman who was a heterosexual contact of a healthy Kenyan man with HTLV-III antibodies. Six of seven homosexual men with AIDS-related complex were seropositive for HTLV-III antibodies. In three of these, AIDS has since developed over a period of 6 to 12 months.

Table 1. HTLV-III Antibodies in Hospital Employees and Patients.

		No. Positive for HTLV-III Antibody		
Group	No.	ELISA	Western blot	% positive
Patients with AIDS	22	12	22	100
Patients with AIDS-related complex	7	6	6	86
Hospital employees				
Accidental exposures	33*	0	0	0
Endoscopists	9†	0	0	0
Pathologists	8	0	0	0
Research investigators	20	0	0	0
Others‡	15	0	0	0

*Thirty needle sticks, one splattering of an eye with blood, and two blood spills on an open cut.

†Seven gastroenterologists and two endoscopy nurses.

‡Physicians, nurses, and medical students with extensive exposure to patients with AIDS.

Victims of Accidental Inoculations Involving Patients with AIDS

Thirty-one needle-stick accidents involving 30 persons who were thus exposed to material from patients with AIDS were reported to the Massachusetts General Hospital Infection Control Unit between August 1982 and April 1984. At the New York Medical College, 24 needle-stick accidents in 22 persons were reported during this period. These subjects have remained healthy, and 30 consented to serologic study for HTLV-III antibodies. All 30 had single needle-stick exposures that punctured the skin. Another employee reported that her eye was splattered with blood from a patient with AIDS, and two others had blood contamination of an open hand wound. Of the 33 accident victims studied, 23 were women and 10 were men. Their ages ranged from 22 to 46 years (mean, 30). The mean duration between accident and serologic testing was eight months (range, 0.5 to 20 months). Several of these persons also had repeated occupational exposures to specimens from patients with AIDS. Serologic determinations were performed in 11 of the patients with AIDS who were involved in the needle-stick accidents, and all their serum samples were positive for HTLV-III antibody. In contrast, all 33 accident victims were seronegative for HTLV-III (Table 1).

Other Potentially High-Risk Employees

Serum samples from eight pathologists who performed autopsies (average, four per pathologist) and processed biopsy specimens from patients with AIDS between December 1981 and November 1983 were tested for HTLV-III antibodies. Most had repeated exposures because they were working with material from several patients who had AIDS. All the pathologists were seronegative, despite the fact that all three of the autopsy subjects with AIDS for whom premortem serum samples were available were seropositive for HTLV-III.

Seven gastroenterologists and two endoscopy nurses were evaluated. All had performed endoscopies in patients with AIDS between September 1982 and October 1983. In addition, many had had repeated exposures to several different patients with AIDS or AIDS-related complex. The patients with AIDS in whom these procedures were performed and for whom serum samples were available were all seropositive for HTLV-III (5 of 5), whereas the endoscopists were seronegative. One surgeon and one bronchoscopist with multiple exposures to biopsy specimens and secretions from patients with AIDS and AIDS-related complex over a two-year period were also seronegative for HTLV-III.

Twenty research scientists and technicians were

studied. All worked with blood specimens from patients with AIDS, and many with other AIDS specimens, including urine, semen, throat washes, and biopsy or autopsy tissue. All had handled specimens from many patients with AIDS or AIDS-related complex, often performing in vitro studies with such material. Exposures were repeated over a period of one to three years. All were seronegative for HTLV-III.

Discussion

Previous seroepidemiologic studies have suggested that the infectious agent that is responsible for AIDS is transmitted by sexual routes and by blood products in a pattern reminiscent of hepatitis B virus infection.[14,15] Hepatitis B infections among hospital personnel as a result of needle-stick accidents or other exposures to blood products from infected patients are well-documented.[16-19] The incidence of hepatitis B after needle-stick exposure to blood from persons positive for hepatitis B surface antigen is 10 to 15 percent; if the donor is positive for hepatitis B e antigen, the incidence is 19 percent.[19] In contrast, nosocomial cases of AIDS have not been clearly established. According to published reports, AIDS has developed in four health-care workers without known risk factors.[20,21] The source of AIDS in these subjects is unclear, and none were known to have had contact with patients with the syndrome. All the hospital personnel who had parenteral exposure to the blood of patients with AIDS at our hospitals are clinically well, including 22 persons who have been observed for over a year. A recent study of the results of immunologic testing of 12 of the exposed persons from the Valhalla study center (all studied at least six months after exposure; mean, 10.3 months) found no differences in the counts of white cells, lymphocytes, T lymphocytes, or T-cell subsets between the exposed persons and 30 co-worker controls who specifically denied such exposures.[22]

The identification of a human retrovirus, HTLV-III, as the likely etiologic agent of AIDS will allow better definition of the means of transmission and of the subjects at risk. We have studied hospital employees who were thought to be at particular risk despite the institution of strict isolation procedures for blood and secretions. These employees include nurses, physicians, and technicians who had accidental needlesticks while obtaining specimens from patients with AIDS, as well as endoscopists potentially exposed to gastrointestinal secretions and pathologists exposed to autopsy tissue from patients with AIDS. In addition, serum samples from workers in research laboratories who were repeatedly handling specimens from patients with AIDS were studied. The precautions employed for hospitalized patients were designed to avoid percutaneous or mucosal contact with any suspected infectious material (blood, urine, feces, semen, saliva) according to established guidelines.[23-25] Particular attention was directed to the avoidance of accidental wounds and the proper disposal of needles. In the laboratory, containment procedures included the use of laminar-flow safety cabinets and of mechanical pipettes, the wearing of gowns and gloves, and the use of effective disinfectants.[26]

It is reassuring that not a single HTLV-III seroconversion was observed among the hospital employees evaluated by ELISA and Western blot techniques. However, these results do not indicate that precautions within hospitals should be relaxed. The numbers studied are small, and the natural history of antibody development to HTLV-III is unclear. Persons involved in accidents will continue to be serially monitored for HTLV-III seroconversion over a more prolonged period. Our results do suggest that the isolation procedures currently recommended for AIDS[22-24] are adequate and that the risk of transmission within hospitals is low. Moreover, accidental needle-stick exposure appears to provide little additional risk of HTLV-III transmission.

We are indebted to Ms. Theresa Flynn, R.N., for her help in collecting data and to Ms. Janet Steele for preparing the manuscript.

References

1. Popovic M, Sarngadharan MG, Read E, Gallo RC. Detection, isolation, and continuous production of cytopathic retroviruses (HTLV-III) from patients with AIDS and pre-AIDS. Science 1984; 224:497-500.
2. Gallo RC, Salahuddin SZ, Popovic M, et al. Frequent detection and isolation of cytopathic retroviruses (HTLV-III) from patients with AIDS and at risk for AIDS. Science 1984; 224:500-2.
3. Schüpbach J, Popovic M, Gilden RV, Gonda MA, Sarngadharan MG, Gallo RC. Serological analysis of a subgroup of human T-lymphotropic retroviruses (HTLV-III) associated with AIDS. Science 1984; 224:503-5.
4. Sarngadharan MG, Popovic M, Bruch L, Schüpbach J, Gallo RC. Antibodies reactive with human T-lymphotropic retroviruses (HTLV-III) in the serum of patients with AIDS. Science 1984; 224:506-8.
5. Barré-Sinoussi F, Chermann JC, Rey F, et al. Isolation of a T-lymphotropic retrovirus from a patient at risk for acquired immune deficiency syndrome (AIDS). Science 1983; 220:868-71.
6. Sarngadharan MG, Markham PD, Gallo RC. Human T lymphotropic viruses: primary etiologic agents for adult T-cell leukemia and AIDS. In: Fields BN, ed. Virology. New York: Raven Press (in press).
7. Groopman JE, Salahuddin SZ, Sarngadharan MG, et al. HTLV-III in saliva of people with AIDS-related complex and healthy homosexual men at risk for AIDS. Science 1984; 226:447-9.
8. Zagury D, Bernard J, Leibowitch J, et al. HTLV-III in cells cultured from semen of two patients with AIDS. Science 1984; 226:448-51.
9. Ho DD, Schooley RT, Rota TR, et al. HTLV-III in the semen and blood of a healthy homosexual man. Science 1984; 226:451-3.
10. Update: acquired immunodeficiency syndrome (AIDS) — United States. MMWR 1983; 32:389-91.
11. Update on acquired immune deficiency syndrome (AIDS) — United States. MMWR 1982; 31:507-14.
12. Krause RM. Koch's postulates and the search for the AIDS agent. Rev Infect Dis 1984; 6:270-9.
13. Towbin H, Staehlin T, Gordon J. Electrophoretic transfer of proteins from polyacrylamide gels to nitrocellulose sheets: procedure and some applications. Proc Natl Acad Sci 1979; 76:4350-4.
14. Jaffe HW, Choi K, Thomas PA, et al. National case-control study of Kaposi's sarcoma and *Pneumocystis carinii* pneumonia in homosexual men. 1. Epidemiologic results. Ann Intern Med 1983; 99:145-51.
15. Rogers MF, Morens DM, Stewart JA, et al. National case-control study of Kaposi's sarcoma and *Pneumocystis carinii* pneumonia in homosexual men. 2. Laboratory results. Ann Intern Med 1983; 99:151-8.
16. Lauer JL, VanDrunen NA, Washburn JW, Balfour HH Jr. Transmission of hepatitis B virus in clinical laboratory areas. J Infect Dis 1979; 140: 513-6.
17. Pantelick EL, Steere AC, Lewis HD, Miller DJ. Hepatitis B infection in hospital personnel during an eight-year period: policies for screening and pregnancy in high risk areas. Am J Med 1981; 70:924-7.
18. Dienstag JL, Ryan DM. Occupational exposure to hepatitis B virus in hospital personnel: infection or immunization? Am J Epidemiol 1982; 115: 26-39.

19. Werner BG, Grady GF. Accidental hepatitis-B-surface-antigen-positive inoculations: use of e antigen to estimate infectivity. Ann Intern Med 1982; 97:367-9.
20. An evaluation of the acquired immunodeficiency syndrome (AIDS) reported in health-care personnel — United States. MMWR 1983; 32:358-60.
21. Belani A, Dunning R, Dutta D, et al. AIDS in a hospital worker. Lancet 1984; 1:676.
22. Wormser GP, Joline C, Duncanson F, Cunningham-Rundles S. Needle-stick injuries during the care of patients with AIDS. N Engl J Med 1984; 310:1461.
23. Acquired immune deficiency syndrome (AIDS): precautions for clinical and laboratory staffs. MMWR 1982; 31:577-60.
24. Acquired immunodeficiency syndrome (AIDS): precautions for health-care workers and allied professionals. MMWR 1983; 32:450-1.
25. Conte JE Jr, Hadley WK, Sande M, et al. Infection-control guidelines for patients with the acquired immunodeficiency syndrome (AIDS). N Engl J Med 1983; 309:740-4.
26. Spire B, Barré-Sinoussi F, Montagnier L, Chermann JC. Inactivation of lymphadenopathy associated virus by chemical disinfectants. Lancet 1984; 2:899-901.

ORIGINAL ARTICLE

VACUOLAR MYELOPATHY PATHOLOGICALLY RESEMBLING SUBACUTE COMBINED DEGENERATION IN PATIENTS WITH THE ACQUIRED IMMUNODEFICIENCY SYNDROME

Carol K. Petito, M.D., Bradford A. Navia, M.D., Eun-Sook Cho, M.D., Barry D. Jordan, M.D., Daniel C. George, B.S., and Richard W. Price, M.D.

Abstract Twenty of 89 consecutive patients with the acquired immunodeficiency syndrome (AIDS) in whom autopsies were performed over a 3½-year period had a vacuolar myelopathy that was most severe in the lateral and posterior columns of the thoracic cord. Light and electron microscopy showed that vacuoles were surrounded by a thin myelin sheath and appeared to arise from swelling within myelin sheaths. Signs and symptoms referable to the spinal-cord lesions, including paraparesis, often accompanied by spasticity or ataxia (or both), were present in all five patients with marked pathological changes, in five of seven patients with moderate changes, and in two of eight patients with mild changes. Fourteen patients were demented. The clinical presentation was sufficiently distinctive to provide a guide for antemortem diagnosis. Possible causes of the vacuolar changes include uncharacterized viral infection or a metabolic derangement related to selective nutritional deficiency.

CENTRAL nervous system involvement frequently complicates the acquired immunodeficiency syndrome (AIDS). Approximately 30 percent of patients with AIDS have clinically apparent central nervous system dysfunction, and 80 percent have neuropathological abnormalities at postmortem examination.[1-5] We describe here the clinical and neuropathological features of a previously uncharacterized vacuolar myelopathy that was found in 20 of 89 patients with AIDS who were examined at autopsy at New York Hospital and at Memorial Sloan–Kettering Cancer Center over a 3½-year period.

Methods

Brains and spinal cords from 89 patients with AIDS in whom autopsies were performed between September 1980 and May 1984 were studied according to a protocol previously described.[2] Microscopic sections of spinal cord included mid-thoracic and lumbosacral levels and, often, upper thoracic or upper cervical levels; cervical cord from C2 to C8 was not examined. Pieces of lateral columns from the formalin-fixed thoracic cords of two patients were post-fixed in 2 percent osmium tetroxide, embedded in plastic, and sectioned for light and electron microscopy. Seven spinal cords were assessed for infectious agents with the avidin–biotin conjugate immunoperoxidase method.[6] Primary antiserums included rabbit anti-herpes simplex virus type 2 (DAKO, Santa Barbara, Calif.), which cross-reacts with herpes simplex virus type 1; human herpes zoster convalescent serum with high-titer anti-varicella zoster virus activity[7]; goat antihuman cytomegalovirus serum (Polysciences, Warrington, Pa.); convalescent human anti-*Toxoplasma gondii* serum (courtesy of Dr. Henry Murray, New York Hospital); and rabbit anti-adenovirus (anti-hexon antigen with broad adenovirus reactivity; courtesy of Dr. David Brigate, Hershey Medical Center, Hershey, Pa.). Known positive and negative control tissue was similarly assayed.

The charts of the patients with myelopathy were reviewed with particular focus on neurologic symptoms and signs, systemic complications of AIDS, medications, and nutritional status.

From the Departments of Pathology (Neuropathology) and Neurology, New York Hospital–Cornell Medical Center, Memorial Sloan–Kettering Cancer Center, and the University of Medicine and Dentistry of New Jersey–New Jersey Medical School.

Supported in part by a research grant (A0159) from the New York State AIDS Institute. Dr. Price is a recipient of an Irma T. Hirschl Career Scientist Award.

Results

Clinical

The 20 patients with a vacuolar myelopathy were divided into three groups according to the pathological severity of the myelopathy — Grade I: mild, eight patients; Grade II: moderate, seven patients; and Grade III: marked, five patients (Table 1). There were 19 men and 1 woman with an average age at the time of death of 39 years (range, 26 to 55). Fifteen patients were homosexual, three were intravenous drug addicts, one had both risk factors, and one denied any known risk factor. The average duration of clinical AIDS was 8 months (range, 2 to 17) if the onset of AIDS was designated as the time of presentation with the first opportunistic infection, Kaposi's sarcoma, or in one patient, the unexplained development of central nervous system dysfunction. Nearly all patients had severe weight loss and were emaciated at the time of death.

Serum albumin levels were decreased in all of 16 patients. Serum levels of transaminases and alkaline phosphatase were mildly to markedly abnormal in 16 of 17 patients. No correlation was found between the degree of hepatic dysfunction and the severity of spinal-cord lesions. Seven of 17 patients had a history of treated syphilis, and 2 of 11 had a positive serologic test for syphilis. Serum B_{12} levels were normal in 12 patients; serum folic acid levels were normal in 11 patients and below normal (1.7 ng per milliliter) in 1. The radioassays used (Corning Medical or Becton Dickinson) measured "true" cobalamin.[8] Bone-marrow biopsies disclosed megaloblasts in two of nine patients, both of whom had normal serum B_{12} and folic acid levels.

Opportunistic infections manifested during life or found at autopsy included *Pneumocystis carinii* pneumonia and infections from disseminated cytomegalovirus, oral or gastrointestinal *Candida albicans*, *Mycobacterium avium-intracellulare*, orogenital herpes simplex virus, *Giardia lamblia*, cryptosporidium, sal-

Table 1. Clinical Features and Systemic and Brain Autopsy Findings in 20 Patients with AIDS and Pathologically Defined Myelopathy.*

Pathological Severity	No. of Patients	Risk Factors	Mean Age	Mean Duration of AIDS	Major Systemic Conditions	Mean Duration of CNS Dysfunction	Leg Weakness	Ataxia	Incontinence	Dementia	Brain Disorder
		(no. of patients)	yr	mo	(no. of patients)	mo	no. of patients				(no. of patients)
Grade III (severe)	5	Homosexual (3) Drug abuse (2)	33	10	PCP (5) CMV (4) *C. albicans* (4) *M. avium* (5) HSV (1)	4	5	4	4	4	MGN (3) Vacuolation (3) Gliosis (3)
Grade II (moderate)	7	Homosexual (6) Drug abuse (1)	40	10	PCP (6) CMV (5) *C. albicans* (5) *M. avium* (3) HSV (2) Kaposi's (3) *C. neoformans* (1)	4	5	3	5	5	MGN (5) Vacuolation (1) Gliosis (4)
Grade I (mild)	8	Homosexual (6) Homosexual, drug abuse (1) Undefined (1)	42	6	PCP (7) CMV (6) *C. albicans* (4) *M. avium* (4) HSV (3) Kaposi's (1)	1	1	1	3	5	MGN (7) Vacuolation (1) Gliosis (2)

*CNS denotes central nervous system; PCP, *Pneumocystis carinii* pneumonia; CMV, cytomegalovirus; *M. avium*, *M. avium-intracellulare;* HSV, herpes simplex virus; Kaposi's, Kaposi's sarcoma; MGN, microglial nodule encephalitis; and drug abuse, intravenous drug abuser.

monella, and shigella. Four patients had Kaposi's sarcoma.

Eighteen patients had central nervous system signs or symptoms. The average duration was four months in patients with moderate or severe myelopathy and one month in those with mild myelopathy (overall range, three weeks to eight months). Nine of these patients had been admitted at some point for evaluation of progressive neurologic symptoms. The neurologic evaluation was often incomplete, and evaluation was difficult in patients with overwhelming systemic disease. Three patients had unremarkable myelograms (one with Grade II and two with Grade III myelopathy).

It was sometimes difficult to correlate spinal-cord abnormalities with symptoms and signs in individual patients, since many patients had coexisting peripheral neuropathy or more rostral central nervous system lesions. All five patients with Grade III myelopathy had symptoms and signs that could be attributed to spinal-cord dysfunction. All five had leg weakness. Three had a progressive paraparesis, with spasticity in two and absent reflexes in the third. The fourth patient had a progressive spastic monoparesis of the left leg. The fifth presented with a spastic monoparesis, and quadriparesis developed six months later. Ataxia and incontinence occurred in four patients, and painful, burning paresthesias in one.

Five of the seven patients with Grade II myelopathy had leg weakness and incontinence. Two had spastic paraparesis and ataxia; one each had paraparesis without documented spasticity or ataxia, quadriparesis with areflexia and bilateral extensor plantar responses, and generalized weakness not further characterized. A sixth patient had bilateral extensor plantar responses but no clear documentation of weakness. Three patients had impaired proprioception, although only one had paresthesias.

Motor signs were rare in the eight patients with mild myelopathy. Only one patient had severe generalized weakness accompanied by both upper and lower motor neuron signs. A second patient was ataxic. Three patients were incontinent.

Progressive dementia occurred in 14 of the 20 patients (4 of 5 patients with Grade III myelopathy, 5 of 7 with Grade II, and 5 of 8 with Grade I). Mild memory loss, impaired concentration, slowness, and a blunted affect appeared first and typically progressed over several months, with increasing lethargy, psychomotor retardation, a global cognitive impairment, and in some patients, mutism or coma. Structural lesions that could cause or contribute to dementia were found in only 5 of the 14 patients and included diffuse vacuolation of the centrum semiovale (3 patients) and multiple (3+) microglial nodules (2 patients). Four patients had multifocal myoclonus or terminal generalized seizures or both.

Neuropathology

The spinal cords, subdural spaces, and epidural spaces were grossly normal except in a few patients with severe myelopathy. Their lower thoracic cords were gray and slightly expanded in the posterior and lateral columns.

The myelopathy was defined microscopically as vacuolation in the spinal white matter in association with lipid-laden macrophages, whose presence was required to exclude confusion with a postmortem artifact. The vacuoles were distributed throughout the white matter, were most extensive at the middle to lower thoracic levels, and tended to be more numerous in the lateral than in the posterior columns. Antero-

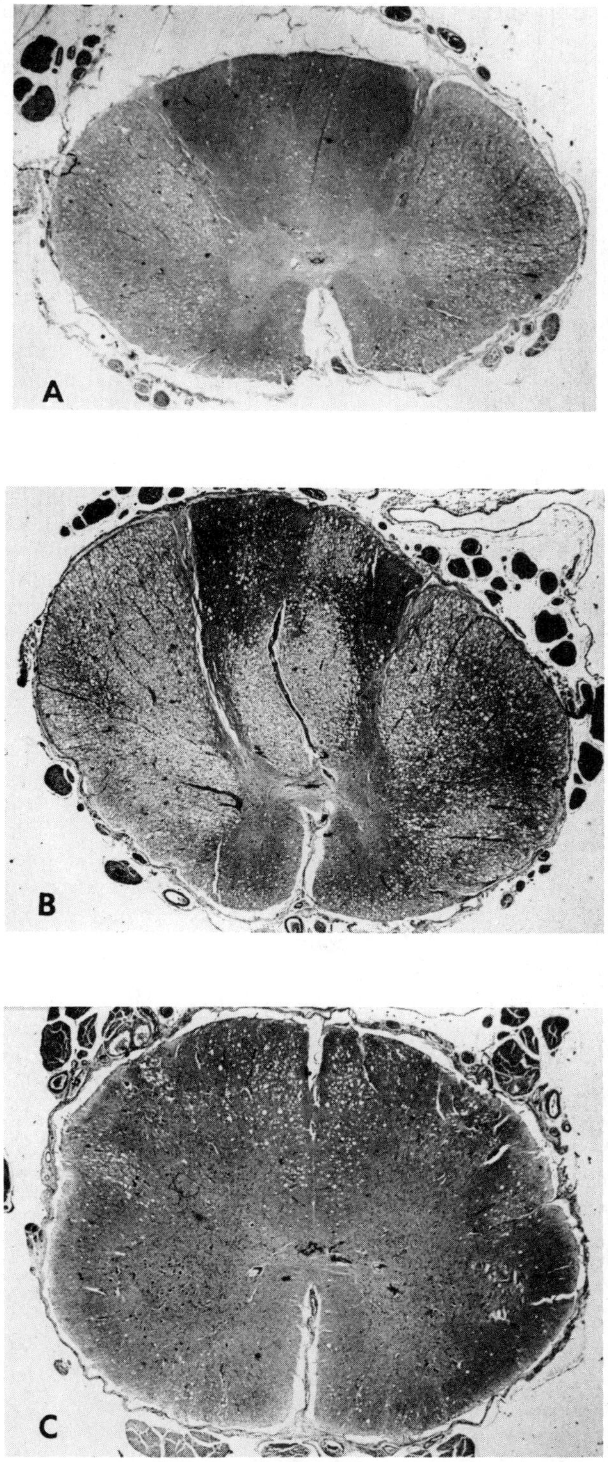

Figure 1. Vacuolation of the Spinal Cord in a Patient with AIDS.

The lower thoracic spinal cord (B) shows marked, confluent vacuolation in the posterior and lateral columns and mild to moderate vacuolation in the anterior columns. The upper thoracic cord (A) and lumbar spinal cord (C) are less severely involved and contain numerous but nonconfluent vacuoles throughout the white matter that are most numerous in the lateral and posterior columns (hematoxylin–eosin stain, ×7.92).

lateral and anterior columns were the least involved. The vacuolation was symmetrical in patients with mild changes but was often asymmetrical in the moderately or markedly severe cases. The vacuolation was not confined to specific anatomic tracts. Five patients had marked changes (Grade III) characterized by areas of confluent vacuolation in the posterior and lateral columns of the mid-thoracic cord. Numerous nonconfluent vacuoles were present at upper-thoracic and at lumbosacral levels (Fig. 1). Seven patients had moderate changes (Grade II) characterized by numerous but nonconfluent vacuoles (similar in severity to the illustrations in Fig. 1A and 1C). Eight patients had mild changes (Grade I) with no more than 15 vacuoles per transverse section.

A thin myelin sheath surrounded the vacuoles (Fig. 2 and 3). Occasionally, the thinned myelin sheath was in continuity with the sheath of a normally myelinated axon, suggesting that the vacuoles had formed by intramyelin swelling. Axons were usually normal in areas of mild to moderate vacuolation but were disrupted in areas of severe vacuolation. Wallerian degeneration was found in the lateral corticospinal tracts of several of these patients. Some of the axons with intramyelin vacuoles were shrunken on electron microscopy. Axons without myelin sheaths could not be found. Intraaxonal vacuoles were not seen. Lipid-laden macrophages were present in small numbers and were usually located within the vacuoles (Fig. 2) or, as seen by electron microscopy, within myelin sheaths. Reactive astrocytes were rare. Inflammation, organisms, and intranuclear viral inclusions were not seen. Immunohistochemical studies performed on the spinal cords of seven patients were negative for herpes simplex virus, varicella zoster virus, cytomegalovirus, *T. gondii,* and adenovirus.

Five patients had central chromatolysis of anterior-horn motor neurons, and two patients had a few microglial nodules in the spinal-cord gray matter. A single section of proximal femoral nerve in four of six patients showed focal loss of myelin and axons.

Five patients had vacuolation in the brain, similar microscopically to that in the spinal cords. Four of these patients had moderate or marked vacuolation in the spinal cord. The white-matter vacuoles were located in the cerebral and cerebellar hemispheres and brain stem in one patient, in the centrum semiovale in two patients, and in the brain stem in two patients. The corticospinal tracts in the cervical or upper thoracic spinal cord in these five patients were normal or only mildly vacuolated, thereby excluding Wallerian degeneration as the cause of the more severe myelopathy present at the lower thoracic levels.

Brain weight was measured in 14 patients and averaged 1287 g (range, 1125 to 1500). There was no correlation between brain weight and pathologic processes in the brain or spinal cord or between brain weight and the presence or absence of dementia. The microglial nodule encephalitis described elsewhere[1,2] was found in 15 of 20 patients and was associated with cytomegalovirus inclusions in 2 patients, chronic healed toxoplasmosis and cytomegalovirus in 1, and cryptococcal meningitis in 1. An additional patient had chronic and subacute toxoplasmosis and acute candida abscesses. Two brains were grossly and microscopically normal, one showed acute hypoxic–ischemic encephalopathy, and one had only diffuse white-matter vacuolation as described above. Pertinent negative findings included the absence of Alzheimer type II astrocytes, of microcavitation in the basal ganglia or cerebral cortex, of neurofibrillary tangles, and of senile plaques.

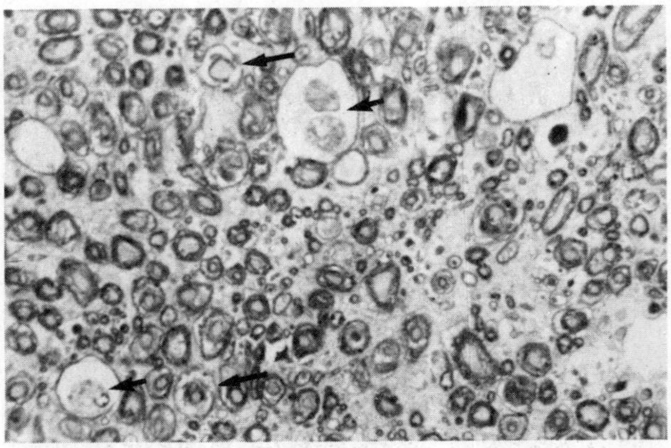

Figure 2. A 1-μm Plastic-Embedded Section from the Lateral Column of a Patient with Moderately Severe Myelopathy, Showing Vacuoles Surrounded by a Thin Myelin Sheath.

Two vacuoles contain lipid-laden macrophages (short arrows). A few myelin sheaths, two of which are indicated by long arrows, show mild intramyelin swelling. The remaining myelinated axons appear normal or show myelin changes consistent with postmortem artifacts (toluidine blue stain, ×1085).

Discussion

This study describes the clinical and pathological features of a previously uncharacterized vacuolar myelopathy in patients with AIDS. This myelopathy is common; it was found in 22 percent of consecutive autopsies of patients with AIDS. The pathological changes were most prominent in the lateral and posterior columns at the thoracic level and appeared to be initiated by focal swellings within the myelin sheath. Axonal destruction was evident only in areas of more intense vacuolation. Long-tract degeneration of the spinal cord, reported recently in a 36-year-old man with AIDS,[9] may represent the same disorder as that found in our patients.

The clinical findings correlated with the severity of the myelopathy and were sufficiently distinct in many patients to provide a guide to antemortem diagnosis. A steadily progressive spastic–ataxic paraparesis, which usually continued to evolve over several weeks to months, and urinary incontinence were most characteristic of patients with a severe myelopathy. Signs and symptoms were similar but less frequent in patients with Grade II myelopathy, but clear myelopathic signs were infrequent in the eight patients with Grade I myelopathy.

Dementia was common in these patients. Although an association between the dementia and the myelopathy is suggested by the similar character of the dementia in each of the patients and the concomitant development and progression of the paraparesis and dementia, no correlation was evident between the incidence and severity of the dementia and the severity of the myelopathy. The absence of serious abnormalities in the brains of many of the demented patients with AIDS and myelopathy, as well as ongoing review of our autopsy cases, suggests that AIDS dementia is not necessarily due to microglial nodule encephalitis.

The cause of the myelopathy is unknown. There were no apparent differences with respect to systemic infections or neoplasms, medications, or clinical laboratory findings between these patients and the remainder of patients with AIDS seen in our institutions or described elsewhere[1,10] (and unpublished data). There was no evidence for cord compression or Wallerian degeneration due to structural lesions. Pathological features caused by conventional infectious agents, including inflammation, microglial nodules, microorganisms, and intranuclear viral inclusions, were not present, and immunohistochemical studies for the antigens of herpes simplex virus, varicella zoster virus, cytomegalovirus, *T. gondii*, and adenovirus were negative.

None of our patients were exposed to the toxic agents that may produce intramyelin swellings or spinal-cord lesions,[11-16] except for six patients who received isoniazid. Metabolic disorders associated with spinal-cord lesions, including hepatic disease with portacaval shunt,[17,18] nicotinic acid deficiency (pellagra),[19,20] and severe nutritional deficiencies,[21,22] can be excluded as possible causes. The myelopathy in these disorders is a dying-back or a Wallerian-type degeneration rather than white-matter vacuolation.

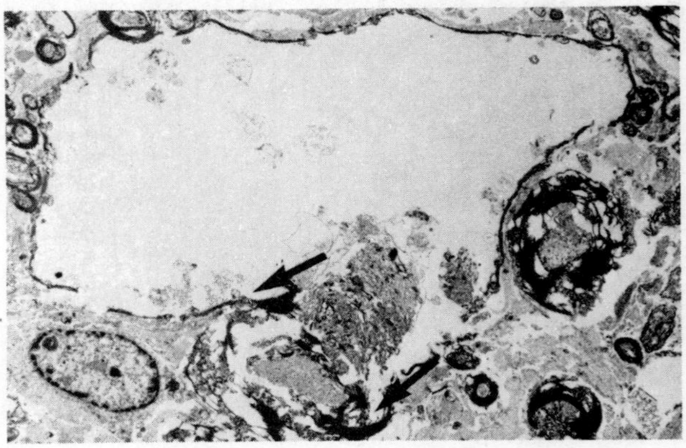

Figure 3. Electron Micrograph from an Area of Marked Vacuolation, Demonstrating a Vacuole Surrounded by a Thin Myelin Sheath.

The arrows indicate points at which the myelin sheath is split by the intramyelin swelling (×2720).

Furthermore, the brains of our patients showed no evidence of hepatic encephalopathy or hepatocerebral degeneration.

The pathologic changes in the spinal cords of the patients most closely resembled subacute combined degeneration due to vitamin B_{12} deficiency[23] or, rarely, folic acid deficiency.[24] Both deficiencies cause spongy vacuolation of myelin due to intramyelin swelling that predominantly affects the posterior and lateral columns, although the most severe lesions in subacute combined degeneration are in posterior columns at cervical or upper thoracic levels.[23,25] The clinical manifestations of B_{12} deficiency resemble AIDS myelopathy and include a progressive spastic paraparesis and ataxia that may be accompanied by dementia and polyneuropathy.[26,27] However, sensory symptoms are more common in B_{12} deficiency and occur early in the course, whereas bladder or bowel dysfunction is a late development.

Subacute combined degeneration may occur without serum B_{12} deficiency and has been reported in association with systemic lupus erythematosus[28] and with a familial defect in cobalamin metabolism.[29] It may be produced by prolonged exposure to nitrous oxide in human beings[30] and other primates.[31] Nitrous oxide may inhibit methionine synthetase, a B_{12}-dependent enzyme, since subacute combined degeneration following nitrous oxide exposure may be prevented by supplementation of dietary methionine.[31] Precipitation or exacerbation of subacute combined degeneration by folic acid administration to B_{12}-deficient patients may be due to a shunting of methionine away from methylation reactions that are important for myelin integrity and function. A similar mechanism may precipitate subacute combined degeneration when folic acid is given to patients who are not B_{12}-deficient but are malnourished and have a possible methionine deficiency.[32] Perturbations of metabolic pathways related to B_{12} and methionine may have been responsible for the myelopathy in our patients with AIDS, since their disease so closely resembled that seen with B_{12} deficiency yet their serum B_{12} and folic acid levels were normal.

Infection of the spinal cord by a previously uncharacterized agent warrants etiologic consideration in this group of severely immunocompromised patients, who may be susceptible to infection by a virus of low pathogeneity in the normal host. A report of a similar myelopathy in a patient with systemic lupus erythematosus and normal serum B_{12} levels suggests a possible precedent in a patient without AIDS.[28] One possible pathogen is human retrovirus, since recent data strongly implicate lymphadenopathy-associated virus[33] or human T-cell lymphotrophic virus III (HTLV-III)[34] as the causative agent for AIDS, and since another type of retrovirus, found in mice, infects the central nervous system without eliciting an inflammatory response.[35] In contrast to AIDS myelopathy, however, the murine retrovirus infection produces a spongiform encephalopathy of gray-matter structures with intracytoplasmic vacuolation in neurons and glial cells.[36,37] Although this pathologic process was not seen in the spinal cords or brains of any of our patients with AIDS, the recent identification of HTLV-III in the brains of patients with AIDS indicates the potential neurotropism of this virus.[38] Clarification of its relation to AIDS myelopathy awaits further study.

Note added in proof: Since submission of this article, the abstracted case report of Goldstick et al.[9] has been published in full.[39]

We are indebted to Dr. J. Lindenbaum for his helpful suggestions and to Drs. J. Gold, R. Roberts, and S. Nielsen for data and serum samples.

References

1. Snider WD, Simpson DM, Nielsen S, Gold JWM, Metroka C, Posner JB. Neurological complications of acquired immune deficiency syndrome: analysis of 50 patients. Ann Neurol 1983; 14:403-18.
2. Nielsen SL, Petito CK, Urmacher CD, Posner JB. Subacute encephalitis in acquired immune deficiency syndrome: a post-mortem study. Am J Clin Pathol 1984; 82:678-82.
3. Jordan BD, Navia BA, Petito C, Cho L, Price RW. Neurological syndromes complicating AIDS. Front Radiat Ther Oncol 1985; 19:82-7.
4. Britton CB, Miller JR. Neurologic complications in acquired immunodeficiency syndrome (AIDS). Neurol Clin 1984; 2:315-39.
5. Anders K, Verity MA, Cancilla PA, Vinters HV. Acquired immune deficiency syndrome (AIDS): neuropathologic studies. J Neuropathol Exp Neurol 1984; 43:315.
6. Hsu S-M, Raine L, Fanger H. Use of avidin-biotin-peroxidase complex (ABC) in immunoperoxidase techniques: a comparison between ABC and unlabeled antibody (PAP) procedures. J Histochem Cytochem 1981; 29:577-80.
7. Horten B, Price RW, Jimenez D. Multifocal varicella-zoster virus leukoencephalitis temporally remote from herpes zoster. Ann Neurol 1981; 9: 251-66.
8. Kolhouse JF, Kondo H, Allen NC, Podell E, Allen RH. Cobalamin analogues are present in human plasma and can mask cobalamin deficiency because current radioisotopic dilution assays are not specific for true cobalamin. N Engl J Med 1978; 299:785-92.
9. Goldstick L, Mandybur TI, Means E. Spinal cord long tract degeneration in AIDS. J Neuropathol Exp Neurol 1984; 43:294.
10. Fauci AS, Macher AM, Longo DL, et al. Acquired immunodeficiency syndrome: epidemiologic, clinical, immunologic and therapeutic considerations. Ann Intern Med 1984; 100:92-106.
11. Powell HC, Lampert PW. Hexachlorophene toxicity. In: Vinken PJ, Bruyn GW, eds. Handbook of clinical neurology. Vol. 37. New York: Elsevier, 1979:479-509.
12. Watanabe I, Hodges GR, Dworzack DL, Kepes JJ, Duensing GF. Neurotoxicity of intrathecal gentamicin: a case report and experimental study. Ann Neurol 1978; 4:564-72.
13. Hodges GR, Watanabe I. Chemical injury of the spinal cord of the rabbit after intracisternal injection of gentamicin: an ultrastructural study. J Neuropathol Exp Neurol 1980; 39:452-75.
14. Cammer W. Toxic demyelination: biochemical studies and hypothetical mechanisms. In: Spencer PS, Schaumburg HH, eds. Experimental and clinical neurotoxicology. Baltimore: Williams & Wilkins, 1980:239-56.
15. Shiraki, Hirotsugu. Neuropathological aspects of the etiopathogenesis of subacute myelo-optico-neuropathy (SMON). In: Vinken PJ, Bruyn GW, eds. Handbook of clinical neurology. Vol. 37. New York: Elsevier, 1979:141-98.
16. Hoover DM, Carlton WW, Henrikson CK. Ultrastructural lesions of clioquinol toxicity in beagle dogs. Food Cosmet Toxicol 1981; 19:200-7.
17. Victor M, Adams RD, Cole M. The acquired (non-Wilsonian) type of chronic hepatocerebral degeneration. Medicine (Baltimore) 1965; 44:345-96.
18. Pant SS, Rebeiz JJ, Richardson EP. Spastic paraparesis following portocaval shunts. Neurology (Minneap) 1968; 18:134-41.
19. Leigh D. Pellagra and the nutritional neuropathies: a neuropathologic review. J Ment Sci 1952; 98:130-42.
20. Still CN. Nicotinic acid and nicotinamide deficiency: pellagra and related disorders of the nervous system. In: Vinken PJ, Bruyn GW, eds. Handbook of clinical neurology. Vol. 28. New York: Elsevier, 1976:59-104.
21. Denny-Brown D. Neurological conditions resulting from prolonged and severe dietary restriction. Medicine (Baltimore) 1947; 26:41-113.
22. Grieve S, Jacobson S, Proctor NSF. A nutritional myelopathy occurring in the Bantu on the Witwatersrand. Neurology (Minneap) 1967; 17:1205-12.

23. Pant SS, Asbury AK, Richardson EP Jr. The myelopathy of pernicious anemia. Acta Neurol Scand (Suppl) 1968; 44:4-36.
24. Robertson DM, Dinsdale HB, Campbell RJ. Subacute combined degeneration of the spinal cord: no association with vitamin B_{12} deficiency. Arch Neurol 1971; 24:203-7.
25. Agamanolis DP, Victor M, Harris JW, Hines JD, Chester EM, Kark JA. An ultrastructural study of subacute combined degeneration of the spinal cord in vitamin B_{12}-deficient rhesus monkeys. J Neuropathol Exp Neurol 1978; 37:273-99.
26. Shulman R. Psychiatric aspects of pernicious anemia: a prospective controlled investigation. Br Med J 1967; 3:266-70.
27. Roos D. Neurological symptoms and signs in a selected group of partially gastrectomized patients with particular reference to B_{12} deficiency. Acta Neurol Scand 1974; 50:719-52.
28. Johnson RT, Richardson EP Jr. The neurological manifestations of systemic lupus erythematosus. Medicine (Baltimore) 1968; 47:337-69.
29. Shinnar S, Singer HS. Cobalamin C mutation (methylmalonic aciduria and homocystinuria in adolescence: a treatable case of dementia and myelopathy. N Engl J Med 1984; 311:451-4.
30. Layzer RB. Myeloneuropathy after prolonged exposure to nitrous oxide. Lancet 1978; 2:1227-30.
31. Scott JM, Dinn JJ, Wilson P, Wrir DG. Pathogenesis of subacute combined degeneration: a result of methyl group deficiency. Lancet 1981; 334-7.
32. Scott JM, Weir DG. The methyl folate trap. Lancet 1981; 337-40.
33. Barré-Sinoussi F, Chermann JC, Rey F, et al. Isolation of a T-lymphotropic retrovirus from a patient at risk for acquired immune deficiency syndrome (AIDS). Science 1983; 220:868-70.
34. Gallo RC, Salahuddin SZ, Popovic M, et al. Frequent detection and isolation of cytopathic retroviruses (HTLV-III) from patients with AIDS and at risk for AIDS. Science 1984; 224:500-3.
35. Oldstone MBA, Lampert PW, Lee S, Dixon FJ. Pathogenesis of the slow disease of the central nervous system associated with WM 1504 E virus. 1. Relationship of strain susceptibility and replication to disease. Am J Pathol 1977; 88:193-212.
36. Oldstone MBA, Jensen F, Dixon FJ, Lampert PW. Pathogenesis of the slow disease of the central nervous system associated with wild mouse virus. Virology 1980; 107:180-93.
37. Swarz JR, Brooks BR, Johnson RT. Spongiform polioencephalomyelopathy caused by a murine retrovirus. II. Ultrastructural localization of virus replication and spongiform changes in the central nervous system. Neuropathol Appl Neurobiol 1981; 7:365-80.
38. Shaw GM, Harper ME, Hahn BH, et al. HTLV-III infection in brains of children and adults with AIDS encephalopathy. Science 1985; 227:177-81.
39. Goldstick L, Mandybur TI, Bode R. Spinal cord degeneration in AIDS. Neurology 1985; 35:103-5.

ORIGINAL ARTICLE

QUALITATIVE ANALYSIS OF IMMUNE FUNCTION IN PATIENTS WITH THE ACQUIRED IMMUNODEFICIENCY SYNDROME

Evidence for a Selective Defect in Soluble Antigen Recognition

H. Clifford Lane, M.D., Joel M. Depper, M.D., Warner C. Greene, M.D., Ph.D., Gail Whalen, B.S., Thomas A. Waldmann, M.D., and Anthony S. Fauci, M.D.

Abstract We studied purified subpopulations of lymphocytes from patients with the acquired immunodeficiency syndrome (AIDS) in order to determine whether intrinsic defects in lymphocyte function, aside from those due to alterations in lymphocyte numbers, were present. Mitogen-stimulated DNA synthesis, production of gamma interferon, production of interleukin-2, and expression of interleukin-2 receptors, although variably decreased in unseparated cell populations, were normal in populations of purified T-cell subsets. In contrast, DNA synthesis in response to the soluble protein antigen tetanus toxoid was decreased in both unseparated and purified T-cell subpopulations. Cell-mixing experiments demonstrated that the hyporesponsiveness of the unfractionated lymphocytes from patients with AIDS was not due to active suppression. We conclude that the lymphocytes of patients with AIDS, although capable of undergoing a normal degree of blast transformation and lymphokine production after mitogenic stimulation, have an intrinsic defect in their ability to recognize and respond to soluble antigen.

The acquired immunodeficiency syndrome (AIDS) has become one of the most challenging problems in modern medicine. The variety of infections seen in patients with this illness bespeaks an immune system that is incapable of protecting the host against the most indolent of environmental organisms. The unusually high occurrence of Kaposi's sarcoma in patients with AIDS underscores the role of the immune system in protecting the host against malignant processes and will possibly provide a window that will allow us to understand this particular function of the immune system to a greater degree. In addition to infectious and malignant processes, patients with AIDS have been reported to have a wide variety of autoimmune phenomena — suggesting that these patients have immunoregulatory defects at multiple levels of the immune system.

The etiologic agents of this syndrome are a family of human retroviruses — including human T-cell lymphotropic virus Type III (HTLV-III) and lymphadenopathy-associated virus (LAV) — that are cytotropic and cytopathic for T lymphocytes.[1,2] The precise way in which these viruses cause the profound immune-deficiency state characteristic of AIDS is not well delineated. Recent reports suggest that these viruses act in vitro through mechanisms that are selective for the helper/inducer subpopulation of T cells.[3]

The immune systems of patients with AIDS are characterized by a profound decrease in the ratio of helper to suppressor cells, due predominantly to a defect in the number of circulating T lymphocytes bearing the helper/inducer phenotype (T4 or Leu-3).[4-16] It is thought that this decrease in the number of helper lymphocytes is responsible for the variety of immunologic abnormalities that have been described in this syndrome. These abnormalities include decreased blast transformation to mitogens and antigens,[4-16] decreased lymphokine production,[14,15] decreased expression of interleukin-2 receptors,[17] decreased alloreactivity,[5,11,12] and a decreased ability to provide help to B lymphocytes.[9,18] However, it is unclear whether these abnormalities are due to decreased numbers of lymphocytes or to intrinsic defects of the lymphocytes.

Two separate studies have examined the ability of purified lymphocyte subsets from patients with AIDS to help or suppress mitogen-stimulated immunoglobulin production.[9,18] In both studies the helper T lymphocytes appeared to be qualitatively defective, whereas the suppressor T lymphocytes functioned normally.

In this study, we have evaluated the ability of purified subsets of T lymphocytes from patients with AIDS to undergo blast transformation in response to mitogenic lectins or the soluble protein antigen tetanus toxoid. Moreover, we have evaluated four components of mitogenic responses that have been implicated in the pathogenesis of abnormal immune responses in patients with AIDS — namely, interleukin-2 production, expression of interleukin-2 receptors, gamma interferon production, and suppressor phenomena. Our findings suggest that the underlying immune defect in AIDS is a selective, qualitative inability of the helper/inducer T-cell subpopulation to respond to soluble antigen.

Methods

Patients

The 12 patients selected for this study all had clinically defined AIDS according to the surveillance definition established by the Centers for Disease Control.[19] Eleven of the 12 patients were homosexual men. Six of these had Kaposi's sarcoma only; three had completely recovered from an initial bout of *Pneumocystis carinii* pneumonia; one had Kaposi's sarcoma and had completely recovered from an initial bout of *P. carinii* pneumonia; and one had Kaposi's sarcoma and had recovered from a lymphocytic menin-

From the Laboratory of Immunoregulation, National Institute of Allergy and Infectious Diseases; the Metabolism Branch, National Cancer Institute; and Critical Care Medicine, Clinical Center, National Institutes of Health, Bethesda, Md.

gitis. The remaining patient was a man with transfusion-associated AIDS who had recovered completely from an initial bout of *P. carinii* pneumonia. The age range of the group was 22 to 55. Healthy normal volunteers 21 to 38 years of age served as control subjects.

Cell Populations

Unfractionated peripheral-blood mononuclear cells were obtained by Hypaque–Ficoll separation of peripheral blood or buffy coats obtained by the technique of manual plasmapheresis.[20] All procedures were carried out according to peer-reviewed protocols of the National Institutes of Health.

Peripheral-blood mononuclear cells forming rosettes with sheep red cells previously treated with S-2-aminoethylisothiuronium bromide hydrobromide (AET; Sigma Chemical, St. Louis) were obtained by Hypaque–Ficoll separation and subsequent lysis of the red cells with ammonium chloride.[21]

T4+ or T8+ lymphocytes were obtained by positive selection. Erythrocyte-rosette–positive cells were treated with 0.05 ml of OKT4 or OKT8 monoclonal antibody (Ortho Pharmaceuticals, Raritan, N.J.) per 10^6 cells. The suspensions were incubated at 4°C for 45 minutes, washed three times, and then rosetted with ox red cells that had been coated with goat antimouse immunoglobulin (Boehringer Mannheim Biochemicals, Indianapolis) and rosette-positive cells obtained as described above. Cells obtained in this manner contained 5 percent or less of the opposite cell type.

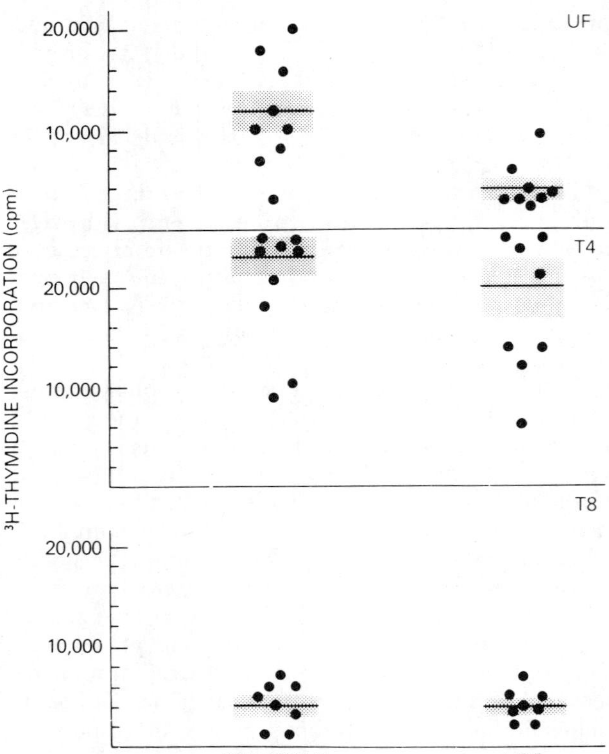

Figure 1. Proliferative Responses of Unfractionated Cells, Purified T4 Cells, and Purified T8 Cells from Patients with AIDS and from Controls to the Nonspecific Signal Delivered by Pokeweed Mitogen.

Data points indicate the mean net number of counts per minute of triplicate cultures from individual patients. The shaded areas represent the means ±SEM Data for the unfractionated cells are shown in the upper graph, for T4 cells in the middle graph, and for T8 cells in the lower graph. The diminished responses seen in AIDS unfractionated cells are not seen when purified T-cell subsets are studied.

Functional Assays

Proliferative responses were measured in 96-well, round-bottomed microtiter plates (Costar Data Packaging, Cambridge, Mass.). Each well contained 50,000 cells of the type being tested; 10,000 irradiated autologous AET-negative cells to serve as a source of monocytes or macrophages; and one of the following: no mitogen or antigen at all; 2 μg of phytohemagglutinin per milliliter (Wellcome Research Laboratories, Beckenham, England); a 1:200 dilution of pokeweed mitogen (Gibco Laboratories, Grand Island, N.Y.); 5 μg of tetanus toxoid per milliliter (Lederle Laboratories, Pearl River, N.Y.); or 50,000 allogeneic irradiated AET-negative cells. All cultures were performed in a final volume of 200 μl. The culture medium was RPMI-1640 containing 15 percent human serum from subjects who had blood group A. Proliferative responses were measured by the incorporation of [^{3}H]thymidine over a four-hour pulse with 2 μCi of [^{3}H]thymidine (New England Nuclear, Boston). Proliferative responses to phytohemagglutinin were measured on Day 3, and those to pokeweed mitogen, tetanus toxoid, or alloantigen were measured on Day 5 or 6.

Lymphokine Production and Measurement of Tac Antigen Expression

Cultures containing 2×10^6 cells of the type being tested, 4×10^5 irradiated AET-negative cells, and 10 μg of phytohemagglutinin were performed in 24-well, flat-bottomed culture dishes (Costar) containing 1 ml of RPMI-1640 and 10 percent fetal-calf serum (Dutchland Laboratories, Denver, Pa.). Supernatants and cells were harvested at 48 hours. Biofluids (Rockville, Md.) assayed the gamma-interferon activity in the supernatant by measuring the ability of the supernatants to inhibit the cytopathic effect of vesicular stomatitis virus on WISH cells.[22] The expression of interleukin-2 receptors was measured by binding of monoclonal [^{3}H]anti-Tac antibody (anti-interleukin-2 receptor antibody).[23,24] Binding data were normalized to the number of molecules of anti-Tac bound per viable cell at the time of assay. Interleukin-2 activity in supernatants was measured in a standard proliferation assay using murine CTLL cells as previously described.[25]

Results

The proliferative responses to pokeweed mitogen of unfractionated peripheral-blood mononuclear cells, purified T4 cells, and purified T8 cells from eight patients with AIDS and eight simultaneous controls are shown in Figure 1. Although there was a significant difference in the mean proliferative responses of the unfractionated cells in the controls and the patients (12,000 vs. 4000, $P<0.01$), the proliferative responses for both the T4 cells (23,200 vs. 20,000, $P>0.05$) and the T8 cells (4000 vs. 4000, $P>0.05$) were essentially the same. Similar data (not shown) were obtained with the use of the pure T-cell mitogen phytohemagglutinin.

The integrity of the mechanisms that allow the individual lymphocyte subsets to mount proliferative responses to mitogen was confirmed by studies of the expression of interleukin-2 receptors, interleukin-2 production, and gamma interferon production (Table 1). Although interleukin-2 receptor expression was decreased in the unfractionated cells of patients with AIDS, this decrease was not statistically significant. No differences were seen in the T4 or T8 subsets of patients and controls.

Having demonstrated that cultures of T4 cells from patients with AIDS were capable of proliferating normally in response to mitogens, we turned our attention

Table 1. Mitogen-Induced Expression of Interleukin-2 (IL-2) Receptors and Lymphokine Production.*

Cells	IL-2 Receptors		IL-2 Production		γ-Interferon Production	
	control	AIDS	control	AIDS	control	AIDS
	molecules bound†		*units/ml*		*units/ml*	
Unfractionated	58.5±6.2	45.6±8	3.2±1.3	4.0±2.6	334±83	343±152
T4	39.7±9.9	47.0±14	3.5±1.4	2.9±0.7	528±366	676±175
T8	28.7±9.8	41.2±10	0.5±0.5	1.8±1.0	520±187	1217±461

*All cultures were stimulated with 2 μg of phytohemagglutinin per milliliter. Data are expressed as means ±SEM for five separate experiments.

†Values are numbers of molecules (anti-Tac) bound per cell $\times 10^{-3}$.

to determining whether or not the decreased proliferation in response to mitogen that was seen in cultures of unfractionated cells from patients with AIDS was due to suppressor activity of the other cells in the unfractionated pool. In order to assess such suppressor activity, one cocultures cells with suspected suppressor activity with an indicator population of cells that, on their own, exhibit a normal level of responsiveness. For these experiments, we chose mitogen-stimulated unfractionated cells from control subjects or T4 cells from patients with AIDS as our indicator populations. This allowed us to assess not only whether there was enhanced suppressor activity in any subset of mononuclear cells from the patients but also whether their T4 cells were especially susceptible to suppressor influences. As can be seen from Table 2, the addition of T8 cells, B cells plus monocytes, irradiated T4 cells, or unfractionated cells from patients or controls either to unfractionated peripheral-blood mononuclear cells from a control or to T4 cells from a patient did not suppress and, in some instances, even slightly enhanced the net proliferative responses. Similar data (not shown) were obtained in three other experiments.

In contrast to the findings in the study of lymphocyte responses to mitogen, lymphocytes from patients with AIDS failed to respond normally to the soluble protein antigen tetanus toxoid either as unfractionated cells or as purified populations of T4 cells (Fig. 2). Lymphocytes from only one patient exhibited any proliferation at all in response to tetanus toxoid. This patient was unique in that his only clinical manifestation of AIDS was Kaposi's sarcoma limited to the lymph nodes. The capacity to respond to soluble antigen is a unique property of T4 cells, and thus neither T8 cells from controls nor those from patients responded. Studies of interleukin-2 receptor expression and interleukin-2 production in response to tetanus toxoid were attempted in parallel with the studies on proliferation. The responses of both controls' and patients' lymphocytes were so low, however, that no meaningful comparisons could be made.

In the next series of experiments, the ability of unfractionated peripheral-blood mononuclear cells, purified T4 cells, or purified T8 lymphocytes to proliferate in response to alloantigen was examined (Table 3). As in the case of the mitogen-stimulated cultures, enhanced proliferative responses were seen when purified T4 lymphocytes were examined. Although the response of the T4 cells from patients with AIDS was still less than that of the control cells, this subset was at least capable of recognizing and proliferating in response to alloantigen.

In the final series of experiments, designed to assess the degree of functional in vivo lymphocyte activation, unfractionated cells and T-lymphocyte subsets from patients with AIDS and from controls were examined for their degree of spontaneous proliferation. In these experiments unfractionated cells from patients exhibited substantially more spontaneous proliferation than did the unfractionated cells from controls (Fig. 3). This increased proliferation was noted not only in unfractionated cells but also in unseparated T cells, purified T4 cells, and purified T8 cells.

Discussion

This study has demonstrated that the helper/inducer T lymphocytes of patients with AIDS respond

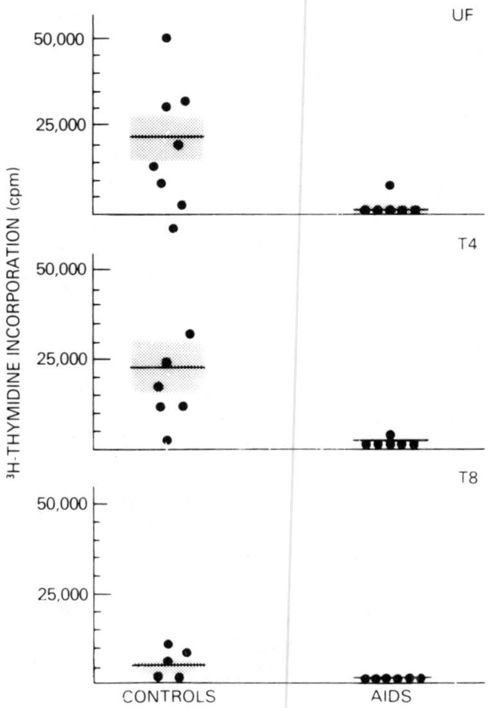

Figure 2. Proliferative Responses of Unfractionated Cells, Purified T4 Cells, and Purified T8 Cells from Patients with AIDS and from Controls to the Antigen-Specific Signal Delivered by Tetanus Toxoid.

Data points indicate the mean net number of counts per minute of triplicate cultures from individual patients. The shaded areas represent the means ±SEM Data for the unfractionated cells are shown in the upper graph, for T4 cells in the middle graph, and for T8 cells in the lower graph. The diminished responses seen in AIDS unfractionated cells are also present in purified T4 cells.

Table 2. Suppressor Activity in Mononuclear-Cell Subpopulations from Patients with AIDS and from Controls.*

Indicator Cells	Test Cells		
	Cell type added	Control†	AIDS†
		cpm incorporated	
Unfractionated peripheral-blood mononuclear cells from a control subject	None (base line)	22,100	22,100
	T8	33,000	26,000
	Irradiated T4‡	27,000	21,200
	$T4^-/T8^-$ E-rosette$^+$ cells	18,100	19,700
	B cells plus monocytes	45,400	38,800
T4 cells from a patient	None (base line)	17,000	17,000
	T8	28,800	22,300
	Irradiated T4‡	15,200	26,100
	$T4^-/T8^-$ E-rosette$^+$ cells	18,400	27,500
	B cells plus monocytes	28,100	36,300

*Fifty thousand test cells were added to 50,000 indicator cells from either a control subject or a patient with AIDS. All cultures were stimulated with 2 μg of phytohemagglutinin per milliliter.

†Values indicate tritiated thymidine incorporation as measured on Day 3.

‡Cells received 1500 R before culture.

normally to mitogen and are capable of proliferating in response to alloantigen; however, they exhibit a selective qualitative defect in the ability to respond to soluble antigen. This may represent the initial critical immune defect in patients with AIDS. The helper/inducer T lymphocyte is the central cell type in the immune system and is responsible for the induction and regulation of virtually all cellular immune functions at both the T-cell and the B-cell levels.[26] One of its primary unique immune functions among those of the T-cell repertoire is its ability to recognize and proliferate in response to soluble protein antigens. This recognition capability coupled with the ability of the helper/inducer cell to recruit other immune cells into action is thought to be the essence of the specificity of the immune system. The striking intactness of the ability of these purified lymphocyte subsets to respond to such nonspecific stimuli as phytohemagglutinin or pokeweed mitogen with DNA synthesis and lymphokine production suggests that the critical immunologic lesion in this syndrome is an inability of the T lymphocyte to recognize and be triggered by a specific stimulus, rather than an inability to mount an effector function after cell triggering.

This selective defect in antigen reactivity is comparable to a defect observed in patients with AIDS and patients with hemophilia A that suggested a qualitative defect in the helper/inducer cells that give rise to an autologous mixed-lymphocyte response.[27,28] Insofar as the autoreactive cell is believed to represent a subset of the antigen-reactive cells in the human system, these data are in agreement.[29]

The data presented here demonstrating intact interleukin-2 production, gamma interferon production, and Tac expression are in contrast to those of numerous other reports.[14,15,17] The main distinguishing feature of this report is that purified subsets were studied in addition to unfractionated cells and that the patients selected for these studies were often at the earliest phase of the clinically defined AIDS spectrum — that is, they were patients with only Kaposi's sarcoma and with total lymphocyte counts generally above 1000 cells per cubic millimeter. Thus, immunologic abnormalities due to secondary infections or to alterations in lymphocyte number rather than function were minimized.

A decrease in the proliferative responses of unfractionated cells that is not seen in purified subpopulations of cells could conceivably be due either to a selective alteration in the function of the responding subset or to an active suppressor influence expressed by a suppressor subset. Accordingly, mixing experiments were done to determine the ability of different subsets of cells from patients with AIDS to suppress either autologous or allogeneic proliferative responses. The inability of both unfractionated cells and T-cell subsets from patients to suppress either AIDS or normal lymphocytes in optimal systems provides strong evidence that the basic defect in the AIDS immune system is a lack of help rather than an overabundance of suppression.

In this study as well as in previous ones, purified populations of T8 lymphocytes functioned normally when provided with appropriate inducer signals in the form of either lymphokines or allogeneic helper/inducer T cells. This relative intactness of T8 function with a selective defect in T4 function fits well with the current hypothesis that AIDS is due to a human retrovirus (HTLV-III or LAV) with a selective tropism for the T4 lymphocyte.[2,3,30,31]

The marked elevation in spontaneous T-lymphocyte proliferation probably represents an in vivo state of activation of the T lymphocyte in patients with AIDS. This correlates with the earlier observations that patients with this syndrome have an increased percentage of cells in the peripheral blood that bear surface markers of activation.[10] Data not presented here show that this elevation in spontaneous lymphocyte proliferation is a property of B cells as well as T cells. The fact that this elevation in spontaneous proliferation has not been seen in all patients with AIDS

Table 3. Alloreactivity of AIDS and Control Lymphocyte Subsets.*

Cells	Control†	AIDS†
	cpm incorporated	
Unfractionated	9,200±1,900	2,300±670
T4	16,500±7,500	6,160±1,900
T8	2,060±670	240±100

*Data are expressed as means ±SEM for four separate experiments.

†Values indicate tritiated thymidine incorporation as measured on Day 3.

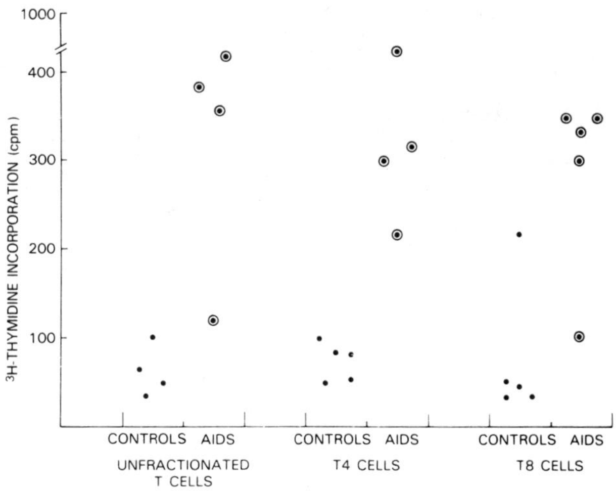

Figure 3. Spontaneous DNA Synthesis for Unfractionated T Cells, T4 Cells, and T8 Cells from Controls (●) and Patients with AIDS (◉).

suggests that it is a secondary rather than a primary phenomenon and that it may be related to opportunistic viral infection.

The precise mechanism underlying the selective qualitative defect in the ability of the helper/inducer T-cell subpopulation to respond to soluble antigen is currently under investigation. The ability of a soluble antigen to induce a proliferative response is the end result of a complex series of interactions of antigen, helper/inducer T cells, and monocyte/macrophages. Although we believe that the most likely explanation for the observed phenomena is at the level of the T4 cell itself — either a selective depletion of the antigen-reactive subset of T4 cells or virus-induced distortion of surface recognition sites — there may be a monocyte/macrophage defect as well. This possibility is supported by the fact that epidermal Langerhans' cells from patients with AIDS are defective in Ia antigen expression.[32] In this regard, if a macrophage defect has a role in the unresponsiveness of T4 cells from such patients, it would have to be at the level of antigen presentation rather than interleukin-1 production, since mitogen-induced responses are intact.

A defect of such selectivity as that described here for the antigen-reactive T4 subset is unprecedented in previously recognized immunodeficiency states. Further delineation of this defect should be useful in understanding the full nature of the impact of T-cell–tropic viruses on the human immune system, as well as in establishing the precise nature of the immunopathology of AIDS. Finally, such insight will be critical in our attempts to develop therapies for the progressive and fatal immune deficiency of this syndrome.

We are indebted to Ms. Susan P. Allyn, Ms. Sandra E. Higgins, Ms. Penny Svetlik, and Ms. Nancy Peffer for technical assistance, to Ms. Ann London and Ms. Lori Schlaffer for editorial assistance, and to Drs. Edward P. Gelmann and Ronald G. Steis for help in the clinical care of the patients.

References

1. Barré-Sinoussi F, Chermann JC, Rey F, et al. Isolation of a T-lymphotropic retrovirus from a patient at risk for acquired immune deficiency syndrome (AIDS). Science 1983; 220:868-71.
2. Gallo RC, Salahuddin SZ, Popovic M, et al. Frequent detection and isolation of cytopathic retroviruses (HTLV-III) from patients with AIDS and at risk for AIDS. Science 1984; 224:500-2.
3. Klatzmann D, Barré-Sinoussi F, Nugeyre MT, et al. Selective tropism of lymphadenopathy associated virus (LAV) for helper-inducer T lymphocytes. Science 1984; 225:59-63.
4. Gottlieb MS, Schroff R, Schanker HM, et al. *Pneumocystis carinii* pneumonia and mucosal candidiasis in previously healthy homosexual men: evidence of a new acquired cellular immunodeficiency. N Engl J Med 1981; 305:1425-31.
5. Masur H, Michelis MA, Greene JB, et al. An outbreak of community-acquired *Pneumocystis carinii* pneumonia: initial manifestation of cellular immune dysfunction. N Engl J Med 1981; 305:1431-8.
6. Siegal FP, Lopez C, Hammer GS, et al. Severe acquired immunodeficiency in male homosexuals, manifested by chronic perianal ulcerative herpes simplex lesions. N Engl J Med 1981; 305:1439-44.
7. Stahl RE, Friedman-Kien A, Dubin R, Marmor M, Zolla-Pazner S. Immunologic abnormalities in homosexual men: relationship to Kaposi's sarcoma. Am J Med 1982; 73:171-8.
8. Mildvan D, Mathur U, Enlow RW, et al. Opportunistic infections and immune deficiency in homosexual men. Ann Intern Med 1982; 96:700-4.
9. Lane HC, Masur H, Edgar LC, Whalen G, Rook AH, Fauci AS. Abnormalities of B-cell activation and immunoregulation in patients with the acquired immunodeficiency syndrome. N Engl J Med 1983; 309:453-8.
10. Schroff RW, Gottlieb MS, Prince HE, Chai LL, Fahey JL. Immunological studies of homosexual men with immunodeficiency and Kaposi's sarcoma. Clin Immunol Immunopathol 1983; 27:300-14.
11. Ammann AJ, Abrams D, Conant M, et al. Acquired immune dysfunction in homosexual men: immunologic profiles. Clin Immunol Immunopathol 1983; 27:315-25.
12. Cunningham-Rundles S, Michelis MA, Masur H. Serum suppression of lymphocyte activation *in vitro* in acquired immunodeficiency disease. J Clin Immunol 1983; 3:156-65.
13. Lane HC. Immunologic abnormalities. In: Fauci AS, ed. Acquired immunodeficiency syndrome: epidemiologic, clinical, immunologic, and therapeutic considerations. Ann Intern Med 1984; 100:98-9.
14. Murray HW, Rubin BY, Masur H, Roberts RB. Impaired production of lymphokines and immune (gamma) interferon in the acquired immunodeficiency syndrome. N Engl J Med 1984; 310:883-9.
15. Ciobanu N, Welte K, Kruger G, et al. Defective T-cell response to PHA and mitogenic monoclonal antibodies in male homosexuals with acquired immunodeficiency syndrome and its *in vivo* correction by interleukin 2. J Clin Immunol 1982; 3:332-40.
16. Lane HC, Masur H, Gelmann EP, et al. Correlation between immunologic function and clinical subpopulations of patients with the acquired immune deficiency syndrome. Am J Med 1985; 78:417-22.
17. Prince HE, Kermani-Arab V, Fahey JL. Depressed interleukin 2 receptor expression in acquired immune deficiency and lymphadenopathy syndromes. J Immunol 1984; 133:1313-7.
18. Benveniste E, Schroff R, Stevens RH, Gottlieb MS. Immunoregulatory T cells in men with a new acquired immunodeficiency syndrome. J Clin Immunol 1983; 3:359-67.
19. Update on acquired immune deficiency syndrome (AIDS) — United States. MMWR 1982; 31:507-14.
20. Lane HC, Whalen G, Fauci AS. Antigen-induced human T cell help: precursor frequency, radiation sensitivity, and allogeneic effects. J Clin Invest 1983; 72:636-47.
21. Pellegrino MA, Ferrone S, Dierich MP, Reisfield RA. Enhancement of sheep red blood cell human lymphocyte rosette formation by the sulfhydryl compound 2-aminoethylisothiouronium bromide. Clin Immunol Immunopathol 1975; 3:324-33.
22. Stewart WE. The interferon system. 2nd ed. New York: Springer-Verlag, 1981:13-26.
23. Depper JM, Leonard WJ, Waldmann TA, Greene WC. A monoclonal antibody which recognizes the human receptor for T cell growth factor: functional effects and use as a probe to investigate receptor regulation. In: Pick E, ed. Lymphokines. Vol. 9. New York: Academic Press, 1984:127-52.
24. Depper JM, Leonard WJ, Krönke M, Waldmann TA, Greene WC. Augmented T cell growth factor expression in HTLV-1-infected human leukemic T cells. J Immunol 1984; 133:1691-5.
25. Depper JM, Leonard WJ, Krönke M, et al. Regulation of interleukin-2 receptor expression: effects of phorbol diester, phospholipase-C, and reexposure to antigen or lectin. J Immunol (in press).
26. Reinherz EL, Kung PC, Goldstein G, Schlossman SF. Further characterization of the human inducer T cell subset defined by monoclonal antibody. J Immunol 1979; 123:2894-6.
27. Gupta S, Safai B. Deficient autologous mixed lymphocyte reaction in Kap-

osi's sarcoma associated with deficiency of Leu-3^{+} responder T cells. J Clin Invest 1983; 71:296-300.

28. Smolen JS, Bettelheim P, Köller U, et al. Defect in intercellular communication in patients with hemophilia. Fed Proc 1984; 43:1922.
29. Hausman PB, Stites DP, Stobo JD. Antigen-reactive T cells can be activated by autologous macrophages in the absence of added antigen. J Exp Med 1981; 153:476-81.
30. Dalgleish AG, Beverley PCL, Clapham PR, Crawford DH, Greaves MF, Weiss RA. The CD4 (T4) antigen is an essential component of the receptor for the AIDS retrovirus. Nature 1984; 312:763-7.
31. Klatzmann D, Champagne E, Chamaret S, et al. T-lymphocyte T4 molecule behaves as the receptor for human retrovirus LAV. Nature 1984; 312: 767-8.
32. Belsito DV, Sanchez MR, Baer RL, Valentine F, Thorbecke GJ. Reduced Langerhans' cell Ia antigen and ATPase activity in patients with the acquired immunodeficiency syndrome. N Engl J Med 1981; 310:1279-82.

ORIGINAL ARTICLE

TARGET PLATELET ANTIGEN IN HOMOSEXUAL MEN WITH IMMUNE THROMBOCYTOPENIA

RAPHAEL B. STRICKER, M.D., DONALD I. ABRAMS, M.D., LAURENCE CORASH, M.D., AND MARC A. SHUMAN, M.D.

Abstract A syndrome of isolated immune thrombocytopenic purpura (ITP) has recently been described in homosexual men. We have identified an antiplatelet antibody in the serum of 29 of 30 homosexual men with isolated ITP. The antibody binds to a platelet membrane antigen of 25,000 daltons, and binding is effected by the $F(ab)_2$ portion of the immunoglobulin. Similar antibody activity was not detected in serum from 30 nonhomosexual patients with either ITP or nonimmune thrombocytopenia. The 25,000-dalton antigen was not found on other hematopoietic cells, and it was distinct from the core protein of the AIDS-associated retrovirus. In contrast, serum antibody reacted with a 25,000-dalton antigen associated with cultured herpes simplex virus Types I and II. In these experiments the antigen appeared to be derived from green-monkey kidney cells in which the herpes simplex viruses were grown. Identical antigenic activity was also demonstrated in uninfected human skin fibroblasts. We conclude that ITP in homosexual men is accompanied by a serum antibody directed against a platelet antigen of 25,000 daltons. The nature of the antigen and the relation of the serum antibody to ITP require further study.

THROMBOCYTOPENIA has emerged as a major hematologic abnormality associated with the acquired immunodeficiency syndrome (AIDS) and AIDS-related conditions. Recently, a group of homosexual men with isolated immune thrombocytopenic purpura (ITP) has been identified.[1,2] Although increased levels of circulating immune complexes have been found in the serum of these patients,[3] the pathogenesis of platelet destruction in this form of ITP remains unclear.

Recent studies have identified target platelet antigens in idiopathic immune thrombocytopenia[4,5] and in drug-induced immune thrombocytopenia[6] by means of immunoprecipitation or immunoblotting. In this study, we have attempted to define the target platelet antigen in homosexual men with ITP.

METHODS

Patient Population

Serum samples were obtained from 30 consecutive homosexual men with ITP treated at the AIDS Clinic of San Francisco General Hospital and the Hematology Clinic of the University of California, San Francisco. Serum samples were also obtained from the following groups of patients: 18 nonhomosexual adult patients with ITP, 12 patients with nonimmune thrombocytopenia, and 16 homosexual men with normal platelet counts and either the lymphadenopathy syndrome or AIDS. AIDS was defined according to the surveillance criteria of the Centers for Disease Control — i.e., a disease indicative of an underlying cellular immunodeficiency when no known cause of reduced resistance to the disease is present.[7] All serum samples were frozen at −70°C before use.

Platelet Antibody

Platelet-associated immunoglobulin was detected by means of a fluorescence-activated flow cytometric assay. Platelets were isolated from acid–citrate–dextrose-anticoagulated whole blood by differential centrifugation. They were then washed once in phosphate-buffered saline containing glucose and resuspended in 1 percent ammonium oxalate to lyse contaminating red cells. After three washes in calcium-free Tyrode's buffer, the platelets were fixed with 1 percent paraformaldehyde and reacted with biotin-conjugated goat antihuman $F(ab)_2$ directed against IgG, IgM, and IgA (Tago, Burlingame, Calif.). The cells were then incubated with an avidin–fluorescein isothiocyanate label (Tago), washed, and passed through a flow cytometer (Becton Dickinson), and the mean fluorescence was determined. A normal range was defined, and each sample was compared with its own negative control by means of goat antirabbit $F(ab)_2$ conjugated to biotin. Platelet-associated immunoglobulin was expressed as mean platelet fluorescence on a logarithmic scale. A sample was defined as positive if the mean fluorescence was 2 SD above the mean in the control population.

Target-Cell Preparation

Platelets were isolated from a single normal O-positive donor as described above. After the final wash in Tyrode's buffer, the platelets were solubilized in 2 percent sodium dodecyl sulfate sample buffer containing 5 mM EDTA, 0.05 M imidazole, 1 percent (vol/vol) aprotinin, 15 percent glycerol, and 0.005 percent bromphenol blue dye at a final concentration of 10^9 per milliliter (1 mg of protein per milliliter).

Platelets from three homosexual patients with ITP and from patients with Glanzmann's thrombasthenia or Bernard–Soulier syndrome were prepared in a similar manner. In addition, 1-ml aliquots containing 1×10^9 control platelets were subjected to digestion with trypsin,[8] 1 mg per milliliter for 30 minutes at 37°C, or thrombin,[9] 5 U per milliliter for 90 minutes at room temperature, before solubilization in sodium dodecyl sulfate. Supernatants from the treated platelets were electrophoresed on sodium dodecyl sulfate–polyacrylamide gels to verify the adequacy of the trypsin or thrombin treatment.

Erythrocytes were obtained from the same control donor. Red-cell ghosts were prepared by washing in 0.9 percent saline, followed by solubilization in 2 percent sodium dodecyl sulfate at a concentration of 10^7 per milliliter (1 mg of protein per milliliter). B cells were obtained by Ficoll–Hypaque separation from control blood, followed by removal of T cells by rosetting with sheep red cells.[10] The residual B cells were solubilized at 1 mg per milliliter in 2 percent sodium dodecyl sulfate. Granulocytes were prepared by sucrose gradient separation,[10] and membrane fractions were solubilized in 2 percent sodium dodecyl sulfate.

Cultured green-monkey kidney (Vero) cells and human skin fibroblasts were obtained from the American Type Culture Collection (Rockville, Md.). The cells were washed extensively in phosphate-buffered saline before solubilization in sample buffer at a concentration of 1 mg per milliliter. Cytopathic testing for viral infection was negative before solubilization.

From the Cancer Research Institute and the Departments of Medicine and Laboratory Medicine, University of California, San Francisco, and the Department of Medicine, San Francisco General Hospital.

Whole-virus preparations of herpes simplex virus Types I and II and Epstein–Barr virus were obtained from Cambridge Medical Diagnostics (Billerica, Mass.). The herpes simplex viruses were isolated from infected Vero cells, and the Epstein–Barr virus was derived from the human Burkitt's lymphoma line P3H3. Cytomegalovirus isolated from an infected human lung cell line, WI38, was obtained from the American Type Culture Collection. The viral antigens were solubilized in sample buffer at 1 mg per milliliter. Human AIDS-associated retrovirus,[11] kindly provided by Dr. Jay Levy, was prepared in sample buffer at the same concentration. All samples were stored at −70°C before use.

Immunoblot Technique

Sodium dodecyl sulfate–polyacrylamide gel electrophoresis was performed according to the method of Laemmli.[12] Fifty microliters of cell samples was subjected to electrophoresis in 5 to 15 percent linear-gradient polyacrylamide gels under nonreducing conditions. Low-molecular-weight standards (Bio-Rad, Richmond, Calif.) were subjected to electrophoresis simultaneously with the samples. Electrophoresis was stopped when the dye front was 1 cm from the bottom of the gel.

Immunoblotting was performed according to the method of Towbin et al.[13] Samples separated on gradient gels were electrophoretically transferred to nitrocellulose paper (pore size, 0.1 μm [Sartorius, Hayward, Calif.]) in a Bio-Rad Transblot apparatus. The transfer was performed at 30 V for 16 hours. It was crucial that the pore size of the nitrocellulose be smaller, since proteins of lower molecular weight were not recovered when the pore size was 0.45 μm. After transfer, the nitrocellulose was cut into strips, and the low-molecular-weight standards were stained with 0.05 percent amido black. Thirty to 40 protein bands ranging in molecular weight from 10,000 to 300,000 daltons were routinely visible on the nitrocellulose.

The rest of the nitrocellulose strips were incubated in 5 percent (wt/vol) gelatin in TRIS-buffered saline for one hour at 37°C to block background binding. A lower gelatin concentration or substitution of 10 percent fetal-calf serum gave unacceptable background staining. The strips were then incubated with test serum, IgG, or $F(ab)_2$ diluted 1:100 in TRIS-buffered saline with 1 percent (wt/vol) gelatin for two hours at room temperature. After the washing in TRIS-buffered saline, the nitrocellulose was incubated with biotin-conjugated goat $F(ab)_2$ antihuman IgG, IgM, and IgA (Tago) diluted 1:500 in TRIS-buffered saline–1 percent gelatin for one hour. After washing, the strips were placed in an avidin–peroxidase solution (Cappel, Malvern, Pa.) diluted 1:500 in TRIS-buffered saline–1 percent gelatin for one hour. Color development was performed, with 4-chloronaphthol used as substrate.[14]

In cases in which $F(ab)_2$ binding was investigated, the biotin-conjugated second antibody was a mixture of goat $F(ab)_2$ antihuman kappa and lambda light chains (Tago). It was found that the goat antibody raised against human heavy chains did not recognize $F(ab)_2$ digests of immunoglobulin; in contrast, the anti-kappa/lambda antibody bound to both whole immunoglobulin and $F(ab)_2$ fragments on the blots. In serum from five patients, blotting with monospecific biotin-conjugated goat antibody against human IgG, IgM, or IgA (Tago) was used to demonstrate antibody binding by specific immunoglobulin classes.

Immunoglobulin and $F(ab)_2$ Preparation

Staphylococcal protein A–Sepharose CL6B (Pharmacia, Piscataway, N.J.) was used to purify IgG from serum.[15] Protein concentration was measured by the Bio-Rad modification of the Lowry technique.[16] The IgG was stored at −20°C until use.

$F(ab)_2$ fragments were prepared by a modification of the method of Madsen and Rodkey[17]: 10 mg of IgG in phosphate-buffered saline was dialyzed against 0.1 M sodium acetate, pH 4.5, for three hours at 4°C. Freshly prepared porcine pepsin (Sigma, St. Louis) suspended in the same buffer at 4 mg per milliliter was added to give a final concentration of 2 percent (wt/wt) pepsin per milligram of total globulin. The solution was then incubated overnight at 37°C and dialyzed against phosphate-buffered saline, pH 7.4, for eight hours. The digestion products were incubated with staphylococcal protein A bacterial adsorbent (Miles Scientific, Naperville, Ill.) for 30 minutes at 4°C. The beads were centrifuged, and the supernatant free of IgG and Fc fragments was again analyzed for protein concentration. The yield of $F(ab)_2$ by this technique was 50 to 80 percent. Samples of IgG and $F(ab)_2$, also subjected to electrophoresis with sodium dodecyl sulfate–polyacrylamide gels, demonstrated that residual IgG was absent from the $F(ab)_2$ preparations. The $F(ab)_2$ was stored at −20°C until use.

Antibody Elution from Platelets

Ether elution of platelet-associated antibody was performed according to the method of von dem Borne et al.[18] Patient platelets were isolated as described above. After the final wash in Tyrode's buffer, 10^8 platelets were resuspended in 1 ml of phosphate-buffered saline, and 2 ml of diethyl ether was added. After being shaken for 2 minutes, the sample was incubated for 30 minutes at 37°C. The platelets were then centrifuged at $3000 \times g$ for 10 minutes, and the ether and stromal layers were removed. The eluate was frozen at −70°C until use.

In the fluorescence-activated cell-sorter assay, 100 μl of eluate was diluted in 900 μl of phosphate-buffered saline and incubated with control platelets for one hour, followed by second-antibody and fluorescence labeling as described above. When used for immunoblotting, the eluate was diluted 1:100 in TRIS-buffered saline–1 percent gelatin and incubated for two hours with the nitrocellulose.

Results

The characteristics of the patients studied are shown in Table 1. Of the 30 homosexual men with ITP, all had elevated platelet-associated immunoglobulin as demonstrated with the cell-sorter technique. The platelet counts ranged from 7000 to 105,000 at the time of study, with a mean of 43,000. Sixteen patients were taking prednisone; none had undergone splenectomy at the time of initial evaluation. None of the patients had AIDS or evidence of sepsis, and no medication other than steroids was being taken. White-cell counts and hemoglobin levels were normal in all patients.

The control group consisted of 18 nonhomosexual patients with ITP, as well as 12 patients with thrombocytopenia due to thrombotic thrombocytopenic purpura, disseminated intravascular coagulation, hypersplenism, Hodgkin's disease, or aplastic anemia. All patients with ITP had elevated platelet-associated immunoglobulin, whereas those with nonimmune thrombocytopenia had normal platelet-associated antibody. Ten of the patients with ITP were taking steroids at the time that serum was obtained.

A third group consisted of 16 homosexual men with either lymphadenopathy syndrome (5 patients) or AIDS as manifested by *Pneumocystis carinii* pneumonia (6 patients) or Kaposi's sarcoma (5 patients). The platelet counts of these patients were normal at the time of study. Platelet-associated immunoglobulin was measured in two men with lymphadenopathy syndrome and three with AIDS; it was elevated in all five patients despite normal platelet counts. None of the patients were taking steroids; their other medications are listed in Table 1.

Figure 1 shows a typical immunoblot using control serum (Lane A) or serum from a homosexual man with ITP (Lane B). All blots contained a band at 150,000 daltons. This band was also present when test

Table 1. Patient Diagnoses, Treatment, and Laboratory Findings.*

Patient Group	Associated Conditions	Therapy	Mean Platelet Count	Elevated PAIg†	Antibody to 25,000-dalton Antigen
			cells/μl	*no. with feature/no. tested*	
ITP‡					
Homosexual (30)	None	Prednisone (16)	43,000	30/30	29/30
Nonhomosexual (18)	SLE (4), infection (3), CLL (1); ITP, idiopathic (8) or drug-induced (2)	Prednisone (10)	25,000	18/18	0/18
Nonimmune thrombocytopenia (12)	DIC (5), TTP (3), hypersplenism (2), Hodgkin's disease (1), aplastic anemia (1)	Prednisone (3), heparin (5), plasmapheresis (3), oxymetholone (1), MOPP (1)	47,000	0/12	0/12
Lymphadenopathy or AIDS (16)	*Pneumocystis carinii* pneumonia (6), Kaposi's sarcoma (5)	TMP/SMX (5), pentamidine (1)	192,000	5/5	15/16

*Values in parentheses represent numbers of patients. ITP denotes immune thrombocytopenic purpura, and AIDS acquired immunodeficiency syndrome; SLE denotes systemic lupus erythematosus, CLL chronic lymphocytic leukemia, DIC disseminated intravascular coagulation, and TTP thrombotic thrombocytopenic purpura; MOPP denotes mechlorethamine–vincristine (Oncovin)–prednisone–procarbazine, and TMP/SMX trimethoprim–sulfamethoxazole.

†PAIg denotes platelet-associated immunoglobulin.

‡The criteria for inclusion in this category were clinical findings compatible with a diagnosis of immune thrombocytopenia and the presence of anti-platelet antibodies.

serum was omitted, and represented IgG in the control platelet preparation. A second band was present at 45,000 daltons in all blots after incubation with test serum. This represents nonspecific binding of IgG to actin in the platelet preparation. In Lane B, an additional band is seen at 25,000 daltons. This band was detected with serum from 29 of 30 homosexual men with ITP, but not with serum from any of the 30 nonhomosexual patients with ITP or nonimmune thrombocytopenia. It was also seen in 15 of 16 homosexual men with lymphadenopathy syndrome or AIDS. Antibody binding was detected on control platelets and autologous platelets from the patients with ITP, as well as platelets from the patients with Glanzmann's thrombasthenia and Bernard–Soulier syndrome (data not shown). The class of antibody was studied in five patients: three had only IgG binding to the 25,000-dalton antigen, one had IgG and IgM binding, and one had IgG and IgA.

Neither trypsin hydrolysis nor thrombin stimulation of target platelets abolished antibody binding to the 25,000-dalton antigen, suggesting that the binding site is not secreted and is an integral part of the platelet membrane. Binding did not occur with red-cell ghosts (Lane C), B lymphocytes, T lymphocytes, or polymorphonuclear leukocytes. In addition, the antigen was not found on human erythroleukemia cells[19] or spleen cells (data not shown). Megakaryocytes were not tested.

In contrast, Figure 2 shows the results of blotting with various viral preparations. Binding to an identical 25,000-dalton band occurred in samples of both herpes simplex I (Lane B) and II, but not in preparations of Epstein–Barr virus (Lane C) or cytomegalovirus. Serum reactivity with the core protein of AIDS-associated retrovirus is clearly seen in Lane D, but this band migrates at 27,000 daltons in our system and appears to be distinct from the target platelet antigen. Antibody also bound to a 25,000-dalton antigen on green-monkey kidney cells and human skin fibroblasts (Lanes E and F). Since the kidney cells were shown to be negative for herpes simplex I and II, we believe that the antigen on the herpes simplex blots was derived from the cells in which the virus was grown, and not from the virus itself. Other bands recognized by the test serum included those of Epstein–Barr nuclear antigen (80,000 daltons) and an uncharacterized 20,000-dalton protein in the Epstein–Barr virus preparation (Lane C), proteins of 41,000 and 68,000 daltons in the AIDS virus preparation (Lane D), and an as yet uncharacterized protein of 55,000 daltons in both the Vero cells and fibroblasts (Lanes E and F).

Figure 3 shows the results of blotting studies using serum (Lane A), whole IgG (Lane B), and $F(ab)_2$ fragments (Lanes C through E). In all four homosexual men with ITP who were tested, binding to the target 25,000-dalton antigen occurred with both IgG and $F(ab)_2$ fragments. $F(ab)_2$ binding could be dem-

Table 2. Clinical Course of a Homosexual Man with ITP, Showing Correlation of Platelet Count with Platelet-Associated Immunoglobulin (PAIg) and Serum Antibody against a 25,000-dalton Antigen.

	Treatment	Platelet Count	PAIg*	Antibody* Testing
May	Prednisone	8,000	Pos	Pos
June	Prednisone	12,000	ND	Pos
July	Splenectomy			
Before operation		6,000	ND	Pos
After operation (July 12)		327,000	ND	Pos
August	None	264,000	Neg	Neg
September	None	160,000	ND	Pos
October	None	20,000	Pos	Pos

*Pos denotes positive, Neg negative, and ND not done.

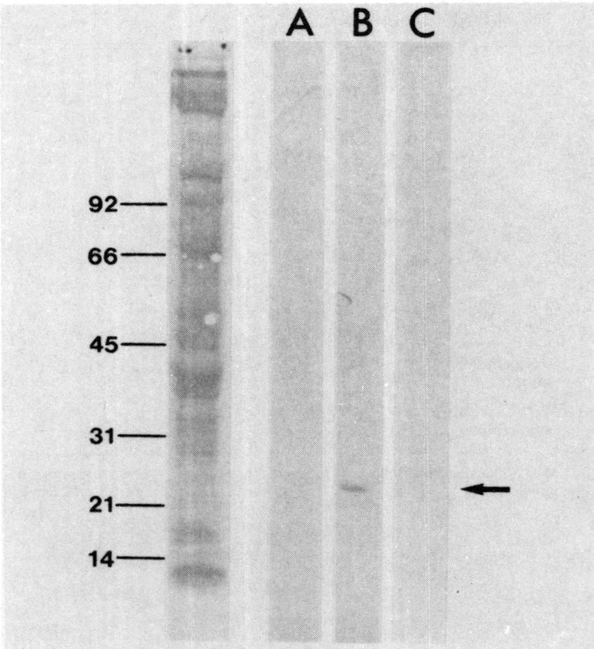

Figure 1. Identification of Antibody against 25,000-dalton Platelet Antigen in Serum from Homosexual Men with ITP.

Solubilized cells were subjected to sodium dodecyl sulfate–polyacrylamide gel electrophoresis, transferred to nitrocellulose, and incubated in stepwise fashion with test serum, biotin-conjugated goat $F(ab)_2$ antihuman immunoglobulin, and avidin–peroxidase as described in Methods.

The left lane shows amido black stain of platelet proteins transferred to nitrocellulose, with molecular-weight markers; Lane A, platelets incubated with control serum; Lane B, platelets incubated with serum from a patient; and Lane C, the same serum incubated with red-cell ghosts. Note target platelet antigen at 25,000 daltons (arrow) recognized by antibody from the patient's serum. The antigen is not seen on red-cell ghosts.

onstrated only with anti-light-chain antibody (and not with antibody against intact IgG), effectively ruling out the possibility of residual IgG binding in the $F(ab)_2$ preparation. Thus, antibody activity was mediated by the $F(ab)_2$ portion of the IgG. Ether eluates from each of two patients tested also bound to the 25,000-dalton antigen (Lanes F and G).

The clinical course in one homosexual patient with ITP is shown in Table 2. This patient had severe thrombocytopenia unresponsive to prednisone therapy. Tests for platelet-associated immunoglobulin and serum antibody against the 25,000-dalton platelet antigen were positive. The patient underwent splenectomy, and his platelet count rose to 327,000 per microliter. Subsequently, studies for both the platelet-associated immunoglobulin and serum antibody became negative. However, by two months after surgery, the platelet count had dropped to 160,000 and platelet antibody was again detectable by immunoblotting. Relapse occurred one month later, with a platelet count of 20,000 per microliter and elevated platelet-associated immunoglobulin. Testing for serum antibody remained positive.

Discussion

We have used a sensitive immunoblot technique to demonstrate serum-antibody binding to a particular platelet antigen. In 29 of 30 homosexual men with ITP, serum antibody bound to a target antigen of 25,000 daltons. This antibody activity was not detected in nonhomosexual patients with ITP or in patients with nonimmune thrombocytopenia. Furthermore, the antibody was shown to bind via the $F(ab)_2$ portion of the molecule, indicating that it is an autoantibody and not an immune complex. The 25,000-dalton antigen appears to be an integral part of the platelet membrane rather than an adsorbed antigen, since it resists trypsin hydrolysis and thrombin stimulation of platelets. Previously, Phillips[8] showed that trypsin treatment of platelet membranes resulted in increased expression of a 26,000-dalton protein, which remains uncharacterized. Whether this component and the antigen that we identified are similar has not yet been determined.

In 1982 Morris et al.[1] described a group of 11 homosexual men with thrombocytopenia, elevated platelet-associated immunoglobulin, and increased bone marrow megakaryocytes consistent with a diagnosis of ITP. A follow-up report by Walsh et al.[3] described 33 additional patients with thrombocytopenia. Although 10 of these patients had AIDS, the other 23 had a syndrome that was indistinguishable from idiopathic immune thrombocytopenia. The authors postulated

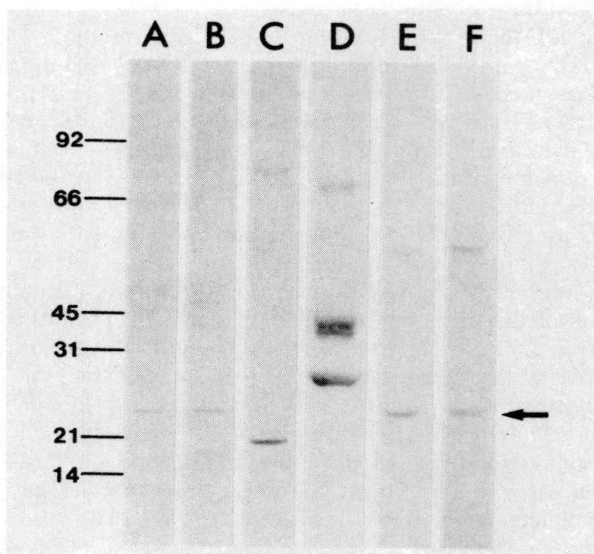

Figure 2. Immunoblot Using Serum of a Homosexual Patient with ITP.

Serum was incubated with autologous platelets — Lane A; herpes simplex virus Type I — Lane B; Epstein–Barr virus — Lane C; AIDS-associated retrovirus — Lane D; uninfected green-monkey kidney (Vero) cells — Lane E; and human skin fibroblasts (uninfected) — Lane F. Note that antibody binds to 25,000-dalton antigen (arrow) on the platelets, herpesvirus, Vero cells, and fibroblasts, but not on the Epstein–Barr virus or AIDS-associated retrovirus.

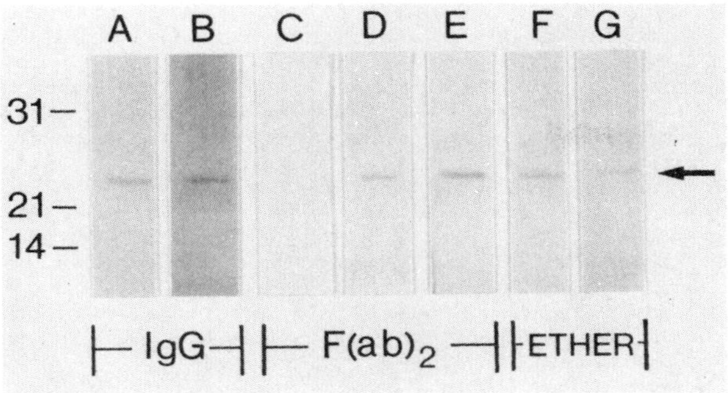

Figure 3. Immunoblot Characterization of Antibody against 25,000-dalton Antigen.

Platelets were electrophoresed and transferred to nitrocellulose as described in Methods. The nitrocellulose was then incubated with various preparations of patients' antibody: Lane A, serum from a homosexual patient with ITP; Lane B, IgG (2 mg per milliliter) purified from patient serum; Lane C, control $F(ab)_2$ fragment (2.5 mg per milliliter); Lanes D and E, $F(ab)_2$ fragments (2.5 mg per milliliter) from two patients; and Lanes F and G, ether eluates from platelets of the two patients represented in Lanes D and E. Reactivity with 25,000-dalton antigen did not occur with control $F(ab)_2$ but did occur with patient IgG, $F(ab)_2$, and ether eluates (arrow).

that the mechanism of thrombocytopenia was related to immune-complex–mediated platelet destruction, on the basis of their observation that circulating immune complexes measured by a polyethylene glycol assay were increased in 88 percent of homosexual patients with ITP but normal in five controls with ITP. However, Trent[20] and Lurhuma[21] and their colleagues have shown increased circulating immune complexes in 89 percent (102 of 115) of patients with "classic" ITP, using the C1q assay. Using this assay, we found elevated circulating immune complexes in 64 percent (7 of 11) of our homosexual patients with ITP (unpublished data). Thus, elevated circulating immune complexes appear to be a common feature of ITP in homosexual and heterosexual patients.

Walsh et al. also noted that the "immune complex" fraction of serum isolated by polyethylene glycol precipitation bound to target platelets in 79 percent of patients.[3] However, there is doubt whether the polyethylene glycol assay is specific for circulating immune complexes, since free IgG or IgM may also be precipitated when high serum concentrations are present.[22,23] Since patients with AIDS-related syndromes have increased immunoglobulin levels,[24] the polyethylene glycol technique may precipitate autoantibody together with immune complexes in these patients. Thus, although circulating immune complexes may be elevated in homosexual men with ITP, direct evidence is lacking that thrombocytopenia results from these complexes.

Whether the antibody against the 25,000-dalton platelet antigen is responsible for thrombocytopenia in these patients has not yet been demonstrated. The presence of antibody against this antigen on the surface of platelets suggests at least a partial explanation for thrombocytopenia, since antibody-coated platelets have been shown to be phagocytosed by leukocytes.[25] Thus, accelerated destruction of these autoantibody-coated platelets by the reticuloendothelial system would be expected. In addition, the presence of serum antibody against the 25,000-dalton antigen seemed to parallel disease activity in the single patient studied longitudinally (Table 2). The role of this antibody in the pathogenesis of ITP requires further evaluation.

The possible derivation of the platelet autoantibody in our patients is intriguing. The antibody recognizes the same antigen in fibroblasts and monkey kidney cells, as well as on herpes simplex virus cultured in the kidney cells. An attractive hypothesis based on these observations is that in some patients with herpetic infections, the cellular 25,000-dalton protein may become incorporated into viral proteins or adsorbed to the virus. The protein may thus be altered, rendering it immunogenic. Alternatively, the 25,000-dalton protein may be synthesized by the herpesvirus and some mammalian cells. Antibodies raised against the virus after infection may then secondarily react with host cells, including platelets. Similar mechanisms of autoimmunity have been postulated in other forms of viral infection.[26,27] The role of the AIDS-associated retrovirus in development of the autoantibody also requires clarification.

Finally, the absence of thrombocytopenia among patients with AIDS or lymphadenopathy syndrome whose serum contains antiplatelet antibody is unexplained. As noted in Table 1, five such patients with normal platelet counts had increased amounts of platelet-associated immunoglobulin. A possible explanation is related to the finding of Bender et al.[28] that Fc-receptor–mediated clearance is defective in patients with AIDS. Thus, these patients may have increased antibody bound to their platelets but decreased clearance, as described by Kelton et al.[29] in other diseases. An alternative explanation is that compensated thrombocytolysis is present in these cases, since borderline platelet counts were recorded in three of the five patients at the time that serum was obtained, and subsequently thrombocytopenia developed in all three patients. Further studies of platelet-associated antibody and Fc-receptor–mediated clearance in nonthrombocytopenic patients with AIDS or AIDS-related conditions should help to clarify this issue.

In summary, we have identified a platelet autoantibody in the serum of 29 of 30 homosexual men with ITP. The antibody binds to an antigen of 25,000 daltons that appears to be a part of the platelet membrane. The nature of the target platelet antigen and the relation of the serum antibody to the pathogenesis of ITP in homosexual men require further study.

We are indebted to Jay Levy, M.D., and Joel Chasis, M.D., for helpful discussion, to Dr. Margaret Johnson (Medical Center of Delaware, Newark, Del.) for providing platelets from the patients with Bernard–Soulier syndrome, and to Margaret Rheinschmidt, Mary Rossi, Ramila Philip, and Bobak Banapour for technical assistance.

References

1. Morris L, Distenfeld A, Amorosi E, Karpatkin S. Autoimmune thrombocytopenic purpura in homosexual men. Ann Intern Med 1982; 96:714-7.
2. Abrams DI, Volberding PA, Linker CA, et al. Immune thrombocytopenic purpura in homosexual men: clinical manifestations and treatment results. Blood 1983; 62:108a. abstract.
3. Walsh CM, Nardi MA, Karpatkin S. On the mechanism of thrombocytopenic purpura in sexually active homosexual men. N Engl J Med 1984; 311:635-9.
4. Mason D, McMillan R. Platelet antigens in chronic idiopathic thrombocytopenic purpura. Br J Haematol 1984; 56:529-34.
5. Beardsley DS, Spiegel JE, Jacobs MM, Handin RI, Lux SE IV. Platelet membrane glycoprotein IIIa contains target antigens that bind anti-platelet antibodies in immune thrombocytopenias. J Clin Invest 1984; 74:1701-7.
6. Chong BH, Berndt MC, Koutts J, Castaldi PA. Quinidine-induced thrombocytopenia and leukopenia: demonstration and characterization of distinct antiplatelet and antileukocyte antibodies. Blood 1983; 62:1218-23.
7. Selik RM, Haverkos HW, Curran JW. Acquired immune deficiency syndrome (AIDS) trends in the United States, 1978-1982. Am J Med 1984; 76:493-500.
8. Phillips DR. Effect of trypsin on the exposed polypeptides and glycoproteins in the human platelet membrane. Biochemistry 1972; 11:4582-8.
9. Berndt MC, Phillips DR. Purification and preliminary physicochemical characterization of human platelet membrane glycoprotein V. J Biol Chem 1981; 256:59-65.
10. Andersson LC, Gahmberg CG. Surface glycoproteins of human white blood cells: analysis by surface labeling. Blood 1978; 52:57-67.
11. Levy JA, Hoffman AD, Kramer SM, Landis JA, Shimabukuro JM, Oschiro LS. Isolation of lymphocytopathic retroviruses from San Francisco patients with AIDS. Science 1984; 225:840-2.
12. Laemmli UK. Cleavage of structural proteins during the assembly of the head of bacteriophage T4. Nature 1970; 227:680-5.
13. Towbin H, Staehelin T, Gordon J. Electrophoretic transfer of proteins from polyacrylamide gels to nitrocellulose sheets: procedure and some applications. Proc Natl Acad Sci USA 1979; 76:4350-4.
14. Hawkes R. Identification of concanavalin A-binding proteins after sodium dodecyl sulfate–gel electrophoresis and protein blotting. Anal Biochem 1982; 123:143-6.
15. Kessler SW. Use of protein A-bearing staphylococci for the immunoprecipitation and isolation of antigens from cells. Methods Enzymol 1981; 73: 442-59.
16. Lowry OH, Rosebrough NJ, Farr AL, Randall RJ. Protein measurement wiRiesz E, Engelfriet CP. Autoimmune thrombocytopenia: detection of platelet autoantibodies with the suspension immunofluorescence test. Br J Haematol 1980; 45:319-27.
19. Martin P, Papayannopoulou T. HEL cells: a new human erythroleukemia cell line with spontaneous and induced globin expression. Science 1982; 216:1233-5.
20. Trent RJ, Clancy RL, Danis V, Basten A. Immune complexes in thrombocytopenic patients: cause or effect? Br J Haematol 1980; 44:645-54.
21. Lurhuma AZ, Riccomi H, Masson PL. The occurrence of circulating immune complexes and viral antigens in idiopathic thrombocytopenic purpura. Clin Exp Immunol 1977; 28:49-55.
22. Digeon M, Laver M, Riza J, Bach JF. Detection of circulating immune complexes in human sera by simplified assays with polyethylene glycol. J Immunol Methods 1977; 16:165-83.
23. IUIS/WHO Working Group. Use and abuse of laboratory tests in clinical immunology: critical considerations of eight widely used diagnostic procedures. Clin Immunol Immunopathol 1982; 24:122-38.
24. Amman AJ, Abrams D, Conant M, et al. Acquired immune dysfunction in homosexual men: immunologic profiles. Clin Immunol Immunopathol 1983; 27:315-25.
25. McMillan R. Chronic idiopathic thrombocytopenic purpura. N Engl J Med 1981; 304:1135-47.
26. Billings PB, Hoch SO, White PJ, Carson DA, Vaughan JH. Antibodies to the Epstein–Barr virus nuclear antigen and to rheumatoid arthritis nuclear antigen identify the same polypeptide. Proc Natl Acad Sci USA 1983; 80:7104-8.
27. Fujinami RS, Oldstone MBA, Wroblewska Z, Frankel ME, Koprowski H. Molecular mimicry in virus infection: crossreaction of measles virus phosphoprotein or of herpes simplex virus protein with human intermediate filaments. Proc Natl Acad Sci USA 1983; 80:2346-50.
28. Bender BS, Quinn TC, Lawley TJ, Smith W, Brinkman C, Frank MM. Acquired immune deficiency syndrome (AIDS): a defect in Fc-receptor specific clearance. Clin Res 1984; 32:511A. abstract.
29. Kelton JG, Carter CJ, Rodger C, et al. The relationship among platelet-associated IgG, platelet lifespan, and reticuloendothelial cell function. Blood 1984; 63:1434-8.

ORIGINAL ARTICLE

PATIENTS AT RISK FOR AIDS-RELATED OPPORTUNISTIC INFECTIONS

Clinical Manifestations and Impaired Gamma Interferon Production

HENRY W. MURRAY, M.D., JANICE K. HILLMAN, M.D., BERISH Y. RUBIN, PH.D., CATHERINE D. KELLY, B.A., JONATHAN L. JACOBS, M.D., LISA W. TYLER, B.A., DARIA M. DONELLY, B.A., SUSAN M. CARRIERO, B.S., JAMES H. GODBOLD, PH.D., AND RICHARD B. ROBERTS, M.D.

Abstract We studied 81 men (79 homosexuals and 2 drug abusers) with persistent lymphadenopathy to determine whether those at risk for AIDS-related opportunistic infections could be identified prospectively. (Sixty-nine of 76 [91 percent] had antibodies to human T-cell lymphotropic virus Type III [HTLV-III], and 76 of 79 [96 percent] had abnormal T4/T8 cell ratios.) During the follow-up period (mean ±SEM, 12.9±0.5 months; range, 8 to 19), infections developed in none of 38 patients with lymphadenopathy alone and in only 1 of 15 (7 percent) with antecedent herpes zoster infection; however, 13 of 28 (46 percent) with lymphadenopathy accompanied by constitutional symptoms or oral candidiasis or both had opportunistic infections within the follow-up period. Among the results of various T-cell assays, only antigen-stimulated lymphocyte proliferation and gamma interferon generation, which were absent or barely measurable in those in whom AIDS ultimately developed, were of prognostic value. T cells from 15 patients, 11 of whom had constitutional symptoms or thrush, failed to generate antigen-induced gamma interferon; infections developed in 10 of these 15 (67 percent) within a mean of 8.2 months. These results suggest that patients with AIDS-related complex who are at risk for opportunistic infections within a year can be identified by correlating clinical manifestations with antigen-stimulated T-cell responses — in particular, with the production of gamma interferon.

AMONG the numerous T-cell defects identified in patients with the acquired immunodeficiency syndrome (AIDS),[1] the failure to generate gamma interferon[2] seems likely for several reasons to be relevant to the immunopathogenesis of AIDS-related opportunistic infections. For example, gamma interferon is probably the key T-cell-derived lymphokine that induces macrophages and other potential host defense cells to exert enhanced antimicrobial activity against both intracellular and extracellular pathogens.[3-10] In addition, gamma interferon also appears to have a pivotal regulatory role in a variety of other cellular immune reactions,[11] including those involved in antigen-stimulated T-cell activation.[12-15] Given this background and the earlier demonstration that T lymphocytes from patients with AIDS who have opportunistic infections typically fail to generate any gamma interferon in response to specific microbial antigen,[2] we initiated this study of patients at risk for AIDS with two goals in mind: first, to determine whether we could prospectively identify persons with the "AIDS prodrome" (AIDS-related complex) who already had the immunophenotype of fully established AIDS (absent antigen-induced production of gamma interferon in vitro[2]), and secondly, to test the hypothesis that such patients are at immediate risk for the development of AIDS-related opportunistic infections.

From the Divisions of Infectious Diseases and Immunology, Department of Medicine, Cornell University Medical College; the New York Blood Center; and the Biostatistics Laboratory of Memorial Sloan–Kettering Cancer Center, New York.

Supported by research grants (CA 35018, CA 38661, AI 21510, and Clinical Research Center grant RR47) from the National Institutes of Health, (AO 129) a grant from the New York State AIDS Institute, and a grant from the Will Rogers Memorial Fund.

METHODS

Patient Selection and Clinical Definitions

Between April 1983 and June 1984, 85 men screened at this hospital for possible AIDS were found to have unexplained generalized lymphadenopathy.[16] The latter was defined as the presence of enlarged lymph nodes (>1 cm) at two or more noncontiguous, extrainguinal sites for at least three months.[16] For each patient, the following were also recorded: unexplained oral candidiasis (thrush), herpes zoster within the previous year, and unexplained systemic constitutional symptoms including (1) intermittent or continuous fever (>38°C) for more than one month, (2) repeated night sweats, (3) debilitating fatigue, (4) persistent diarrhea, and (5) a loss of body weight of 10 percent or more. To reduce the likelihood that patients with clinically inapparent opportunistic infections (unrecognized AIDS) might have inadvertently been enrolled, anyone in whom an opportunistic infection developed in the first 12 weeks of testing was omitted from this analysis. Four of the 85 patients were excluded on this basis.

T-Lymphocyte Enumeration and Immunologic Testing

All testing was performed at the time patients were originally entered into the study. Peripheral-blood T cells, helper T cells, and suppressor T cells were identified with use of the monoclonal antibodies OKT3, OKT4, and OKT8 in a standard indirect immunofluorescence assay.[2] Serum antibody to human T-cell lymphotropic virus Type III (HTLV-III)[17] was measured in a spectrophotometric enzyme-linked immunosorbent assay (ELISA) by Dr. Jacob C. Holper (Litton Bionetics, Laboratory Products Division, Charleston, S.C.). Standard preparations of candida, mumps, trichophytin, tetanus-toxoid, and purified-protein-derivative antigens were used to test for cutaneous anergy. Peripheral-blood mononuclear cells separated by the Ficoll–Hypaque technique and cultivated in RPMI-1640 medium containing antibiotics and 15 percent heat-inactivated normal heterologous serum were used for assays of lymphocyte proliferation and gamma interferon generation.[2] Proliferative activity was determined by the incorporation of [^{3}H]thymidine by 0.5×10^5 cells after stimulation with optimal doses either of mitogens (concanavalin A [30 μg per milliliter], phytohemagglutinin [10 μg per milliliter]) for three days, or of one or more previously encountered microbial antigens for six days.[2] The latter included *Toxoplasma gondii* lysate antigen (15 μg per milliliter) for patients with positive results on the Sabin–Feldman dye test,[2] cytomegalovirus antigen (1:250 dilution of antigen purchased from MA Bioproducts, Walkersville, Md.) for patients with titers of serum complement-fixation antibody ≥1:8, and *Candida albicans* sonicate antigen (15 μg per milliliter) for those with oral candidiasis or positive skin tests for candida.[2] For gamma interferon generation, mononuclear cells (3×10^6 per milliliter) were stimulated for 48 hours with either (1) concanavalin A (30 μg per milliliter) or (2) *T. gondii* (50 μg per milliliter) or cytomegalovirus (1:50 dilution) antigens depending on the patient's antibody titer.[2] The culture supernatants were tested for antiviral activity with a standard cytopathic-effect-inhibition bioassay that employed WISH cells and vesicular stomatitis virus.[2] The antiviral activity of supernatants (lymphokines) stimulated by concanavalin A and *T. gondii* antigen was completely neutralized by a monoclonal antihuman gamma interferon antibody[2,3,5,18] that neutralizes neither alpha nor beta interferon.[18] For supernatants stimulated by cytomegalovirus antigen, this antibody did not consistently neutralize all antiviral activity; therefore, in assaying all antigen-stimulated lymphokines, we employed a radioimmunoassay test kit (Centocor, Malvern, Pa.) that specifically measures only gamma interferon.[19,20] Gamma interferon activity was measured against a National Institutes of Health laboratory standard for gamma interferon (Gg 23-901-530, Biological Response Modifiers Program) and is expressed in National Institutes of Health units.[2,18] As in a previous study,[2] a level below 10 U per milliliter was considered to be undetectable. In our laboratory, mean (±SEM) gamma interferon production in healthy seropositive controls is comparable in response to both *T. gondii* (986±149 U per milliliter) and cytomegalovirus antigens (773±140 U per milliliter), and in 58 experiments, none of 19 controls have generated less than 100 U per milliliter in response to either antigen. Thus, we consider 100 U per milliliter to be the lower limit of normal gamma interferon production in response to these two antigens, and responses to *T. gondii* or cytomegalovirus antigen have been grouped together as responses to "antigen." Heterosexual, age-matched laboratory personnel served as controls for each patient tested.

Statistical Analysis

Analyses of variance were performed on variables with continuous data. Scheffé's multiple-comparisons procedure was used to look for differences between groups when the analyses of variance indicated significant differences.[21] Kaplan–Meier curves were generated to describe the risk for AIDS in the various groups; log-rank tests were used to test for differences between groups.[22]

Results

Clinical and Laboratory Features

All 81 patients with lymphadenopathy were men,

Table 1. Clinical Features and T-Lymphocyte Subpopulations and Function in 81 Patients with Generalized Lymphadenopathy.*

	All Patients†	Group 1 (Lymphadenopathy Alone)	Group 2 (Lymphadenopathy plus Zoster, Thrush, or Symptoms)	Normal Values‡
No. of patients	81	38	43	—
Age — yr	35.4±1.4	35.5±1.3	34.9±1.2	—
Lymphadenopathy — mo§	10.8±1.8	11.1±2.2	10.3±1.6	—
(range)	3–72	3–72	3–48	—
Seropositivity for HTLV-III (%)	69/76 (91)	29/35 (83)	40/41 (98)	—
Cutaneous anergy (%)	15/48 (31)	5/16 (31)	10/32 (31)	—
Lymphocytes/mm³				
Total lymphocytes	1,514±80	1,591±99	1,448±121	1,834±82
T cells	1,049±64	1,006±84	1,081±96	1,478±59
T4+ cells	271±20	304±29	243±26	853±53
T8+ cells	750±52	729±63	766±77	579±45
T4/T8 ratio	0.42±0.03	0.46±0.04	0.40±0.04	1.6±0.1
Lymphocyte proliferation — cpm¶ (no. of patients)				
Mitogens				
PHA	27,524±2,556 (55)	27,085±3,465 (30)	28,011±4,026 (25)	75,601±6,396
Concanavalin A	5,625±1,299 (43)	7,285±1,815 (14)	4,887±1,701 (29)	35,155±3,966
Antigens				
T. gondii	7,657±5,659 (13)	15,998±1,444 (5)	2,445±2,152 (8)	64,869±8,051
Cytomegalovirus	4,223±1,415 (32)	11,079±4,962 (8)	2,017±792 (24)	51,891±10,143
C. albicans	8,646±2,691 (27)	10,972±5,001 (7)	7,851±3,247 (20)	36,411±5,473
Gamma interferon generation — U/ml				
Mitogen (no. of patients)	861±137 (78)	972±199 (37)	765±190 (41)	1,401±160
No. <10 U/ml (%)	3/78 (4)	0/37 (0)	3/41 (7)	
Antigen (no. of patients)	286±65 (81)	421±102 (38)	177±74 (43)	843±106
No. <10 U/ml (%)	15/81 (19)	2/38 (5)	13/43 (30)	
Follow-up — mo	12.9±0.5	12.8±0.6	13.0±0.5	
Range	8–19	8–18	8–19	
No. who contracted AIDS (%)	14/81 (17)	0/38 (0)	14/43 (33)	

*Plus–minus values are means ±SEM. HTLV-III denotes human T-cell lymphotropic virus Type III, PHA, phytohemagglutinin; *T. gondii*, *Toxoplasma gondii*; *C. albicans*, *Candida albicans*; and AIDS, acquired immunodeficiency syndrome.

†Except for lymphocytes and T8+ cells, results for lymphocyte enumeration, proliferation, and gamma interferon production for the total group, Group 1, and Group 2 are significantly different from control values (P<0.05). For Group 1 vs. Group 2, antigen-stimulated proliferation and gamma interferon production, the proportion (%) who produced <10 U of gamma interferon per milliliter in response to antigen (undetectable levels) and the proportion of patients in whom AIDS with opportunistic infections developed are significantly different (P<0.05).

‡For lymphocyte enumeration, values are for 34 healthy controls. Ranges (per cubic millimeter): total lymphocytes, 800 to 3200; T4+ cells, 328 to 1466; T8+ cells, 231 to 868; and T4/T8 cell ratio, 0.84 to 3.40. Normal values for lymphocyte proliferation are from 19 to 61 experiments using cells from 5 to 36 healthy controls for each stimulus. Ranges (cpm): phytohemagglutinin, 23,482 to 188,000; concanavalin A, 6000 to 153,487; *T. gondii*, 8250 to 152,685; cytomegalovirus, 10,500 to 113,943; and *Candida albicans*, 6725 to 105,834. Normal values for gamma interferon production in response to mitogen (concanavalin A): 300 to 10,000 U per milliliter (22 controls, 63 experiments); and in response to antigen (*T. gondii* or cytomegalovirus): 100 to 3800 U per milliliter (19 controls, 58 experiments).

§Duration of lymphadenopathy before entry into study.

¶Means of triplicate determinations corrected for the number of background counts per minute in unstimulated cultures.

79 were homosexual, and 2 were narcotic-drug abusers. At the time of enrollment and immunologic testing, 38 patients had lymphadenopathy alone, and 43 had lymphadenopathy accompanied by oral thrush, constitutional symptoms, or a recent episode of localized herpes zoster infection (Table 1). Sixty-nine of 76 patients (91 percent) were seropositive for HTLV-III, and 15 of 48 (31 percent) were anergic. Among 79 patients the following were also present: lymphopenia in 10 (13 percent); decreased numbers of T cells and T4+ cells in 22 (28 percent) and 48 (61 percent), respectively; increased numbers of T8+ cells in 28 (35 percent); and abnormal T4/T8 cell ratios (<0.84) in 76 (96 percent). In the entire group, mean lymphocyte proliferation and gamma interferon generation in response to all nonspecific mitogens and specific antigens were significantly lower than in the controls ($P<0.05$). Analysis of individual data, however, indicated normal proliferative responses to at least one mitogen in 60 percent of the patients tested and normal gamma interferon production in response to concanavalin A in 73 percent. Upon antigen stimulation, proliferative activity and gamma interferon generation were in the normal range in 27 and 37 percent of the patients, respectively. Overall, cells from 15 of the 81 patients failed to produce detectable levels of gamma interferon (<10 U per milliliter) in response to specific microbial antigen. During the follow-up period, which averaged 12.9±0.5 months (range, 8 to 19), the course in 14 patients progressed to full-blown AIDS as evidenced by various opportunistic infections; Kaposi's sarcoma subsequently developed in 3 of the 14.

Since patients with the AIDS prodrome who have clinical manifestations other than or in addition to lymphadenopathy (e.g., oral candidiasis, herpes zoster, or constitutional symptoms) appear to be at a higher risk for AIDS,[23-25] the 81 patients were next divided into two groups on the basis of their clinical findings.

Comparison of the Two Groups

Group 1 consisted of patients with lymphadenopathy alone, and Group 2, patients with lymphadenopathy accompanied by herpes zoster, oral thrush, or constitutional symptoms. Patients in both groups were similar with respect to all the variables shown in Table 1, with the exception of antigen-stimulated proliferative activity and gamma interferon production ($P<0.05$). Totally absent or barely detectable proliferative activity (<1000 cpm) in response to all antigens tested was observed in 16 of 28 Group 2 patients (57 percent) as compared with 2 of 13 Group 1 patients (15 percent), and 13 of 43 in Group 2 (30 percent) as compared with 2 of 38 in Group 1 (5 percent) did not produce gamma interferon in response to antigen. In addition, all 14 patients in whom opportunistic infections developed were in Group 2.

Five patients in Group 1 and two with herpes zoster in Group 2 also had thrombocytopenia, with platelet counts between 36,000 and 122,000 per cubic millimeter. This abnormality,[26] however, was not associated with impaired T-cell function, since cells from each of the seven (none of whom went on to the development of AIDS) generated normal levels of gamma interferon (≥300 U per milliliter) in response to concanavalin A, and antigen-induced production of gamma interferon was also normal (≥100 U per milliliter) in six of the seven patients with thrombocytopenia.

Analysis of Group 2 Patients

The finding that all those in whom infections developed were in Group 2 prompted the division of these 43 patients into four categories according to clinical manifestations. As shown in Table 2, patients with lymphadenopathy who had antecedent herpes zoster closely resembled those with lymphadenopathy alone (Group 1, Table 1) with respect to all the previously analyzed variables, including antigen-induced production of gamma interferon, which was normal in 9 of the 15 patients with herpes zoster (60 percent). In contrast, patients with constitutional symptoms or oral candidiasis or both were strikingly more deficient in T-cell proliferation and gamma interferon generation ($P<0.05$), especially in response to antigen. Among the 28 patients with thrush or symptoms — the group that contained 13 of the 14 who contracted opportunistic infections — antigen-stimulated gamma

Table 2. T-Cell Number and Function in 43 Group 2 Patients.*

	Conditions Accompanying Lymphadenopathy			
	Zoster	Constitutional Symptoms†	Oral Thrush	Symptoms† & Thrush
No. of patients	15	14	10	4
Cutaneous anergy (%)	3/11 (27)	4/12 (33)	1/5 (20)	2/4 (50)
T4+ cells/mm^3	332±63	231±30	249±46	157±44
Range	87–873	68–453	25–445	55–268
T4/T8 cell ratio	0.42±0.08	0.40±0.06	0.40±0.07	0.29±0.09
Range	0.11–1.36	0.05–0.78	0.10–0.79	0.15–0.51
Normal proliferative responses to				
Mitogen (%)	12/15 (80)	4/13 (31)	4/10 (40)	0/4 (0)
Antigen (%)	5/9 (56)	2/11 (18)	0/6 (0)	0/4 (0)
Gamma interferon production (U/ml)				
Mitogen	1292±442	734±291	165±40	167±88
Antigen	426±100	37±16	63±38	12±7
No. who contracted AIDS (%)	1/15 (7)	6/14 (43)	4/10 (40)	3/4 (75)

*Age, duration of lymphadenopathy and other clinical manifestations, seropositivity for HTLV-III, and number of lymphocytes, T cells, and T8+ cells were all similar for the four groups shown. Plus–minus values are means ±SEM.

†Constitutional symptoms in the 18 patients who had them included fever in 16 patients, fatigue in 9, weight loss in 9, and night sweats in 8. Fourteen patients had >1 of these symptoms.

Table 3. Patients with Lymphadenopathy and with Constitutional Symptoms or Thrush Who Did and Who Did Not Contract AIDS-Related Opportunistic Infections.*

Patient No.	Symptoms or Thrush	T4+ Cells per mm^3	T4/T8 Ratio	Gamma Interferon Production: Mitogen	Gamma Interferon Production: Antigen	Opportunistic Infections (Mo after Study)
				units/ml		
Patients with infections						
1	OT	29	0.25	300	<10	PCP (3)
2	OT	382	0.31	60	<10	PCP (4)†
3	Sx + OT	131	0.51	300	<10	Histoplasmosis (5)‡
4	Sx	169	0.43	600	<10	PCP (5)
5	OT	204	0.39	300	22	PCP (5)
6	Sx	68	0.07	300	15	PCP (6)
7	Sx	341	0.25	300	<10	PCP (8)
8	OT	95	0.18	2000	<10	PCP (9)
9	Sx + OT	20	0.04	200	<10	MAI (10)‡
10	Sx + OT	174	0.15	ND	16	MAI (10)‡
11	Sx	376	0.45	3000	<10	HSV (11)‡
12	Sx	171	0.25	30	24	PCP (12)
13	OT	319	0.31	30	<10	Toxoplasmosis (12)‡
Mean ±SEM		191±35	0.28±0.04	618±262	6±3	7.7±0.9 months
Range		20–382	0.04–0.51	30–3000	<10–24	3–12 months
Patients without infections (n = 15)§						
Mean ±SEM		259±33	0.40±0.06	396±198	73±34	None
Range		25–453	0.10–0.79	<10–3000¶	<10–500¶	—

*OT denotes oral thrush, Sx constitutional symptoms, PCP *Pneumocystis carinii* pneumonia, MAI *Mycobacterium avium-intracellulare*, ND not done, and HSV herpes simplex virus. All 13 patients whose conditions progressed to become AIDS were seropositive for HTLV-III.

†Kaposi's sarcoma also subsequently developed in this patient.

‡Patients 3, 9, 10, and 13 had disseminated infections. Patient 11 had chronic perianal and oral ulcerations caused by herpes simplex virus and esophagitis, which responded to treatment with acyclovir.

§Of the 15 patients, 5 had oral thrush, 9 had constitutional symptoms, and 1 had both. All 15 were seropositive to HTLV-III.

¶In response to mitogen (concanavalin A) or antigen, 3 and 2 of these 15 patients, respectively, did not generate detectable levels of gamma interferon (<10 U per milliliter).

interferon secretion was normal in only 2 patients (7 percent) and absent in 11 (39 percent).

Since the presence of constitutional symptoms and oral thrush appeared to be associated with progression to AIDS, we analyzed this group of 28 patients further to determine what findings might permit more specific prospective identification of those at particularly high risk (Table 3). This analysis of the 13 patients who contracted opportunistic infections and the 15 patients who did not indicated no significant differences with respect to prestudy duration of lymphadenopathy, thrush, or symptoms, HTLV-III seropositivity, absolute numbers of T cells or T4+ cells, T4/T8 cell ratios mean mitogen-stimulated lymphocyte proliferation or gamma interferon production, or duration of follow-up. The 13 patients in whom AIDS developed, however, were more often anergic (5 of 10 vs. 2 of 11), and had appreciably more severe defects in T-cell responses to microbial antigen. For 7 of the 9 patients (78 percent) who were tested in this group of 13, proliferative activity in response to antigen was totally absent (range, 0 to 870 cpm) (as compared with 1 of the 10 tested among the 15 patients [range, 0 to 15166 cpm] who remained free of infections), and cells from 9 of the 13 (69 percent) failed to generate detectable levels of antigen-induced gamma interferon (Table 3). This latter finding, characteristic of patients with established AIDS and opportunistic infections,[2] was present in only 2 of the 15 patients (13 percent) with symptoms or thrush who did not contract an infection. Responses to nonspecific mitogen stimulation were not helpful in discriminating among those at risk, since 8 of the 13 patients whose condition progressed to become AIDS generated normal levels of concanavalin A–induced gamma interferon (Table 3).

Prognostic Value of Clinical Manifestations and Antigen-Stimulated Gamma Interferon Production

Of 38 patients with lymphadenopathy alone (Group 1), none went on to contract an opportunistic infection during the study period of 8 to 18 months (Table 4). *Pneumocystis carinii* pneumonia (without intervening thrush or constitutional symptoms) developed in 1 of 15 patients with herpes zoster nine months after study, and two months later Kaposi's sarcoma developed in the same patient. This patient was one of the two with herpes zoster whose cells generated <10 U of gamma interferon per milliliter in response to antigen. The remaining 13 patients who had opportunistic infections all had preceding thrush or constitutional symptoms or both. For the entire group of 81 patients, none of 54 whose cells produced normal (≥100 U per milli-

Table 4. Clinical Manifestations, Antigen-Induced Gamma Interferon Production, and Development of Opportunistic Infections in 81 Patients with the AIDS Prodrome and Generalized Lymphadenopathy.

	Lymphadenopathy: Alone	Lymphadenopathy: Zoster	Lymphadenopathy: Thrush & Symptoms	Opportunistic Infections
				no. (%)
No. of patients	38	15	28	14/81 (17)
Antigen-stimulated gamma interferon production (U/ml)				
≥100	20	9	2	0/31 (0)
≥50<100	5	2	2	0/9 (0)
≥25<50	8	2	4	0/14 (0)
≥10<25	3	0	9	4/12 (33)
<10	2	2	11	10/15 (67)
AIDS developed — no. (%)	0/38 (0)	1/15 (7)	13/28 (46)	

liter) or moderately decreased (≥25<100 U per milliliter) levels of antigen-induced gamma interferon acquired an infection (Table 4). In contrast, 4 of 12 patients (33 percent) with severely impaired but detectable production (≥10<25 U per milliliter) and 10 of 15 (67 percent) who did not generate gamma interferon (<10 U per milliliter) contracted opportunistic infections within 8.2±0.9 months (range, 3 to 12). Overall, 14 of 22 patients (64 percent) who had herpes zoster, thrush, or other symptoms and whose cells generated <25 U of gamma interferon per milliliter acquired infections, whereas none of 59 whose cells produced ≥25 U per milliliter had infections, irrespective of clinical manifestations (Table 4). On the basis of the preceding results, Figure 1 shows the probability of the development of opportunistic infections as a function of clinical manifestations and of gamma interferon production in response to specific antigen.

Additional Follow-up Data

The five patients with absent antigen-stimulated production of gamma interferon who did not contract an infection during the study period have now been followed for a total of 17 to 21 months. The clinical status of four of these five patients has not changed: one has lymphadenopathy alone, and one each has herpes zoster, constitutional symptoms, and thrush. Eleven months after initial evaluation, however, the fifth patient, who originally had lymphadenopathy alone, experienced weight loss and fever, and six months later he acquired an opportunistic infection (candida esophagitis).

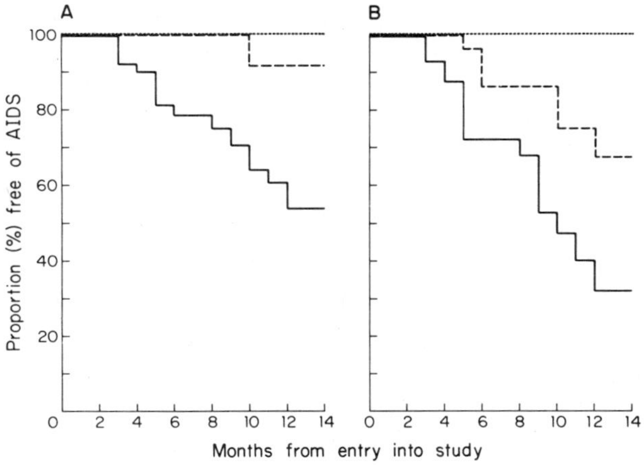

Figure 1. The Probability of Remaining Free of AIDS-Related Opportunistic Infections over Time as a Function of Clinical Manifestations (A) and the Capacity to Produce Gamma Interferon in Response to Specific Antigen in Vitro (B).

Panel A shows the results in patients with lymphadenopathy alone (dotted line), lymphadenopathy plus herpes zoster (dashed line), and lymphadenopathy plus constitutional symptoms or oral thrush (solid line). Panel B indicates the results in patients whose gamma interferon generation was normal (≥100 U per milliliter) or moderately impaired (≥25<100 U per milliliter) (dotted line), severely impaired but detectable (≥10<25 U per milliliter) (dashed line), or undetectable (<10 U per milliliter) (solid line).

Discussion

Since more than 90 percent of patients with AIDS die within 12 months of their first major infection,[2] the ability to identify prospectively with reasonable accuracy the persons likely to contract AIDS-related opportunistic infections would logically serve to intensify the evaluation of both potential antiviral agents[27-30] and experimental regimens aimed at immunoprophylaxis. The results of this study suggest that it is possible, by correlating clinical manifestations with in vitro T-cell responses to specific antigen, to identify a subpopulation of patients with the AIDS prodrome who are at definite and immediate risk for AIDS and opportunistic infections. This group appears to comprise principally those with lymphadenopathy accompanied by oral candidiasis or constitutional symptoms, and may represent more than one third of patients with the prodrome who have sought medical attention or have been recruited for study.[16] At the same time, our results also suggest that patients with lymphadenopathy alone or lymphadenopathy associated with herpes zoster or thrombocytopenia are not nearly as deficient in T-cell responses, and in parallel fashion, do not appear to be at a similar immediate risk for the development of opportunistic infections. Patients with lymphadenopathy alone, however, may first acquire constitutional symptoms or oral thrush before their condition progresses to become AIDS.[25] Thus, long-term follow-up will be required before we can correlate the base-line T-cell responses of our Group 1 patients and remaining patients with herpes zoster with the likelihood either that they will enter a high-risk category or that AIDS will develop directly without an intervening symptomatic stage.

Although a substantial proportion (46 percent) of our 28 patients with thrush or constitutional symptoms or both contracted AIDS-related infections, 15 others (54 percent) with these same clinical manifestations did not, despite similar durations of follow-up and the presence of at least one and typically several T-cell defects. However, the data in Table 3 suggest that it was still possible to identify nearly all those in this group who were at high risk by their barely measurable, or more often undetectable, responses to a previously encountered microbial antigen. Other assays performed in parallel were generally not helpful in identifying those destined to contract opportunistic infections in the period immediately after the study. There were, for example, no significant differences between the results in Group 1 (no infections) and Group 2 with respect to cutaneous anergy, lymphocyte responses to nonspecific stimulation with T-cell mitogens, numbers of T lymphocytes, or T4/T8 cell ratios. Although 4 of the 14 patients whose condition progressed to become AIDS had <100 T4+ cells per cubic millimeter, four others had normal numbers of T4+ cells (Table 3), and there was no correlation overall between the number of T4+ cells and the development of opportunistic infections. Since we have not routinely examined lymph nodes histologically[31,32] or performed other in vitro assays to evaluate the immunologic status of patients with the AIDS prodrome,[24,25,31-39] it also remains possible that analyses other than those of antigen-stimulated lymphocyte proliferation and gamma interferon generation may prove useful as indicators of a high risk for the development of AIDS. Nonetheless, given the broad immunoregulatory effects of gamma interferon,[11] the failure of the T cells of a patient with the prodrome to produce this molecule in response to specific antigen is, in our opinion, compelling evidence that the profound defect in cellular immune mechanisms typical of fully established AIDS[2] is probably present.

Despite our emphasis on the implications of the absence of in vitro production of antigen-stimulated gamma interferon, 4 of the 15 patients whose levels were undetectable have thus far remained free of infections, and 4 of the 14 who contracted opportunistic infections had detectable, albeit extremely low, levels (e.g., 15 to 24 U per milliliter) (Table 3). Thus, although the correlation between progression to AIDS and absent gamma interferon production is high, it is not absolute. In addition, 1 of the 14 patients had preceding herpes zoster but not thrush or constitutional symptoms. Both observations serve to reemphasize the innate immunologic and clinical heterogeneity of patients with the prodrome who have been observed by other investigators.[23,25,31,34,36,38,40] Nevertheless, the data summarized in Table 4 appear to support a clear relation between (1) the type of prodromal clinical manifestation, (2) T-cell competence as judged by specific antigen-induced gamma interferon secretion, and (3) the risk of contracting AIDS-related opportunistic infections.

Finally, despite the fact that a large number of patients with the AIDS prodrome have now been studied at various institutions, there is still considerable debate about the actual overall risk for the development of either AIDS-related opportunistic infections or Kaposi's sarcoma.[23-25,31,41,42] Although the results of our study appear clear and are consistent with other reports from New York City,[23-25] it seems most prudent to conclude that there is still more to be learned about the natural history of the AIDS prodrome (AIDS-related complex) and to determine which of the plethora of currently available immunologic assays will prove accurate in identifying patients at definite risk for AIDS. Our findings indicate the importance of considering both clinical manifestations and specific antigen-induced T-cell responses.

We are indebted to Drs. Lawrence Downs, Ronald Grossman, Lorenzo Lavorgna, John Montana, Lawrence Nathanson, Kenneth Unger, and Daniel Williams for allowing us to study their patients; to Mary Lou Aprile, R.N., for her assistance; and to Susan Messina and Linda Schaefer for preparing the manuscript.

References

1. Seligmann M, Chess L, Fahey JL, et al. AIDS — an immunologic reevaluation. N Engl J Med 1984; 311:1286-92.
2. Murray HW, Rubin BY, Masur H, Roberts RB. Impaired production of lymphokines and immune (gamma) interferon in the acquired immunodeficiency syndrome. N Engl J Med 1984; 310:883-9.
3. Nathan CF, Murray HW, Wiebe ME, Rubin BY. Identification of interferon-γ as the lymphokine that activates human macrophage oxidative metabolism and antimicrobial activity. J Exp Med 1983; 158:670-89.
4. Nathan CF, Prendergast TJ, Wiebe ME, et al. Activation of human macrophages: comparison of other cytokines with interferon-γ. J Exp Med 1984; 160:600-5.
5. Murray HW, Rubin BY, Rothermel CD. Killing of intracellular *Leishmania donovani* by lymphokine-stimulated human mononuclear phagocytes: evidence that interferon-γ is the activating lymphokine. J Clin Invest 1983; 72:1506-10.
6. Rothermel CD, Rubin BY, Murray HW. γ-interferon is the factor in lymphokine that activates human macrophages to inhibit intracellular *Chlamydia psittaci* replication. J Immunol 1983; 131:2542-4.
7. Wisseman CL Jr, Waddell A. Interferonlike factors from antigen- and mitogen-stimulated human leukocytes with antirickettsial and cytolytic actions on *Rickettsia prowazekii*: infected human endothelial cells, fibroblasts, and macrophages. J Exp Med 1983; 157:1780-93.
8. Ockenhouse CF, Schulman S, Shear HL. Induction of crisis forms in the human malaria parasite *Plasmodium falciparum* by γ-interferon-activated monocyte-derived macrophages. J Immunol 1984; 133:1601-8.
9. James SL, Natovitz PC, Farrar WL, Leonard EJ. Macrophages as effector cells of protective immunity in murine schistosomiasis: macrophage activation in mice vaccinated with radiation-attenuated cercariae. Infect Immun 1984; 44:569-75.
10. Kiderlen AF, Kaufmann SHE, Lohman-Matthes M-L. Protection of mice against the intracellular bacterium *Listeria monocytogenes* by recombinant immune interferon. Eur J Immunol 1984; 14:964-7.
11. Vilcek J, Gray PW, Rinderknecht E, Sevastopoulos CG. Interferon-gamma: a lymphokine for all seasons. In: Pick E, ed. Lymphokines. Vol. 11. New York: Academic Press (in press).
12. Basham TY, Merigan TC. Recombinant interferon-γ increases HLA-DR synthesis and expression. J Immunol 1983; 130:1492-4.
13. Heagy W, Kelley VE, Strom TB, et al. Decreased expression of human class II antigens on monocytes from patients with acquired immune deficiency syndrome: increased expression with interferon-γ. J Clin Invest 1984; 74:2089-96.
14. Unanue ER, Beller DI, Lu CY, Allen PM. Antigen presentation: comments on its regulation and mechanism. J Immunol 1984; 132:1-5.
15. Frasca D, Adorini L, Landolfo S, Doria G. Enhancing effect of IFN-γ on helper T cell activity and IL 2 production. J Immunol 1985; 134:3907-11.
16. Persistent, generalized lymphadenopathy among homosexual males. MMWR 1982; 31:249-51.
17. Gallo RC, Salahuddin SZ, Popovic M, et al. Frequent detection and isolation of cytopathic retroviruses (HTLV-III) from patients with AIDS and at risk for AIDS. Science 1984; 224:500-3.
18. Rubin BY, Bartal AH, Anderson SL, Millet SK, Hirshaut Y, Feit C. The anticellular and protein-inducing activities of human γ interferon preparations are mediated by the interferon. J Immunol 1983; 130:1019-20.
19. Chang TW, McKinney S, Liu V, Kung PC, Vilček J, Le J. Use of monoclonal antibodies as sensitive and specific probes for biologically active human γ-interferon. Proc Natl Acad Sci USA 1984; 81:5219-22.
20. Vilček J, Henricksen-Destefano D, Robb RJM, Le J. Interleukin 2 as the inducing signal for interferon-gamma in peripheral blood leukocytes stimulated with mitogen or antigen. In: Kirchner H, Schnellekens H, eds. The biology of the interferon system — 1984. Amsterdam: Elsevier (in press).
21. Snedecor GW, Cochran WG. Statistical methods. 7th ed. Ames, Iowa: Iowa State University Press, 1980.
22. Lee ET. Statistical methods for survival data analysis. Belmont, Calif.: Lifetime Learning Publications, 1980.
23. Klein RS, Harris CA, Small CB, Moll B, Lesser M, Friedland GH. Oral candidiasis in high-risk patients as the initial manifestation of the acquired immunodeficiency syndrome. N Engl J Med 1984; 311:354-8.
24. Mathur-Wagh U, Enlow RW, Spigland I, et al. Longitudinal study of persistent generalised lymphadenopathy in homosexual men: relation to acquired immunodeficiency syndrome. Lancet 1984; 1:1033-8.
25. Metroka CE, Cunningham-Rundles S, Pollack MS, et al. Generalized lymphadenopathy in homosexual men. Ann Intern Med 1983; 99:585-91.
26. Walsh CM, Nardi MA, Karpatkin S. On the mechanism of thrombocytopenic purpura in sexually active homosexual men. N Engl J Med 1984; 311:635-9.
27. Mitsuya H, Popovic M, Yarchoan R, Matsushita S, Gallo RC, Broder S. Suramin protection of T cells in vitro against infectivity and cytopathic effect of HTLV-III. Science 1984; 226:172-4.
28. McCormick JB, Getchell JP, Mitchell SW, Hicks DR. Ribavirin suppresses replication of lymphadenopathy-associated virus in cultures of human adult T lymphocytes. Lancet 1984; 2:1367-9.
29. Rozenbaum W, Dormont D, Spire B, et al. Antimoniotungstate (HPA 23)

treatment of three patients with AIDS and one with prodrome. Lancet 1985; 1:450-1.

30. Ho DD, Hartshorn KL, Rota TR, et al. Recombinant human interferon alpha-A suppresses HTLV-III replication in vitro. Lancet 1985; 1:602-4.
31. Byrnes RK, Chan WC, Spira TJ, Ewing EP Jr, Chandler FW. Value of lymph node biopsy in unexplained lymphadenopathy in homosexual men. JAMA 1983; 250:1313-7.
32. Guarda LA, Butler JJ, Mansell P, Hersh EM, Reuben J, Newell GR. Lymphadenopathy in homosexual men: morbid anatomy with clinical and immunologic correlations. Am J Clin Pathol 1983; 79:559-68.
33. Zolla-Pazner S, William D, El-Sadr W, Marmor M, Stahl R. Quantitation of β_2-microglobulin and other immune characteristics in a prospective study of men at risk for acquired immune deficiency syndrome. JAMA 1984; 251:2951-5.
34. Stahl RE, Friedman-Kien A, Dubin R, Marmor M, Zolla-Pazner S. Immunologic abnormalities in homosexual men: relationship to Kaposi's sarcoma. Am J Med 1982; 73:171-8.
35. deShazo RD, Andes WA, Nordberg J, Newton J, Daul C, Bozelka B. An immunologic evaluation of hemophiliac patients and their wives: relationships to the acquired immunodeficiency syndrome. Ann Intern Med 1983; 99:159-64.
36. Reuben JM, Hersh EM, Mansell PW, et al. Immunological characterization of homosexual males. Cancer Res 1983; 43:897-904.
37. Grieco HM, Reddy MM, Kothari HB, Lange M, Buimovici-Klein E, William D. Elevated β_2-microglobulin and lysozyme levels in patients with acquired immune deficiency syndrome. Clin Immunol Immunopathol 1984; 32:174-84.
38. deShazo RD, Penico JP, Pankey GA, et al. Studies in homosexual patients with and without lymphadenopathy: relationships to the acquired immune deficiency syndrome. Arch Intern Med 1984; 144:1153-8.
39. Lopez C, Fitzgerald PA, Siegal FP, Landesman S, Gold JW, Krown S. Deficiency of interferon-alpha generating capacity is associated with susceptibility to opportunistic infections in patients with AIDS. Ann NY Acad Sci (in press).
40. Fahey JL, Prince H, Weaver M, et al. Quantitative changes in T helper or T suppressor/cytotoxic lymphocyte subsets that distinguish acquired immune deficiency syndrome from other immune subset disorders. Am J Med 1984; 76:95-100.
41. Abrams DI, Lewis BJ, Beckstead JH, Casavant CA, Drew WL. Persistent diffuse lymphadenopathy in homosexual men: endpoint or prodrome? Ann Intern Med 1984; 100:801-8.
42. Ioachim HL, Lerner CW, Tapper ML. Lymphadenopathies in homosexual men: relationships with the acquired immune deficiency syndrome. JAMA 1983; 250:1306-9.

SPECIAL REPORT

THE WALTER REED STAGING CLASSIFICATION FOR HTLV-III/LAV INFECTION

Robert R. Redfield, D. Craig Wright, and Edmund C. Tramont

BEFORE the identification of the human T-cell lymphotropic virus Type III/lymphadenopathy-associated virus (HTLV-III/LAV) as the cause of the acquired immunodeficiency syndrome (AIDS), the clinical recognition of this disease depended on the occurrence of secondary opportunistic infections and certain neoplastic processes.[1] However, focusing on the late complications of HTLV-III infections severely limits the clinical appreciation of the spectrum of disease as related to the causative agent. Although the natural history of HTLV-III infection is only partially defined, it is clear that patients with AIDS represent only a minority of the patients who have been infected. The clinical presentation of patients with HTLV-III infections can range from asymptomatic (with viremia or antibody or both), through chronic generalized lymphadenopathy, to subclinical and clinical T-cell deficiency.[2] The clinical presentation of patients with HTLV-III infection depends on the integrity of the T helper cell and T-cell immunity.[3]

There are many unique problems that military personnel with HTLV-III/LAV infection face in a military environment. For example, all military recruits receive live-virus vaccines against such diseases as vaccinia, rubella, measles, adenovirus infection, and poliomyelitis and may fall victim to the attenuated virus itself (Redfield RR, et al.: unpublished data); all military personnel receive multiple vaccines to which they may respond suboptimally[4]; military personnel may be deployed to areas where they are at risk of acquiring such diseases as malaria, leishmaniasis, and trypanosomiasis, to which they may succumb more easily; and all military personnel are potential blood donors in the field.

Recently, the U.S. Army has adopted a staging classification for HTLV-III/LAV infection (Fig. 1) to provide uniformity within its health care system for routine clinical evaluations of patients with such infections; to facilitate an understanding of the natural history of these infections; and to help evaluate the clinical response to antiviral treatment regimens directed against HTLV-III/LAV. This staging scheme is applicable to adults only; newborns, infants, and young children may require a different classification because of differences in base-line functional T-cell indexes.

Stage WR0 designates high-risk contacts — e.g., recipients of blood products and sexual contacts of persons with documented HTLV-III/LAV infection (HTLV-III antibody or HTLV-III virus isolation or both). Stages WR1 through WR6 require documentation of HTLV-III infection by demonstration of HTLV-III antibody on Western blot or comparable confirmation assay using virus-specific antigens or HTLV-III virus isolation or both. Stage WR5 is defined by the occurrence of complete anergy or thrush or both (see below).

HTLV-III infections with symptoms (temperature higher than 38°C [100.5°F] for three weeks, unexplained loss of more than 10 percent of body weight over a period of three months, night sweats for three weeks, or chronic diarrhea for more than one month) should be further designated by the addition of the letter B (e.g., WR5B). Many patients in this category can be documented as having an occult opportunistic infection that can be diagnosed by a careful and complete evaluation.

The occurrence of Kaposi's sarcoma is designated by adding the letter K after the appropriate stage (e.g., WR4K, WR5BK). Current evidence suggests that this neoplastic process can occur without severe T-helper-cell depletion. Patients with neurologic disease (demyelinating disease, encephalopathy, or neuropathy) secondary to infection of the nervous system

STAGE	HTLV III ANTIBODY AND/OR VIRUS ISOLATION	CHRONIC LYMPHADENOPATHY	T HELPER CELLS/mm3	DHS	THRUSH	O.I.
WR 0	-	-	>400	NL	-	-
WR 1	+	-	>400	NL	-	-
WR 2	+	+	>400	NL	-	-
WR 3	+	±	<400	NL	-	-
WR 4	+	±	<400	P	-	-
WR 5	+	±	< 400	C AND/OR +		-
WR 6	+	±	< 400	PC	±	+

Figure 1. The Walter Reed Staging Classification for HTLV-III/LAV Infection.

The essential criteria for assignment to each stage are indicated by hatched hexagons. DHS denotes delayed hypersensitivity; NL, normal; P, partial cutaneous anergy, which is defined as an intact cutaneous response to only one of the four test antigens (see text); C, complete cutaneous anergy to the four test antigens; and O.I., opportunistic infection.

The views of the authors do not purport to reflect the position of the Department of the Army or the Department of Defense.

by HTLV-III virus itself are designated by adding the letters CNS to the appropriate stage (e.g., WR4CNS). The occurrence of neoplasms other than Kaposi's sarcoma is designated by adding the letter N after the appropriate stage (e.g., WR4N).

HTLV-III antibody is defined as antibody to the structural proteins of HTLV-III as determined by Western blot techniques. HTLV-III virus isolation can also be used to document HTLV-III infection, particularly in patients in stage WR1 who are seronegative but viremic. Chronic lymphadenopathy is defined as the presence of lymph nodes in two or more extrainguinal sites at least 1 cm in diameter that persist for more than three months. T helper cells (OKT4 or Leu-3+) are counted and expressed as the number of cells per cubic millimeter (methods previously described[2]). Quantitative depletion must persist for at least three months for a patient to be classified in stage WR3.

Delayed hypersensitivity is defined as an intact cutaneous response (induration of at least 5 mm) to at least two of the following four test antigens: tetanus, trichophyton, mumps, and candida. Thrush is defined as clinical oral candidiasis (creamy-white, curd-like patches on the tongue or other oral mucosal surfaces, which are removable by scraping), including a positive potassium hydroxide preparation or Gram stain showing masses of hyphae, pseudohyphae, and yeast forms.

Opportunistic infections include *Pneumocystis carinii* pneumonia, central nervous system or disseminated toxoplasmosis, chronic cryptosporidiosis, candida esophagitis, disseminated histoplasmosis, central nervous system or disseminated cryptococcosis, disseminated atypical mycobacterial disease, extrapulmonary tuberculosis, disseminated nocardiosis, disseminated cytomegalovirus, or chronic mucocutaneous herpes simplex. Other disseminated or chronic, not-self-limited infections with agents in which cellular immunity has a pivotal role in host defense (e.g., viral, parasitic, fungal, mycobacterial, and certain other bacterial agents) should be anticipated as causing opportunistic disease in patients with stages WR5 and WR6. Kaposi's sarcoma does not itself fulfill the criteria for stage WR6.

This classification scheme is based on two central observations: the fact that the T helper cell is the principal target cell of HTLV-III,[5] and the clinical observation that the functional integrity of the T helper cell determines the clinical presentation.[6] Preliminary studies in 39 sequential patients followed for more than 18 months demonstrated that the patients entered in stages WR3 to WR6 had a slow but progressive course to the next stage or death. However, it should be stressed that the use of the word "stage" does not imply that all patients (particularly those in stages WR1 and WR2) will have progressive disease. Many questions about clinical progression are currently unanswered; this staging classification is designed to facilitate their resolution.

References

1. Gallo RC, Salahuddin SZ, Popovic M, et al. Frequent detection and isolation of cytopathic retroviruses (HTLV-III) from patients with AIDS and at risk for AIDS. Science 1984; 224:500-3.
2. Redfield RR, Markham PD, Salahuddin SZ, et al. Frequent transmission of HTLV-III among spouses of patients with AIDS-related complex and AIDS. JAMA 1985; 253:1571-3.
3. Fauci AS, Macher AM, Longo DL, et al. Acquired immunodeficiency syndrome: epidemiologic, clinical, immunologic, and therapeutic considerations. Ann Intern Med 1984; 100:92-106.
4. Lane CH, Depper JM, Greene WC, Whalen G, Waldmann TA, Fauci AS. Qualitative analysis of immune function in patients with the acquired immunodeficiency syndrome: evidence for a selective defect in soluble antigen recognition. N Engl J Med 1985; 313:79-84.
5. Dalgleish AG, Beverly PCL, Clapham PR, Crawford DH, Greaves MF, Weiss RA. The CD4 (T4) antigen is an essential component of the receptor for the AIDS retrovirus. Nature 1985; 312:763-7.
6. Redfield RR, Salahuddin SZ, Markham PD, et al. The clinical spectrum of HTLV-III disease at Walter Reed Army Medical Center. Presented at the International Conference on the Acquired Immunodeficiency Syndrome, Atlanta, Ga., April 16, 1985.

CORRESPONDENCE

AIDS WITH *MYCOBACTERIUM AVIUM–INTRACELLULARE* LESIONS RESEMBLING THOSE OF WHIPPLE'S DISEASE

To the Editor: The defect in cellular immunity primarily affecting the male homosexual population and associated with opportunistic systemic infections and Kaposi's sarcoma is currently the subject of intense medical interest.[1] Many of these patients have evidence of disseminated infection with the *Mycobacterium avium–intracellulare* complex (MAC), leading to widespread organ infiltration with foamy macrophages containing large numbers of acid-fast bacilli.[2-4] We have recently observed a patient who had the acquired immunodeficiency syndrome (AIDS) with MAC and unusual small-bowel lesions with the histopathological appearance of Whipple's disease.

A 30-year-old white male homosexual was admitted with AIDS and advanced Kaposi's sarcoma diagnosed on cervical lymph-node biopsy. The patient had spiking fever, diarrhea, weakness, and abdominal pain secondary to a massively enlarged spleen. Multiple lesions of the skin and oral mucosa consistent with Kaposi's sarcoma were present. The peripheral blood showed anemia and marked lymphopenia. A bone-marrow examination revealed ill-defined granulomas with large numbers of acid-fast bacilli, which on culture grew out resistant MAC. The patient died a short time later.

On post-mortem examination, there was an unusual small-bowel lesion characterized by prominent folds in the small-bowel mucosa, with elevated yellowish grains and nodules on the surface of the villi. Microscopical study of the bowel lesion revealed foamy macrophages infiltrating the entire intestinal mucosa with isolated small residual intestinal mucus-secreting glands similar to the appearance in Whipple's disease (Fig. 1A, 1B and 1C). The mucosal macrophages and regional lymph nodes were filled with foamy macrophages that were heavily crowded with acid-fast organisms consistent with MAC (Fig. 1D). The macrophages and intracellular organisms in the small bowel were strongly positive on staining with periodic acid–Schiff (PAS). The presence of massively enlarged lymph nodes suggested the possibility that this bowel lesion might be the portal of entry for MAC.

Since the bowel lesions in this patient with AIDS and MAC had a histologic appearance similar to Whipple's disease involving the intestinal mucosa, it might be reasonable to presuppose a similar cell-mediated immune defect. The cellular response in Whipple's disease is generally described as an infiltrative one in which the macrophage is predominant. The mucosa shows a marked decrease in the number of plasma cells, suggesting an alteration in the mucosal immune barrier.[5] Dobbins[6] has reported evidence for an immune defect in patients with Whipple's disease. There is a decreased percentage of T lymphocytes, with diminished lymphocyte responsiveness to phytohemagglutinin and concanavalin A and borderline skin anergy to antigens. Detailed studies of the helper/suppressor lymphocyte ratios have not been done in Whipple's disease, to our knowledge. The presence of the Whipple bacillus within the macrophage makes one wonder why it survives intracellularly. Most bacterial pathogens are rapidly digested by the macrophage after phagocytosis; however, the Whipple bacillus requires a lymphokine from T lymphocytes, macrophage-activating factor, to kill the intracellular bacteria.[6-8] The absence of this factor may also have a key role in survival of MAC within the macrophage in patients with AIDS. This leads one to the conclusion that a similar defect in cell-mediated immunity may be present in AIDS with MAC and in Whipple's disease, the common factor being defective macrophage processing of bacterial antigen.

Robert L. Strom, M.D.
Robert P. Gruninger, M.D.
Hennepin County Medical Center
Minneapolis, MN 55415

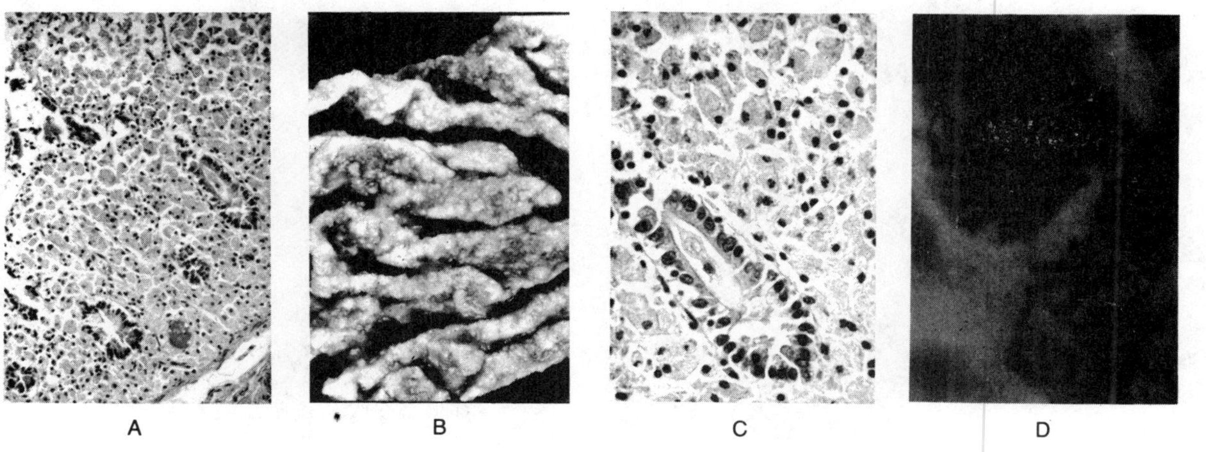

Figure 1. Small-Bowel Lesions in a Patient with AIDS with the *Mycobacterium avium–intracellulare* Complex (MAC).
Part A shows the intestinal lesion of AIDS with MAC. Part B shows the intestinal mucosa replaced by foamy macrophages (the muscularis mucosa is in the lower right-hand corner). Part C is a high-power view of foamy macrophages containing intracellular MAC bacteria, and Part D is an oil-immersion view of intracellular MAC bacteria.

References

1. Centers for Disease Control Task Force on Kaposi's Sarcoma and Opportunistic Infections. Epidemiologic aspects of the current outbreak of Kaposi's sarcoma and opportunistic infections. N Engl J Med 1982; 306:248-52.
2. Greene JB, Sidhu GS, Lewin S, et al. *Mycobacterium avium-intracellulare*: a cause of disseminated life-threatening infection in homosexuals and drug abusers. Ann Intern Med 1982; 97:539-46.
3. Zakowski P, Fligiel S, Berlin OGW, Johnson BL Jr. Disseminated *Mycobacterium avium-intracellulare* infection in homosexual men dying of acquired immunodeficiency. JAMA 1982; 248:2280-2.
4. Sohn CC, Schroff RW, Kliewer KE, Lebel DM, Fligiel S. Disseminated *Mycobacterium avium-intracellulare* infection in homosexual men with acquired cell-mediated immunodeficiency: a histologic and immunologic study of two cases. Am J Clin Pathol 1982; 79:247-52.
5. Dobbins WO III, Ruffin JM. A light- and electron-microscopy study of bacterial invasion in Whipple's disease. Am J Pathol 1967; 51:225-42.
6. Dobbins WO III. Is there an immune deficit in Whipple's disease? Dig Dis Sci 1981; 26:247-52.
7. Keren DF. Whipple's disease: a review emphasizing immunology and microbiology. CRC Crit Rev Clin Lab Sci 1981; 14:75-108.
8. Unanue ER. The regulation of lymphocyte functions by the macrophage. Immunol Rev 1978; 40:227-55.

To the Editor: In patients with AIDS, diarrhea and malabsorption are associated with a spectrum of formerly uncommon bacterial and parasitic infections that present new problems in differential diagnosis. Duodenal biopsy in a 30-year-old man with Kaposi's sarcoma, lymphadenopathy, and malabsorption revealed villi distended by macrophages filled with PAS-positive rods, consistent with Whipple's disease in histologic and electron microscopical appearance (Fig. 1).[1] Symptoms were not, however, relieved by tetracycline, as expected in Whipple's disease. Subsequent blood and sputum cultures grew *Mycobacterium avium*, yet despite antimycobacterial drugs, the patient's condition deteriorated and he died with multiple infections.

At autopsy sections of his intestine were compared with sections from patients with classical Whipple's disease and from a macaque with intestinal *M. avium* infection. When trypsinized sections were incubated with bacterial typing antiserums, patterns of cross-reactivity detected by indirect immunofluorescence were quite different from the characteristic pattern previously reported in tissue from patients with Whipple's disease.[3,4] Acid-fast stains were positive in the patient with AIDS and the macaque but negative in the patients with Whipple's disease. Villous lymphatics in the patient with AIDS were not distended as in Whipple's disease, despite extensive involvement of mesenteric lymph nodes by macrophages filled with bacteria. Thus, PAS-positive macrophages filling the lamina propria of intestinal villi can no longer be considered pathognomonic of Whipple's disease. Whipple's disease diagnosed solely on the basis of the postmortem histologic pattern in a Haitian woman with AIDS and cardiac Kaposi's sarcoma[5] probably should have been diagnosed as systemic *M. avium* infection instead.

In previously reported cases of disseminated *M. avium* infection in human beings,[6,7] intestinal involvement was discovered post mortem, when autolytic changes may have obscured the Whipple's-like villus

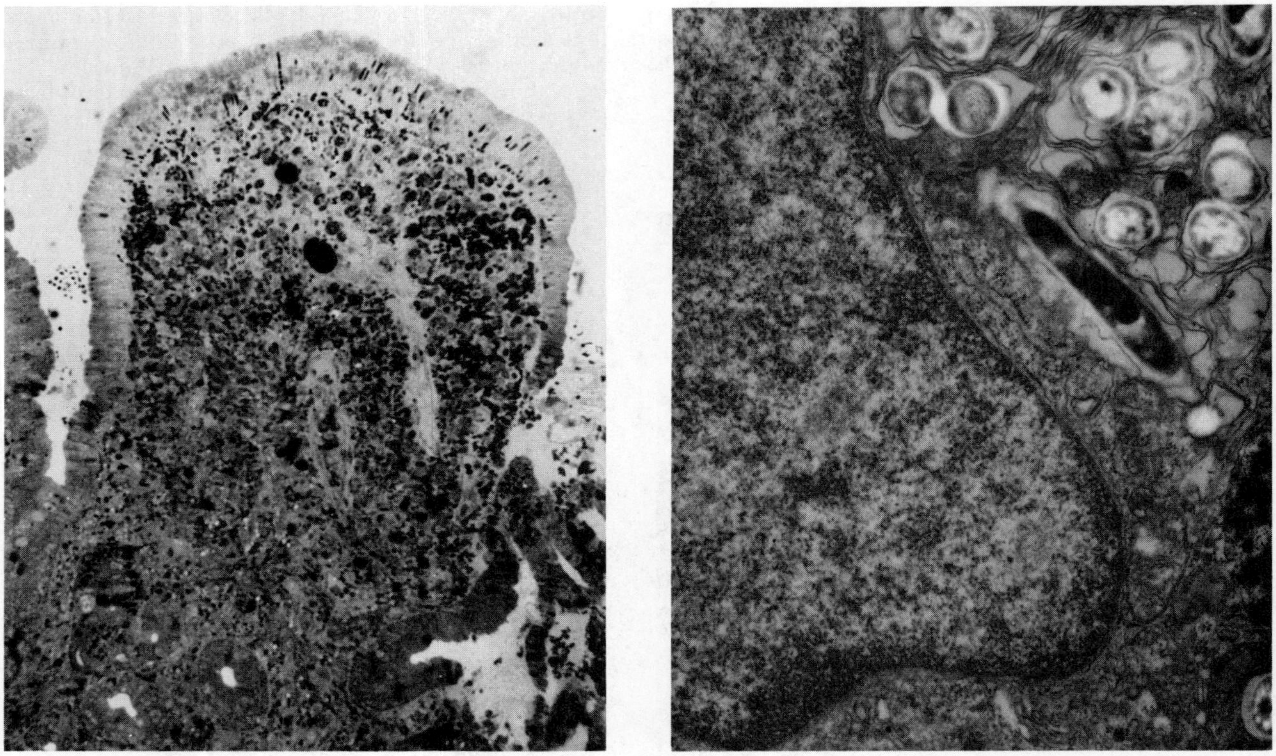

Figure 1. Endoscopic Duodenal Biopsy Specimen of a Patient with AIDS and *M. avium* Infection.

Part A shows villi distended by foamy macrophages (toluidine blue–stained section embedded in plastic, ×120). The macrophages shown in B contain intracytoplasmic lamellar membranous inclusions and bacilliform microorganisms resembling those seen in Whipple's disease[2] (transmission electron micrograph, ×16,700).

appearance, which has, however, been seen in primates.[8] Small-bowel biopsy specimens are of use in the diagnosis of diarrhea in patients with AIDS but must be interpreted with caution because of the varied presentations of opportunistic infections in immunosuppressed patients. Both Whipple's disease and *M. avium* infection appear to be conditions in which the elimination of intracellular bacteria by macrophages is impaired. Similar histologic patterns can be discriminated on the basis of the clinical setting, acid-fast staining, antibacterial staining patterns, culture data, and ultimately, the response to antibiotics.

ROBERT I. ROTH, M.D.
ROBERT L. OWEN, M.D.
University of California, San Francisco
School of Medicine
San Francisco, CA 94143

DAVID F. KEREN, M.D.
University of Michigan School of Medicine
Ann Arbor, MI 48109

REFERENCES

1. Owen RL, Roth RI, St. Hilaire RJ, Keren DF. Pseudo Whipple's disease — intestinal infection with *Mycobacterium avium-intracellulare (M. avium)* in acquired immune deficiency syndrome (AIDS). Gastroenterology 1983; 84:1267. abstract.
2. Trier JS, Phelps PC, Eidelman S, Rubin CE. Whipple's disease: light and electron microscope correlation of jejunal mucosal histology with antibiotic treatment and clinical status. Gastroenterology 1965; 48:684-707.
3. Keren DF, Weisburger WR, Yardley JH, Salyer WR, Arthur RR, Charache P. Whipple's disease: demonstration by immunofluorescence of similar bacterial antigens in macrophages from three cases. Johns Hopkins Med J 1976; 139:51-9.
4. Bhagavan BS, Hofkin GA, Cochran BA. Whipple's disease: morphologic and immunofluorescence characterization of bacterial antigens. Hum Pathol 1981; 12:930-6.
5. Autran B, Gorin I, Leibowitch M, et al. AIDS in a Haitian woman with cardiac Kaposi's sarcoma and Whipple's disease. Lancet 1983; 1:767-8.
6. Greene JB, Sidhu GS, Lewin S, et al. *Mycobacterium avium-intracellulare:* a cause of disseminated life-threatening infection in homosexuals and drug abusers. Ann Intern Med 1982; 97:539-46.
7. Sohn CC, Schroff RW, Kliewer KE, Lebel DM, Fligiel S. Disseminated *Mycobacterium avium-intracellulare* infection in homosexual men with acquired cell-mediated immunodeficiency: a histologic and immunologic study of two cases. Am J Clin Pathol 1983; 79:247-52.
8. Sesline DH, Schwartz LW, Osburn BI, et al. *Mycobacterium avium* infection in three rhesus monkeys. J Am Vet Med Assoc 1975; 167:639-45.

TUBERCULIN TESTING FOR PERSONS WITH POSITIVE SEROLOGIC STUDIES FOR HTLV-III

To the Editor: Persons who are seropositive for HTLV-III are at high risk for the development of T-cell immunosuppression of varying degrees of severity,[1] and those who are concurrently infected with *Mycobacterium tuberculosis* (i.e., those with positive tuberculin skin tests) may therefore also be at high risk for contracting and then transmitting tuberculosis. In the setting of a rapidly spreading AIDS epidemic, preventive therapy with isoniazid in persons seropositive for HTLV-III and with a positive tuberculin skin test could be of major public health importance. Such chemoprophylaxis is likely to be effective, since tuberculosis responds very well to standard treatment with antibiotics, even among patients with AIDS.[2]

From January 1980 through October 1985, the Florida Department of Health documented 90 cases of tuberculosis associated with AIDS. From January 1980 through June 1983, 17 of 25 such reported cases (65 percent) occurred among Haitian immigrants, and 7 of 25 (28 percent) occurred among persons born in the United States. Since July 1983, 28 of 65 such cases (43 percent) have occurred among Haitians and 29 of 65 (44.6 percent) have occurred among U.S. natives. In Florida, therefore, cases of tuberculosis associated with AIDS seem to be increasing both in their total number and in the number and percentage of patients who are U.S. natives. It is likely that the number of cases of tuberculosis related to HTLV-III immunosuppression exceeds that associated with AIDS, since tuberculosis tends to precede the syndrome by months or years.[2] Furthermore, it is possible that some cases of tuberculosis related to HTLV-III immunosuppression are never followed by severe opportunistic infections or tumors diagnostic of AIDS. These factors, at least in part, may explain the recent abrupt increase in the incidence of tuberculosis (43 percent) among persons born in the United States and residing in southeast Florida.[3] Furthermore, the incidence of tuberculosis may increase in other areas of the United States and in other parts of the world (e.g., developing countries) where tuberculosis infection is prevalent and the rates of HTLV-III infection and AIDS are rising.

Tuberculosis is the only AIDS-related infection that is spread to normal persons by the aerosol route and is preventable by chemoprophylaxis. We believe that persons with a confirmed positive HTLV-III serologic test (especially those in high-risk groups for AIDS) should be advised to have a tuberculin skin test. If the skin test is positive or if there has been a documented positive skin test in the past, such person should be offered isoniazid prophylaxis (especially if T-cell testing already shows immunosuppression). Even if they decline, the positive skin test will still represent valuable base-line information if further subclinical T-cell immunodeficiency, AIDS-related complex, or AIDS subsequently developed in persons seropositive for HTLV-III. At this point, although their tuberculin skin test may have become falsely negative (in itself a bad prognostic sign), they will already have been identified as being infected and can be given isoniazid prophylactically to reduce their relatively high risk of contracting and then transmitting tuberculosis. Such chemoprophylaxis may help to control the spread of tuberculosis in areas of high AIDS risk, and in the individual patient at risk for AIDS it may prevent the T-cell immunosuppression of tuberculosis[4] from being superimposed on the T-cell immunosuppression of HTLV-III infection.

ARTHUR E. PITCHENIK, M.D.
University of Miami Medical School and
Veterans Administration Medical Center

JANICE BURR, M.D.
Dade County Florida Department of Public Health
Miami, FL 33125

CLIFFORD H. COLE, M.D., M.P.H.
Florida Department of Health
and Rehabilitative Services
Jacksonville, FL 32231

REFERENCES

1. Francis DP, Jaffe HW, Fultz PN, et al. The natural history of infection with

the lymphadenopathy-associated virus human T-lymphotropic virus type III. Ann Intern Med 1985; 103:719-21.

2. Pitchenik AE, Cole C, Russell BW, Fischl MA, Spira TJ, Snider DE Jr. Tuberculosis, atypical mycobacteriosis, and the acquired immunodeficiency syndrome among Haitian and non-Haitian patients in south Florida. Ann Intern Med 1984; 101:641-5.
3. Tuberculosis Register of the State of Florida, 1985.
4. Katz P, Goldstein RA, Fauci AS. Immunoregulation in infection caused by *Mycobacterium tuberculosis*: the presence of suppressor monocytes and the alteration of subpopulations of T lymphocytes. J Infect Dis 1979; 140:12-21.

Clinical Studies

Epstein–Barr Virus, Cytomegalovirus, and Herpes Virus Related to AIDS

ORIGINAL ARTICLE

DEFECTIVE REGULATION OF EPSTEIN–BARR VIRUS INFECTION IN PATIENTS WITH ACQUIRED IMMUNODEFICIENCY SYNDROME (AIDS) OR AIDS-RELATED DISORDERS

Deborah L. Birx, M.D., Robert R. Redfield, M.D., and Giovanna Tosato, M.D.

Abstract Patients with the acquired immunodeficiency syndrome (AIDS) acquire undifferentiated B-cell lymphomas that are similar to African Burkitt's lymphoma and contain Epstein–Barr virus (EBV). Using an in vitro assay system that measures a complex of cellular responses to EBV-infected lymphocytes, we found that B cells from 7 patients with AIDS and from 10 patients with AIDS-related disorders produced abnormally low numbers of immunoglobulin-secreting cells ($P<0.001$ as compared with normal controls) and that T-cell suppression, which was greater than 80 percent in EBV-seropositive normal controls, was absent. Instead, the patients' T cells markedly increased immunoglobulin production induced by EBV. In further studies, we determined that the mean frequency of circulating EBV-infected B cells capable of spontaneous outgrowth in vitro was 13 per 10^6 B cells in 7 patients with AIDS and 21 per 10^6 B cells in 10 patients with AIDS-related disorders — figures that were significantly higher than the mean in normal controls ($P<0.001$). Thus, patients with AIDS or AIDS-related disorders may be predisposed to the development of EBV-containing lymphomas, because they have a profound defect of T-cell immunity to EBV and abnormally high numbers of EBV-infected B cells in the circulation.

UNDIFFERENTIATED lymphomas similar or identical to Burkitt's lymphoma have been reported with increasing frequency in patients with the acquired immunodeficiency syndrome (AIDS).[1-7] Like the African Burkitt's tumors, some of the undifferentiated lymphomas occurring in patients with AIDS have been reported to contain Epstein–Barr virus (EBV) DNA and to display characteristic chromosomal translocations.[2,6,8-11]

Infection with EBV in association with environmental cofactors — possibly endemic malaria, for example — has been proposed as having a critical role in the development of African Burkitt's lymphoma.[12] Children from Uganda with high antibody titers to EBV are at high risk for Burkitt's lymphoma,[13] and during infection with *Plasmodium falciparum* malaria, T-cell immunity to EBV is altered so that EBV-infected B cells proliferate abnormally in vitro.[14] It was hypothesized that the development of African Burkitt's lymphoma is a multistep process that requires EBV infection as a necessary first event, leading to the long-lasting presence in the organism of B cells latently infected with EBV. Environmental cofactors would subsequently lead to an expansion of the pool of EBV-infected B cells in vivo. Since EBV-infected B cells are long-lived and replicating, the probability of the occurrence of genetic aberrations would increase.[12]

To assess whether similar events may occur in patients with AIDS or AIDS-related disorders, we have studied T-cell immunity to EBV and analyzed the frequencies of EBV-infected B cells in a group of patients with these illnesses.

Methods

Study Population

The study population consisted of 7 patients with AIDS, 10 patients with AIDS-related disorders, and 18 age-matched normal controls. All the patients with AIDS or AIDS-related disorders had serum antibody to human T-cell lymphotropic virus Type III/lymphadenopathy-associated virus (HTLV-III/LAV).[15] All the patients and controls had antibodies to EBV.[16] Selected clinical and laboratory features of these patients are shown in Table 1. None of the patients were studied during an episode of acute infection, and none had taken any medication for one week preceding the in vitro study.

From the Department of Allergy and Immunology, Walter Reed Army Medical Center, Washington, D.C.; the Department of Viral Diseases, Walter Reed Institute of Research, Washington, D.C.; and the Division of Biochemistry and Biophysics, Office of Biologics Research and Review, Food and Drug Administration, Bethesda, Md.

Cell Cultures and Assays for Immunoglobulin Production and Spontaneous Immortalization

Unseparated mononuclear cells and cell subsets enriched for B and T cells were purified from peripheral blood by standard techniques.[17] T-cell regulation of EBV-infected B cells was examined as previously described.[17] Briefly, B cells were cultured in 96-well round-bottomed microtiter plates (Costar, Cambridge, Mass.) with or without EBV (B95-8 strain), either alone or mixed with autologous T cells at various cell densities. At the end of a 14-day culture period, the number of immunoglobulin-secreting cells generated in culture was assessed by a reverse hemolytic-plaque assay.

The frequencies of precursors of spontaneously transforming B cells were determined by limiting-dilution analysis of multiple B-cell microcultures, as previously described.[18] Briefly, B cells were cultured at serial (at least 20) two-fold reductions in cell densities with a feeder layer of normal allogeneic, irradiated (3000 R) T cells in flat-bottomed microtiter plates (Costar). Spontaneous outgrowth was assessed weekly from the 4th through the 10th week of incubation by visual examination, according to the criteria previously described.[19] The frequencies of precursors of transforming B cells were calculated by Poisson analysis[20] and were corrected for the fraction of cells positive for surface immunoglobulin in the B-cell population.

Testing for the EBV-induced nuclear antigen EBNA, for the HTLV-III/LAV-related antigen P-15, and for cell-surface determinants was performed by immunofluorescence with use of appropriate human serum samples and monoclonal antibodies (Biotech Research Laboratories, Ortho Diagnostics, and Becton Dickinson).

Geometric means, standard errors of the mean, and Student's t-test were calculated by conventional formulas.

Results

Previous studies have demonstrated that EBV-seropositive normal people have regulatory T cells in their peripheral blood that inhibit the growth and differentiation of autologous B cells activated by EBV in culture. Blood from EBV-seronegative

Table 1. Clinical and Laboratory Features of Patients with AIDS or AIDS-Related Disorders.*

Patient No.	Date of Diagnosis	Age	Clinical Features	Lymphocytes	B Cells	T4/T8 Ratio	Antibody Titer to EBV-VCA†
				no./mm³			
AIDS							
1	3/84	34	PCP, CR, OC, disseminated TB	1037	101	0.1	1:160
2	3/84	19	PCP, OC	782	189	0.5	1:640
3	10/83	35	PCP, molluscum contagiosum	364	140	0.3	1:640
4	2/84	28	PCP, OC	360	109	0.1	1:320
5	1/84	29	PCP, OC	504	91	0.3	1:320
6	12/84	31	PCP, OC, CR	486	80	0.1	1:320
7	11/84	34	PCP, cryptococcal meningitis	325	104	0.2	1:640
Means (×÷SEM)				506 (1.18)	112 (1.11)	0.19 (1.28)	1:390 (1.20)
AIDS-related disorders							
1	8/83	29	LN	540	108	2.0	1:320
2	2/84	30	LN	832	127	1.7	1:160
3	10/83	23	LN, OC, anergic	1541	529	0.3	1:160
4	11/83	25	LN, OC	972	219	0.6	1:640
5	6/83	24	LN, anergic	2520	148	0.6	1:640
6	6/84	29	LN	1824	295	0.8	1:640
7	7/84	29	LN	1056	133	2.3	1:640
8	8/84	30	LN	1820	333	0.8	1:640
9	9/83	25	LN, anergic	1488	372	0.3	1:640
10	9/84	31	LN, OC, anergic	2156	306	0.6	1:320
Means (×÷SEM)				1343 (1.16)	226 (1.19)	0.8 (1.26)	1:425 (1.20)
Controls (n = 9) Means (×÷SEM)				1710 (1.10)	112 (1.21)	2.2 (1.13)	1:201 (1.33)

*EBV denotes Epstein–Barr virus, VCA viral capsid antigen, PCP *Pneumocystis carinii* pneumonia, CR cryptosporidiosis, OC oral candidiasis, TB tuberculosis, and LN lymphadenopathy lasting for more than six months in two non-inguinal sites. Anergic denotes negative skin-test reactions to purified protein derivative, tetanus toxoid, trichophyton, candida, and mumps.

†All patients had antibodies to the EBV-induced nuclear antigen EBNA; two patients with AIDS and three patients with an AIDS-related disorder also had low levels of antibodies to the early antigen complex.

persons characteristically lacks these inhibitory T cells.[17,21] B cells (5×10^4) from 11 EBV-seropositive normal controls, cultured in the presence of EBV, generated a geometric mean (×÷SEM) of 3121 ×÷ 1.11 immunoglobulin-secreting cells after 14 days in culture. In contrast, the same B cells (5×10^4), cultured with autologous T cells (25×10^4) generated an average of only 536 ×÷ 1.26 immunoglobulin-secreting cells, indicating an inhibition of more than 80 percent (Fig. 1). The degree of T-cell suppression depended on the number of T cells added (Table 2). Parallel experiments performed with EBV-seropositive blood from 7 patients with AIDS and 10 patients with AIDS-related disorders yielded different results (Fig. 1). After 14 days in culture, EBV-infected B cells (5×10^4) from patients with AIDS produced an average of only 22 ×÷ 3.35 immunoglobulin-secreting cells, and those from patients with AIDS-related disorders only 281 ×÷ 1.44 — values significantly lower than normal ($P<0.001$ for each group of patients). Also, autologous cocultures of B (5×10^4) and T (25×10^4) cells from these patients generated an average of 336 ×÷ 3.27 immunoglobulin-secreting cells in patients with AIDS and 1737 ×÷ 1.32 in patients with AIDS-related disorders, indicating the absence of T-cell suppression. Instead, in each experiment the T cells had an enhancing effect on EBV-induced immunoglobulin production, which depended on the number of T cells added (Table 2). This T-cell effect could not be attributed to B-cell contamination, since 14-day cultures of T cells (25×10^4) from patients with AIDS and AIDS-related disorders produced only 2.0 ×÷ 1.9 and 73.6 ×÷ 1.4 immunoglobulin-secreting cells, respectively, in the presence of EBV. Thus, B cells from patients with AIDS or AIDS-related disorders produced abnormally low numbers of immunoglobulin-secreting cells when exposed to EBV in vitro. In addition, unlike normal EBV-immune T cells that suppress autologous B cells infected with EBV, T cells from these patients failed to inhibit EBV-induced immunoglobulin production. These experiments suggest that T-cell immunity to EBV is markedly defective in these patients.

We asked whether these in vitro abnormalities in regulation might be reflected in patients with AIDS or AIDS-related syndromes by an increased number of EBV-infected B cells in vivo. During acute EBV-induced infectious mononucleosis, many of the circulating B cells are infected with EBV, and after primary infection, circulating B cells continue to be infected

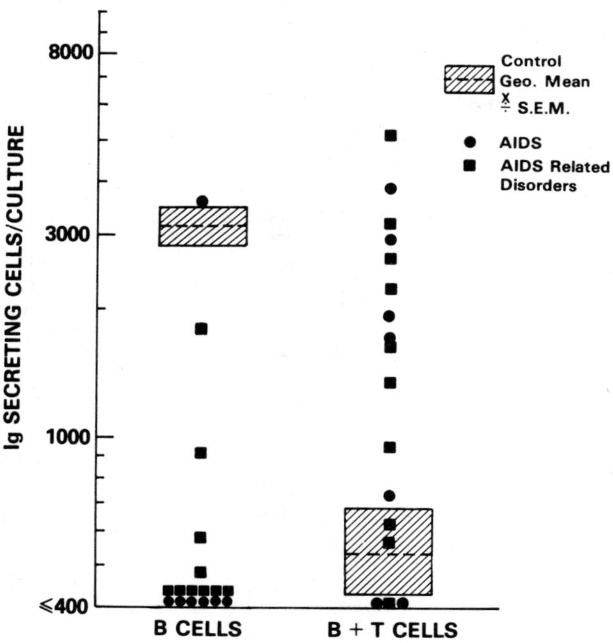

Figure 1. Comparison of Numbers of Immunoglobulin-Secreting Cells Generated in EBV-Stimulated Cultures from Controls and Patients with AIDS or AIDS-Related Disorders.

The individual data points represent the responses of 7 patients with AIDS and 10 patients with AIDS-related disorders; the hatched areas represent the geometric mean (×÷SEM) response in 11 EBV-seropositive normal controls. EBV-infected B cells (5×10^4) were cultured for 14 days either alone or in a mixture with autologous T cells (25×10^4). In the absence of exogenous EBV, B cells from the patients with AIDS and AIDS-related disorders produced 14.6 ×÷ 2.7 and 6.5 ×÷ 1.8 immunoglobulin-secreting cells, respectively, at 14 days.

with EBV, although with a low frequency.[18,22,23] These circulating EBV-carrying B cells can transform spontaneously in vitro, and their frequency can be determined in normal blood by statistical analysis of multiple limiting-dilution cultures.[18] A representative experiment to determine the frequency of precursors of spontaneously transforming cells from the blood of a patient with an AIDS-related disorder is shown in Figure 2. In this determination, 1 in 62,000 B cells transformed spontaneously, indicating that at least 16 B cells per 10^6 circulating B cells were infected with EBV in this patient. Using this method, we determined the frequencies of spontaneous B-cell growth in the blood of 7 patients with AIDS and 10 patients with AIDS-related disorders; these frequencies were compared with those found in 17 normal EBV-seropositive controls. In the controls, the mean frequency of spontaneous transformation was 1.8 ×÷ 1.29 per 10^6 circulating B cells, and the range was between less than 1 and 9.1 per 10^6 B cells (Fig. 3). In contrast, the mean frequency of spontaneous cell outgrowth was 13.1 ×÷ 1.80 per 10^6 circulating B cells in patients with AIDS and 20.7 ×÷ 1.37 per 10^6 circulating B cells in patients with AIDS-related disorders. These differences in frequencies between controls and patients were significant ($P<0.001$) for each patient group. Since the mean number of circulating B cells per cubic millimeter in the patients was not significantly lower than that in the controls, these results indicate that these patients generally have significantly more spontaneously transforming B cells in the blood than normal healthy persons.

Some patients with AIDS are infected with human T-cell lymphotropic virus Type I (HTLV-I) in addition to HTLV-III/LAV.[24] Since HTLV-I is a T-cell–transforming retrovirus,[25] it was possible that a few of the spontaneously transforming cell clones from patients with AIDS or AIDS-related disorders were of T-cell lineage and did not reflect spontaneous outgrowth of EBV-infected B cells. Also, since EBV-infected B-cell lines have been infected with HTLV-III/LAV in vitro,[26] it is conceivable that a similar event can occur in vivo, and as a consequence, the spontaneously transforming B cells from patients infected with HTLV-III/LAV could simultaneously harbor EBV and HTLV-III/LAV. To address these questions, 25 clonal populations of spontaneous transformants (8 obtained from a patient with AIDS and 17 from two patients with AIDS-related disorders) were expanded for further investigation. All the clones had evidence of EBV infection, since in each case more than 80 percent of the cells were positive for EBNA. None of the clones expressed the HTLV-III/LAV–related antigen P-15, indicating that HTLV-III/LAV was absent. The H-9 cell line, either infected or not infected with HTLV-III/LAV, served as a control. All 25 clones expressed surface immunoglobulin and the B-cell–related antigen B-2, whereas the T-cell–specific markers T11, T4, T8, and the monocyte marker M3 were absent. Thus, all the clones tested were likely to be the product of spontaneous in vitro outgrowth of EBV-infected B cells, and they were not coinfected with HTLV-III/LAV.

Discussion

In this report, we have demonstrated that patients

Table 2. Enhancement of EBV-Induced B-Cell Activation by T Lymphocytes from Patients with AIDS or AIDS-Related Disease.*

Study Group (No.)	B Cells Alone	B Cells + Autologous T Cells		
		25×10^4	10×10^4	5×10^4
	mean (×÷SEM)†			
Controls (11)	3121 (1.11)	536 (1.26)	1045 (1.28)	1836 (1.20)
Patients with AIDS (7)	22 (3.35)	336 (3.27)	295 (3.22)	200 (3.17)
Patients with AIDS-related disease (10)	281 (1.44)	1737 (1.32)	1092 (1.31)	874 (1.31)

*B cells (5×10^4) were cultured with EBV either alone or with autologous T cells at various cell densities (25, 10, and 5×10^4) in 96-well round-bottomed microtiter plates (Costar, Cambridge, Mass.).

†Mean (×÷SEM) number of immunoglobulin-secreting cells per culture generated after 14 days of incubation.

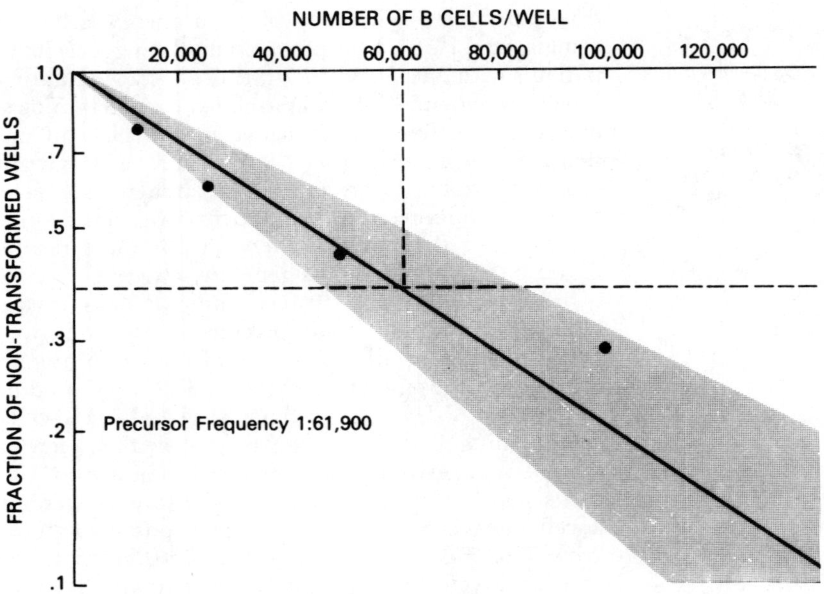

Figure 2. Representative Limiting-Dilution Analysis of Spontaneous B-Cell Outgrowth in a Patient with an AIDS-Related Disorder.

Multiple replicate cultures of B cells established in the presence of a feeder layer of irradiated (3000 R) normal T cells were assessed at 4 to 10 weeks for the presence or absence of outgrowth. The plot of numbers of B cells per culture against the log of the fraction of negative cultures yielded a straight line, indicating that the technique is valid for the detection of outgrowth by the progeny of a single limiting precursor. The shaded area indicates the 95 percent confidence interval.

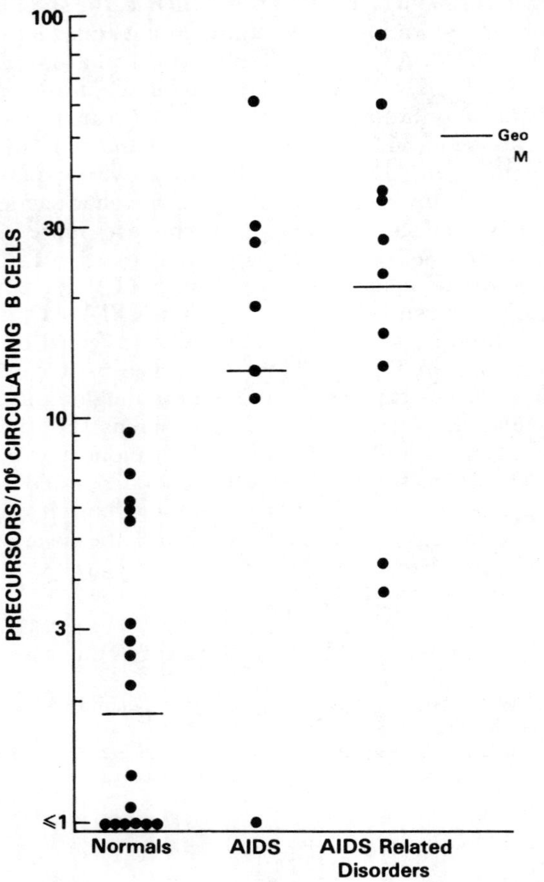

Figure 3. Frequencies of Precursors of Spontaneous B-Cell Outgrowth in Normal Subjects, Patients with AIDS, and Patients with AIDS-Related Disorders.

Limiting-dilution cultures of peripheral-blood B cells were assessed for the occurrence of spontaneous outgrowth after 4 to 10 weeks in culture, and the results analyzed by Poisson's statistics. The individual data points represent the frequency of spontaneously transforming cells per 10^6 circulating B cells.

with AIDS or AIDS-related disorders have a defect in the regulation of EBV-infected B cells. In addition, we have shown that such patients have abnormally high numbers of circulating EBV-infected B cells.

EBV causes a latent infection in more than half of all adults worldwide.[27] This is associated with the presence of small numbers of EBV-infected B cells in the circulation that can proliferate progressively when cultured in vitro.[18,28,29] Such progressive proliferations of EBV-infected B cells are rare in vivo, probably because the healthy carrier acquires specific T-cell immune responses that constantly control the EBV-infected B cells.[17,21,28] To assess T-cell immunity to EBV in patients with AIDS or AIDS-related disorders, we have used immunoglobulin secretion as a marker for B-cell activation by EBV, and we have compared immunoglobulin production by EBV-infected B cells cultured alone or mixed with autologous T cells.[17] In this system, T cells from normal persons who are EBV-seropositive, but not from those who are seronegative, profoundly inhibit immunoglobulin production by the autologous EBV-infected B cells.[17] In contrast to these findings in controls, B cells from patients with AIDS or AIDS-related disorders produced abnormally low numbers of immunoglobulin-secreting cells after 14 days in culture with EBV; also, autologous cocultures of T cells with the same EBV-activated B cells resulted in enhancement, rather than suppression, of immunoglobulin production. The inability of T cells from patients with AIDS or AIDS-related disorders to suppress autologous B cells infected with EBV cannot be considered a normal response to an active or reactivated EBV infection itself, since patients with acute EBV-induced infectious mononucleosis or with chronic active EBV infection have a profound T-cell inhibition of EBV-activated B cells.[17,18]

Previous studies of lymphocyte function in AIDS have demonstrated that the B cells are hyperactive, with increased numbers of cells spontaneously secreting immunoglobulin.[30] Since EBV activates only resting B lymphocytes,[31] it is not surprising that B cells from patients with AIDS or AIDS-related disorders produced abnormally low numbers of immunoglobulin-secreting cells with exogenous EBV. A possible explanation for the T-cell defect in patients with AIDS or AIDS-related disorders is that the T cells are intrinsically defective. It is known that T8-positive lymphocytes include the effector cells for inhibition of EBV-activated B cells, but it is believed that a subset of T4-positive cells is a necessary additional component of this immune response.[32] Patients with AIDS or AIDS-related disorders, including those described in this report, have abnormally low numbers of T4-positive cells in their blood, and a variety of immune functions attributed to this T-cell subset have been described as abnormal in such patients.[30,33-36] In contrast, the number of T8-positive cells and at least some of their functions are believed to be generally preserved.[35,36] It is possible, therefore, that a defect involving a subset of T4-positive T cells is responsible for the abnormal regulation of EBV-infected B cells in patients with AIDS or AIDS-related diseases.

Whatever its cause, defective in vitro T-cell regulation of EBV-infected B cells may offer an explanation for the presence of abnormally high numbers of EBV-infected B cells in the blood of patients with AIDS or AIDS-related conditions. The frequencies of EBV-infected B cells reported here should be considered minimal estimates, since our assay system detects only infected B-cell precursors capable of long-term growth when transferred in vitro. It is likely that a proportion of the EBV-infected B cells is lost because of manipulations and culture conditions. In addition, some of the infected cells may be productively infected with EBV[8] and incapable of long-term growth in vitro, or they may be coinfected with HTLV-III/LAV[26] and destroyed by the retrovirus. We have considered the possibility that a proportion of the spontaneously transforming B cells may have been coinfected with EBV and HTLV-III/LAV. Although not all spontaneously transforming B-cell clones were examined, none of 25 from three patients had evidence of HTLV-III/LAV infection, suggesting that B cells latently infected with EBV are uncommonly coinfected with HTLV-III/LAV in a stable manner.

The existence of abnormally large numbers of EBV-infected B cells in the circulation has been proposed to be an important step in the development of African Burkitt's lymphoma.[12] Since such B cells are long-lived and may undergo many more cell divisions than the B cells not infected with EBV, the probability of the occurrence of chromosomal aberrations would be increased.[12] Patients with AIDS or AIDS-related disorders may be similarly predisposed to the development of EBV-positive lymphomas by a sequence of events that include EBV infection, decreased regulation of EBV-infected B cells, and an increased pool of such cells.

The possibility of a more direct role of HTLV-III/LAV in the induction of Burkitt's lymphoma can also be raised. Allograft recipients have only rarely been reported to have acquired Burkitt's lymphoma, even though their immunodeficiency may be associated with defects in immunity to EBV. Also, recent epidemiologic evidence has shown that serum samples collected from children in the West Nile district of Uganda between 1972 and 1973 contained low-level antibody titers to HTLV-III/LAV, suggesting that infection with this or a related retrovirus has been endemic in Africa for years.[37] Finally, it has been reported that HTLV-III/LAV can infect EBV-positive B cells.[26] It is interesting, therefore, to speculate that HTLV-III/LAV may have a role in the pathogenesis of both African and AIDS EBV-positive lymphomas, and may act directly on B cells containing EBV.

The views of the authors do not purport to reflect the opinions of the Department of Defense.

We are indebted to Dr. C. Wright for his valuable help with the patients; to S.E. Pike, T. Hase, B. Reed, and R.E. Cunningham for technical assistance; to Drs. R. Gallo and H. Stricker for providing the anti-HTLV-III/LAV monoclonal antibody; to Drs. R. Yarchoan, R.M. Blaese, and T. Fleisher for constructive discussions; and to E. Kirshbaum for excellent assistance in the preparation of the manuscript.

References

1. Doll DC, List AF. Burkitt's lymphoma in a homosexual. Lancet 1982; 1:1026-7.
2. Zeigler JL, Drew WL, Miner RC, et al. Outbreak of Burkitt's-like lymphoma in homosexual men. Lancet 1982; 2:631-3.
3. Shibuya A, Saitoh K, Tsuneyoshi H, Tanaka S. Burkitt's lymphoma in a haemophiliac. Lancet 1983; 2:1432.
4. Levine AM, Meyer PR, Begandy MK, et al. Development of B-cell lymphoma in homosexual men: clinical and immunologic findings. Ann Intern Med 1984; 100:7-13.
5. Zeigler JL, Beckstead JA, Volberding PA, et al. Non-Hodgkin's lymphoma in 90 homosexual men: relation to generalized lymphadenopathy and the acquired immunodeficiency syndrome. N Engl J Med 1984; 311:565-70.
6. Petersen JM, Tubbs RR, Savage RA, et al. Small noncleaved B cell Burkitt-like lymphoma with chromosome t (8;14) translocation and Epstein–Barr virus nuclear-associated antigen in a homosexual man with acquired immune deficiency syndrome. Am J Med 1985; 78:141-8.
7. Boring CC, Brynes RK, Chan WC, et al. Increase in high-grade lymphomas in young men. Lancet 1985; 1:857-9.
8. Magrath IT, Erikson J, Whang-Peng J, et al. Synthesis of kappa light chains by cell lines containing an 8;22 chromosomal translocation derived from a male homosexual with Burkitt's lymphoma. Science 1983; 222:1094-8.
9. Whang-Peng J, Lee EC, Sieverts H, Magrath IT. Burkitt's lymphoma in AIDS: cytogenetic study. Blood 1984; 63:818-22.
10. Chaganti RSK, Jhanwar SC, Koziner B, Arlin Z, Mertelsmann R, Clarkson BD. Specific translocations characterize Burkitt's-like lymphoma of homosexual men with the acquired immunodeficiency syndrome. Blood 1983; 61:1265-8.
11. Lind SE, Gross P, Andiman WA, Stone GC, Schooley RT, Harris NL. Malignant lymphoma presenting as Kaposi's sarcoma in a homosexual man with the acquired immunodeficiency syndrome. Ann Intern Med 1985; 102:338-40.
12. Klein G, Klein E. Evolution of tumours and the impact of molecular oncology. Nature 1985; 315:190-5.
13. de-Thé G, Geser A, Day NE, et al. Epidemiological evidence for causal relationship between Epstein–Barr virus and Burkitt's lymphoma from Ugandan prospective study. Nature 1978; 274:756-61.
14. Whittle HC, Brown J, Marsh K, et al. T-cell control of Epstein–Barr virus-infected B cells is lost during *P. falciparum* malaria. Nature 1984; 312:449-50.
15. Sarngadharan MG, Popovic M, Bruch L, Schüpbach J, Gallo RC. Antibodies reactive with human T-lymphotropic retroviruses (HTLV-III) in the serum of patients with AIDS. Science 1984; 224:506-8.
16. Henle W, Henle G, Horwitz CA. Epstein–Barr virus diagnostic tests in infectious mononucleosis. Hum Pathol 1974; 5:551-65.
17. Tosato G, Magrath IT, Blaese RM. T cell-mediated immunoregulation of Epstein Barr virus- (EBV) induced B lymphocyte activation in EBV-seropositive and EBV-seronegative individuals. J Immunol 1982; 128:575-9.

18. Tosato G, Straus S, Henle W, et al. Characteristic T cell dysfunction in patients with chronic active Epstein–Barr virus infection (chronic infectious mononucleosis). J Immunol 1985; 134:3082-8.
19. Tosato G, Blaese RM, Yarchoan R. Relationship between immunoglobulin production and immortalization by Epstein Barr virus. J Immunol 1985; 135:959-64.
20. Taswell C. Limiting dilution assays for the determination of immunocompetent cell frequencies. I. Data analysis. J Immunol 1981; 126: 1614-9.
21. Moss DJ, Rickinson AB, Pope JH. Long-term T-cell-mediated immunity to Epstein–Barr virus in man. I. Complete regression of virus-induced transformation in cultures of seropositive donor leukocytes. Int J Cancer 1978; 22:662-8.
22. Rocchi G, de Felici A, Ragona G, Heintz A. Quantitative evaluation of Epstein–Barr-virus-infected mononuclear peripheral blood leukocytes in infectious mononucleosis. N Engl J Med 1977; 296:132-4.
23. Robinson JE, Smith D, Niederman J. Plasmacytic differentiation of circulating Epstein–Barr virus-infected B lymphocytes during acute infectious mononucleosis. J Exp Med 1981; 153:235-44.
24. Essex M, McLane MF, Lee TH, et al. Antibodies to cell membrane antigens associated with human T-cell leukemia virus in patients with AIDS. Science 1983; 220:859-62.
25. Popovic M, Sarin PS, Robert-Guroff M, et al. Isolation and transmission of human retrovirus (human T-cell leukemia virus). Science 1983; 219:856-9.
26. Montagnier L, Gruest J, Chamaret S, et al. Adaptation of lymphadenopathy associated virus (LAV) to replication in EBV-transformed B lymphoblastoid cell lines. Science 1984; 225:63-6.
27. Henle W, Henle G. Seroepidemiology of the virus. In: Epstein MA, Achong BG, eds. The Epstein–Barr virus. Berlin: Springer-Verlag, 1979: 61-78.
28. Tosato G, Blaese RM. Epstein–Barr virus infection and immunoregulation in man. Adv Immunol 1985; 37:99-149.
29. Gerber P, Whang-Peng J, Monroe JH. Transformation and chromosome changes induced by Epstein–Barr virus in normal human leukocyte cultures. Proc Natl Acad Sci USA 1969; 63:740-7.
30. Lane HC, Masur H, Edgar LC, Whalen G, Rook AH, Fauci AS. Abnormalities of B-cell activation and immunoregulation in patients with the acquired immunodeficiency syndrome. N Engl J Med 1983; 309:453-8.
31. Åman P, Ehlin-Hendriksson B, Klein G. Epstein–Barr virus susceptibility of normal human B lymphocyte populations. J Exp Med 1984; 159:208-20.
32. Konttinen YT, Bluestein HG, Zvaifler NJ. Regulation of the growth of Epstein–Barr virus-infected B cells. I. Growth regression by E rosetting cells from VCA-positive donors is a combined effect of autologous mixed leukocyte reaction and activation of $T8^+$ memory cells. J Immunol 1985; 134:2287-93.
33. Gottlieb MS, Schroff R, Schanker HM, et al. *Pneumocystis carinii* pneumonia and mucosal candidiasis in previously healthy homosexual men: evidence of a new acquired cellular immunodeficiency. N Engl J Med 1981; 305:1425-31.
34. Masur H, Michelis MA, Greene JB, et al. An outbreak of community-acquired *Pneumocystis carinii* pneumonia: initial manifestation of cellular immune dysfunction. N Engl J Med 1981; 305:1431-8.
35. Benveniste E, Schroff R, Stevens RH, Gottlieb MS. Immunoregulatory T cells in men with a new acquired immunodeficiency syndrome. J Clin Immunol 1983; 3:359-67.
36. Lane HC, Depper JM, Greene WC, Whalen G, Waldmann TA, Fauci AS. Qualitative analysis of immune function in patients with the acquired immunodeficiency syndrome: evidence for a selective defect in soluble antigen recognition. N Engl J Med 1985; 313:79-84.
37. Saxinger WC, Levine PH, Dean AG, et al. Evidence for exposure to HTLV-III in Uganda before 1973. Science 1985; 227:1036-8.

ORIGINAL ARTICLE

REPLICATION OF EPSTEIN–BARR VIRUS WITHIN THE EPITHELIAL CELLS OF ORAL "HAIRY" LEUKOPLAKIA, AN AIDS-ASSOCIATED LESION

JOHN S. GREENSPAN, B.D.S., PH.D., DEBORAH GREENSPAN, B.D.S., EVELYNE T. LENNETTE, PH.D., DONALD I. ABRAMS, M.D., MARCUS A. CONANT, M.D., VIBEKE PETERSEN, B.S., AND U. KARL FREESE, M.D.

Abstract We conducted a study to identify the viruses in tissue specimens of oral "hairy" leukoplakia, a lesion that is found in immunosuppressed male homosexuals and that is associated with the subsequent development of the acquired immunodeficiency syndrome. When stained for papillomavirus core antigen, 49 of 67 biopsy specimens (73 percent) yielded positive results in epithelial-cell nuclei. Electron microscopy showed papillomavirus-like particles in all of 25 specimens, and the herpes-type virus described in a previous report was seen in 23 of the 25 specimens. Three specimens had both types of particle in the same individual epithelial cells. Immunofluorescence for herpes simplex virus, varicella–zoster virus, and cytomegalovirus gave negative results in all cases, but 19 of 20 specimens showed intense nuclear staining in epithelial cells for the viral capsid antigen of Epstein–Barr virus (EBV). DNA hybridization using EBV probes in Southern blots demonstrated EBV DNA in all of 13 specimens and found 200 or more viral DNA molecules per cellular genome in 11 of the 13. The whole EBV genome was also demonstrated in the specimens and found to be in linear virion form. We conclude that EBV replicates within the epithelial cells in hairy leukoplakia.

VIRAL leukoplakia of the tongue in immunosuppressed male homosexuals (oral "hairy" leukoplakia) is a newly described lesion that is associated with the subsequent development of the features of the acquired immunodeficiency syndrome (AIDS), most often with *Pneumocystis carinii* pneumonia. The clinical appearance is of a slightly raised, poorly demarcated lesion with a corrugated or "hairy" surface. The lesions range from a few millimeters to 3.5 by 2 cm in size, they do not rub off, and they usually produce no symptoms. Initial studies suggested that the lesions contained papillomavirus as well as a virus of the herpes group.[1] In this report, we present evidence that both papillomavirus and Epstein–Barr virus (EBV) are present within the epithelial cells of hairy leukoplakia, and that the cells contain EBV DNA and viral capsid antigen. It is highly unusual to find intact EBV particles and EBV viral capsid antigen within the cells of biopsy specimens. Our observations indicate that EBV replicates within oral hairy leukoplakia lesions in human beings.

METHODS

Patients

The study population, which has been described previously,[1] consisted of patients referred to the Oral Medicine Clinic at the University of California, San Francisco, by the university's AIDS Clinical Research Center or by physicians and dentists in the San Francisco area. Patients gave medical and social histories response to standard questionnaires and had complete physical and oral examinations. When white lesions were found in the mouth, smears and cultures for candida were performed and, when the patients' permission was granted, biopsy examinations were done.

Immunologic Studies

Delayed-hypersensitivity skin testing and assessment of peripheral-blood lymphocytes for the numbers of T4 and T8 cells and for T4/T8 ratios were performed as described previously.[1]

Oral Biopsy

Incisional biopsy specimens of lesions with clinical features of hairy leukoplakia were obtained under local anesthesia from 67 patients, none of whom had AIDS at the time of the biopsy. Routine histopathology and staining with periodic acid–Schiff were performed on samples fixed in formol–saline and embedded in paraffin. Some samples were frozen for viral immunostaining and DNA hybridization. Samples for electron microscopy were fixed with 3 percent glutaraldehyde, postfixed in 1 percent buffered osmic acid, and embedded in epon; thin sections were stained with lead citrate.

Because the biopsy specimens were small, staining for papillomavirus antigen was the only procedure performed on all of them. When available, remaining portions of the tissues were usually large enough for assignment, at most, to only one additional testing procedure. Thus, staining for herpesvirus antigens was performed on 20 samples, EBV DNA hybridization on 13, and electron microscopical examination on 25. From six of the patients whose lesion specimens were stained for herpesviruses, and from six of those whose underwent EBV DNA hybridization, specimens of clinically normal buccal mucosa were also obtained for the same test. Additional appropriate control specimens were collected for each procedure. For the staining of papillomavirus antigen, the controls were paraffin-embedded biopsy specimens from 10 oral warts or condylomata (positive controls), 5 cases of epithelial hyperplasia, 3 cases of lichen planus, and 2 of fibroepithelial hyperplasia. For the staining of herpesviruses, controls were frozen specimens from oral mucosal lesions from two patients with pemphigoid, one with pemphigus, two with erythema multiforme, two with epithelial hyperplasia, two with epithelial dysplasia, and two with lichen planus.

Papillomavirus Antigen

Peroxidase–antiperoxidase immunocytochemical staining for the papillomavirus core antigen was performed as described previously.[1] In addition to the control specimens described above, controls for the staining reagents consisted of human fetal diploid lung cells infected with either herpes simplex 1 or 2, cytomegalovirus, or varicella–zoster virus, as well as a lymphoma cell line (P3HR1) known to produce EBV.

From the Department of Stomatology, School of Dentistry, the Departments of Pathology, Dermatology, Medicine, and the Cancer Research Institute, School of Medicine, and the AIDS Clinical Research Center, University of California, San Francisco; Virolab Inc., Berkeley, Calif.; and the Deutsches Krebsforschungszentrum, Heidelberg, Federal Republic of Germany.

Supported by grants from the University of California Taskforce on AIDS and the Deutsche Forschungsgemeinschaft "SFB 31."

Presented in part at the First International Symposium on AIDS-Associated Syndromes, Irvine, California, December 11, 1984, and in part at the International Conference on AIDS, Atlanta, Georgia, April 16, 1985.

Tissue Staining for the Herpesviruses

Cryostat sections (5 μm thick) of biopsy specimens from patients with hairy leukoplakia or other oral lesions were stained by a direct immunofluorescence assay that used three types of rabbit hyperimmune serum conjugated to fluorescein–isothiocyanate to detect herpes simplex virus 1 and 2 and varicella–zoster virus. Cytomegalovirus and EBV antigens were sought by anticomplement indirect immunofluorescence, as described previously,[2] that used human serum samples with the following specificities: three samples were EBV-positive and cytomegalovirus-negative, three were cytomegalovirus-positive and EBV-negative, and one was EBV-negative and cytomegalovirus-negative. In addition, serum samples from three patients with infectious mononucleosis that were cytomegalovirus-negative were used to identify the particular EBV antigens found in the hairy leukoplakia tissue. The antigens sought were the viral capsid antigen, the early-antigen diffuse component, and the early-antigen restricted component.[3] All three of the serum samples were negative for EBV-associated nuclear antigen. One was positive for the viral capsid antigen and negative for the early antigen; the second was positive for the viral capsid antigen and the early-antigen diffuse component, but negative for the restricted component; and the third was positive for the viral capsid antigen and the restricted component but negative for the diffuse component.

The results of the EBV staining were confirmed by indirect immunofluorescence with use of three mouse monoclonal antibodies specific for EBV viral capsid antigen and the early-antigen restricted and diffuse components (molecular weights, 160,000, 50,000 to 55,000, and 85,000, respectively), purchased from Biotech Research Laboratories, Rockville, Maryland.

DNA Hybridization

EBV DNA was sought in 13 biopsy specimens taken from the hairy leukoplakia tongue lesions and in biopsy specimens taken from normal buccal mucosa from six of the patients with those lesions. The specimens were frozen in liquid nitrogen, pulverized, and thawed in lysis buffer (75 mM TRIS-HCl [pH 8.5], 25 mM EDTA, and 3 percent Sarkosyl). DNA was purified from the lysates by treatment with sodium dodecyl sulfate and pronase, followed by phenol extraction, RNase digestion, and dialysis.[4] Extraction of DNA and subsequent digestion with restriction endonucleases, separation of fragments by gel electrophoresis, and Southern blot transfer to nitrocellulose paper were carried out essentially as described previously.[5] Small fragments of DNA generated by digestion with restriction endonucleases were separated by size by gel electrophoresis, denatured to single-stranded form, and transferred to nitrocellulose paper by capillary blotting (which preserves the spatial relations generated by electrophoretic separation). Single-stranded, radioactive DNA probes were then used to detect, by specific hybridization, homologous nonradioactive DNA sequences blotted on the paper. Bound radioactivity was detected by autoradiography with x-ray film.

Two types of probe were used: recombinant plasmid probes and high-complexity nonrecombinant probes, both of which were radioactively labeled with ^{32}P by nick-translation.[6] The recombinant probes, which were hybridized to nitrocellulose blots that contained DNA from lesion or control biopsy specimens, were pBgl 2-U,[7] which is specific for the large internal repeat sequence of the EBV genome, and p961-20, which contains sequences homologous to the two linear ends of the EBV virion DNA. Since the large internal repeat sequence is present at more than 10 copies per EBV genome, it is detected more readily than the other sequences. As a result, the pBgl 2-U probe is sensitive for very low amounts of EBV DNA (Fig. 1). The radiolabeled high-complexity probes[8] were generated from DNA extracted from hairy leukoplakia lesions and were hybridized to nitrocellulose blots that contained an overlapping set of restriction-enzyme–digested recombinant plasmids with large cloned inserts that collectively represented the entire EBV genome[9,10] (Fig. 2).

EBV Serology

IgG antibodies to EBV viral capsid antigen, and to the early-antigen diffuse and restricted components, were measured by

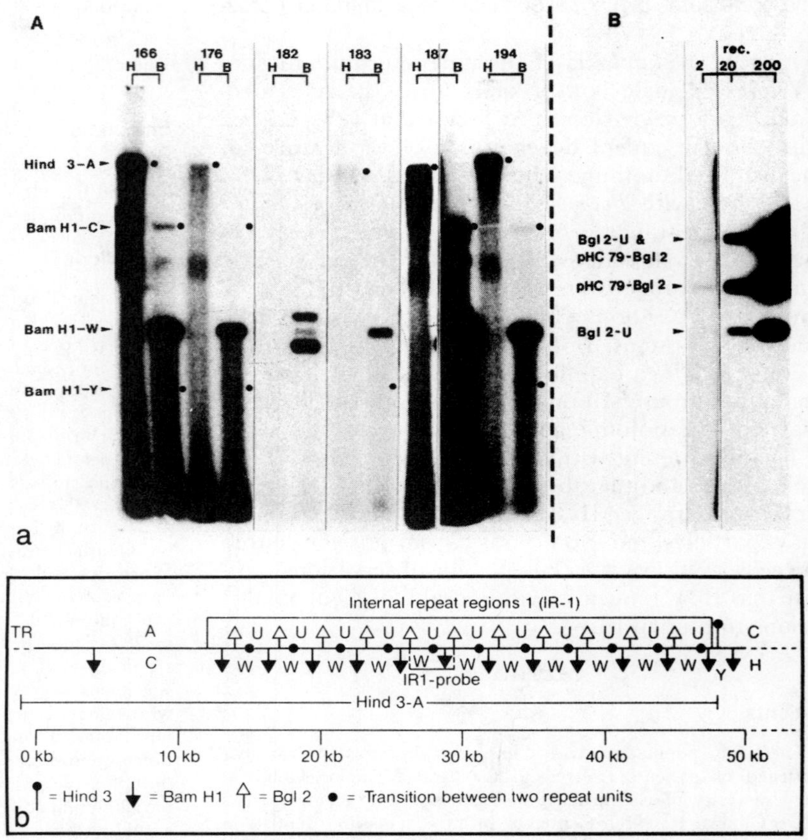

Figure 1. Detection of Epstein–Barr Virus DNA in Hairy Leukoplakia Tissue by Southern Blot Hybridization.

Panel A shows a Southern blot of DNA extracted from 6 of 13 specimens (No. 166 to 194) of hairy leukoplakia tissue digested by either *Hin*dIII (H) or *Bam*HI (B), subjected to electrophoresis on a 0.5 percent agarose gel, and hybridized with the ^{32}P-labeled large internal repeat (IR-1) sequence probe, pBgl 2-U. The location of the IR-1 fragment within the EBV genome is indicated on the map (Fig. 1b; kb denotes kilobase). Each slot was loaded with 0.5 μg of restriction-enzyme–digested DNA extracted from a hairy leukoplakia specimen. The predicted and hybridizing EBV fragments are indicated at the left margin of this panel or within the panel by dots. Panel B in Figure 1a, which depicts reconstruction experiments, shows three lanes of a *Bgl*II digest that are representative of 2, 20, and 200 copies of the pBgl 2-U clone per 10 μg of cellular DNA per slot. The DNA was hybridized with the pBgl 2-U probe in order to provide standards for quantitation of the results shown in Panel A.

the method of Henle et al.[3] Antibodies to the EBV-associated nuclear antigen were measured by the anticomplement indirect immunofluorescence assay with the use of guinea pig complement and rabbit anti-guinea pig C3 conjugated to fluorescein–isothiocyanate.[11] In addition to the serum samples collected from 30 patients with hairy leukoplakia, control samples were obtained from 10 apparently healthy male homosexuals and 10 heterosexual men (five healthy and five with recurrent aphthous ulcers) who visited our clinics.

Results

Clinical Findings

Between October 1981 and December 1984, 90 cases of hairy leukoplakia were diagnosed in our clinic, including the 37 previously reported.[1] The clinical appearances (Fig. 3) of the lesions were as we have described.[1] Eighty of the patients did not have AIDS, according to the Centers for Disease Control definition,[12] at the time of biopsy. Ten patients did have features of AIDS at the time of diagnosis of hairy leukoplakia; of these, four had *P. carinii* pneumonia and six had Kaposi's sarcoma. Among the 80 patients who did not have AIDS, it has since developed in 20 (25 percent). These include 16 patients with *P. carinii* pneumonia, of whom 6 have died; 2 patients with Kaposi's sarcoma; and 2 with other life-threatening opportunistic infections, of whom 1 has died. Of the remaining 60 patients, 58 do not have AIDS as of this writing and 2 have been lost to follow-up. The 20 cases of AIDS developed 1 to 33 months (mean, 7.3 months) after the time of diagnosis of hairy leukoplakia.

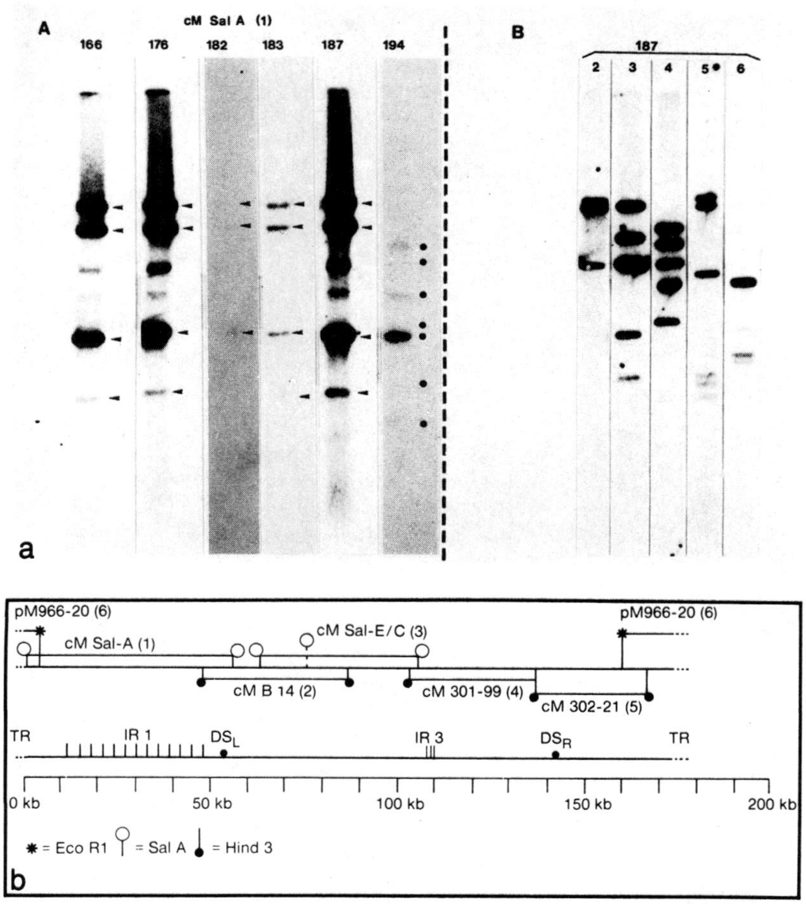

Figure 2. Detection of the Whole Genome of EBV in Hairy Leukoplakia Tissue by Southern Blot Hybridization

Panel A shows high-complexity probe hybridization of ^{32}P-labeled DNA from six specimens of hairy leukoplakia (166 to 194, top) with restriction-enzyme–digested plasmid cM Sal-A (1) recombinant DNA (0.05 pmol). A *Sal*I/*Bgl*II digest of cM Sal-A was used for specimens 164 to 187, and a *Bam*HI digest of the same clone was used for specimen 194. The map region of the EBV genome that is represented within this clone is shown in Figure 2b. Panel B shows high-complexity probe hybridization of ^{32}P-labeled DNA from hairy leukoplakia specimen 187 with DNA (0.05 pmol) from each of the following: a *Sal*I digest of cMB14 (2), an *Eco*RI digest of cM Sal-E/C (3), a *Bam*HI digest of cM301-99 (4), a *Hind*III digest of cM302-21 (5), and a *Sal*I, *Bgl*II, *Hind*III triple digest of pM966-20.

Immunologic Findings

Sixty-nine patients who had no features of AIDS at the time of diagnosis of hairy leukoplakia had skin tests for four antigens: purified protein derivative, candida, mumps, and trichophytin. Twenty-eight had no response; 16 responded to one antigen, 21 to two antigens, 4 to three, and none to all four. Thirty of the same group of 69 patients underwent assessment of T4/T8 ratios in peripheral blood; all 30 had a ratio of less than 1.3, and 28 had a ratio of less than 1.

Candida was found in a smear and culture from a scraping of the hairy leukoplakia lesion in 47 of the 80 patients studied. It was also found in sections stained with periodic acid–Schiff in 33 of the 67 patients from whom biopsy specimens were taken. As in our previous study,[1] we found very few cases (6 of 47) in which the lesion regressed after antifungal therapy.

Histopathology

Biopsy specimens for hairy leukoplakia diagnosis were obtained from 67 patients. All showed the histologic appearance of hairy leukoplakia described previously.[1] The histologic characteristics resembled those of flat wart of the skin and were remarkable for three features: fine keratin projections (in many cases), koilocytosis of prickle cells, and little, if any, subepithelial inflammatory-cell infiltration.

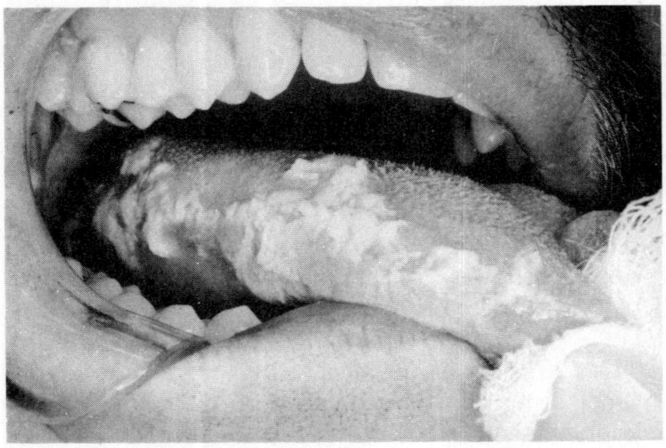

Figure 3. Clinical Appearance of a Severe Case of Oral Hairy Leukoplakia.

Note the extensive raised white areas, with projections, on the lateral and dorsal surface of the tongue. The patient developed *P. carinii* pneumonia three months after this photograph was taken.

Ultrastructure

Electron microscopical examination of specimens from 25 patients, which involved the viewing of at least 150 epithelial cells, revealed (in each specimen) some prickle cells with individual structures whose appearance resembled that of individual papillomavirus particles in genital condylomata, reported in some studies.[13,14] These structures were polygonal particles, approximately 46 to 52 nm in diameter, with a poorly defined internal structure. They were observed only within nuclei. Arrays resembling those of typical papillomavirus particles[15] were seen in a few specimens (Fig. 4). Twenty-three of the 25 specimens showed numerous particles of the herpes-type virus described previously.[1] These were 100-nm naked capsids within the prickle-cell nuclei, accompanied in nine cases by numerous arrays of ill-defined particles (65 to 75 nm in diameter). Enveloped virions (150 to 200 nm in diameter) were seen in the cytoplasm and in the intercellular spaces. Both herpes-type virus particles and papillomavirus-like particles were seen in the same epithelial cells in three specimens (Fig. 5).

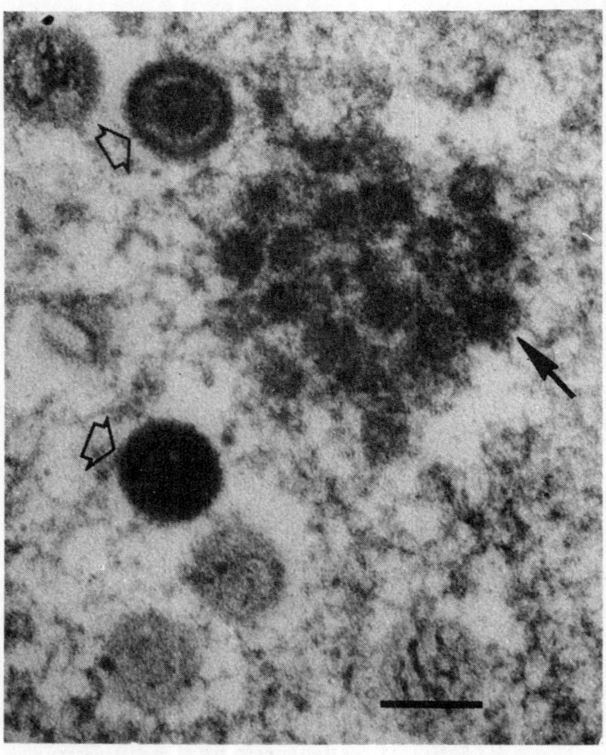

Figure 4. Array of Papillomavirus-Like Particles in the Nucleus of an Epithelial Cell in Hairy Leukoplakia (Solid Arrow).

The individual particles are 46 to 52 nm in diameter. The open arrowheads point to herpes-type particles, presumed to be Epstein–Barr virus, which are 100 nm in diameter. The bar represents 100 nm (×143,640).

Papillomavirus Antigen

Of the 67 hairy leukoplakia biopsy specimens tested, 49 (73 percent) showed positive staining. Six of the 10 oral warts and condylomata, none of the 10 other oral mucosal lesions, and none of the 6 unaffected buccal mucosal specimens from patients with hairy leukoplakia showed positive staining. None of the cell lines that contained the herpes-group viruses showed staining.

Herpesvirus Antigens

Direct immunofluorescence staining of cryosections of the hairy leukoplakia tissue for herpes simplex 1 and 2 and varicella–zoster virus yielded negative results. Staining for cytomegalovirus by anticomplement indirect immunofluorescence that used three reference serum samples positive for cytomegalovirus and negative for EBV also gave uniformly negative results. No staining was obtained with any of the four EBV-negative serum samples. Staining of all control biopsy specimens was negative for all herpesviruses.

Staining for EBV in the hairy leukoplakia tissue was consistently positive and striking in appearance. Nineteen of 20 specimens showed intense nuclear staining in epithelial cells with each of the six reference serum samples that were positive for EBV. The stained cells were confined to the prickle-cell and koilocytotic-cell layers. On cryostat sections, the cells appeared as a well-defined area of fluorescence, usually less than six to eight cells deep (Fig. 6). Among the specimens from the six patients from whom both lesion (tongue) and nonlesion (buccal) tissues were available, positive staining for EBV was seen in the lesion specimens from five. Interestingly, electron microscopical examination of the single EBV-negative specimen showed only the papillomavirus-like particles.

We further determined that the EBV antigen seen in the sections was predominantly the viral capsid antigen, since serum with antibodies only to that antigen produced the characteristic intense staining depicted in Figure 6. Serum that was positive for both the viral capsid antigen and the early-antigen dif-

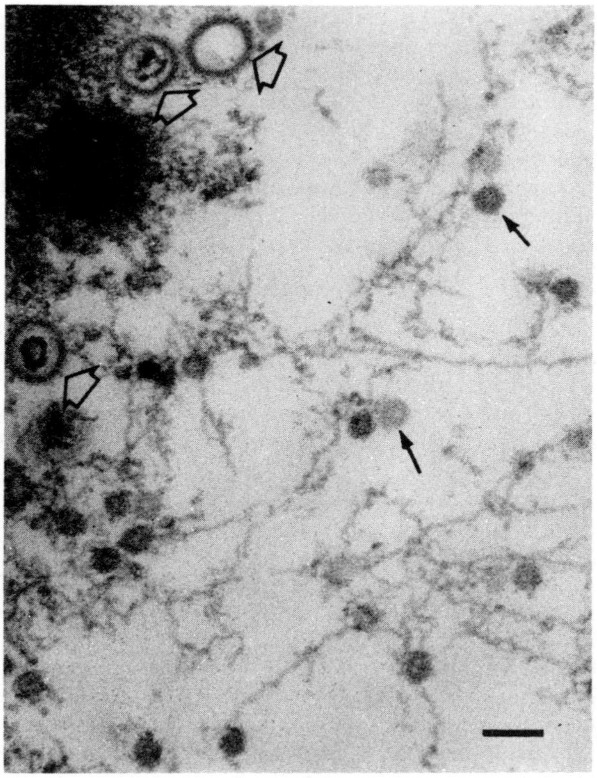

Figure 5. Papillomavirus-Like and Herpes-Type Viral Particles in the Nucleus of a Single Epithelial Cell in Hairy Leukoplakia.

The solid arrows indicate 48-nm papillomavirus-like particles, and the open arrows identify 100-nm herpes-type particles, presumed to be Epstein–Barr virus. The bar represents 100 nm (×83,075).

fuse component produced an additional but subtler staining pattern: many of the brightly stained nuclei showed a halo of speckled staining, which is characteristic of staining for the diffuse antigen component seen in all lymphoblastoid cells that are positive for the early antigen (not shown). Indirect immunofluorescence staining that used mouse monoclonal antibodies against EBV viral capsid antigen and the early-antigen diffuse component confirmed the presence of both antigens in all three specimens tested. The early-antigen restricted component was found in two of three specimens; the staining in the third was too faint to ascertain its presence or absence.

EBV in Hairy Leukoplakia Tissue

EBV DNA

When nitrocellulose-filter (Southern) blots of the DNA extracted from 13 lesions were hybridized with the ^{32}P-labeled pBgl 2-U probe for the large internal repeat region of EBV DNA, the typical EBV-specific pattern of bands was revealed (Fig. 1a, Panel A). The reconstruction hybridization, with amounts of large internal repeat sequences of DNA that were equivalent to 2, 20, and 200 EBV genome copies per cell in the 10-μg cellular DNA per slot (Fig. 1a, Panel B), indicated (by comparison with Panel A) that more than 200 viral molecules per cellular genome were present within 11 of the lesion specimens, and that less than 200 molecules per genome were present in the remaining two specimens (samples 182 and 183, Fig. 1a, Panel A). The hybridization of the analogous blot of the DNA extracted from the six specimens of unaffected buccal mucosal tissue showed no reaction in five instances (data not shown). In the sixth, the DNA from control tissue was inadvertently mixed with that from the lesion DNA and the result was falsely positive.

Genome of EBV

To determine whether regions other than the large internal repeat region (recognized by pBgl 2-U) of the EBV genome were present in the DNA from the lesions, high-complexity ^{32}P-labeled probes generated from the DNA of each lesion specimen were hybridized to Southern blots. The blots contained fragments of cloned EBV DNA that together constituted the complete genetic information of the virus (Fig. 2). Since the high-complexity probes showed hybridiza-

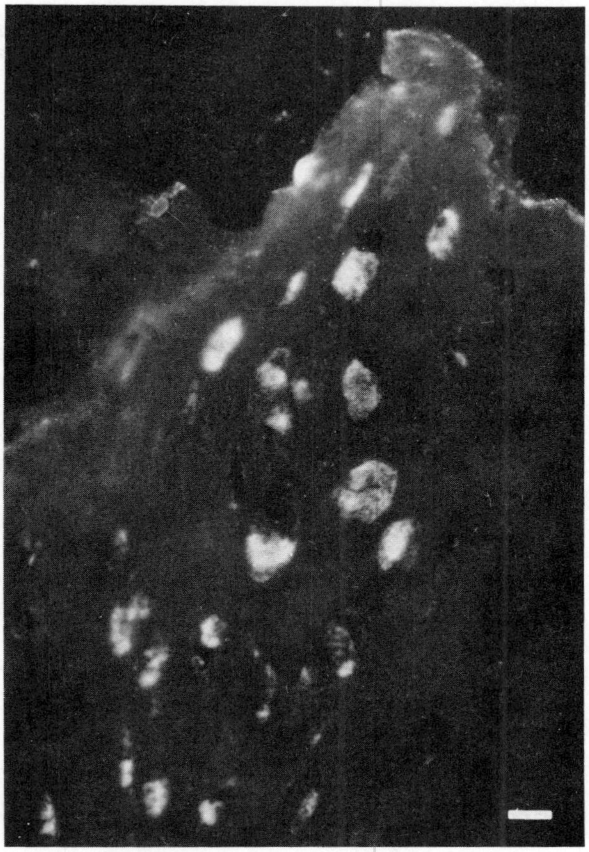

Figure 6. Anticomplement Indirect Immunofluorescence Staining for Epstein–Barr Virus Viral Capsid Antigen, Using Serum from a Patient with Infectious Mononucleosis.

A 5-μm cryostat section is shown. An identical staining pattern was obtained when mouse monoclonal antibody against viral capsid antigen was used. The bar represents 6 μm (×1000).

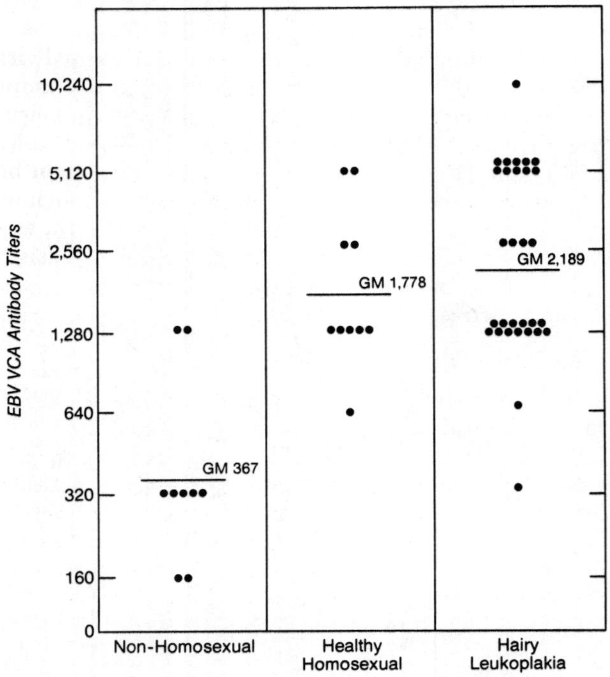

Figure 7. Titers of Serum IgG Antibodies to Epstein–Barr Virus Viral Capsid Antigen (EBV VCA) in Patients with Hairy Leukoplakia and Nonhomosexual and Healthy Homosexual Control Subjects.

GM denotes geometric mean.

tion with restriction fragments from many positions — from all parts of the EBV genome — it is reasonable to conclude that the entire EBV genome is present in hairy leukoplakia tissue.

Linear EBV Virion DNA

To determine whether the hairy leukoplakia tissue contained linear EBV DNA molecules (as would be expected in a lytic infection that generates mature EBV particles), we hybridized Southern blots of DNA from the lesions with the ^{32}P-labeled recombinant EBV DNA probe p961-20, which recognizes both ends of the linear form of the viral genome. In four of the six specimens tested, the resulting hybridization revealed the typical stepladder pattern of both ends of linear EBV virion DNA, digested with restriction endonucleases *Hind*III or *Bam*HI (data not shown). Two specimens were negative because of the lower sensitivity of the p961-20 probe as compared with the internal repeat probe (data not shown).

EBV Serology

The results of the EBV serologic tests (Fig. 7) revealed a sharp difference between the geometric means of the IgG antibody titers to the viral capsid antigen of the heterosexuals (geometric mean, 367) and those of the apparently healthy homosexuals (geometric mean, 1778). We found that the mean titers among the apparently healthy homosexuals were about five times higher than those among the heterosexuals. The patients with hairy leukoplakia appeared to be a subgroup of the homosexual group, since their antibody titers to the viral capsid antigen (geometric mean, 2198) were noticeably higher than those of either of the other groups. There were no biologically important differences among the three groups in the titers of antibodies to the early-antigen diffuse and restricted components or to the EBV-associated nuclear antigens.

Discussion

EBV is associated with several clinical disorders that affect at least two types of target cells. It is generally considered to be a lymphotropic virus because of its causative role in infectious mononucleosis, its close association with Burkitt's lymphoma, and the ease with which it can infect B lymphocytes in vitro.[4,16,17] The presence of EBV-associated nuclear antigen and EBV DNA in four epithelial cancers — nasopharyngeal carcinoma,[4] carcinoma of the palatine tonsil,[18] supraglottic laryngeal carcinoma,[19] and thymic carcinoma[20] — makes it clear that EBV can infect epithelial tissues. In these tumors, as well as in peripheral-blood lymphocytes from patients with acute infectious mononucleosis, the virus transforms the cells and becomes latent. Although the viral genome and its expression can be demonstrated readily by DNA hybridization and immunofluorescence of the EBV-associated nuclear antigen, electron microscopical studies of the tissues have failed to detect the viral particles.[21-25] Cell lines derived from Burkitt's lymphoma tumors and a small number of lymphoblastoid lines can be induced to enter a productive viral infection cycle, but usually only after laboratory manipulations. Although it is possible that latently infected B lymphocytes are the reservoirs for EB infectious viruses, it is not likely. EBV replication in peripheral-blood lymphocytes appears to be under stringent host regulation, both in vivo and in vitro. Yet copious amounts of extracellular virus can be found in the saliva of patients with acute infectious mononucleosis and in patients who are immunosuppressed.[26-28] The source of the infectious virus in these conditions and in asymptomatic carriers[29] remains an enigma.

Attempts to identify a possible reservoir in the oropharynx have yielded noteworthy results. Lemon[30] and Sixbey[31] and their colleagues showed that both EBV DNA and transcript RNA can be demonstrated in desquamated epithelial cells recovered from the oropharynx in patients with infectious mononucleosis. The presence of EBV DNA in the nuclei of such cells clearly indicates their susceptibility to the virus. Although structural components, such as viral capsid antigen or complete virus particles, were not demonstrated, the presence of EBV-specific RNA indicates viral gene expression. The source of the desquamated cells is not known. More recently, Wolf and colleagues[32] have cited the results of in situ hybridization and reassociation kinetics studies to suggest the presence of EBV genomes in three postmortem or biopsy specimens of parotid gland.

From our study of patients with oral hairy leukoplakia, we have strong evidence that EBV can and does replicate in the epithelial cells of the tongue, although we have no evidence to suggest that this occurs in persons other than these profoundly immunosuppressed patients. Immunofluorescence staining of the lesions with reference-specific serum samples identified the herpes-type virus to be EBV and not herpes simplex virus, varicella–zoster virus, or cytomegalovirus. The EBV was associated with the lesions only, since healthy buccal mucosal specimens from the same patients were negative for the virus, and the complete EBV genome, in its linear virion form, was found in the lesion but not in the normal buccal mucosa. The infection was permissive of EBV replication, as indicated by the production of EBV viral capsid antigen and the presence of large numbers of viral particles in both the nuclei and cytoplasm of the infected cells (seen by electron microscopy). The results of DNA hybridization were entirely in agreement with those obtained by immunofluorescence staining. Varying amounts of EBV DNA — in most cases more than 200 EBV genome equivalents per cell — were detected in the hairy leukoplakia lesions. Such high numbers of copies of EBV indicate that the virus was actively replicating within the lesions.

Evidence that suggests the possible coexistence of papillomavirus and EBV in the same cell is another intriguing finding of this study. Hairy leukoplakia may provide an opportunity to explain and study another facet of EBV pathogenesis. In our series, 73 percent of the lesion biopsy specimens stained positively for papillomavirus antigen. Using immunostaining that was specific for EBV and papillomavirus antigen, as well as EBV DNA hybridization, we found that five of six specimens examined for both viruses showed evidence of the presence of both. In the case in which only papillomavirus-like particles were evident, the patient's titer of antibody against EBV viral capsid antigen was comparatively low (1:320). To date, no hairy leukoplakia lesions have been found to contain EBV only.

These findings raise the following questions. First, is the coexistence of the two viruses fortuitous? Second, does infection of any one epithelial cell of the tongue by the two viruses occur successively? For example, papillomavirus might facilitate the persistence, entry, or subsequent replication of EBV in this particular site. There are also in vitro data that suggest that EBV may replicate actively in epithelial cells during terminal differentiation.[33] Our observations show that EBV is able to replicate in a specific site in the epithelium of the tongue in vivo. Papillomavirus is also known to replicate in terminally differentiating cells. The existence of occasional EBV-negative cases of hairy leukoplakia does not exclude the possibility that EBV is involved in the pathogenesis of the lesion in most cases. A similar situation is found with African Burkitt's lymphoma; 1 of 27 specimens in one series[22] and 1 of 15 in another[34] were EBV-negative.

The small size of the biopsy specimens allowed viral culture of only a few of them. Preliminary attempts have yielded negative results for herpes simplex virus, varicella–zoster virus, and cytomegalovirus. We are also attempting cultivation of EBV. The relation between hairy leukoplakia and the AIDS-associated retroviruses[35-37] is currently under investigation, as is the role of the Langerhans cell in the pathogenesis of the lesion.

We are indebted to Drs. Jeffrey Felton, Troy E. Daniels, David Purtillo, Harald zur Hausen, Jay A. Levy, Sol Silverman, Jr., and John Ziegler for advice and comments; to Yvonne de Souza and Brigitte Gewahl for technical assistance; to Marjorie Standow and Debra Stephenson for clinical assistance; to Carol Fiuren and Lin Moses for assistance in preparing the manuscript; to Evangeline Leash for editing the manuscript; and to the staffs of the San Francisco General Hospital AIDS Service, the UCSF AIDS Clinical Research Center, the UCSF AIDS Specimen Bank, and the San Francisco Men's Health Study.

References

1. Greenspan D, Greenspan JS, Conant M, Petersen V, Silverman S Jr, de Souza Y. Oral "hairy" leucoplakia in male homosexuals: evidence of association with both papillomavirus and a herpes-group virus. Lancet 1984; 2:831-4.
2. Ziegler JL, Drew WL, Miner RC, et al. Outbreak of Burkitt's-like lymphoma in homosexual men. Lancet 1982; 2:631-3.
3. Henle W, Henle G, Horwitz CA. Infectious mononucleosis and Epstein–Barr virus-associated malignancies. In: Lennette EH, Schmidt NJ, eds. Diagnostic procedures for viral, rickettsial and chlamydial infections. 5th ed. Washington, D.C.: American Public Health Association, 1979:441-70.
4. zur Hausen H, Schulte-Holthausen H, Klein G, et al. EBV DNA in biopsies of Burkitt tumours and anaplastic carcinomas of the nasopharynx. Nature 1970; 228:1056-8.
5. Bornkamm GW, Hudewentz J, Freese UK, Zimber U. Deletion of the nontransforming Epstein–Barr virus strain P3HR-1 causes fusion of the large internal repeat to the DS_L region. J Virol 1982; 43:952-68.
6. Rigby PWJ, Dieckmann M, Rhodes C, Berg P. Labeling deoxyribonucleic acid to high specific activity *in vitro* by nick translation with DNA polymerase I. J Mol Biol 1977; 113:237-51.
7. Desgranges C, Bornkamm GW, Zeng Y, et al. Detection of Epstein–Barr viral DNA internal repeats in the nasopharyngeal mucosa of Chinese with IgA/EBV-specific antibodies. Int J Cancer 1982; 29:87-91.
8. Peden K, Mounts P, Hayward GS. Homology between mammalian cell DNA sequences and human herpesvirus genomes detected by a hybridization procedure with high-complexity probe. Cell 1982; 31:71-80.
9. Polack A, Hartl G, Zimber U, et al. A complete set of overlapping cosmid clones of M-ABA virus derived from nasopharyngeal carcinoma and its similarity to other Epstein–Barr virus isolates. Gene 1984; 27:279-88.
10. Baer R, Bankier AT, Biggin MD, et al. DNA sequence and expression of the B95-8 Epstein–Barr virus genome. Nature 1984; 310:207-11.
11. Reedman BM, Klein G. Cellular localization of an Epstein–Barr virus (EBV)-associated complement-fixing antigen in producer and non-producer lymphoblastoid cell lines. Int J Cancer 1973; 11:499-520.
12. Acquired immunodeficiency syndrome (AIDS) update — United States. MMWR 1983; 32:309-11.
13. Dunn AEG, Ogilvie MM. Intranuclear virus particles in human genital wart tissue: observations on the ultrastructure of the epidermal layer. J Ultrastruct Res 1968; 22:282-95.
14. Oriel JD, Almeida JD. Demonstration of virus particles in human genital warts. Br J Vener Dis 1970; 46:37-42.
15. Williams MG, Howatson AF, Almeida JD. Morphological characterization of the virus of the human common wart (*Verruca vulgaris*). Nature 1961; 189:895-7.
16. Henle G, Henle W. The virus as the etiologic agent of infectious mononucleosis. In: Epstein MA, Achong BG, eds. The Epstein–Barr virus. New York: Springer-Verlag, 1979:297-320.
17. Diehl V, Henle G, Henle W, Kohn G. Demonstration of a herpes group virus in cultures of peripheral leukocytes from patients with infectious mononucleosis. J Virol 1968; 2:663-9.
18. Břicháček B, Hirsch I, Šíbl O, Vilikusová E, Vonka V. Presence of Epstein–Barr virus DNA in carcinomas of the palatine tonsil. JNCI 1984; 72:809-11.

19. *Idem.* Association of some supraglottic laryngeal carcinomas with EB virus. Int J Cancer 1983; 32:193-7.
20. Leyvraz S, Henle W, Chahinian AP, et al. Association of Epstein–Barr virus with thymic carcinoma. N Engl J Med 1985; 312:1296-9.
21. Nonoyama M, Huang CH, Pagano JS, Klein G, Singh S. DNA of Epstein–Barr virus detected in tissue of Burkitt's lymphoma and nasopharyngeal carcinoma. Proc Natl Acad Sci USA 1973; 70:3265-8.
22. Lindahl T, Klein G, Reedman BM, Johansson B, Singh S. Relationship between Epstein–Barr virus (EBV) DNA and the EBV-determined nuclear antigen (EBNA) in Burkitt lymphoma biopsies and other lymphoproliferative malignancies. Int J Cancer 1974; 13:764-72.
23. Epstein MA, Achong BG, Barr YM. Virus particles in cultured lymphoblasts from Burkitt's lymphoma. Lancet 1964; 1:702-3.
24. Nadkarni JS, Nadkarni JJ, Klein G, Henle W, Henle G, Clifford P. EB viral antigens in Burkitt tumor biopsies and early cultures. Int J Cancer 1970; 6:10-7.
25. Gazzolo L, de-Thé G, Vuillaume M, Ho HC. Nasopharyngeal carcinoma. II. Ultrastructure of normal mucosa, tumor biopsies, and subsequent epithelial growth *in vitro*. JNCI 1972; 48:73-86.
26. Miller G, Niederman JC, Andrews L-L. Prolonged oropharyngeal excretion of Epstein–Barr virus following infectious mononucleosis. N Engl J Med 1973; 288:229-32.
27. Niederman JC, Miller G, Pearson HA, Pagano JS, Dowaliby JM. Infectious mononucleosis: Epstein–Barr-virus shedding in saliva and the oropharynx. N Engl J Med 1976; 294:1355-9.
28. Cheeseman SH, Henle W, Rubin RH, et al. Epstein–Barr virus infection in renal transplant recipients: effects of antithymocyte globulin and interferon. Ann Intern Med 1980; 93:39-42.
29. Rickinson A. Epstein–Barr virus in epithelium. Nature 1984; 310:99-100.
30. Lemon SM, Hutt LM, Shaw JE, Li J-LH, Pagano JS. Replication of EBV in epithelial cells during infectious mononucleosis. Nature 1977; 268:268-70.
31. Sixbey JW, Nedrud JG, Raab-Traub N, Hanes RA, Pagano JS. Epstein–Barr virus replication in oropharyngeal epithelial cells. N Engl J Med 1984; 310:1225-30.
32. Wolf H, Haus M, Wilmes E. Persistence of Epstein–Barr virus in the parotid gland. J Virol 1984; 51:795-8.
33. Sixbey JW, Vesterinen EH, Nedrud JG, Raab-Traub N, Walton LA, Pagano JS. Replication of Epstein–Barr virus in human epithelial cells infected *in vitro*. Nature 1983; 306:480-3.
34. Olweny CLM, Atine I, Kaddu-Mukasa A, et al. Epstein–Barr virus genome studies in Burkitt's and non-Burkitt's lymphomas in Uganda. JNCI 1977; 58:1191-6.
35. Barré-Sinoussi F, Chermann JC, Rey F, et al. Isolation of a T-lymphotropic retrovirus from a patient at risk for acquired immune deficiency syndrome (AIDS). Science 1983; 220:868-71.
36. Popovic M, Sarngadharan MG, Read E, Gallo RC. Detection, isolation, and continuous production of cytopathic retroviruses (HTLV-III) from patients with AIDS and pre-AIDS. Science 1984; 224:497-500.
37. Levy JA, Hoffman AD, Kramer SM, Landis JA, Shimabukuro JM, Oshiro LS. Isolation of lymphocytopathic retroviruses from San Francisco patients with AIDS. Science 1984; 225:840-2.

ORIGINAL ARTICLE

TREATMENT OF SERIOUS CYTOMEGALOVIRUS INFECTIONS WITH 9-(1,3-DIHYDROXY-2-PROPOXYMETHYL)GUANINE IN PATIENTS WITH AIDS AND OTHER IMMUNODEFICIENCIES

COLLABORATIVE DHPG TREATMENT STUDY GROUP

Abstract The drug 9-(1,3-dihydroxy-2-propoxymethyl)-guanine (DHPG) was used to treat serious cytomegalovirus infections in 26 patients with underlying immunodeficiency (including 22 with the acquired immunodeficiency syndrome).

In 17 of 22 patients in whom cytomegalovirus was virologically confirmed, clinical status improved or stabilized, although in 4 of them the status of some affected organs deteriorated or did not improve. Fourteen of 18 patients with adequate viral-culture data had clearing of cytomegalovirus from all cultured sites. Patients with cytomegalovirus pneumonia often responded poorly; four of seven died before completing 14 days of DHPG therapy. The condition of 11 of 13 patients with cytomegalovirus retinitis and 5 of 8 with gastrointestinal disease stabilized or improved. However, clinical and virologic relapses occurred in 11 of 14 patients (79 percent) when DHPG was discontinued. Neutropenia was the most frequent adverse reaction.

We conclude that DHPG offers promise for the therapy of severe cytomegalovirus infections in some immunodeficient patients, but further study will be necessary to establish its efficacy and safety.

CYTOMEGALOVIRUS infections are a major cause of morbidity and mortality in patients with the acquired immunodeficiency syndrome (AIDS),[1] as well as in other patients with decreased cellular immunity, such as those receiving organ or bone marrow transplants and those with neoplasms. The incidence of cytomegalovirus infection among patients with AIDS is high,[2] and the infection can take many forms, including retinitis,[2,3] pneumonia,[2] colitis,[4] and various syndromes. Cytomegalovirus is also well recognized as a major pathogen in recipients of bone marrow[5,6] and renal[7,8] transplants.

9-(1,3-Dihydroxy-2-propoxymethyl)guanine (DHPG, Syntex Research, Palo Alto, Calif.) inhibits viral replication in vitro,[9,10] including the activity of all human herpesviruses and therefore cytomegalovirus.[10-12] The drug is also known as BW759U (Burroughs–Wellcome, Research Triangle Park, N.C.), 2′NDG (Merck Sharp and Dohme, Rahway, N.J.), and BIOLF-62 (ENS Bio-Logicals, Toronto, Ont.). In cytomegalovirus-infected cells, DHPG is phosphorylated to DHPG-monophosphate by a cellular deoxyguanosine kinase (Matthews TR: personal communication), then further phosphorylated to the triphosphate by other cellular enzymes. DHPG appears to be phosphorylated about 10-fold more in virus-infected cells affording some selectivity to the compound. DHPG-triphosphate competitively inhibits binding of deoxyguanosine triphosphate to DNA polymerase, inhibiting DNA synthesis and also terminating DNA elongation.

The toxicologic profile of DHPG in animals is essentially radiomimetic. Inhibition of spermatogenesis, bone marrow depression, and atrophy and necrosis of gastrointestinal mucosa occur in a dose-related fashion.

METHODS

Patients

Between May 3 and December 15, 1984, 26 patients received DHPG on a "compassionate use" basis for treatment of severe (life- or sight-threatening) cytomegalovirus infections (Table 1). Informed consent was obtained before treatment from all patients or their legal guardians. All patients had underlying immunodeficiencies (22 with AIDS, 2 with bone marrow transplants, 1 with severe combined immunodeficiency, and 1 receiving alkylating agents for myeloproliferative syndrome).

The patients' concurrent diseases and sites of cytomegalovirus involvement are listed in Table 1. The diagnosis of cytomegalovirus retinitis was made on clinical grounds that had been defined at each study center: a positive culture (from any site) for cytomegalovirus, no other likely explanation of the retinal findings, and funduscopic features typical of cytomegalovirus retinitis — generally with inflammation manifested as areas of white, fluffy lesions, often with associated hemorrhage, tending to follow a vascular pattern of distribution. For sites other than the retina, a diagnosis in most cases was based on a positive cytomegalovirus culture from the putative site, but in some cases, on histologic findings of inclusions consistent with cytomegalovirus disease. In retrospect, all cytomegalovirus cultures for four patients (No. 15, 17, 22, and 29), including base-line cultures, were negative. These patients were included in the analysis of the safety of DHPG but excluded from the analysis of efficacy.

This study excluded pregnant women, patients receiving an antimetabolite, interferon, or another nucleoside analogue, and transplant recipients in whom a trial reduction of dosages of immunosuppressive drugs was feasible.

Supported by a grant from Syntex Research.

In accordance with *Journal* policy, Drs. Koretz, Buhles, Brewin, and Roe state that they were employed by Syntex Research (the manufacturer of DHPG) at the time of the study.

The members of the Collaborative DHPG Treatment Study Group were Stuart H. Koretz, M.D., Ph.D. (study director), William C. Buhles, D.V.M., Ph.D., Austin Brewin, M.D., and Robert L. Roe, M.D., Institute of Clinical Medicine, Syntex Research, Palo Alto, Calif.; Thomas Merigan, M.D. (study chairman), Jack Bissett, M.D., and Mark P. Eisenberg, M.D., Stanford University Hospital, Stanford, Calif.; H. Clifford Lane, M.D., Henry Masur, M.D., and Anthony S. Fauci, M.D., National Institutes of Health, Bethesda, Md.; Richard Pollard, M.D., Debbie Matzke, M.D., and Keith Ramsey, M.D., University of Texas Medical Branch, Galveston; Peter Mansell, M.D., and Gerald Bodey, M.D., M.D. Anderson Hospital, Houston, Tex.; Steven Mehalko, M.D., R.K. Davies Hospital, San Francisco; John Mills, M.D., Howard Brodie, M.D., and Connie Wofsy, M.D., San Francisco General Hospital, San Francisco; Clyde Crumpacker, M.D., and Steven Marlowe, M.D., Beth Israel Hospital, Boston; Thomas Issekutz, M.D., Izaac Walton Killam Hospital, Halifax, N.S.; Donald Kotler, M.D., Michael Lange, M.D., and George McKinley, M.D., St. Lukes Hospital, New York; Eskild A. Petersen, M.D., University of Arizona, Tucson; Stanley Plotkin, M.D., Children's Hospital, Philadelphia; Richard Whitley, M.D., and David Barnes, M.D., University of Alabama, Birmingham; Prof. V. Faber, University of Copenhagen, Copenhagen, Denmark; Donald Rubin, M.D., and Ian Frank, M.D., University of Pennsylvania, Philadelphia; Douglas Dieterich, M.D., New York University, New York; and W. Lawrence Drew, M.D., Ph.D., Mt. Zion Hospital, San Francisco.

DHPG (Syntex Research) was administered in doses of 5 mg per kilogram of body weight (2.5 mg per kilogram in one patient), infused intravenously over 1 hour at 8- to 12-hour intervals, for a median of 14 days. Efficacy was assessed clinically and by follow-up cultures for cytomegalovirus. The criteria for a favorable clinical response in patients with retinitis were improved visual acuity, healing of lesions, and no extension of existing lesions or development of new lesions; in those with colitis, reduction in the severity of diarrhea; in those with pneumonia, improved blood oxygenation or improved appearance of the chest film; and in those with esophagitis, decreased esophageal pain. Drug safety was evaluated by clinical assessment and laboratory tests, including complete blood counts, renal and liver chemistries, urinalyses, and other tests when clinically indicated. Abnormal findings considered by the attending physician to be unrelated to DHPG were excluded from the analysis.

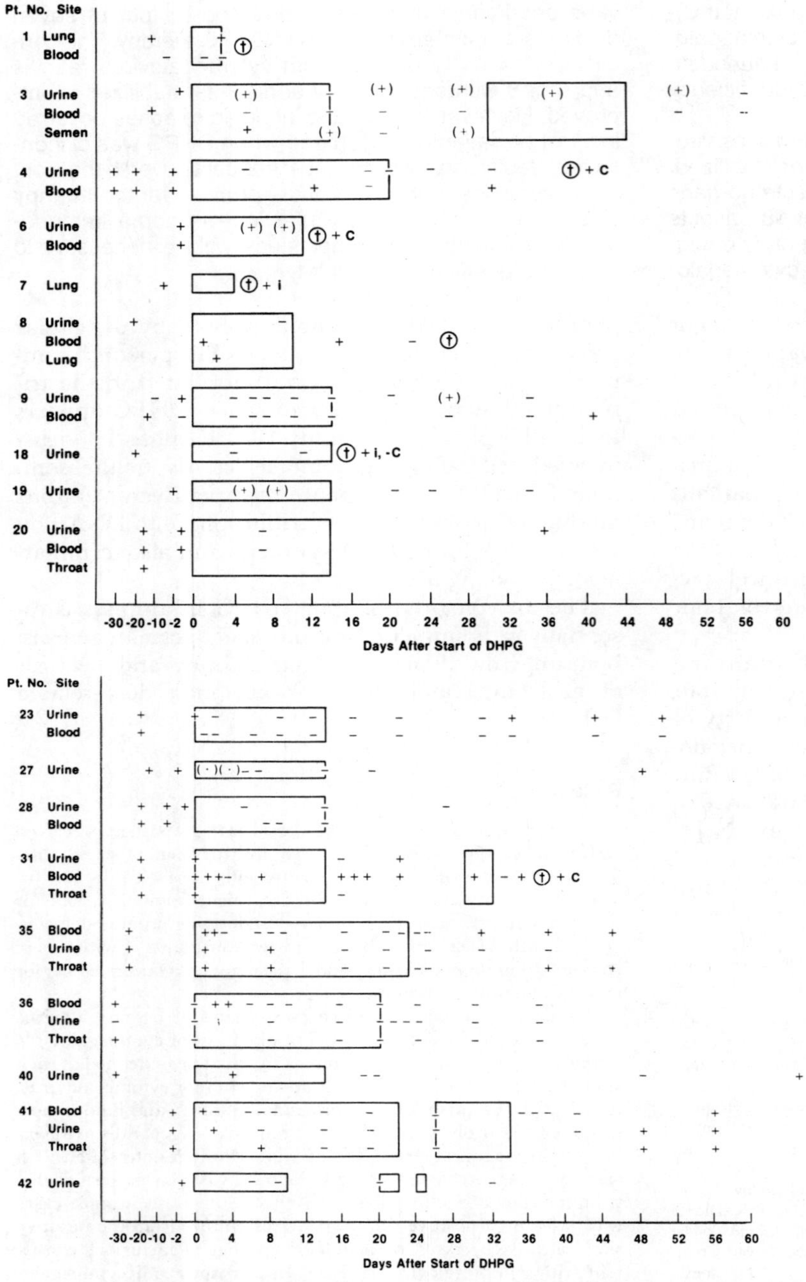

Figure 1. Results of Viral Cultures for Cytomegalovirus before, during, and after Treatment with DHPG.

Cultures are shown as + (positive) or − (negative). (+) denotes a positive culture with a marked reduction in the number of plaque-forming units per milliliter, as compared with base line.

† denotes death, +i viral inclusions present at autopsy, and +C and −C cytomegalovirus cultures at autopsy (positive or negative). Treatment periods are represented as rectangles.

Viral Studies

Viral cultures were performed on various body-fluid and tissue samples, used diploid human fibroblasts, and were rated as positive if a cytopathic effect typical of cytomegalovirus occurred, but they were not otherwise standardized among the 13 participating laboratories. Negative cultures were held at least four weeks before they were finally read. In five laboratories, the results from culture isolates were confirmed by immunofluorescence staining. In four laboratories evaluating cultures from 11 patients, the viral titers in specimens were quantified by serial dilutions and plaque-counting techniques.

Results

Clinical and Virologic Findings

Figure 1 summarizes virologic data for the 19 patients who had positive base-line cultures for cytomegalovirus and at least one follow-up culture. The seven patients excluded from Figure 1 had inadequate viral cultures. In four of these seven (No. 15, 17, 22, and 29), all cultures were negative, including base-line cultures. In the other three patients (No. 21, 34, and 39), although base-line cultures were positive, no follow-up cultures were obtained. In five patients (No. 3, 6, 9, 19, and 27), quantitative cultures for cytomegalovirus revealed that the numbers of infectious cytomegalovirus units decreased in titer after DHPG treatment, before the cultures became negative. For example, in Patient 3 viral titers in urine decreased from 163 pfu (plaque-forming units) per milliliter before treatment to 5 pfu per milliliter and then to less than 1 pfu per milliliter (negative), and titers in semen decreased from 1.5×10^6 pfu per milliliter to 9500 pfu per milliliter and then below 62.5 pfu per milliliter.

Table 2 summarizes the clinical responses to treatment of the three most common sites of cytomegalovirus involvement (retina, gastro-

Table 1. Clinical Characteristics of 26 Immunodeficient Patients with Cytomegalovirus (CMV) Infection.

Patient No.*	Sex/Age	Concurrent Disease†				CMV Infection Site‡			
		KS	PCP	Thrush	Other	Retina	Lung	GI	Other
1	F/29						C		
3	M/41	+			HSV proctitis	F			
4	M/45			+		F	C	C	CNS-C
6	M/51	+	+	+	MAC		H		
7	M/30	+				F	C		
8	M/38				HSV, perianal	F	C		
9	M/38	+		+				C	
15	M/35			+	HSV proctitis	F			
17	M/36				HSV, perianal	F			
18	M/3 mo		+				H		
19	M/35	+				F			
20	M/40			+		F			
21	M/31					F			
22	M/5								Wasting
23	M/28		+	+			C		
27	M/33							H	Liver-C
28	M/31				Cryptosporidiosis	F			
29	F/31						H		
31	M/40			+		F		H	
34	M/40		+	+	MAC			H	
35	M/31			+		F		C	
36	F/60					F			
39	M/34				MAC				CNS-C
40	M/52		+	+	MAC			C	
41	M/38	+		+	Cryptosporidiosis	F		C	
42	M/44		+		Crypto	F			

*Numbers are not consecutive, because the numbers not listed here had been assigned to other patients not ultimately treated with DHPG.

All patients had underlying AIDS except for Patient 1 (metastatic malignant melanoma, chemotherapy, autologous bone marrow transplant), Patient 18 (severe combined immunodeficiency), Patient 22 (acute myelogenous leukemia, allogeneic bone marrow transplant), and Patient 36 (myeloproliferative syndrome treated with alkylating agents).

†KS denotes Kaposi's sarcoma, PCP *Pneumocystis carinii* pneumonia, HSV herpes simplex virus, MAC *Mycobacterium avium complex*, and Crypto cryptococcal meningitis.

‡GI denotes gastrointestinal tract, CNS central nervous system, F diagnosis based on funduscopy, C diagnosis based on culture, and H diagnosis based on histopathology.

intestinal tract, and lung). The total number of sites of involvement (28) exceeds the number of patients because some patients had multiple sites.

Of the 22 patients in whom diagnosis was virologically confirmed, 13 had stabilization or improvement of all reported sites of cytomegalovirus involvement; 4 had improvement of at least one site but no apparent improvement of at least one other site; and 5 died before the completion of the standard 14-day treatment, with no or minimal apparent benefit. Despite favorable initial clinical responses, many patients ultimately died (17 of the 26, as of March 1, 1985).

The retina was the most frequent site of cytomegalovirus disease in this series. Of 13 patients with retinitis and positive viral cultures, 9 (69 percent) had clinical improvement, manifested by increased visual acuity, decreased retinal inflammation, or both. In two additional patients (15 percent), the retinitis stabilized. Two patients, one of whom died five days after the initiation of DHPG treatment, had no improvement. Of the 11 patients whose retinitis either stabilized or improved, 9 had clearing of cytomegalovirus from all cultured sites; 1 had clearing from the urine and throat but persistence of virus in the blood; and 1 did not have virologic follow-up. Follow-up data were available for 7 of these 11 patients. Five (71 percent) had relapses of retinitis two to six weeks after completing the initial course of DHPG treatment. Virologic relapse occurred in association with clinical relapse in three of these patients, and the virologic status of the other two is unknown.

Thus, in patients with cytomegalovirus retinitis, a clinical response commonly occurred and a good correlation was observed between clinical and virologic responses to DHPG treatment. Unfortunately, clinical and virologic relapses were frequent.

Eight patients had cytomegalovirus involving the gastrointestinal tract — most often, colitis with severe diarrhea and weight loss, or esophagitis with severe dysphagia and weight loss. Five of the eight patients had a favorable clinical response to DHPG treatment, manifested by decreased diarrhea (colitis) or decreased esophageal pain (esophagitis); follow-up cultures became negative in four of the five patients and were unevaluable in one patient because of fungal contamination. One patient (No. 4) had cessation of virus shedding and clinical improvement

Table 2. Clinical and Virologic Response to Cytomegalovirus (CMV) to DHPG.

CMV Infection Site	No. of Sites*	Clinical Response		Mean Dose	Mean Therapy Duration	Virologic Response†		
						cleared	persisted	unknown
		no. of patients		*mg/kg/day*	*days*	*no. of patients*		
Retina	13	Favorable	11	10.9 (10–15)	15.6 (13–21)	9	1	1
		None	2	13.3 (10–15)	14.7 (4–30)	0	1	1
Gastrointestinal tract	8	Favorable	5	10.5 (7.5–15)	18.8 (14–30)	4	0	1
		None	3	11.7 (10–15)	18.3 (14–21)	2	1	0
Lung	7	Favorable	3	15 (15–15)	14.6 (10–21)	2	0	1
		None	4	11.3 (10–15)	8.0 (3–14)	1	2	1

*Patients in whom the diagnosis could not be virologically confirmed are excluded from this table. The total number of sites is larger than the study population (26) because some patients had more than one site of cytomegalovirus disease.

†"Cleared" denotes cytomegalovirus cultures from all culture sites converted to negative; "Persisted," cytomegalovirus cultures from at least one cultured site remained positive; and "Unknown," viral-culture data were inadequate for assessment of virologic response.

of pneumonia and retinitis but not of central nervous system symptoms or colitis; another (No. 35) had negative viral cultures and improvement of retinitis but not of colitis. A single patient (No. 31) with gastrointestinal involvement (colitis) had persistence of positive blood cultures despite DHPG treatment. Perforation of his colon necessitated partial colectomy on the fifth day of DHPG treatment. The resected segment had evidence of cytomegalovirus colitis.

Like the patients with cytomegalovirus retinitis, the patients with gastrointestinal involvement had a high rate of relapse occurring after the completion of DHPG treatment. Four of the five patients who improved during the initial course of therapy had clinical relapses two weeks to 3½ months after DHPG was discontinued. In three of these patients with relapses, cultures of blood or urine that had become negative for cytomegalovirus during the initial course of DHPG treatment became positive 12 to 60 days after DHPG was discontinued. Follow-up culture data for the fourth patient were unavailable. Two patients with gastrointestinal recurrence were treated again; a favorable response occurred in one, and the results of the treatment in the other are pending.

Of the seven patients with cytomegalovirus pneumonia and positive base-line cultures for cytomegalovirus, four (No. 1, 6, 7, and 18) died of respiratory failure before completing a 14-day course of DHPG. All four had culture or histologic evidence of active cytomegalovirus disease at the time of death (although Patient 18 had clearing of cytomegalovirus from his urine before he died, and post-mortem cultures from multiple sites were negative despite the presence of inclusions consistent with cytomegalovirus). The three patients with pneumonia who survived for at least 14 days after DHPG treatment (No. 4, 8, and 23) died of pulmonary failure 3, 1½, and 7 weeks (respectively) after completing treatment. Patient 4 had clearing of cytomegalovirus from urine cultures during DHPG therapy but died of severe, recurrent cytomegalovirus pneumonia three weeks after DHPG was stopped, and Patient 23 had a urine culture showing recurrence before he died.

Of the 26 patients who were treated under the compassionate-use protocol, 17 are known to have died as of March 1, 1985. None of the deaths were attributed to DHPG. Five patients died before completing a 14-day course of DHPG — four of cytomegalovirus pneumonia and one of an unspecified cardiopulmonary event. Four other patients died with fulminating cytomegalovirus disease two days to three weeks after discontinuing DHPG. One patient (No. 31), who died two days after completion of treatment, had positive blood cultures while receiving DHPG. The other three all had clearing of the virus during treatment, with subsequent relapse. Six additional patients died five days to 2½ months after the completion of DHPG treatment, and death was attributed to causes other than cytomegalovirus, although two of these patients (No. 9 and 23) had had virologic relapse before they died. Finally, two patients (No. 20 and 27) died of unspecified causes six to eight weeks after completing DHPG treatment; both had had virologic relapse before death.

Adverse Reactions

Neutropenia that was reversible developed or worsened in six patients and recurred in one patient who had been retreated with DHPG. Eosinophilia was observed in three patients. Elevation of one or more serum liver enzymes occurred in six patients, but these elevations generally reached maximum values of only twice the base-line values or twice the upper limit of normal. The platelet count decreased in one patient but recovered partly during DHPG treatment. Edema occurred in two patients, and nausea in one. One patient had myalgias and headaches, and one had anorexia and disorientation, in association with DHPG treatment. One patient, who had had a prior psychotic episode, experienced hallucinations; one had a rash, which resolved when cloxacillin was discontinued; and two had phlebitis. The two patients with adverse central nervous system reactions had normal renal function.

Discussion

These preliminary findings suggest that DHPG treatment of immunodeficient patients with severe cytomegalovirus infections may result in clinical and virologic improvement, particularly in patients with extrapulmonary sites of involvement. Eighty-four percent of patients with retinal involvement and 62 percent of those with gastrointestinal involvement had clinical improvement in association with DHPG treatment. However, patients with cytomegalovirus pneumonia fared less well; 57 percent died before completing a two-week course of DHPG. The time required for an antiviral effect may be too long to allow much likelihood of benefit in some patients with advanced cytomegalovirus pneumonia. Whether patients with cytomegalovirus pneumonia would do better with earlier initial treatment and long-term maintenance therapy after the initial course of treatment needs to be evaluated.

Relapse occurred in all three subgroups (retinitis, pneumonia, and gastrointestinal disease). Eleven of 14 patients (79 percent) who were followed after DHPG was discontinued eventually had a relapse, and in many cases both clinical and virologic relapses occurred. Several patients have had favorable responses to second courses of therapy (Koretz S: unpublished data), and more recently, attempts have been made to devise a maintenance regimen to prevent relapse.

The existence or emergence of DHPG-resistant strains of cytomegalovirus is a possibility, given the clinical course in Patient 31, in whom DHPG treatment failed to result in complete virologic clearing. If DHPG is given over the long term or in repeated intermittent doses, it will be necessary to evaluate patients' responses for evidence of viral resistance to DHPG.

In this open study, assessments of clinical responses could have been markedly influenced by a number of potential sources of bias, including subjective factors. For these reasons, we place special emphasis on the data on viral cultures, which serve as an independent, objective measure of efficacy. The high degree of concordance between clinical and virologic responses and relapses strongly supports the overall validity of the clinical assessments.

The most serious adverse drug reaction in this series was neutropenia, not an unexpected problem with an agent capable of interfering with host-cell DNA metabolism. The neutropenia generally appeared to be dose-related and reversible. It may limit the ability of some patients to tolerate a therapeutic course of DHPG. Patients with AIDS appear to be especially susceptible to the development of neutropenia, which may be aggravated by such drugs as trimethoprim–sulfamethoxazole.[13] Whether neutropenia related to DHPG is less common in patients without AIDS remains to be determined.

To date, attempts to treat cytomegalovirus infections with other antiviral agents have been disappointing. In immunosuppressed patients, vidarabine (adenine arabinoside),[14-16] alpha-interferon,[17] acyclovir,[18,19] and the combination of vidarabine and human leukocyte interferon[20] have been used to treat cytomegalovirus infections, with little benefit at tolerated doses. Thus, our results with DHPG are encouraging. However, it must be emphasized that our results are preliminary, and that further analysis of efficacy and safety will be necessary before the therapeutic utility of this investigational drug can be established.

We are indebted to Dr. Phillip Smith and Dr. Alan Palestine (National Institutes of Health), Dr. James O'Donnell (University of California, San Francisco), Dr. Robert E. Neger (R.K. Davies Hospital, San Francisco), Dr. Everett Ai (Presbyterian Hospital, San Francisco), Barbara Mastre, R.N., and Ms. Nanette Goldman (Syntex Research, Palo Alto).

Note added in proof: Since submission of this paper, one subsequent patient, not among these 26, has died with persistent neutropenia and sepsis possibly due to DHPG. In addition, several reports of small series of patients treated with DHPG have appeared.[21-24] The results in general have been similar to those reported here.

References

1. Macher AM, Reichert CM, Straus SE, et al. Death in the AIDS patient: role of cytomegalovirus. N Engl J Med 1983; 309:1454.
2. Lerner CW, Tapper ML. Opportunistic infection complicating acquired immune deficiency syndrome: clinical features of 25 cases. Medicine (Baltimore) 1984; 63:155-64.
3. Palestine AG, Rodrigues MM, Macher AM, et al. Ophthalmic involvement in acquired immunodeficiency syndrome. Ophthalmology (Rochester) 1984; 91:1092-9.
4. Meiselman MS, Cello JP, Margaretten W. Cytomegalovirus colitis: report of the clinical, endoscopic, and pathologic findings in two patients with the acquired immune deficiency syndrome. Gastroenterology 1985; 88: 171-5.
5. Winston DJ, Gale RP, Meyer DV, Young LS. Infectious complications of human bone marrow transplantation. Medicine (Baltimore) 1979; 58:1-31.
6. Meyers JD, Flournoy N, Thomas ED. Nonbacterial pneumonia after allogeneic marrow transplantation: a review of ten years' experience. Rev Infect Dis 1982; 4:1119-32.
7. Peterson PK, Balfour HH Jr, Marker SC, Fryd DS, Howard RJ, Simmons RL. Cytomegalovirus disease in renal allograft recipients: a prospective study of the clinical features, risk factors and impact on renal transplantation. Medicine (Baltimore) 1980; 59:283-300.
8. Glenn J. Cytomegalovirus infections following renal transplantation. Rev Infect Dis 1981; 3:1151-78.
9. Field AK, Davies ME, DeWitt C, et al. 9-{[2-hydroxy-1-(hydroxymethyl)-ethoxy]methyl}guanine: a selective inhibitor of herpes group virus replication. Proc Natl Acad Sci USA 1983; 80:4139-43.
10. Mar E-C, Cheng Y-C, Huang E-S. Effect of 9-(1,3-dihydroxy-2-propoxymethyl)guanine on human cytomegalovirus replication in vitro. Antimicrob Agents Chemother 1983; 24:518-21.
11. Martin JC, Dvorack CA, Smee DE, Matthews TR, Verheyden JPH. 9-[(1,3-dihydroxy-2-propoxy)methyl]guanine: a new potent and selective antiherpes agent. J Med Chem 1983; 26:759-61.
12. Tocci MJ, Livelli TJ, Perry HC, Crumpacker CS, Field AK. Effects of the nucleoside analog 2′-nor-2′-deoxyguanosine on human cytomegalovirus replication. Antimicrob Agents Chemother 1984; 25:247-52.
13. Gordin FM, Simon GL, Wofsy CB, Mills J. Adverse reactions to trimethoprim-sulfamethoxazole in patients with the acquired immunodeficiency syndrome. Ann Intern Med 1984; 100:495-9.
14. Pollard RB, Egbert PR, Gallagher JG, Merigan TC. Cytomegalovirus retinitis in immunosuppressed hosts. I. Natural history and effects of treatment with adenine arabinoside. Ann Intern Med 1980; 93:655-64.
15. Ch'ien LT, Cannon NJ, Whitley RJ, et al. Effect of adenine arabinoside on cytomegalovirus infections. J Infect Dis 1974; 130:32-9.
16. McCracken GH Jr, Luby JP. Cytosine arabinoside in the treatment of congenital cytomegalic inclusion disease. J Pediatr 1972; 80:488-93.
17. Chou SW, Dylewski JS, Gaynon MW, Egbert PR, Merigan TC. Alpha-interferon administration in cytomegalovirus retinitis. Antimicrob Agents Chemother 1984; 25:25-8.
18. Balfour HH Jr, Bean B, Mitchell CD, Sachs GW, Boen JR, Edelman CK. Acyclovir in immunocompromised patients with cytomegalovirus disease: a controlled trial at one institution. Am J Med 1982; 73(1A):241-8.
19. Wade JC, Hintz M, McGuffin RW, Connor JD, Meyers JD. Treatment of cytomegalovirus pneumonia with high-dose acyclovir. Am J Med 1982; 73(1A):249-56.
20. Meyers JD, McGuffin RW, Bryson YJ, Cantell K, Thomas ED. Treatment of cytomegalovirus pneumonia after marrow transplant with combined vidarabine and human leukocyte interferon. J Infect Dis 1982; 146:80-4.
21. Shepp DH, Dandliker PS, de Miranda P, et al. Activity of 9-[2-hydroxy-1-(hydroxymethyl)ethoxymethyl]guanine in the treatment of cytomegalovirus pneumonia. Ann Intern Med 1985; 103:368-73.
22. Felsenstein D, D'Amico DJ, Hirsch MS, et al. Treatment of cytomegalovirus retinitis with 9-[2-hydroxy-1-(hydroxymethyl)ethoxymethyl]guanine. Ann Intern Med 1985; 103:377-80.
23. Bach MC, Bagwell SP, Knapp NP, Davis KM, Hedstrom PS. 9-(1,3-Dihydroxy-2-propoxymethyl)guanine for cytomegalovirus infections in patients with the acquired immunodeficiency syndrome. Ann Intern Med 1985; 103:381-2.
24. Masur H, Lane HC, Palestine A, et al. Effect of 9-(1,3-dihydroxy-2-propoxymethyl)guanine on serious cytomegalovirus disease in eight immunosuppressed homosexual men. Ann Intern Med 1986; 104:41-4.

ORIGINAL ARTICLE

SEVERE ACQUIRED IMMUNODEFICIENCY IN MALE HOMOSEXUALS, MANIFESTED BY CHRONIC PERIANAL ULCERATIVE HERPES SIMPLEX LESIONS

FREDERICK P. SIEGAL, M.D., CARLOS LOPEZ, PH.D., GLENN S. HAMMER, M.D., ARTHUR E. BROWN, M.D., STEPHEN J. KORNFELD, M.D., JONATHAN GOLD, M.D., JOSEPH HASSETT, M.D., SHALOM Z. HIRSCHMAN, M.D., CHARLOTTE CUNNINGHAM-RUNDLES, M.D., PH.D., BERNARD R. ADELSBERG, M.D., DAVID M. PARHAM, M.D., MARTA SIEGAL, M.A., SUSANNA CUNNINGHAM-RUNDLES, PH.D., AND DONALD ARMSTRONG, M.D.

Abstract Four homosexual men presented with gradually enlarging perianal ulcers, from which herpes simplex virus was cultured. Each patient had a prolonged course characterized by weight loss, fever, and evidence of infection by other opportunistic microorganisms including cytomegalovirus, *Pneumocystis carinii,* and *Candida albicans.* Three patients died; Kaposi's sarcoma developed in the fourth. All were found to have depressed cell-mediated immunity, as evidenced by skin anergy, lymphopenia, and poor or absent responses to plant lectins and antigens in vitro. Natural-killer-cell activity directed against target cells infected with herpes simplex virus was depressed in all patients. The absence of a history of recurrent infections or of histologic evidence of lymphoproliferative or other neoplastic diseases suggests that the immune defects were acquired.

CHRONIC ulcerating lesions caused by herpes simplex viruses (HSV) are unusual even in patients with severe immunologic defects. These lesions occur in advanced lymphoproliferative disease, after immunosuppression for organ transplantation, during treatment with high doses of corticosteroids, and in certain primary immunodeficiency disorders.[1-8] In four previously healthy homosexual men we found chronic perianal ulcers infected with HSV. Immunologic evaluation confirmed the presence of apparently acquired cellular immunodeficiency. The course in these patients was characterized by severe, unrelenting opportunistic infections, leading to death in three patients.

METHODS

Subjects

The four patients were referred to Mount Sinai Hospital or to Memorial Hospital for diagnosis or treatment. Controls were normal male and female volunteers 20 to 50 years old.

Immunologic Studies

Mononuclear cells were obtained from heparinized venous blood and characterized by cell markers as previously described.[9] Hybridoma-derived reagents defining Leu-1, present on all normal human T lymphocytes, and Leu-2a, characteristic of a suppressor/cytotoxic subset, were kindly provided by Dr. Robert L. Evans.[10] Responses to phytohemagglutinin,, concanavalin A, pokeweed mitogen, and antigens from microbial pathogens were measured by cellular DNA synthesis.[11] Natural-killer-cell function was determined by comparing the cells' cytotoxicity among uninfected ^{51}Cr-labeled human-foreskin fibroblasts with their cytotoxicity among HSV-infected fibroblasts.[12] Delayed skin hypersensitivity was tested with recall antigens that usually elicted a response in normal adults (*Candida albicans*, streptokinase-streptodornase, mumps, and tetanus toxoid). Immune complexes were detected with a modification of the Raji-cell assay for Patient 1[13] and precipitation with 3.5 percent polyethylene glycol for the other three patients.[14] Specimens for viral culture were transported in Hanks' salts and incubated with a panel of cell types. Cytopathic effects in human embryonic kidney were observed within 24 to 48 hours when a specimen was positive for HSV. Commercial antiserums were used to characterize direct immunofluorescence for HSV in biopsy specimens.

From the divisions of Clinical Immunology and Infectious Diseases, the Mount Sinai Medical Center, and the Clinical Immunology and Infectious Diseases Services, Memorial Sloan-Kettering Cancer Center, New York.

Supported in part by grants (AI-16186 and CA-08748) from the U.S. Public Health Service, by the American Cancer Society, the Chemotherapy Foundation, and the Irma T. Hirschl Charitable Trust.

PATIENTS

Patient 1

A 26-year-old white homosexual man first noted perianal pain and vesiculation in January 1980. During the following spring, ulcerations gradually developed and fever and weight loss began. At presentation elsewhere the patient was anemic. Results of marrow and liver biopsies were negative. Antibiotics were administered. A large perianal ulcer had formed by July, and hepatosplenomegaly and generalized lymphadenopathy were observed when he was admitted to Memorial Hospital. Cultures taken from the ulcer bed indicated HSV Type 2; sigmoidoscopy revealed proctitis and an anterior anal ulcer. Chest x-ray films showed an infiltrate of the right upper lobe. Skin anergy was noted. Further evaluation for suspected inflammatory bowel disease or lymphoma was negative. By August, the patient had lost approximately half his original weight, and fever and perianal ulceration continued. Exploratory laparotomy with splenectomy and biopsies of the liver, small intestine, and lymph nodes showed only lymphocyte depletion. Satellite ulcers appeared on the buttocks. Parenteral nutritional supplements, transfusions, and antibiotics were given, but without benefit. In October, the chest films were unchanged. Persistently positive cultures for HSV, abnormal liver-function tests, and an enlarging ulcer led to a trial of an experimental antiviral compound 2′-fluoro, 5-iodoaracytosine (FIAC). Rectal bleeding developed; colonscopy revealed vesicles and ulcers, but biopsies were nondiagnostic and cultures were negative for HSV and other pathogens. Human-leukocyte interferon, broad-spectrum antibiotics, and trimethoprim-sulfamethoxazole (TMP-SMZ) were given for increasing dyspnea with bilateral pulmonary infiltrates. Renal failure and encephalopathy developed, and the patient died in October.

Autopsy revealed herpetic proctitis and colitis, with viral dissemination to the posterior columns of the spinal cord. *Pneumocystis carinii* was present in the lungs. Intranuclear and intracytoplasmic inclusions typical of cytomegalovirus were present in the adrenals, lungs, colonic smooth muscle, and endothelium underlying the ulcerations. Electron microscopy (kindly performed by Dr. Robert A. Erlandson) showed inclusions compatible with either HSV or cytomegalovirus.

Patient 2

A 32-year-old Hispanic homosexual man had perianal vesicular lesions in July 1979; biopsy suggested cytomegalovirus infection. In

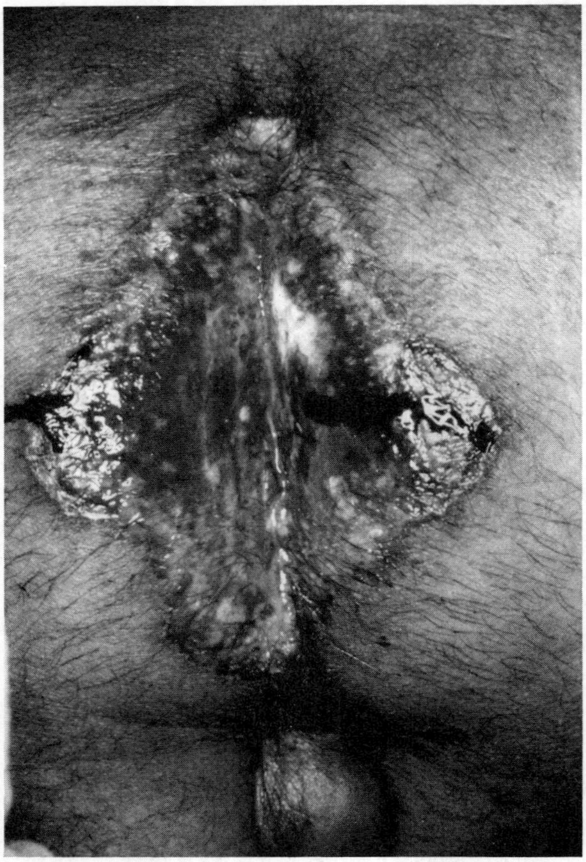

Figure 1. Perianal Ulceration of Patient 3, before Therapy with Vidarabine.

The appearance of the lesion did not change during or after this treatment.

November, he began to have fever, anorexia, gradual weight loss, abdominal pain, and hematochezia. In March 1980, rectal bleeding was severe enough to require transfusion of eight units of blood. Ulceration of the perianal lesion and diffuse lymphadenopathy were noted. The cause of these conditions was not revealed by sigmoidoscopy, gastrointestinal barium studies, examination of stools for bacteria and parasites, abdominal computerized tomography, sonography, or serologic studies; on the basis of inclusions found on rectal biopsy, which suggested lymphogranuloma venereum, tetracycline was given, without effect.

The patient was transferred to the Mount Sinai Hospital in May because of continued fevers and cachexia. He had oral candidiasis, generalized shotty lymphadenopathy, and abdominal tenderness in the left lower quadrant. The perianal ulcer had enlarged to 12 cm. Anemia and leukopenia were noted. Culture and immunofluorescence testing of the ulcer showed only HSV Type 2. Evaluation for lues, gonorrhea, lymphogranuloma venereum, and other pathogens was negative. A biopsy suggested that HSV and cytomegalovirus coexisted in the ulcer. Lymph-node biopsy indicated the absence of germinal centers. Treatment with vidarabine for five days had no effect, nor did a four-day trial of acyclovir (kindly provided by Burroughs–Wellcome). Spiking fevers, rectal bleeding, progressive wasting and lymphopenia did not respond to broad-spectrum antibiotics and transfusions. Terminally, the patient appeared to have a generalized cardiomyopathy; he died on August 8, 1980. Permission for autopsy was denied.

Patient 3

A 28-year-old Colombian homosexual man reported dull pain in the left lower abdominal quadrant and rectal bleeding in May 1980. He was treated surgically for presumed perianal abscess. Postoperative rectal bleeding necessitated transfusions. In June fever (temperature to 40°C) and weight loss began. After additional anal surgery, a perianal ulcer developed and gradually spread. Tetracycline and prednisone were given. However, unrelenting fever, perianal ulceration, and a 12-kg weight loss prompted an extensive but unrevealing evaluation, which included colonoscopy, gastrointestinal contrast studies, marrow biopsy, gallium and liver/spleen scans, abdominal sonography, and standard cultures.

The patient was transferred to the Mount Sinai Hospital in February 1981 because of cachexia and a 20-cm perianal ulcer (Fig. 1). Repeat evaluation for inflammatory bowel disease and lymphoma included exploratory laparotomy and construction of a diverting colostomy. No specific pathologic process was found; node-biopsy specimens were normal. Cultures of the ulcer grew HSV Type 2, which was confirmed by immunofluorescence testing and typical morphologic appearance. Vidarabine was given until central nervous system toxicity developed. In April, the patient was transferred to Memorial Hospital for further treatment with interferon and FIAC; however, the ulcer did not regress and cultures remained positive. Bilateral interstitial pneumonitis and encephalopathy led to his death in June.

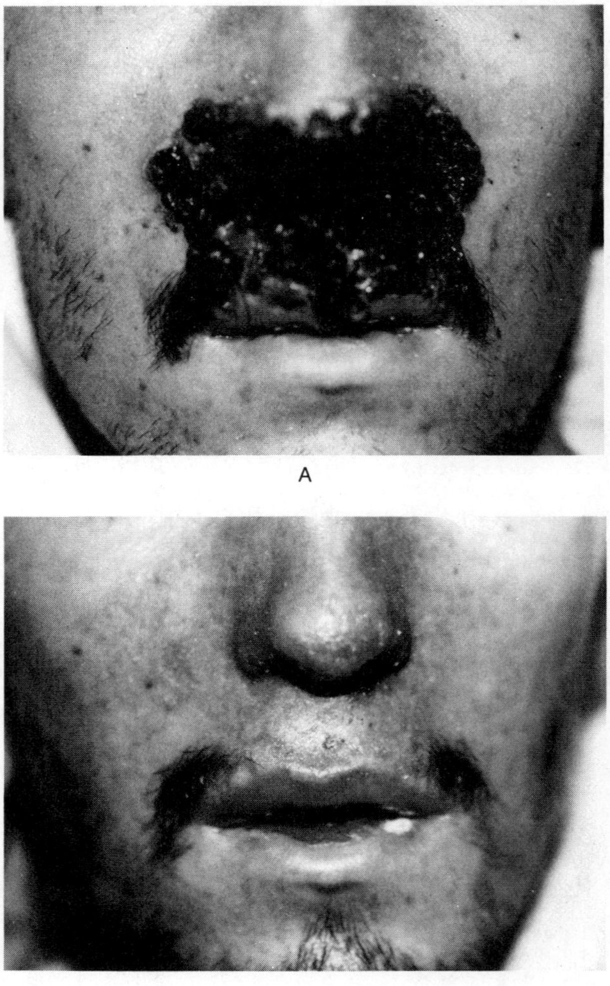

A

B

Figure 2. Nasolabial Lesion of Patient 4.

Panel A shows lesion (completely obstructing both nares) before therapy with acyclovir, and Panel B shows healing three days after treatment.

At autopsy, necrotizing, hemorrhagic bronchopneumonia, hemorrhagic colitis, and cholelithiasis were found. Post-mortem cultures from lung, liver, spleen, lymph nodes, and heart were negative, but herpetic intranuclear inclusions suggestive of cytomegalovirus were seen in the colon, adrenals, stomach, and lungs.

Patient 4

A 22-year-old Hispanic homosexual man had fever (38.5°C) and night sweats in July 1980. Gradual weight loss began. Oral candidiasis was noted in September. By December, an 8-kg weight loss, generalized lymphadenopathy, splenomegaly, anemia, and leukopenia were observed. Chest films showed an infiltrate in the right upper lobe. Evaluation for underlying disease, including gastrointestinal roentgenography, liver biopsy, gallium scanning, abdominal sonography, and colonic and lymph-node biopsies, gave nonspecific or normal results. In January 1981, perianal vesicular lesions first appeared; cultures showed HSV Type 2. Spiking fever, lethargy, anorexia, and weight loss continued, and the perianal lesions formed a gradually enlarging ulcer; ulcerative lesions, from which HSV was cultured, also appeared on the nasolabial fold (Fig. 2A). By April, the patient had lost 22 kg and had severe oral candidiasis. Treatment with amphotericin led to some reduction in the candidal infection; klebsiella bacteremia resolved with antibiotics. Treatment with vidarabine for two weeks did not affect the lesions or other symptoms, but in May acyclovir (Burroughs–Wellcome) given for 10 days led to defervescence and gradual healing of the ulcers (Fig. 2B). The marked lymphopenia and lymphoid dysfunction that had characterized the disease (see Results) were not altered. TMP–SMZ was given in low doses to prevent pneumocystosis. In July, the ulcers recurred and HSV was again cultured. During successful retreatment with acyclovir, bluish nodules on the back and penile shaft were noted. On biopsy, a diagnosis of Kaposi's sarcoma was made.

Results

Serologic data are summarized in Table 1. Patient 1 never had detectable complement-fixing antibodies against HSV, Patients 2 and 4 had unchanging titers, and Patient 3 had a fourfold increment in titer. Serologic evidence of active cytomegalovirus infection was present only in Patient 2. Patient 4 had complement-fixing antibody titers of 1:8 and less than 1:8. There was no evidence of acute or recent infection with varicella-zoster or Epstein–Barr viruses, lymphogranuloma venereum, or toxoplasmosis. Antibody to hepatitis B virus was present in two patients, and hepatitis B surface antigenemia developed late in Patient 1. Other serologic studies, particularly in Patient 1, failed to suggest infection with legionella species, cryptococcosis, histoplasmosis, *Entamoeba histolytica,* toxoplasma, respiratory syncytial viruses, or rubeola virus. Serologic testing for syphilis was negative in all patients.

Skin anergy to recall antigens was present in all subjects (Table 2). Total lymphocyte counts were regularly depressed. Except for a single determination (Patient 1, July 1980), counts did not exceed 1000 and averaged from 200 to 600. The severe lymphopenia limited the studies that could be done. The proportion of cells with T-cell characteristics ranged from normal to depressed in various determinations. The proportion of sheep rosettes tended to be lower than the proportion of cells demonstrable with use of hybridoma-derived antibodies to T cells (anti-Leu-1). Although this finding suggests that a serum inhibitor of rosette formation was present, none was found in Patients 3 or 4. The proportion of T cells exhibiting a suppressor/cytotoxic cell phenotype (Leu-2a) was increased in Patient 3 but not in Patients 2 or 4. Lymphocyte responses to plant lectins were moderately diminished in Patient 1, more severely so in Patients 2 and 3, and progressively depressed in Patient 4. Only Patient 4 had a response to phytohemagglutinin that was within the normal range when he was first studied. Responses to pokeweed mitogen were relatively preserved. In Patient 1, despite only moderate depression of mitogen-induced proliferation, transformation responses to all antigens tested, including HSV and cytomegalovirus, were absent.

Measurements of serum immunoglobulin and immunoelectrophoresis indicated polyclonal hyperimmunoglobulinemia, particularly of IgA. Despite this finding, serum antibody titers were generally low. The proportions of B cells were normal in all subjects. Absolute numbers of B cells, as well as of T cells, were depressed.

We considered the results of the assay of natural-killer-cell function in two ways. (1) HSV-specific natural-killer activity in lytic units per million mononuclear cells was determined directly from the lytic system. The calculation, which is based on a range of ratios of killer cells to target cells, considers all cells isolated from blood.[12] According to this standard, natural-killer activity was normal in Patients 1 and 4; it

Table 1. Evidence of Ulcerative Herpes Simplex and Other Infections among Four Homosexual Men.

Evidence	Infection*							
	HSV	CMV	HBsAg	HBsAb	*Candida albicans*	*Pneumocystis carinii*	Adenovirus	*Entamoeba histolytica*
	no. of patients positive/no. tested							
Positive Culture	4/4	0/4	†	†	2/4	†	1/4	†
Morphologic (active infection)	4/4	3/4	†	†	2/4	1/4	1/4	0/4
Serologic								
Prior exposure	3/4	2/4	0/4	2/4	†	†	0/1	1/4
Active infection (titer rise)	1/4	1/4‡	1/4	0/4	†	†	0/1	0/4

*HSV denotes herpes simplex virus, CMV cytomegalovirus, HBsAg hepatitis B surface antigen, and HBsAb antibody to HBsAg.

†Study was either inappropriate or not performed.

‡Another patient (Patient 4) had a cytomegalovirus titer below 1:8 on complement fixation when first studied; on a repeat study two weeks later the titer was 1:8.

Table 2. Immunologic Findings in Patients and Controls.

Study	Finding*								
	Patients								Controls
	1	*2*	*3*		*4*				*mean ±SD*
Delayed-type skin response	Absent	Absent	Absent		Absent				Present
Meal lymphocyte count	657	435	316		360				1000–4800
T cells (percent)									
Sheep rosettes	70	59, 79	28		69, 55				80±7
Leu-1	ND	89	53		65				78±5
Leu-2a	ND	20	62		29				32±9
Mitogen responses (net cpm †)									
Phytohemagglutinin	11,852	1,509	1,313	613	23,100	968	475	231	29,000±4,400
Concanavalin A	1,683	1,767	674	386	1,372	767	478	576	21,000±6,200
Pokeweed mitogen	5,635	1,148	3,887	766	4,136	1,067	132	589	15,800±5,100
Antigen responses in vitro	Absent	QNS	QNS		QNS				Positive
Mixed leukocyte reaction (net cpm †)	1,505	QNS	QNS		QNS				>5000
Natural killing of HSV-infected target cells ‡	8.2, 1.4	0	0.2–21.7		15.7				111 (52–239)
Serum immunoglobulin (mg/dl)									
IgG	864–1394	2360	1660		1370–1710				500–1500
IgA	322–375	445	435		420–1431				40–300
IgM	133–300	90	230		55–275				40–200
Isohemagglutinin									
Reciprocal									
Titers (anti-A/B)	—/8	8/—	32/8		4/0				>4
B cells (percent IgM-positive)	0	ONS	8		8				6±2
Immune complexes	0	0.20	0.20		0.04	0.04			<0.12

*ND denotes "not determined," and QNS "quantity not sufficient [for determination]."

†Net cpm = (cpm stimulated) − (cpm unstimulated control), where cpm = counts (per minute) of tritiated thymidine incorporated after three days' culture (five days for mixed leukocyte reaction).

‡Killing = (cytotoxicity toward infected targets) − (cytotoxicity toward uninfected targets), expressed a lytic units per milliliter of blood. Normal range = ±2SD on long-transformed data.[12]

was initially very depressed, in Patient 3, but later gradually became normal. (2) Because of the severe deficiency of mononuclear cells, calculation of the lytic units per milliliter of blood, based on cell yields, was also made (Table 2). By this criterion, all subjects had severely depressed natural-killer function; Patient 2 had no measurable activity.

Discussion

Ulcerative lesions caused by HSV are usually observed only in patients with severe deficits of cellular immunity associated with another underlying disease.[1-8] That four patients who were believed not to have been previously immunocompromised had such skin lesions (with three dying after an inexorably downhill course) suggests that some factor common to all the patients was operative. The fact that all were homosexual men was striking. Reports of Kaposi's sarcoma and opportunistic infections similar to those that we observed (e.g., *P. carinii*, *Cryptococcus neoformans*, and cytomegalovirus) suggest that our findings are part of a nationwide epidemic of immunodeficiency among male homosexuals.[15,16]

The most prominent and so far unexplained immunologic finding in these four men was profound lymphopenia. Many of the immunologic deficits that we measured could be attributed to this state of apparent lymphocyte depletion. Skin anergy was present in all subjects. When the responses to in vitro stimulation with plant lectins and antigens could be determined, they showed moderate to marked depressions in lymphocyte proliferative ability. Difficulty in interpretation of these data arises because of the paucity of available lymphoid cells and their dilution by monocytes in the mononuclear-cell isolates. Relative monocytosis in mononuclear-cell preparations is known to lead to poor in vitro proliferative responses.[17] Among the lymphoid cells present, there was specific depression of cells forming sheep-erythrocyte rosettes in two patients and a relative rise in cells bearing the Leu-2a phenotype in one patient. The relative rise implies an increase in the ratio of suppressor to helper cells among the lymphoid-cell populations — a finding that we (unpublished data) and others[18] have observed in cases of infectious mononucleosis. Attempts to rectify the lymphoid-cell responses of one patient in vitro by means of thymic humoral factors[19] were unsuccessful. When these findings were taken together, a severe defect in cellular immunity, which had been suspected on clinical grounds, was confirmed. The defect can be characterized as a progressive state of lymphocyte depletion and consequent dysfunction, in which cellular immunity is principally affected.

The specific host defense against HSV is poorly understood. Although patients with depressed lymphocyte counts or T-lymphocyte-macrophage dysfunction might be expected to have severe illness secondary to HSV, the vast majority of such patients do not. Consequently, it is suspected that other factors play an important part in HSV-specific host defense. The group of patients most frequently reported to be susceptible to ulcerative HSV are those who have had immunosuppression for organ transplantation. Recently, cells that confer "natural" immunity and do not require prior exposure to their specific target cells have been described. Certain natural-killer cells are thought to be involved in the host defense against HSV in mice and in human beings.[12,20] Overwhelming disseminated HSV infection in neonates and in some adults is associated with depressed natural-killer activity of this sort.[12] We measured this type of natural-killer cell in our patients because of their unusual HSV lesions. On a "per-cell" basis, the natural-killer cells in two of the four patients were abnormally hyporesponsive. Moreover, in view of the paucity of mononuclear cells present per unit of blood, the calculated herpes-directed natural-killer activity was severely depressed in all patients. Thus, a common absence of HSV-directed natural-killer activity may be involved in the development of the ulcerative skin lesions.

The cause of the immunodeficiency disorder that we observed is undoubtedly complex. Viral infection, especially in unusually heavy inoculum transmitted by enteric routes, may be an important initiating factor.

Infection by a great many viruses such as measles or rubella can result in depressed delayed-type hypersensitivity.[21] Primary cytomegalovirus infection has been associated with a particularly prolonged cellular immunodeficiency state.[22,23] Exposure to cytomegalovirus is known to be particularly heavy within the homosexual community; a 94 percent prevalence has been defined by anticomplement immunofluorescence.[24] A series of four previously healthy homosexual men with active cytomegalovirus infections complicated by *P. carinii* pneumonia has been reported.[15] In our series, disseminated cytomegalovirus was found at autopsy in Patients 1 and 3, and on biopsy and by seroconversion in Patient 2. Cytomegalovirus must be considered a candidate initiator of the immune defects observed.

Serum immunoglobulins were increased. The consistent elevation of serum IgA levels could reflect the importance of gut-associated lymphoid tissue as a primary site of immunization in this disorder. Battisto and Chase described a state of antigen-specific hyporesponsiveness occurring after oral immunization[25] that has recently been reported to result from the seeding of suppressor cells to non-gut-associated lymphoid tissue.[26] The immune deficit that we observed could likewise result, in part from the route of exposure to viral pathogens.

Since these cases are certainly rare, even among homosexuals, additional factors must be involved in susceptibility. A group may be specifically hyporesponsive to HSV, perhaps because of their genetic background — e.g., HLA-D-linked immune-response genes. Heavy exposure to HSV could lead to chronic infection, and secondary immunodeficiency could then result. At present, no group has been defined that is genetically susceptible to HSV.

Still another possibility is that among men who are homosexual, some have a latent, broad-based cellular immunodeficiency that becomes clinically manifest only because of heavy exposure to certain pathogens in particular combinations. For example, a homosexual male nurse whom we studied recovered from pneumocystis pneumonia but eventually died at another hospital of recurrent pneumocystis and cytomegalovirus pneumonia. He had markedly depressed cellular immunity in vitro and increased proportions of Leu-2a-positive cells among his T lymphocytes. Extensive history taking by one of us (B.R.A.) indicated susceptibility to a variety of infectious agents over the previous 20 years, suggesting a low-grade cell-mediated immunodeficiency.

Severe malnutrition probably accentuated the immune deficits that we observed.[27] By the time these patients came under study, all were anorectic and cachectic and had been chronically ill for many months. Because of the specific immunosuppressive effects of zinc deficiency,[28] plasma zinc levels were determined; they were found to be normal in all four patients, but three were nevertheless given zinc salts empirically. In addition, efforts were made to improve overall protein-calorie intake through oral and parenteral nutritional supplements. Neither of these approaches seemed to alter the patients' clinical courses appreciably.

In view of the relative preservation of immunologic functions early in the course of the illness in Patient 4, immune deficits like those we observed appeared to be progressive with time. It seems possible that earlier recognition and prospective study of such patients will reveal an anomaly in host defense that could illuminate the pathogenesis of this disorder.

There was no obvious contact between the four men. To ascertain whether there was any epidemiologic relation among the viral strains isolated, we submitted samples of the viruses for restriction-endonuclease mapping[29] (by Dr. Bernard Roizman, University of Chicago). The isolates, all Type 2, were found to be unrelated.

We are indebted to Drs. Mark Chapman, Lawrence Ossias, Burton J. Lee, Jose Romeu, Donald T. Evans, and Mark Kunkel for allowing us to study their patients, and Drs. Jose Giron, Joseph Masci, and Roslyn Posner for their help in treating the patients.

Note added in proof: We recently studied a fifth patient, a 45-year-old homosexual man with a nine-month history of hepatitis, gradual wasting, eventual intergluteal herpes simplex ulcers, and probable herpes encephalitis. During the period of study, lymphoid function was initially normal, but it later deteriorated. Lymphopenia developed only late in the course. Natural-killer-cell activity studied while the patient had normal lymphocyte counts was very depressed.

References

1. Rawls WE. Herpes simplex virus. In: Kaplan AS, ed. The herpesviruses. New York: Academic Press 1973:291-325.
2. Stroud GM. Recurrent herpes simplex and steroid dosage. Arch Dermatol 1961; 84:396-401.
3. Bean SF, Fusaro RM, Atypical cutaneous Herpes simplex infection associated with acute myelogenous leukemia. Acta Derm Venereol (Stockh) 1969; 49:94-6.

4. Logan WS, Tindall JP, Elson ML. Chronic cutaneous herpes simplex. Arch Dermatol 1971; 103:606-14.
5. Nishimura K, Nagamoto A, Igarashi M. Extensive skin manifestations of herpesvirus infection in an acute leukemic child. Pediatr 1972; 49: 294-7.
6. Muller SA, Herrmann EC Jr, Winkelmann RK. Herpes simplex infections in hematologic malignancies. Am J Med 1972; 52:102-14.
7. Stone WJ, Scowden EB, Spannuth CL, Lowry SP, Alford RH. Atypical herpesvirus hominis type 2 infection in uremic patients receiving immunosuppressive therapy. Am J Med 1977; 63:511-6.
8. Cupps TR, Straus SE, Waldmann TA. Successful treatment with acyclovir of an immunodeficient patient infected simultaneously with multiple herpesviruses. Am J Med 1981; 70:882-6.
9. Siegal FP. IgG on infants' B lymphocytes: enhanced binding of IgG by IgM-bearing lymphoid cells in early childhood. Scand J Immunol 1976; 5:721-9.
10. Evans RL, Wall DW, Platsoucas CD, et al. Thymus-dependent membrane antigens in man: inhibition of cell-mediated lympholysis by monoclonal antibodies to T_{H2} antigen. Proc Natl Acad Sci USA 1981; 78:544-8.
11. Oppenheim JJ, Schecter B. Lymphocyte transformation. In: Rose NR, Friedman H, eds. Manual of clinical immunology. 2nd ed. Washington, D.C.: American Society for Microbiology 1980:233-45.
12. Ching C, Lopez C. Natural killing of herpes simplex virus type 1-infected target cells: normal human responses and influence of antiviral antibody. Infect Immun 1979; 26:49-56.
13. Cunningham-Rundles C, Brandeis WE, Zacharczuk T, Good RA, Day NK. Quantitation of circulating immune complexes in serum by Raji cells using an enzyme-linked immunosorbent assay. Clin Exp Immunol 1980; 40:411-5.
14. Digeon M, Laver M, Riza J, Bach JF. Detection of circulating immune complexes in human sera by simplified assays with polyethylene glycol. J Immunol Methods 1977; 16:165-83.
15. Gottlieb MS, Schroff R, Schanker HM, et al. *Pneumocystis carinii* pneumonia and mucocutaneous candidiasis in previously healthy homosexual men: evidence of a new severe acquired cellular immunodeficiency. N Engl J Med 1981; 305:1425-31.
16. Kaposi's sarcoma and pneumocystis pneumonia among homosexual men — New York City and California. MMWR 1981; 30:305-8.
17. Berlinger NT, Lopez C, Good RA. Facilitation or attenuation of mixed leukocyte culture responsiveness by adherent cells. Nature 1976; 260:145-6.
18. Reinherz E, O'Brien C, Rosenthal P, Schlossman SF. The cellular basis for viral-induced immunodeficiency: analysis by monoclonal antibodies. J Immunol 1980; 125:1269-74.
19. Pahwa R, Pahwa S, Good RA, Incefy GS, O'Reilly RJ. Rationale for combined use of fetal liver and thymus for immunological reconstitution in patients with variants of severe combined immunodeficiency. Proc Natl Acad Sci USA 1977; 74:3002-5.
20. Lopez C. Herpesvirus infections. In: Safai B, Good RA, eds. Immunodermatology. New York: Plenum Medical Book 1980:539-48.
21. Notkins AL, Mergenhagen SE, Howard RJ. Effect of virus infections on the function of the immune system. Annu Rev Microbiol 1970; 24:525-38.
22. Rinaldo CR Jr, Carney WP, Richter BS, Black PH, Hirsch MS. Mechanisms of immunosuppression in cytomegaloviral mononucleosis. J Infect Dis 1980; 141:488-95.
23. ten Napel CHH, The HH. Acute cytomegalovirus infection and the host immune response. II. Relationship of suppressed *in vitro* lymphocyte reactivity to bacterial recall antigens and mitogens with the development of cytomegalovirus-induced lymphocyte reactivity. Clin Exp Immunol 1980; 39:272-8.
24. Drew WL, Mintz L, Miner RC, Sands M, Ketterer B. Prevalence of cytomegalovirus infection in homosexual men. J Infect Dis 1981; 143:188-92.
25. Battisto JR, Chase MW. Induced unresponsiveness to simple allergenic chemicals. II. Independence of delayed-type hypersensitivity and formation of circulating antibody. J Exp Med 1965; 121:591-606.
26. Winchester RJ. Human and experimental pathology. Theme 18 Summary. Prog Immunol 1980; 4:1263-6.
27. Keusch GT. The effects of malnutrition on host responses and the metabolic sequelae of infections. In: Grieco MH, ed. Infections in the abnormal host. New York: York Medical 1980:210-30.
28. Oleske JM, Westphal ML, Shore S, Gorden D, Bogden JD. Nahmias A. Zinc therapy of depressed cellular immunity in acrodermatitis enteropathica: its correction. Am J Dis Child 1979; 133:915-8.
29. Buchman TG, Roizman B, Adams G, Stover BH. Restriction endonuclease fingerpainting of Herpes simplex virus DNA: a novel epidemiological tool applied to a nosocomial outbreak. J Infect Dis 1978; 138:488-98.

ORIGINAL ARTICLE

HERPES SIMPLEX VIRUS PROCTITIS IN HOMOSEXUAL MEN

Clinical, Sigmoidoscopic, and Histopathological Features

Steven E. Goodell, M.D., Thomas C. Quinn, M.D., Emmanuel Mkrtichian, P.A.-C, Michael D. Schuffler, M.D., King K. Holmes, M.D., Ph.D., and Lawrence Corey, M.D.

Abstract Acute herpes simplex virus (HSV) infection was detected in 23 of 102 consecutively examined, sexually active male homosexuals who presented with anorectal pain, discharge, tenesmus, or hematochezia, as compared with 3 of 75 homosexual men without gastrointestinal symptoms ($P<0.01$). Findings that were significantly more frequent in men with HSV proctitis than in men with proctitis due to other infectious causes included fever (48 percent), difficulty in urinating (48 percent), sacral paresthesias (26 percent), inguinal lymphadenopathy (57 percent), severe anorectal pain (100 percent), tenesmus (100 percent), constipation (78 percent), perianal ulcerations (70 percent), and the presence of diffuse ulcerative or discrete vesicular or pustular lesions in the distal 5 cm of the rectum (50 percent). Serologic evidence indicated that 85 percent of the men with symptomatic HSV proctitis were having their first episode of HSV-2 infection. The diagnosis of HSV proctitis is suggested by the presence of severe anorectal pain, difficulty in urinating, sacral paresthesias or pain, and diffuse ulceration of the distal rectal mucosa.

IN a previous investigation we noted that herpes simplex virus (HSV) was the most common cause of nongonococcal proctitis in sexually active male homosexuals.[1] This paper presents the characteristic symptoms and signs and the histopathological features of HSV proctitis, as determined by a subsequent prospective study of intestinal and anorectal infections in homosexual men.

Methods

Study Design

Between July 1, 1979, and March 31, 1981, all homosexual or bisexual men attending the King County Sexually Transmitted Disease Clinic who had two or more symptoms of proctitis — i.e., anorectal pain, mucopurulent rectal discharge, tenesmus, or hematochezia — for a period of less than four weeks were asked to participate in this investigation. Seventy-five homosexual or bisexual men who had no gastrointestinal or anorectal symptoms, who were not taking antibiotics, and who were attending the clinic were also asked to participate as controls. Controls were selected at random appointments according to a table of random numbers.

At the initial visit, standardized medical histories were taken, and a physical examination and anoscopy were performed. Urethral, pharyngeal, and rectal swabs were obtained for isolation of the neisseria species.[2] Rectal swabs were also obtained for isolation of HSV, *Chlamydia trachomatis, Ureaplasma urealyticum, Mycoplasma hominis*, salmonella, shigella, and campylobacter, according to previously described techniques.[3-6] Anal or rectal lesions were scraped for examination by darkfield microscopy, and lesion scrapings were also submitted for isolation of HSV. A stool specimen was collected within 48 hours of the initial visit; examined for ova and parasites; and cultured for shigella, salmonella, campylobacter, yersinia, and *Vibrio parahemolyticus*.[5,6] Stool filtrates were also inoculated onto duplicate tubes of primary cynomolgus-monkey cells, heteroploid cells (Hep-2), and human diploid fibroblasts — cell lines that allow growth of most of the enteroviruses and adenoviruses.[7] Filtrates were also assayed for *Clostridium difficile* toxin and rotavirus antigen.[8-11] Patients with symptomatic proctitis and abnormal anoscopic findings underwent flexible sigmoidoscopy and rectal biopsy of mucosal lesions. Rectal biopsy specimens were cultured for HSV and *Chlam. trachomatis* and processed for light microscopy. Patients were reexamined at 7 and 21 days after the initial clinic visit. At the initial visit and the visit on the 21st day, serum was drawn for a Venereal Disease Research Laboratory test and for determination of neutralizing antibodies to HSV-1 and HSV-2.

Laboratory and Statistical Methods

HSV isolates were typed with an indirect immunoperoxidase technique.[12] Antibody to HSV was assayed by microneutralization at serum dilutions ranging from 1:4 to 1:256. As previously described, to standardize the microneutralization assay for virus input, the potency of serum for neutralization of HSV-1 and HSV-2 was determined (i.e., pN_1 and pN_2 were calculated for each serum specimen [$pN = \log\{\log \text{virus titer neutralized in each assay} - \log \text{highest neutralizing serum dilution}\} + \log \text{test volume}$]).[13] Antibody specificity to HSV-1 was defined as a value for $pN_1 - pN_2>0.5$, and specificity to HSV-2 as a value for $pN_1 - pN_2<0.05$. A $pN_1 - pN_2$ value between 0.05 and 0.5 was called "indeterminate," a value usually indicating prior infection with both HSV-1 and HSV-2.[14,15]

Statistical comparisons were made by means of Fisher's exact test.

Results

Correlation of Anorectal HSV Infection with Proctitis

During the study period 119 homosexual men with symptoms of diarrhea, anorectal pain, anorectal discharge, tenesmus, or hematochezia consented to being enrolled in the study. In 102 of them there were abnormal anoscopic findings of proctitis, mucosal friability or ulcerations, mucopurulent exudate, or an abnormal rectal biopsy specimen. Seventeen patients had symptoms of enteritis (diarrhea, abdominal pain, and cramping) with no signs of acute proctitis on anoscopy or sigmoidoscopy. Acute HSV infection was documented by isolation of HSV from the rectum or by serology in 23 of the 102 patients with proctitis, as compared with none of the patients with enteritis ($P<0.01$) and 3 of the 75 asymptomatic control patients ($P = 0.01$). Other infectious intestinal pathogens were identified in 59 of the remaining 79 men with abnormal anoscopic findings. Multiple patho-

From the Departments of Medicine, Laboratory Medicine, Microbiology, and Pediatrics, University of Washington and the Seattle Public Health Hospital, Seattle.

Supported by grants (AI-20381, AI-12191, AI-14495, AI-17805, and AM-28180) from the National Institutes of Health and a grant (AM-16059) from the U.S. Public Health Service.

Presented as an abstract at the 21st Interscience Conference on Antimicrobial Agents and Chemotherapy, Chicago, November 1981.

gens (mixed infections) were isolated in 15 of these 59 patients.

Laboratory Diagnosis

HSV was isolated from rectal swabs (14 subjects) or biopsy specimens (1 subject) or both (6 subjects) from 21 symptomatic men. All isolates were typed as HSV-2. Acute-phase and convalescent-phase serum samples were available from 15 of the patients with a positive culture, 13 of whom had seroconversion or a fourfold or greater increase in HSV-2 neutralizing antibody in paired samples. Two other men from whom HSV was not isolated were also classified as having HSV proctitis; both had symptomatic proctitis, ulcerative perianal lesions, no evidence of any concomitant pathogen, and an increase in HSV-2 neutralizing antibody from <1:4 in acute-phase serum to ⩾1:8 in convalescent-phase serum. Seroconversion to HSV-2 occurred in one patient from the asymptomatic control group, and HSV-2 was isolated from the rectum, indicating asymptomatic primary rectal HSV-2 infection. The other two asymptomatic men from whom HSV-2 was isolated had stable titers of HSV-2 neutralizing antibody, suggesting recurrent rectal shedding of HSV-2.[15] HSV-2 was the sole pathogen isolated from 15 of the 23 patients with HSV proctitis. Concomitant pathogens in the other eight patients included *Neisseria gonorrhoeae* (five subjects), *Campylobacter jejuni* (one subject), *Giardia lamblia* (two subjects), and *Entamoeba histolytica* (one subject).

Clinical Manifestations

The mean age of the patients with HSV proctitis was 28 years (range, 15 to 55); 86 percent were white. All reported having anal receptive intercourse. The median number of previous sexual partners was 32,

Table 1. Comparison of Symptoms and Signs in Patients with HSV Proctitis and in Patients with Proctitis Not Attributable to HSV.

	HSV Proctitis (N = 23)	Non-HSV Proctitis (N = 79)
	no. of patients	
Anorectal pain	23*	61
Tenesmus	23*	61
Anal discharge	21	65
Constipation	18*	32
Anal pruritus	17*	36
Hematochezia	14	32
Abdominal pain	2	17
Neurologic symptoms	12*	10
Difficulty in initiating micturition	11*	8
Sacral paresthesias	3*	0
Posterior thigh pain	6*	0
Perianal lesions	16*	6
Inguinal lymphadenopathy	13*	9
Fever	11*	13

*Significantly more frequent (P<0.01, Fisher's exact test).

Table 2. Comparison of Sigmoidoscopic and Histopathological Findings in HSV Proctitis and Non-HSV Proctitis.*

	HSV Proctitis (N = 10)	Non-HSV Proctitis (N = 42)
Sigmoidoscopy		
Positive wipe test	9	27
Focal friability of the rectal mucosa	4	25
Diffuse friability of the rectal mucosa	5†	2
Mucosal friability above 15 cm	1†	14
Diffuse ulceration of the distal rectum	2†	0
Discrete vesiculopustular lesions of the rectum	2†	1
Normal	1‡	15
Histopathology		
Crypt abscesses	5	14
Polymorphonuclear leukocytes in the lamina propria	8	26
Perivascular cuffing with lymphocytes	3†	0
Multinucleated cells	1†	0
Intranuclear inclusions	3†	0

*Only patients in whom HSV was the sole pathogen isolated and who underwent sigmoidoscopy and biopsy are included in this analysis.

†Significantly more frequent (P<0.01, Fisher's exact test).

‡This patient had loss of the mucosal vascular pattern and proctitis on rectal biopsy.

and the mean number of days from the last sexual exposure to the onset of symptoms was 7.0 days.

The symptoms of HSV proctitis are listed in Table 1. The mean duration of symptoms was 21 days (range, 7 to 44). The frequency and duration of symptoms were similar in the 15 patients in whom HSV was the sole pathogen isolated and in those with mixed infections. Anorectal pain, constipation, tenesmus, anal pruritus, difficulty in initiating micturition, sacral paresthesias, posterior thigh pain, fever, and inguinal adenopathy were each reported significantly more frequently by the 23 patients with HSV proctitis than by the 79 patients with proctitis not attributable to HSV (P<0.01 for each comparison). Two patients with HSV proctitis reported that they were impotent during their illness.

External perianal or anal vesicular or ulcerative lesions, usually detected only during anoscopic examination, were present in 16 of the 23 patients with HSV proctitis, as compared with 6 of the 79 patients with proctitis not due to HSV (P<0.01). HSV was isolated from these lesions in 7 of the 16 patients with HSV proctitis. No patient with HSVproctitis had mucocutaneous herpetic lesions outside the perineal area.

Sigmoidoscopic and Histological Findings

Sigmoidoscopic and histological findings were analyzed for 10 patients who underwent sigmoidoscopy and biopsy and in whom HSV was the sole pathogen, and for 42 patients who had proctitis not attributable to HSV. The frequency of rectal mucosal friability, as defined by spontaneous bleeding or a positive wipe test (i.e., mucosal friability or petechiae when touched with a cotton swab), was similar in these two groups (Table 2). Diffuse ulceration of the distal rectum or vesicular lesions of the rectal mucosa were documented in 4 patients with HSV proctitis and in only 1 of 42 patients with proctitis not due to HSV (P<0.01). Of the 10 men with HSV proctitis, 8 had mucosal abnormalities that were limited to the distal 10 cm of the rectum; the abnormalities extended to 20 cm in the sigmoid colon in only 1 patient. In contrast, mucosal friability to 20 cm or more was noted in 14 of 42 patients with proctitis not due to HSV ($P = 0.03$).

Rectal mucosal biopsy specimens were abnormal in 9 of the 10 patients with HSV proctitis (Table 2). The histological characteristics of HSV proctitis included the presence of multinucleated cells, intranuclear inclusions, and lymphocytic infiltration around submucosal vessels (perivascular cuffing) (Fig. 1).

Frequency of Past HSV Infection

None of the patients with HSV proctitis reported a history of known rectal HSV infection, and only one had had genital herpes. The specificity of HSV neutralizing antibody in acute-phase serum was consistent with past HSV-2 infection or was of indeterminate antibody specificity in only 3 (18 percent) of the patients with HSV proctitis, as compared with 23 (58 percent) of 40 of the control patients ($P<0.01$) and 26 (49 percent) of the patients with proctitis not attributable to HSV ($P<0.01$).

Discussion

HSV proctitis appears to be a distinctive clinical and pathologic syndrome that can often be distinguished clinically from other infectious causes of acute proctitis. It is associated with fever, inguinal adenopathy, anorectal pain, tenesmus, constipation, rectal discharge, and hematochezia.[16,17] The severity of rectal pain associated with HSV proctitis is usually greater than that associated with other forms of proctitis, although it is similar to that associated with rectal lymphogranuloma venereum infection.[18] Among homosexual men with intestinal symptoms and signs, neurologic symptoms in the distribution of the sacral roots were noted only in men with HSV proctitis. Difficulty in initiating micturition, posterior thigh pain or paresthesias of the buttock or perineal region, and impotence were reported by 52 percent of men with HSV proctitis, as compared with fewer than 1 percent of 63 heterosexual men and 1.6 percent of 123 women with primary HSV-2 infections who were examined at our clinic for genital herpes.[19] The pathogenesis of these neurologic symptoms is not well understood, although an autonomic-nervous-system dysfunction has been postulated.[20,21] Whether the higher frequency of such symptoms in men with symptomatic HSV proctitis is related to greater or different involvement of the sacral autonomic nerve root, with resulting detrusor muscle dysfunction, or to increased reflex external sphincter tone secondary to severe anorectal pain requires further study.

Mucosal friability on sigmoidoscopic examination was characteristic of all forms of infectious proctitis. However, perianal or anal lesions on anoscopy, vesicular or pustular rectal lesions, and diffuse ulceration of the distal rectum on sigmoidoscopy were each associated with HSV proctitis. These findings were present in 17 of our 23 cases. Rectal mucosal abnormalities 10 cm above the anal verge were noted in only one of our patients with HSV proctitis. In contrast, infections with enteric pathogens, such as shigella, lymphogranuloma venereum strains of *Chlam. trachomatis*, *Camp. jejuni*, *Clost. difficile*, and *E. histolytica* involved both the rectal and sigmoid mucosa, resulting in the clinical syndrome of proctocolitis.

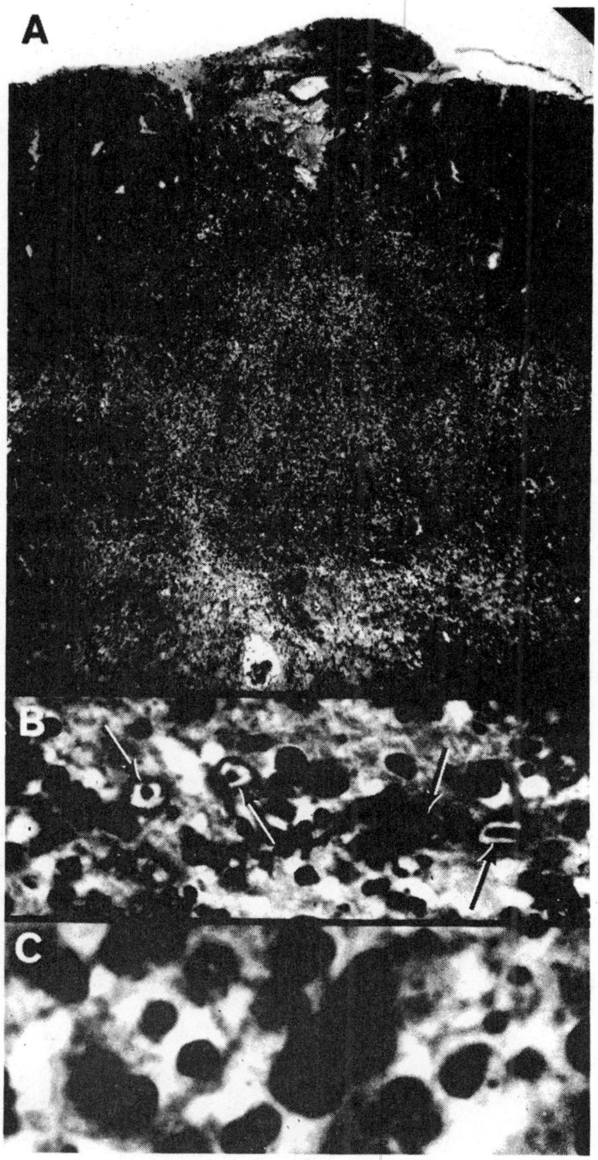

Figure 1. Rectal Biopsy Specimen from a Patient with HSV Proctitis (Hematoxylin and Eosin Stain).

Panel A shows focal ulceration of the rectal mucosa and microabscess formation extending into the submucosa of the rectal wall (×38), B shows intranuclear inclusions (arrows) (×750), and C shows multinucleated cells with ground-glass nuclei in the submucosa (×1500).

Although several symptoms, signs, and histopathological findings, such as intranuclear inclusions and multinucleated cells, were correlated with HSV proctitis, few were pathognomonic, and these were present in a minority of patients. These findings underscore the necessity for viral isolation in order to confirm rectal HSV infection. Although we isolated only HSV-2 in this series, other investigators have also isolated HSV-1 from the rectal mucosa.[22]

Only 10 percent of the homosexual or bisexual men enrolled in this study reported past oral–labial or genital HSV infections, but 68 percent had HSV antibody in acute-phase serum, and 42 percent had neutralizing antibody with HSV-2 or indeterminate specificity. Patients who had HSV proctitis were more likely to be seronegative or to have acute-phase serum with only HSV-1 neutralizing antibody specificity than were the control patients or patients with proctitis not attributable to HSV, indicating that a case of symptomatic HSV proctitis usually represented a first episode of rectal HSV-2 infection.[14,15] However, one of our control patients had virologic and serologic evidence of recent asymptomatic primary rectal HSV infection. The natural history of recurrences of HSV proctitis after the initial episode and the possible effect of antiviral therapy remain to be determined in future studies.

References

1. Quinn TC, Corey L, Chaffee RG, Schuffler MD, Brancato FP, Holmes KK. The etiology of anorectal infections in homosexual men. Am J Med 1981; 71:395-406.
2. Handsfield HH, Sandström EG, Knapp JS, et al. Epidemiology of penicillinase-producing *Neisseria gonorrhoeae* infections: analysis by auxotyping and serogrouping. N Engl J Med 1982; 306:950-4.
3. Wentworth BB, Bonin P, Holmes KK, Gutman L, Wiesner P, Alexander ER. Isolation of viruses, bacteria and other organisms from venereal disease clinic patients: methodology and problems associated with multiple isolations. Health Lab Sci 1973; 10:75-81.
4. Bowie WR, Wang S-P, Alexander ER, et al. Etiology of nongonococcal urethritis: evidence for *Chlamydia trachomatis* and *Ureaplasma urealyticum*. J Clin Invest 1977; 59:735-42.
5. Blaser MJ, Berkowtiz ID, LaForce FM, Cravens J, Reller LB, Wang W-LL. Campylobacter enteritis: Clinical and epidemiologic features. Ann Intern Med 1979; 91:179-85.
6. Quinn TC, Corey L, Chaffee RG, Schuffler MD, Holmes KK. Campylobacter proctitis in a homosexual man. Ann Intern Med 1980; 93:458-9.
7. Lennette EH, Schmidt NJ, eds. Diagnostic procedures for viral, rickettsial and chlamydial infections. 5th ed. New York: American Public Health Association, 1979.
8. Yolken RH, Wyatt RG, Zissis G, et al. Epidemiology of human rotavirus Types 1 and 2 as studied by enzyme-linked immunosorbent assay. N Engl J Med 1978; 299:1156-61.
9. Yolken RH, Kim HW, Clem T, et al. Enzyme-linked immunosorbent assay (ELISA) for detection of human reovirus-like agent of infantile gastroenteritis. Lancet 1977; 2:263-7.
10. Bartlett JG, Moon N, Chang TW, Taylor N, Onderdonk AB. Role of *Clostridium difficile* in antibiotic-associated pseudomembranous colitis. Gastroenterology 1978; 75:778-82.
11. Rifkin GD, Fekety FR, Silva J Jr, Sack RB. Antibiotic-induced colitis: implication of a toxin neutralized by *Clostridium sordellii* antitoxin. Lancet 1977; 2:1103-6.
12. Benjamin DR. Rapid typing of herpes simplex virus strains using the indirect immunoperoxidase method. Appl Microbiol 1974; 28:568-71.
13. Stalder H, Oxman MN, Hermann KL. Herpes simplex virus microneutralization: a simplification of the test. J Infect Dis 1975; 131:423-30.
14. Nahmias AJ, Josey WE, Naib ZM, Luce CF, Duffy A. Antibodies to *Herpesvirus hominis* types 1 and 2 in humans. I. Patients with genital herpetic infections. Am J Epidemiol 1970; 91:539-46.
15. Reeves WC, Corey L, Adams HG, Vontver LA, Holmes KK. Risk of recurrence after first episodes of genital herpes: relation to HSV type and antibody response. N Engl J Med 1981; 305:315-9.
16. Waugh MA. Anorectal *Herpesvirus hominis* infection in men. J Am Vener Dis Assoc 1976; 3:68-70.
17. Goldmeier D. Proctitis and herpes simplex virus in homosexual men. Br J Vener Dis 1976; 56:111-4.
18. Quinn TC, Goodell SE, Mkrtichian E, et al. *Chlamydia trachomatis* proctitis. N Engl J Med 1981; 305:195-200.
19. Corey L, Adams HG, Brown ZA, Holmes KK. Genital herpes simplex virus infections: clinical manifestations, course and complications. Ann Intern Med (in press).
20. Samarasinghe PL, Oates JK, MacLennan IPB. Herpetic proctitis and sacral radiculomyelopathy — a hazard for homosexual men. Br Med J 1979; 2:365-6.
21. Caplan LR, Kleeman FJ, Berg S. Urinary retention probably secondary to herpes genitalis. N Engl J Med 1977; 297:920-1.
22. Levine JB, Saeed M. Herpesvirus Hominis type 1 proctitis. J Clin Gastroenterol 1979; 1:225-7.

CORRESPONDENCE

DEATH IN THE AIDS PATIENT: ROLE OF CYTOMEGALOVIRUS

To the Editor: Pneumocystis carinii pneumonia is considered the most common life-threatening opportunistic infection in patients with the acquired immunodeficiency syndrome (AIDS).[1] However, at the Clinical Center of the National Institutes of Health, *P. carinii* pneumonia is not the principal cause of mortality in our patients with AIDS. Of our first 15 autopsied AIDS cases, 11 patients had a history of one or more antemortem episodes of biopsy-proved *P. carinii* pneumonia. However, therapy with trimethoprim–sulfamethoxazole or pentamidine or both was usually successful in eradicating these infections. At autopsy, residual cysts of *P. carinii* were found in the autopsied lungs of only three patients, and one of those had only rare pneumocysts.

Histopathologically, 14 of our 15 patients' autopsies revealed disseminated cytomegalovirus infections with pulmonary or adrenal involvement or both. In the lungs, cytomegalovirus lesions represented a range from focal to diffuse interstitial pneumonitis with numerous characteristic intranuclear and intracytoplasmic inclusion cells (Fig. 1). In the adrenal glands, hemorrhagic necrotizing cytomegalovirus lesions typically involved the medulla; however, in some cases entire adrenal glands appeared infarcted and hemorrhagic.

Viral blood cultures had been performed for all 15 patients, and MRC-5 human embryonic diploid fibroblasts had been used to identify the typical cytopathic changes associated with cytomegalovirus.[2] The single patient without pathological evidence of cytomegalovirus infection had negative blood cultures for cytomegalovirus. The 14 other patients had numerous positive blood cultures for cytomegalovirus. Initially, cultures required two to three weeks of incubation to become positive. However, subsequent cultures became positive in progressively shorter intervals. In four patients, blood cultures became positive for cytomegalovirus in less than 48 hours, suggesting that a high titer of virus was circulating in their peripheral blood.

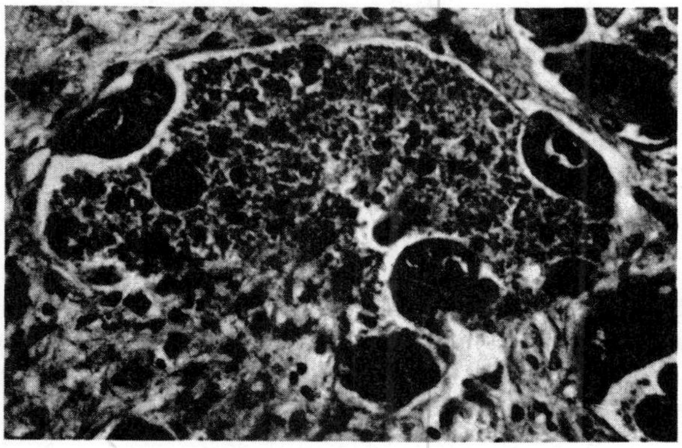

Figure 1. Photomicrograph of Lung at Autopsy, Showing Alveolar Space with Multiple Enlarged Alveolar Epithelial Cells Containing Prominent Oval Intranuclear and Coarse Intracytoplasmic Inclusions Characteristic of Cytomegalovirus (Hematoxylin-Eosin Stain, ×250).

Methenamine silver, toluidine blue, Giemsa, and Fite stains were negative for other organisms.

Many patients with AIDS have terminal courses marked by pneumonia and hypotension. We believe that overwhelming cytomegalovirus viremia and its associated pulmonary and adrenal infections may be major contributors to the death of such patients.

Abe M. Macher, M.D.,
Cheryl M. Reichert, M.D., Ph.D.,
Stephen E. Straus, M.D., Dan L. Longo, M.D.,
Joseph Parrillo, M.D., H. Clifford Lane, M.D.,
and Anthony S. Fauci, M.D.
National Institutes of Health
Bethesda, MD 20205

Alain H. Rook, M.D.,
Jody F. Manischewitz, B.S.,
and Gerald V. Quinnan, Jr., M.D.
National Center for Drugs and Biologics
Bethesda, MD 20205

References

1. Update: acquired immunodeficiency syndrome (AIDS) — United States. MMWR 1983; 32:465-7.
2. Benyesh-Melnick M. Cytomegaloviruses. In: Lennette EH, Schmidt NJ, eds. Diagnostic procedures for viral and rickettsial infections. New York: American Public Health Association, 1969:701-32.

Clinical Studies

Transmission of AIDS and the Blood-Brain Barrier

EDITORIAL

OPPORTUNISTIC INFECTIONS AND KAPOSI'S SARCOMA IN HOMOSEXUAL MEN

DAVID T. DURACK, M.D., D.PHIL

IN the summer of 1981, the Centers for Disease Control (CDC) alerted the medical world to an unexpected outbreak of *Pneumocystis carinii* pneumonia and Kaposi's sarcoma in young homosexual men who had no known reason to contract these uncommon diseases.[1,2] New and surprising though this association may be, enough cases have already been collected to establish its reality. More than 160 examples are now being analyzed at the CDC, and five or six new cases are being reported each week. Recently, eight cases of Kaposi's sarcoma in young homosexual men in New York City were reported in *Lancet.*[3] In this issue, the *Journal* presents for our evaluation further detailed reports of the syndrome of opportunistic infections and Kaposi's sarcoma in homosexual men (three papers, 19 patients, and 32 authors).[4-6]

These salient features have emerged: The patients are typically young homosexual men, most of whom live in large cities and many of whom use drugs; the infectious agents are low-grade pathogens that often cause opportunistic infections in compromised hosts; and the death rate is fearfully high. Two thirds of the patients described in this issue of the *Journal* have died, as have more than one third of the patients on record at the CDC.

This development poses a puzzle that must be solved. Its solution is likely to be interesting and important to many people. Scientists (and the merely curious) will ask, Why this group? Why now, and not before? What does this tell us about immunity and the genesis of tumors? Students of public-health issues will want to put this outbreak into a social perspective. Gay associations, which are often active and well informed on pertinent health issues, will want to take measures to educate and protect their members. Humanitarians will simply want to prevent unnecessary death and suffering.

So far, at least a dozen microbial species have been shown to cause disease in these patients: among viruses, cytomegalovirus and herpes simplex virus; among bacteria, *Myobacterium tuberculosis, M. avium-intracellulare, Klebsiella pneumoniae,* and other gram-negative aerobic bacilli; among fungi, *Candida albicans* and *Cryptococcus neoformans;* and among protozoa, *Pneumocystis carinii, Toxoplasma gondii,* and *Entamoeba histolytica.*

A glance at this list will establish two facts: The gap in host defenses is broad, not limited to those against any one class of microbe, and the pathogens are mostly those to be expected in patients with defective cellular immunity. This clinical evidence of a cellular defect is supported by the demonstration of cutaneous anergy, striking lymphopenia, T-lymphocyte depletion, decreased lymphocyte proliferative responses, and defective natural-killer-cell activity in these patients.[4-6] Humoral immune responses seem to be normal.

The nature and multiplicity of these pathogens and the overwhelming severity of many of the illnesses indicate that the normal defenses are severely compromised. The clinical implication is that homosexuals with syndromes suggesting unusual infections should be investigated promptly and aggressively, like other immunocompromised patients. The physician should anticipate simultaneous multiple infections, poor response to treatment, and a tendency to relapse. Because the mortality is so high, invasive diagnostic procedures such as open-lung biopsy are fully justified. Until the cause of the apparent defect in host defenses is understood, the only available means to reduce mortality is early, specific therapy for each treatable infection. Long-term prophylaxis for pneumocystis pneumonia with trimethoprim plus sulfamethoxazole (as commonly used in children after treatment for lymphocytic leukemia) may be appropriate for patients with this syndrome,[4] whether or not they have already had pneumocystis pneumonia.

The question of cause is obviously central. What clue does the link with homosexuality provide? Homosexual men, especially those who have many partners, are more likely than the general population to contract sexually transmitted diseases.[7] Lesbians are not, and this apparent freedom, whatever its explanation, seems to extend to Kaposi's sarcoma and opportunistic infections. At present, only one woman is included among the patients known to the CDC. Male homosexuals are at increased risk for the acquisition of common viral infections, including those caused by hepatitis B virus, cytomegalovirus, and Epstein–Barr virus, and viruses can cause immunosuppression.[8,9] Notably, many of the patients described by Gottlieb,[4] Masur,[5] and Siegal[6] and their colleagues had an insidious, nonspecific illness marked by malaise, fever, weight loss, lymphadenopathy, and thrush for several months before the onset of more severe opportunistic infections. Were these features manifestations of a primary immunosuppressive viral disease? If so, both neoplasia and infection could be secondary phenomena, with Kaposi's sarcoma acting as an "opportunistic tumor" and the opportunistic infections representing a mode of death rather than the cause of death.

Evidence of previous or current cytomegalovirus infection is a common thread that runs throughout these case reports.[1-6] Cytomegalovirus causes immunosuppression in mice and human beings,[8,9] and this virus can persist is semen for months at a high titer.[10] The pattern of lymphocyte disturbances in these patients is similar to the changes found in patients with cytomegalovirus mononucleosis, which persist for months after recovery.[9] Concurrent cytomegalovirus infection greatly increases the mortality of experimental bacterial and fungal infections in mice.[8] In renal-transplant recipients, Rubin et al.[11] have shown that cytomegalovirus may be associated with leukopenia and may predispose the patient to other opportunistic infections. Accordingly, Gottlieb and his colleagues[4] can argue cogently that cytomegalovirus itself is highly suspect as the cause of this syndrome. On the other hand, more than 90 percent of homosexual men in the community have antibodies indicating previous cytomegalovirus infection.[12] Therefore, positive cultures for cytomegalovirus could represent nothing more than reactivation of latent infection during immunosuppression, as happens predictably in transplant recipients.[11]

What do young Africans, elderly Americans, renal-transplant recipients, and homosexual men have in common? The answer is Kaposi's sarcoma, a tumor that is found in these diverse groups for reasons that we do not yet understand.[13,14] A search for the origins of this unusual neoplasm brings us back to cytomegalovirus, which has been implicated as a possible etiologic factor on the basis of serologic studies.[13] Furthermore, the cytomegalovirus genome has recently been detected in Kaposi's-sarcoma tissue.[15] The final answer on whether cytomegalovirus is a cause or an effect in this setting will carry important implications for tumor biology.

The cytomegalovirus hypothesis suffers from an obvious problem: It does not explain why this syndrome is apparently new. Homosexuality is at least as old as history, and cytomegalovirus is presumably not a new pathogen. Were the homosexual contemporaries of Plato, Michelangelo, and Oscar Wilde subject to the risk of dying from opportunistic infections? Certainly, a few cases caused by unusual microbes would have passed unnoticed among the welter of other deaths caused by common infections before the advent of modern microbiology, but what of recent times? Pneumocystis has been known for almost 30 years, and, given the right specimens and correct stains, it is fairly easy to identify. Present indications are that we are seeing a truly new syndrome, not explainable simply by failure to diagnose earlier cases. Therefore, we must suspect that some new factor may have distorted the host-parasite relation. So-called "recreational" drugs are one possibility. They are widely used in the large cities where most of these cases have occurred, and the only patients in the series reported in this issue who were not homosexual were drug users. Fashions in drug use change frequently, and experimentation with new agents is common. Perhaps one or more of these recreational drugs is an immunosuppressive agent. The leading candidates are the nitrites, which are now commonly inhaled to intensify orgasm. Users of amyl nitrite are more likely than nonusers to have had hundreds of sexual partners and to contract venereal diseases.[16] Preliminary data indicate that this "liberated" subgroup may be at highest risk for immunosuppression.

In our present state of ignorance, some frank speculation seems permissible. Let us postulate that the combined effects of persistent viral infection plus an adjuvant drug cause immunosuppression in some genetically predisposed men. During the early stages, patients may have only a nonspecific illness and minor infections such as thrush. Then Kaposi's sarcoma may develop as an opportunistic tumor (perhaps cytomegalovirus-induced), which is set free by a failure of immune surveillance. Finally, as the defect in cellular immunity becomes progressively more severe, serious opportunistic infections develop. According to this hypothesis, several factors may interact to form a final common pathway of immunosuppression, which then leads to both neoplasia and infection.

The authors of today's three reports deserve congratulations for making a prompt beginning to this investigation. But it is only a beginning. Enumeration of lymphocyte subpopulations, though certainly a fashionable pursuit, seldom seems to provide the final answers; other approaches will be necessary. The CDC, acting with customary dispatch, has commissioned a task force to unravel the tangled threads. Case-control studies to single out possible risk factors, such as promiscuous life styles and nitrite inhalation, are under way. Patients are being HLA-typed (when their lymphocyte counts are not too low for this test) in a search for a possible genetic predisposition. Examination or reexamination of the immunosuppressive potential of recreational drugs has begun. Some of the lymphocyte laboratories have been appropriately stimulated to look for mechanisms. These studies should answer the tantalizing questions raised by this new syndrome, perhaps providing means to protect the persons most at risk, and certainly extending our understanding of host-parasite relations.

References

1. Gottlieb MS, Schanker HM, Fan PT, et al. *Pneumocystis* pneumonia — Los Angeles. MMWR 1981; 30:250-2.
2. Friedman-Kien A, Laubenstein L, Marmor M, et al. Kaposi's sarcoma and *Pneumocystis* pneumonia among homosexual men — New York City and California. MMWR 1981; 30:305-8.
3. Hymes KB, Cheung T, Greene JB, et al. Kaposi's sarcoma in homosexual men — a report of eight cases. Lancet 1981; 2:598-600.
4. Gottlieb MS, Schroff R, Schanker HM, et al. *Pneumocystis carinii* pneumonia and mucosal candidiasis in previously healthy homosexual men: evidence of a new acquired cellular immunodeficiency. N Engl J Med 1981; 305:1425-31.
5. Masur H, Michelis MA, Greene JB, et al. An outbreak of community-acquired *Pneumocystis carinii* pneumonia: initial manifestation of cellular immune dysfunction. N Engl J Med 1981; 305-1431-8.
6. Siegal FP, Lopez C, Hammer GS, et al. Severe acquired immunodeficiency in male homosexuals, manifested by chronic perianal ulcerative herpes simplex lesions. N Engl J Med 1981; 305:1439-44.
7. Darrow WW, Barrett D, Jay K, Young A. The gay report on sexually transmitted diseases. Am J Public Health 1981; 71:1004-11.
8. Hamilton JR, Overall JC Jr, Glasgow LA. Synergistic effect on mortality in mice with murine cytomegalovirus and *Pseudomonas aeruginosa, Staphylococcus aureus,* or *Candida albicans* infections. Infect Immun 1976; 14: 982-9.
9. Carney WP, Rubin RH, Hoffman RA, Hansen WP, Healey K, Hirsch MS. Analysis of T lymphocyte subsets in cytomegalovirus mononucleosis. J Immunol 1981; 126:2114-6.

10. Lang DJ, Kummer JF, Hartley DP. Cytomegalovirus in semen: persistence and demonstration in extracellular fluids. N Engl J Med 1974; 291:121-3.
11. Rubin RH, Cosimi AB, Tolkoff-Rubin NE, Russell PS, Hirsch MS. Infectious disease syndromes attributable to cytomegalovirus and their significance among renal transplant recipients. Transplantation 1977; 24:458-64.
12. Drew WL, Mintz L, Miner RC, Sands M, Ketterer B. Prevalence of cytomegalovirus infection in homosexual men. J Infect Dis 1981; 143:188-92.
13. Giraldo G, Beth E. The relationship of cytomegalovirus to certain human cancers, particularly to Kaposi's sarcoma. In: Giraldo G, Beth E, eds. The role of viruses in human cancer. Vol. 1. Amsterdam: Elsevier North Holland, 1980:57-73.
14. Harwood AR, Osoba D, Hofstader SL, et al. Kaposi's sarcoma in recipients of renal transplants. Am J Med 1979; 67:759-65.
15. Boldogh I, Beth E, Huang ES, et al. Kaposi's sarcoma. IV. Detection of CMV DNA, CMV RNA and CMNA in tumor biopsies. Int J Cancer 1981; 28:469-74.
16. Goode E, Troiden RR. Amyl nitrite use among homosexual men. Am J Psychiatry 1979; 136:1067-9.

MEDICAL INTELLIGENCE

VIROLOGIC STUDIES IN A CASE OF TRANSFUSION-ASSOCIATED AIDS

JEROME E. GROOPMAN, M.D., S. ZAKI SALAHUDDIN, M.S., MANGALASSERIL G. SARNGADHARAN, PH.D., JAMES I. MULLINS, PH.D., JOHN L. SULLIVAN, M.D., CAREL MULDER, D.PHIL., CARL J. O'HARA, M.D., SARAH H. CHEESEMAN, M.D., HARRY HAVERKOS, M.D., PIERRE FORGACS, M.D., NORBERT RIEDEL, PH.D., MARY F. MCLANE, M.S., MYRON ESSEX, PH.D., AND ROBERT C. GALLO, M.D.

THE epidemiology of the acquired immunodeficiency syndrome (AIDS) strongly suggests a transmissible agent, such as a virus, as its cause.[1-3] Transient viral infections in normal hosts with agents such as cytomegalovirus, hepatitis B, and Epstein–Barr virus manifest cellular changes that indicate immunosuppression.[4,5] The high prevalence of such DNA viruses among cohorts at risk for AIDS, such as homosexual men, intravenous drug abusers, Haitians, and hemophiliacs, as well as their transmissibility by sexual, needle, and blood-borne routes, has focused attention on their roles in AIDS.[6-11] These viruses have been proposed either as primary etiologic agents or as important cofactors in susceptibility to another primary AIDS virus.

Human T-cell leukemia viruses (HTLVs) are Type C retroviruses that have also been considered as etiologic agents in AIDS. HTLV Type III has been readily recovered from patients with AIDS, as well as from those with signs and symptoms that often precede AIDS.[12-15] The prevalence of antibody to the p41 antigen of HTLV-III among such patients is higher than 90 percent.[15,16] HTLV-III is cytopathic and tropic for the T4 helper lymphocyte subset, which is reduced in number in patients with AIDS.[13] Such virologic and seroepidemiologic survey data provide compelling circumstantial evidence of an important etiologic role for HTLV-III in AIDS. Studies of HTLV-III in patients without other risk factors who contract AIDS after receiving blood transfusions and in their high-risk blood donors should be of great value in assessing the role of this virus in the pathogenesis of the syndrome. We have studied in detail a patient with transfusion-associated AIDS and a high-risk blood donor for evidence of transmission of one or more of the aforementioned viruses. HTLV-III appears to have been present as a single infectious agent in the patient with AIDS. The high-risk blood donor was asymptomatic and carried HTLV-III in his peripheral-blood cells and saliva. Our study demonstrates that HTLV-III is transmissible through blood products, may be the sole viral agent in the pathogenesis of AIDS, and is associated with a broad clinical spectrum, including an asymptomatic but apparently contagious carrier state.

From the Departments of Medicine and Pathology, New England Deaconess Hospital; and the Department of Cancer Biology, Harvard School of Public Health, Boston; the Departments of Pediatrics, Medicine, Pharmacology, Molecular Genetics, and Microbiology, University of Massachusetts, Worcester, Mass.; the Department of Medicine, Lahey Clinic, Burlington, Mass.; the Centers for Disease Control, Atlanta; the Department of Cell Biology, Litton Bionetics, Inc., Kensington, Md.; and the Laboratory of Tumor Cell Biology, National Cancer Institute, Bethesda, Md.

Supported by grants (CA 18216, CA 34975, CA 37466, and AI 21129) from the National Institutes of Health. Dr. Groopman was the recipient of a Junior Faculty Research Award from the American Cancer Society.

CASE REPORT

Patient with Transfusion-Associated AIDS

A 60-year-old white woman was admitted to the hospital because of weakness, a nonproductive cough, and fever of six weeks' duration. The patient had been in excellent health all her life. Forty-three months before admission, she had undergone a total abdominal hysterectomy for leiomyomata and had received four units of packed red cells. Thirty months before admission, the patient had undergone cholecystectomy but had not received transfusions at that time. She had worked as a social worker and had traveled to Europe in 1976, but had never traveled to Haiti or Africa. She had been widowed and had infrequent vaginal intercourse (less than once a month) with a healthy heterosexual white man. The patient reported that she did not use illicit drugs and had never been given injections except within a hospital setting. Seven months before admission, the patient had noted anorexia, mild nausea, and malaise associated with weight loss. Three months before admission, a chest x-ray film showed bibasilar infiltrates. An extensive evaluation for infectious and neoplastic disorders was unrevealing. At that time, her white-cell count was 5500 per cubic millimeter, with 93 percent neutrophils and 2 percent lymphocytes. One sputum sample grew *Candida albicans*. The patient was empirically treated with erythromycin and clindamycin, which resulted in the clearing of her bilateral pulmonary infiltrates and an improvement in her general clinical condition. One month later, she returned with recurrent bibasilar infiltrates. Bronchoscopy with transbronchial biopsy revealed hemorrhage within the alveolar spaces. Her white-cell count was 3700 per cubic millimeter, with 1 percent lymphocytes. T-cell subset studies were performed with standard techniques[17]; there were 4 percent OKT8 cells and 0 percent OKT4 cells. Skin tests to recall antigens (mumps, candida, and streptokinase–streptodornase) were negative. An open-lung biopsy was performed, and a silver methenamine stain revealed *Pneumocystis carinii*. She was started on intravenous trimethoprim–sulfamethoxazole. Her pulmonary status deteriorated, and pentamidine isethionate was started. Despite antibiotics and mechanical ventilation support, the patient died five weeks after admission. Permission was obtained for autopsy, and tissue was immediately cryopreserved at the time of death. Serum samples had been obtained periodically during her hospital course and stored at −70°C.

High-Risk Blood Donor

Letters were sent to the four blood donors, stating that a recipient of their blood products had contracted AIDS. Informed consent was obtained from the donors, followed by detailed social and medical evaluations. For three of the donors, there were no life-style risk factors for AIDS, the physical examination was normal, and laboratory studies, including studies of T-cell subsets, were also normal. The fourth donor was a sexually active homosexual man who frequently used intravenous drugs. He was asymptomatic but on physical examination had generalized lymphadenopathy of cervical, axillary, and inguinal areas, of unknown duration. He was designated as a high-risk blood donor, according to previously established criteria.[18]

Forty-seven months after his donation of blood to the patient, the high-risk donor underwent lymph-node biopsy, which revealed follicular hyperplasia. Laboratory evaluation at that time revealed a white-cell count of 6300 per cubic millimeter, with 62 percent neutrophils, and 33 percent lymphocytes, a platelet count of 186,000 per cubic millimeter, normal serum chemistry values, and normal liver-function tests. He had normal responses to recall antigens on skin testing with candida, mumps, and streptokinase–streptodornase. Lymph-node and peripheral-blood mononuclear cells were cryopreserved for further studies.

Laboratory Studies

Serum samples were available from the patient with transfusion-associated AIDS and from all four blood donors. Antibodies to HTLV-III were measured by an enzyme-linked immunosorbent assay and by Western blot analysis, as previously described.[15,16] Antibodies to HTLV Types I and II were measured by Western blot analysis.[15] Antibodies to cytomegalovirus, Epstein–Barr virus, hepatitis B virus, varicella zoster, and tetanus toxoid were measured according to previously described methods.[19] Serum acid-labile leukocyte interferon was measured with encephalomyocarditis virus and bovine tracheal fibroblasts.[20] Immunofluorescence studies for Epstein–Barr viral nuclear antigen were performed on tissue imprints of lymph nodes, spleen, lung, and liver from the patient with transfusion-associated AIDS and on peripheral-blood mononuclear cells and lymph-node specimens from the high-risk donor, as previously described.[21] DNA prepared from specimens of the patient's spleen, liver, lymph nodes, and lung and the donor's peripheral-blood mononuclear cells and lymph nodes was studied for the presence of viral nucleic acids by the Southern hybridization technique.[22,23] The DNA was cleaved with restriction endonucleases *Bam*HI, *Pst*I, *Kpn*I, and *Sst*I, subjected to electrophoresis through agarose gels, and transferred to aminophenylthioether paper.[24] Positive controls included DNA from the Raji lymphoblastoid cell line, which is known to contain 50 to 60 copies of Epstein–Barr viral DNA per cell. The negative control was DNA from an Epstein–Barr–negative human T-cell line (8402). The following viral DNA probes were used in our studies: HTLV Type I (pCR), HTLV Type II (pMo II), HTLV Type III (pHT, provided by Dr. F. Wong-Staal, National Cancer Institute, Bethesda, Md.); Epstein–Barr virus (*Bam*HI V fragment, provided by Dr. E. Kieff, University of Chicago), cytomegalovirus (*Eco*RI F, provided by Dr. B. Fleckenstein, University of Erlangen, Erlangen, Germany), herpes simplex virus Type I (pGR 198, provided by Dr. G. Hayward, Johns Hopkins University, Baltimore), hepatitis B virus (pBH20-HBV, provided by Dr. J. Summers, Institute of Cancer Research, Philadelphia), and human parvovirus (pYT 103, provided by Dr. P. Tattersall, Yale University, New Haven, Conn.). RNA was prepared from spleen and lymph-node samples obtained from the patient with transfusion-associated AIDS and was probed for HTLV-III cross-reacting sequences by means of a dot-blot technique.[25] Standard virologic cultures were prepared from urine, semen, buffy-coat, and lymph-node samples from the high-risk donor and from urine, buffy-coat, and lung samples from the patient with AIDS.[10] Cultures of peripheral-blood or lymph-node mononuclear cells grown in the presence of T-cell growth factor were assayed for HTLV-III as previously described.[13] Saliva from the high-risk blood donor was filtered through a 0.45-μm filter (Millipore, Milford, Mass.) and cultured for HTLV-III as previously described.[26]

Results

The laboratory findings in the patient with transfusion-associated AIDS and in the high-risk donor are shown in Table 1. The patient had no known risk factor for AIDS other than blood transfusion. Demonstration of *P. carinii* by open-lung biopsy confirmed the diagnosis of AIDS. The patient had antibody to the p41 antigen of HTLV-III as detected by Western blot analysis but not the enzyme-linked immunosorbent assay (Fig. 1). She was seronegative for antibodies to HTLV Types I and II, cytomegalovirus, Epstein–Barr virus, and hepatitis B virus, but she did have antibody to varicella zoster and tetanus toxoid. The high-risk blood donor was seropositive for antibodies to HTLV-III according to both the enzyme-linked immunosorbent assay and the Western blot analysis (Fig. 1). He had serologic evidence of prior infection with cytomegalovirus, Epstein–Barr virus, and hepatitis B virus. However, he had a normal total lymphocyte count and normal T-cell subsets and was not anergic on skin testing. Neither the enzyme-linked immunosorbent assay nor the Western blot analysis detected antibodies to HTLV-III in the three blood donors who were not at risk for AIDS.

Table 1. Laboratory Studies in a Patient with Transfusion-Associated AIDS and in the High-Risk Donor.*

	Patient with AIDS	High-Risk Donor
White-cell count (mm^3)	3700	6300
Total lymphocytes (mm^3)	37	2100
OKT4 (mm^3)	0	1180
OKT8 (mm^3)	2	715
OKT4/OKT8	0	1.6
IgG (mg/dl)	1410	1960
IgA (mg/dl)	478	512
IgM (mg/dl)	133	151
HTLV-III antibody	+	+
EBNA immunofluorescence	−	−
Viral sequences		
HTLV-III	+	−
HTLV-I	−	−
HTLV-II	−	−
Cytomegalovirus	−	−
Epstein–Barr virus	−	−
Hepatitis B virus	−	−
Herpes simplex virus Type I	−	−
Parvovirus	−	−
Recovery by cocultivation		
HTLV-III, peripheral blood	−	+
HTLV-III, saliva	ND	+

*HTLV-III antibody refers to antibody to the p41 antigen of human T-cell leukemia virus Type III. EBNA denotes Epstein–Barr viral nuclear antigen, and ND not detectable. HTLV-III antibody was detected by the Western electroblot assay. Viral sequences were detected by the Southern hybridization technique or the dot-blot technique; the positive control was an EBV-infected Raji line, as described in the text.

Southern hybridization analysis of DNA from the patient with transfusion-associated AIDS did not demonstrate detectable sequences related to HTLV Types I, II, or III, cytomegalovirus, Epstein–Barr virus, herpes simplex virus Type I, parvovirus, or hepatitis B virus. DNA prepared from peripheral-blood mononuclear cells and lymph-node specimens obtained from the high-risk donor was also negative for these viruses. HTLV-III–related RNA sequences were detected in the spleen of the patient with AIDS. HTLV-III was recovered from cultures of the donor's peripheral-blood cells and saliva but not from the patient's cryopreserved peripheral-blood cells.

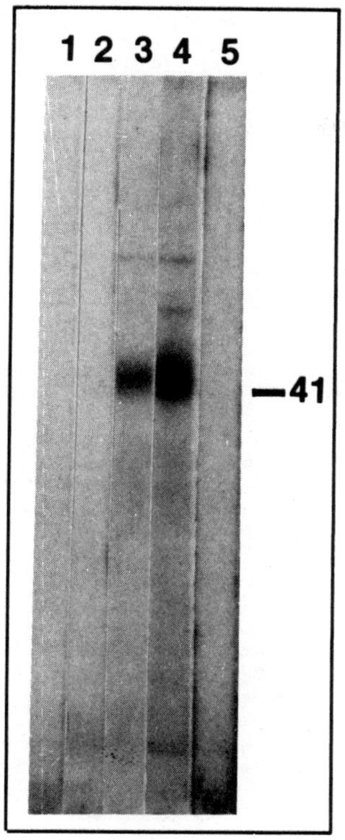

Figure 1. Western Blot Analysis of Antibody to the p41 Antigen of Human T-Cell Leukemia Virus Type III (HTLV-III).

Samples in the first two columns are from healthy heterosexual controls, the sample in the third column is from the patient with transfusion-associated AIDS, the sample in the fourth column is from the high-risk donor, and the sample in the fifth column is from an elderly man with classic Kaposi's sarcoma. The presence of antibody directed against the p41 HTLV-III antigen is indicated by the dark band on the gel. The analysis was performed as previously described.[15]

Discussion

The cause of AIDS has not yet been definitely proved, but accumulating evidence indicates that HTLV-III is the primary etiologic agent.[12-16] Cytomegalovirus, Epstein–Barr virus, and hepatitis B virus are transmissible by parenteral and sexual routes, are associated with transient immunosuppression, are frequent among cohorts at risk for AIDS, and have been proposed as either primary causes or important cofactors in the pathogenesis of the syndrome.[6-10] Cases of transfusion-associated AIDS differ epidemiologically from cases occurring in high-risk cohorts. Patients with transfusion-associated AIDS generally do not have other risk factors for the syndrome and are less likely to have a high background prevalence of herpesviruses. In addition, by studying the blood donors in such cases, one can identify the probable source of AIDS.

In our study there was a striking difference between the seropositivity of the high-risk blood donor and the seronegativity of the patient with transfusion-associated AIDS, with respect to cytomegalovirus, Epstein–Barr virus, and hepatitis B virus. The presence of antibody to varicella zoster and tetanus toxoid in the patient suggests that her humoral immune responses were intact. It is interesting to note that polyclonal hypergammaglobulinemia occurred in the patient without any evidence of prior Epstein–Barr viral infection, contrary to the suggestion of others that such a finding in AIDS can be attributed to stimulation of B lymphocytes by this virus.[8]

Essex and co-workers reported disproportionate seropositivity for antibodies to HTLV-I–encoded membrane antigens among homosexual men with AIDS, as compared with healthy homosexual controls.[27] Jaffe et al. described similar seropositivity among blood donors linked to cases of transfusion-associated AIDS.[28] Recent data indicate that these antibodies are directed against HTLV-III–encoded glycoproteins that cross-react with HTLV-I antigens (Essex M: unpublished data). Barré-Sinoussi and Vilmer and their colleagues have isolated retroviruses from patients with AIDS and related disorders.[29,30] Termed lymphadenopathy-associated or immunodeficiency-associated viruses, they appear by antigenic analysis to be very similar to HTLV-III (Gallo RC, et al.: unpublished data). Feorino and co-workers have isolated lymphadenopathy-associated virus from a patient with transfusion-associated AIDS and from the high-risk blood donor, suggesting its transmissibility by blood products as well.[31]

The demonstration of apparent transmission of HTLV-III by blood transfusion and the inability to detect evidence of infection with other viruses strongly indicate a primary etiologic role for this virus in the pathogenesis of the immunodeficiency syndrome in our patient.

The high-risk blood donor continues to be an asymptomatic carrier of HTLV-III. Epidemiologically, it may be inferred that he has carried the virus since the time of blood donation, more than four years ago. With current techniques of screening for antibody to HTLV-III, such as the enzyme-linked immunosorbent assay, which is applicable to the blood-bank setting, this man would be identified as a possible carrier of the virus, and his blood products would not be used. The mechanism whereby HTLV-III may be chronically carried without clinical symptoms is unknown. The clinical outcome may be related to the viral strain. Recent studies by Shaw et al. demonstrate considerable molecular heterogeneity of HTLV-III isolates from patients with AIDS and related disorders.[32] We are currently comparing the HTLV-III isolates obtained from the high-risk blood donor with the HTLV-III–related RNA sequences detected in the spleen of the woman with tranfusion-associated AIDS, to determine whether molecular changes occurred after transmission of the virus that might be related to the development of the syndrome. An understanding of host and virologic factors that determine different clinical outcomes after HTLV-III infection should be of value in the development of prophylactic (vaccine) and therapeutic strategies in AIDS.

We are indebted to Drs. A. Sliski, J. Lamberson, and D. Webb-Johnson for their assistance in this study.

References

1. Gottlieb MS, Groopman JE, Weinstein WM, et al. The acquired immunodeficiency syndrome. Ann Intern Med 1983; 99:208-20.
2. Fauci AS, Macher AM, Longo DL, et al. Acquired immunodeficiency syndrome: epidemiologic, clinical, immunologic, and therapeutic considerations. Ann Intern Med 1984; 100:92-106.
3. Curran JW, Evatt BL, Lawrence DN. Acquired immune deficiency syndrome: the past as prologue. Ann Intern Med 1983; 98:401-3.
4. Carney WP, Rubin RH, Hoffman RA, Hansen WP, Healey K, Hirsch MS. Analysis of T lymphocyte subsets in cytomegalovirus mononucleosis. J Immunol 1981; 126:2114-6.
5. Tosato G, Magrath I, Koski I, Dooley N, Blaese M. Activation of suppressor T cells during Epstein–Barr-virus-induced infectious mononucleosis. N Engl J Med 1979; 301:1133-7.
6. Gottlieb MS, Schroff R, Shanker H, et al. *Pneumocystis carinii* pneumonia and mucosal candidiasis in previously healthy homosexual men: evidence of a new acquired cellular immunodeficiency. N Engl J Med 1981; 305:1425-31.
7. Siegal FP, Lopez C, Hammer GS, et al. Severe acquired immunodeficiency in male homosexuals, manifested by chronic perianal ulcerative herpes simplex lesions. N Engl J Med 1981; 305:1439-44.
8. Friedman-Kien AE, Laubenstein LJ, Rubenstein PJ, et al. Disseminated Kaposi's sarcoma in homosexual men. Ann Intern Med 1982; 96: 693-700.
9. Drew WL, Conant MA, Miner RC, et al. Cytomegalovirus and Kaposi's sarcoma in young homosexual men. Lancet 1982; 2:125-7.
10. Rogers MF, Morens DM, Stewart JA, et al. National case-control study of Kaposi's sarcoma and *Pneumocystis carinii* pneumonia in homosexual men. Part 2. Laboratory results. Ann Intern Med 1983; 99:151-8.
11. Lederman MM, Ratnoff OD, Scillian JJ, Jones PK, Schacter B. Impaired cell-mediated immunity in patients with classic hemophilia. N Engl J Med 1983; 308:79-83.
12. Popovic M, Sarngadharan MG, Read E, Gallo RC. Detection, isolation, and continuous production of cytopathic retroviruses (HTLV-III) from patients with AIDS and pre-AIDS. Science 1984; 224:497-500.
13. Gallo RC, Salahuddin SZ, Popovic M, et al. Frequent detection and isolation of cytopathic retroviruses (HTLV-III) from patients with AIDS and at risk for AIDS. Science 1984; 224:500-2.
14. Schüpbach J, Popovic M, Gilden RV, et al. Serological analysis of a subgroup of human T-lymphotropic retroviruses (HTLV-III) associated with AIDS. Science 1984; 224:503-5.
15. Sarngadharan MG, Popovic M, Bruch L, Schüpbach J, Gallo RC. Antibodies reactive with human T-lymphotropic retroviruses (HTLV-III) in the serum of patients with AIDS. Science 1984; 224:506-8.
16. Safai B, Sarngadharan M, Groopman JE, et al. Seropepidemiological studies of human T-lymphotropic retrovirus type III in acquired immunodeficiency syndrome. Lancet 1984; 1:1438-40.
17. Fahey JL, Prince H, Weaver M, et al. Quantitative changes in T helper or T suppressor/cytotoxic lymphocyte subsets that distinguish acquired immune deficiency syndrome from other immune subset disorders. Am J Med 1984; 76:95-100.
18. Curran JW, Lawrence DN, Jaffe H, et al. Acquired immunodeficiency syndrome (AIDS) associated with transfusions. N Engl J Med 1984; 310: 69-75.
19. Cheeseman SH, Sullivan JL, Brettler DB, Levine PH. Analysis of cytomegalovirus and Epstein-Barr virus antibody responses in treated hemophiliacs: implications for the study of acquired immunodeficiency syndrome. JAMA (in press).
20. Preble OT, Black RT, Friedman RM, Klippel JH, Vilcek J. Systemic lupus erythematosus: presence in human serum of an ususual acid-labile leukocyte interferon. Science 1983; 216:429-31.
21. Henle W, Henle G, Horowitz CA. Infectious mononucleosis and Epstein–Barr virus-associated malignancies. In: Lennette EH, Schmidt NJ, eds. Diagnostic procedures for viral, ricketsial and chlamydial infections. New York: American Public Health Association, 1979:470.
22. Southern EM. Detection of specific sequences among DNA fragments separated by gel electrophoresis. J Mol Biol 1975; 98:503-17.
23. Youssourian H, Hammer SM, Hirsch MS, Mulder C. Methylation of the viral genome in an *in vitro* model of herpes simplex virus latency. Proc Natl Acad Sci USA 1982; 79:2207-10.
24. Seed B. Diazotizable arylamine cellulose papers for coupling and hybridization of nucleic acids. Nucleic Acids Res 1980; 1799-810.
25. Beltz GA, Jacobs KA, Eichbush TH, Cherbas PT, Kafatos FC. Isolation of multigene families and determination of homologies by filter hybridization methods. Methods Enzymol 1983; 100:266-84.
26. Groopman JE, Salahuddin SZ, Sarngadharan MG, et al. HTLV-III in saliva of people with AIDS-related complex and healthy homosexual men at risk for AIDS. Science 1984; 226:447-9.
27. Essex M, McLane MF, Lee TH, et al. Antibodies to cell membrane antigens associated with human T-cell leukemia virus in patients with AIDS. Science 1983; 220:859-62.
28. Jaffe HW, Francis DP, McLane MF, et al. Transfusion-associated AIDS: serologic evidence of human T-cell leukemia virus infection of donors. Science 1984; 223:1309-12.
29. Barré-Sinoussi F, Chermann JC, Rey F, et al. Isolation of a T-lymphotropic retrovirus from a patient at risk for acquired immune deficiency syndrome (AIDS). Science 1983; 220:868-71.
30. Vilmer E, Barré-Sinoussi F, Rouzioux C, et al. Isolation of a new lymphotropic retrovirus from two siblings with haemophilia B, one with AIDS. Lancet 1984; 1:753-7.
31. Feorino PM, Kalyanaraman VS, Haverkos HW, et al. Lymphadenopathy associated virus infection of a blood donor–recipient pair with acquired immunodeficiency syndrome. Science 1984; 225:69-72.
32. Shaw GM, Hahn BH, Arya SK, et al. Molecular characterization of human T-cell leukemia (lymphotropic) virus type III in the acquired immunodeficiency syndrome. Science (in press).

MEDICAL INTELLIGENCE

COINCIDENT CLASSIC HEMOPHILIA AND "IDIOPATHIC" THROMBOCYTOPENIC PURPURA IN PATIENTS UNDER TREATMENT WITH CONCENTRATES OF ANTIHEMOPHILIC FACTOR (FACTOR VII)

Oscar D. Ratnoff, M.D., Jay E. Menitove, M.D., Richard H. Aster, M.D., and Michael M. Lederman, M.D.

HOME treatment of classic hemophilia with lyophilized concentrates of antihemophilic factor (factor VIII) is now widely practiced. We studied a syndrome resembling chronic idiopathic thrombocytopenic purpura in five patients with severe classic hemophilia who were receiving such therapy. Laboratory studies are summarized in Tables 1 through 3. The presence of increased amounts of platelet-associated IgG, the favorable response in four patients treated with prednisone, and remission after splenectomy in one patient all suggest that the patients' disorder resembled idiopathic thrombocytopenic purpura. In addition, studies in four patients demonstrated evidence of impaired cell-mediated immunity in three.

Case Reports

Patient 1

A 21-year-old man with severe hemophilia (factor VIII titer <0.01 unit per milliliter) was admitted to University Hospitals of Cleveland on December 22, 1981, for study of a petechial rash of three or four weeks' duration. He had been in a home therapy program for five years, using the concentrate of a single manufacturer every three or four weeks. Laboratory studies demonstrated severe thrombocytopenia (30,000 to 36,000 platelets per microliter) and plentiful megakaryocytes in a marrow aspirate. The platelet count rose to 78,000 per microliter upon administration of prednisone (80 mg per day), but that level could not be sustained at lower doses. Splenectomy, with the patient protected by infusions of lyophilized concentrates of factor VIII, was performed on February 2, 1982, and was followed by remission; the platelet count on August 10, 1982, was 293,000 per microliter. The excised spleen weighed 355 g; slight follicular hyperplasia and reactive plasmacytosis of the red pulp were present.

Patient 2

A 30-year-old man with severe hemophilia (factor VIII titer <0.01 unit per milliliter) had been in a home therapy program for six years, giving himself a transfusion containing lyophilized concentrates of factor VIII about once a month. Over the years he had used concentrates prepared by three different manufacturers. He had had episodes of hepatitis after these transfusions at ages 18 and 25 years; before the first episode, he had also received transfusions of cryoprecipitates. In June 1981 the platelet count was 85,000 per microliter, and in January 1982 the count was 43,000 per microliter, but the patient had no unusual bleeding. When he was admitted to the hospital on April 11, 1982, numerous vascular spiders were noted on his thorax and arms. The platelet count was 37,000 per microliter, and a marrow aspirate demonstrated numerous megakaryocytes and erythrocytic hyperplasia. Slight enlargement of the spleen was noted on a liver–spleen scan. In addition, a direct Coombs' test was positive for IgG, and the reticulocyte count was slightly elevated. A partial remission followed the administration of prednisone. A recommendation for splenectomy was rejected by the patient. His platelet count on May 26, 1982, was 81,000 per microliter.

Patient 3

A 16-year-old boy with severe classic hemophilia (factor VIII titer <0.01 unit per milliliter) had been administering his own transfusions at home for five years, using five different lyophilized preparations of factor VIII over this period; he had recently been using factor VIII about once a week. In June 1982 he became aware of a transient punctate red rash on the top of his foot, which recurred several times. Beginning in September he had increasing fatigue. A platelet count on September 23 was 40,000 per microliter, and on October 7 the count was 15,500 per microliter. Results of marrow aspiration were similar to those of Patients 1 and 2. A direct Coombs' test was positive for IgG, and the serum haptoglobin level was severely depressed. Therapy with prednisone was followed by a partial remission, but the platelet count fell within three weeks after discontinuation of treatment and was 55,000 per microliter on December 13, 1982.

Patient 4

An 18-year-old boy with severe classic hemophilia (factor VIII titer <0.01 unit per milliliter) had been in a home therapy program for seven years, self-administering lyophilized factor VIII about once a week. Late in 1981 his physician detected a few cutaneous petechiae. The platelet count was 8000 per microliter, and increased numbers of megakaryocytes were seen in a marrow aspirate. During therapy with prednisone, the patient's platelet count varied from 25,000 to 61,000 per microliter. Therapy was discontinued, and the platelet count on June 29, 1982, was 54,000 per microliter.

Patient 5

A 71-year-old man with severe classic hemophila (factor VIII titer <0.01 unit per milliliter) had been receiving home therapy for nine years. For the first two years, he self-administered cyroprecipitated factor VIII, and since then, lyophilized concentrates of factor VIII. For five years he had mild thrombocytopenia, with platelet counts ranging from 82,000 to 150,000 per microliter. No examination of bone marrow was performed. His mild thrombocytopenia was not treated.

Discussion

The coincidence of chronic "idiopathic" thrombocytopenic purpura and classic hemophilia is most unusual. Hruby[1] has described two such cases. One was in a 19-year-old boy with mild hemophilia (factor VIII titer, 0.10 unit per milliliter) who ultimately responded to splenectomy. In the other, thrombocytopenia was detected when the patient was 14 months of age, and it recurred intermittently during the succeeding five years, ultimately remitting after splenectomy.

From the Department of Medicine, Case Western Reserve University School of Medicine, University Hospitals of Cleveland, Cleveland; and the Blood Center of Southeastern Wisconsin, Milwaukee.

Supported in part by grants (HL01661 and HL13629) from the National Heart, Lung, and Blood Institute, a grant (AM28324) from the National Institute of Arthritis, Diabetes, Digestive and Kidney Diseases, and grants from the American Heart Association and its Northeast Ohio affiliate. Dr. Ratnoff is a Career Investigator of the American Heart Association.

Table 1. Hematologic Values in Patients with Coincident Classic Hemophilia and Chronic "Idiopathic" Thrombocytopenic Purpura.

	Patient Number					Normal Values
	1	2	3	4	5	
Lowest platelet count (/μl)	30,000	37,000	15,500	8000	82,000	150,000–400,00
Platelet IgG (fg/platelet)	5.3*	27.9	32.6	9.8–19.1	15.2	4.3±0.8†
Platelet IgM (fg/platelet)	—	—	13.6	19.5	<0.6	<0.6–1.8
Serum anti-platelet antibodies						
Immunofluorescence	Neg	Neg	Neg	Neg	4+‡	Neg
Chromium release	Neg	Neg	Neg	Neg	4+§	Neg
Hematocrit (%)	47	42	42	41	47	42–52
Reticulocyte count (%)	—	2.4	1.8	—	—	0.5–1.5
Haptoglobin (mg/dl)	—	43.4	2.3	—	—	30–205
Direct Coombs' test	Neg	Pos (IgG)	Pos (IgG)	—	—	Neg
White Cells (/μl)	8100	7100	3900	2800	5600	4800–10,800

*Tested after splenectomy-induced remission (platelet count, 293,000 per microliter). †Mean ±SD.
‡1977; 2+ in 1982. §In 1977; negative in 1982.

This patient (factor VIII titer <0.01 unit per milliliter) had been given a transfusion with commercial lyophilized concentrates of factor VIII when he was about two months old, during surgical correction of pyloric stenosis (Maurer H: personal communication). More recently, Suffredini and Qureshi[2] reported a third case, in a 22-year-old man with severe hemophilia (factor VIII titer <0.01 unit per milliliter) who had been treated for three years with factor VIII concentrates. The patient had a partial remission coincident with prednisone therapy. An instance of acute idiopathic thrombocytopenic purpura in an 18-year-old boy has also been recorded.[3]

The five patients whose cases have been summarized here were all severely affected classic hemophiliacs who had received repeated transfusions with lyophilized preparations of antihemophilic factor. In each, a syndrome developed that resembled idiopathic thrombocytopenic purpura, and four responded to a greater of lesser degree to therapy with prednisone. Splenectomy was performed in one patient and was followed by remission of thrombocytopenia. It is worth noting that the weight of the patient's spleen was greater than is usual in idiopathic thrombocytopenic purpura.[4]

Four of the patients had evidence of mild hepatic

Table 2. Laboratory Values for Hepatic and Immunologic Functions in Patients with Coincident Classic Hemophilia and Chronic "Idiopathic" Thrombocytopenic Purpura.

	Patient Number					Normal Values
	1	2	3	4	5	
SGOT (U/liter)	33–163	110–186	44	39	32–87	<41
SGPT (U/liter)	—	—	—	36	15–102	5–35
Lactic dehydrogenase (U/liter)	319–422	217–278	365	252	179–280	100–225
Alkaline phosphatase (U/liter)	69–95	159	328	—	125	25–115
Alkaline phosphatase (U/liter)	—	—	—	129	—	75–250
Bilirubin (mg/dl)‡	0.8–1.0	1.2	0.5	0.6	0.8	0.1–1.2
Antinuclear antibody	<1:10	Neg	<1:10	—	—	<1:10
Anti-DNA (U/ml)	15.3	0	0	—	—	<15
LE test	Neg	—	—	—	—	Neg
Rheumatoid factor	<1:10	<1:20	<1:20	—	—	<1:20
Immune complexes (μg/ml)†	25.3	32.5	44.0	—	—	<30
CH_{50} (U/ml)	—	320	180	—	—	123–355
C3 (mg/dl)	189	108	11	—	—	83–177
C4 (mg/dl)	34.2	18.5	12.5	—	—	15–45
Serum albumin (g/dl)§	4.5	3.7	4.4	—	—	3.4–5.0
α_1 globulin (g/dl)	0.4	0.6	0.4	—	—	0.2–0.6
α_2 globulin (g/dl)	0.4	0.3	0.3	—	—	0.4–1.1
β globulin (g/dl)	0.9	0.7	1.0	—	—	0.5–1.2
γ globulin (g/dl)	1.7	2.3	3.0	—	—	0.5–1.4
IgG (mg/dl)	1680	2020	3200	—	—	600–1500
IgA (mg/dl)	151	329	374	—	—	85–380
IgM (mg/dl)	239	148	127	—	—	53–375
Fibrinogen-related antigen	—	+1:5	—	—	—	<1:20

*SGOT denotes serum aspartate aminotransferase, SGPT serum alanine aminotransferase, and LE lupus erythematosus.
†Determined by binding to solid-pahse C1q.
‡To convert values for bilirubin to micromoles per liter, multiply by 17.10.
§To convert values for serum albumin to micromoles per liter, multiply by 144.9.

Table 3. Lymphocyte Subpopulations and Results of Functional Assays in Patients with Coincident Classic Hemophilia and Thrombocytopenia.*

	Patient Number				Normal Values†
	1	3	4	5	
Lymphocytes (/μl)	2,400	1,287	1,120	1,104	1519±379
OKT4 cells (%)	25.3	21.7	—	—	45±9
OKT4 cells (%)	—	—	38	43	50±4
OKT8 cells (%)	40.1	56.8	—	—	27±9
OKT8 cells (%)	—	—	38	25	25±2
OKT4/OKT8	0.63	0.38	—	—	1.84±0.70
OKT4/OKT8	—	—	1.0	1.72	2.04±0.24
Natural-killer activity (% killing)	9.8	5.8	—	—	37.8±12.2
Phytohemagglutinin response (cpm)	16,190	33,726	—	—	87,342±15,765
Concanavalin A response (cpm)	16,941	2336	—	—	58,545±13,007

*Lymphocytes bearing OKT4 (helper) and OKT8 (repressor) antigens were counted by flow cytometry. Natural killer activity was detected by ^{51}Cr release from radiolabeled K562 tumor target cells incubated with the subjects' peripheral-blood mononuclear cells (PBMC).[10,11] Lymphocyte proliferative responses were measured by ^{3}H-thymidine incorporation into PBMC that had been cultured for three days with phytohemagglutinin (1 μg per milliliter) or concanavalin A (1 μg per milliliter).[10] The data for Patient 1 have been published elsewhere in a different context.[10]

†Normal values are expressed as means ±SD.

damage (Table 1). Platelet-associated IgG[5] was elevated in four patients, but not in the fifth, who was tested after splenectomy-induced remission (Table 1). The extent to which this reflected an increased concentration of serum IgG (Table 2) is uncertain. One patient had serum antibodies against platlets, as detected by an immunofluorescence test for non-complement-fixing antibodies[6] and by a test for ^{51}Cr release, which is a complement-dependent assay.[7] In addition, two patients had positive direct Coombs' tests for IgG. One of these patients had a slightly elevated reticulocyte count, and the other a decreased concentration of haptoglobin, but neither had the anemia that is typical of Evans's syndrome.

A causal relation between infusions of lyophilized factor VIII and the occurrence of thrombocytopenia has not yet been established. We have not observed concomitant thrombocytopenia in the many patients we have studied who were not treated with lyophilized preparations of factor VIII, but this association could easily have been overlooked. The three cases studied at University Hospitals of Cleveland occurred among 97 patients in home therapy programs in northeastern Ohio, and we know of 60 additional patients in this area who have been treated with lyophilized concentrates but are not receiving home therapy. Similarly, the two cases studied at the Blood Center of Southeastern Wisconsin were among 98 receiving home therapy and an additional 23 who had been treated with lyophilized concentrates under the guidance of the Great Lakes Hemophilia Foundation. The syndrome did not appear to be linked to concentrates prepared by a single manufacturer. The possibility exists that some concentrates may contain an agent or agents that induce what is apparently an immune thrombocytopenia. Whether such an agent is derived from some element of blood or is of infectious origin remains to be determined.

Two recent reports from the Centers for Disease Control[8,9] describe seven patients in whom classic hemophilia was complicated by *Pneumocystis carinii* pneumonia. All had been treated with concentrates of factor VIII. In each of six patients tested, the number and proportion of helper T cells were decreased. Furthermore, in two of these patients lymphocytes did not respond normally to mitogenic stimulation. These changes are similar to those observed in homosexual men with an acquired immunodeficiency syndrome. Among 24 patients with severe hemophilia who were under treatment with lyophilized factor VIII and whom we studied in our laboratories, 14 had impaired cellular immunity.[10,11] Similar changes have been observed in other patients with hemophilia treated with lyophilized factor VIII.[12] Impaired cellular immunity was found in three of the four patients with thrombocytopenia who are described in this report (Table 3). In these persons, the relative number of OKT4 (helper) cells was decreased, and the relative number of OKT8 (suppressor) cells was increased, reversing the normal ratio of OKT4 to OKT8 cells. In addition, natural-killer activity and lymphocyte proliferative responses to mitogens were decreased in Patients 1 and 3.

Whether the impaired cellular immunity observed in our patients was causally related to their thrombocytopenia is unclear. It is perhaps pertinent, however, that Morris et al.[13] have described 11 cases of severe "autoimmune" thrombocytopenic purpura in homosexual men. These studies and our observations suggest a need for careful surveillance of hemophiliacs receiving concentrates of factor VIII for disturbances of immunoregulation.

We are indebted to Dr. Elizabeth Gordon, Dr. Carl Krill, Dr. Charles Ross, Dr. Stewart Adair, and Dr. Joan Gill for referring patients to us for study, to Dr. Bernice Schacter for measurement of natural-killer activity, and to Dr. James Scillian for lymphocyte surface-marker studies.

References

1. Hruby MA. Coexistent hemophilia A and idiopathic thrombocytopenic purpura. J Pediatr 1977; 90:773-5.
2. Suffredini A, Qureshi GD. Concomitant hemophilia and thrombocytopenia. JAMA 1982; 247:2497-8.
3. Wajima T, Maloney TR. Acute idiopathic thrombocytopenic purpura in patients with hemophilia A. Blood 1981; 58: Suppl:208A. abstract.
4. Doan CA, Bouroncle BA, Wiseman BK. Idiopathic and secondary thrombocytopenic purpura: clinical study and evaluation of 381 cases over a period of 28 years. Ann Intern Med 1960; 53:861-76.
5. Kunicki TJ, Koenig MB, Kristopeit SM, Aster RH. Direct quantitation of platelet-associated IgG by electroimmunoassay. Blood 1982. 60:54-8.
6. von dem Borne AEGK, Verheugt FWA, Oosterhof, von Riesz E, Brutel de la Rivière A, Engelfriet CP. A simple immunofluorescence test for detection of platelet antibodies. Br J Haematol 1978; 39:195-207.
7. Aster RH, Enright SE. A platelet and granulocyte membrane defect in paroxysmal nocturnal hemoglobinuria: usefulness for the detection of platelet antibodies. J Clin Invest 1969; 48:1199-210.
8. *Pneumocystis carinii* pneuomonia among persons with hemophilia A. MMWR 1982; 31:365-7.
9. Update on acquired immunodeficiency syndrome (AIDS) among patients with hemophilia A. MMWR 1982; 31:644-6, 652.

10. Lederman MM, Ratnoff OD, Scillian JJ, Jones PK, Schacter B. Impaired cell-mediated immunity in patients with classic hemophilia. N Engl J Med 1983; 308:79-83.
11. Menitove JE, Aster RH, Casper JT, et al. T-lymphocyte subpopulations in patients with hemophilia treated with cryoprecipitate and lyophilized concentrates. N Engl J Med 1983; 308:83-6.
12. Weintrub P, Ammann AJ, Abrams DI, et al. Altered T-cell immunity in hemophiliacs receiving frequent factor VIII concentrate. Blood 1982; 60:Suppl 1:224a. abstract.
13. Morris L, Distenfeld A, Amorosi E, Karpatkin S. Autoimmune thrombocytopenic purpura in homosexual men. Ann Intern Med 1982; 96: 714-7.

MEDICAL INTELLIGENCE

IMMUNOLOGIC DYSFUNCTION IN INFANTS INFECTED THROUGH TRANSFUSION WITH HTLV-III

RANDOLPH F. WYKOFF, M.D., ELLIOTT R. PEARL, M.D., AND FRANK T. SAULSBURY, M.D.

COMPELLING evidence implicates human T-cell lymphotropic virus Type III (HTLV-III) as the etiologic agent of the acquired immunodeficiency syndrome (AIDS).[1-3] HTLV-III has also been associated with a syndrome of persistent lymphadenopathy and with mild immune dysfunction in adults.[4]

We report on three infants with transfusion-acquired HTLV-III infection who had a variety of illnesses. This report confirms that HTLV-III can be transmitted by means of blood transfusion and indicates that infection with the retrovirus can cause a broad spectrum of diseases in infants.

CASE REPORTS

Patient 1

A 3100-g white male infant was transferred to our Neonatal Intensive Care Unit on the second day of life because of a pneumothorax and respiratory distress. He received two blood transfusions during the first week because of anemia. Hepatosplenomegaly was noted at four months of age, but no cause was found. Weight gain ceased at the age of six months. He was readmitted to our hospital at nine months because of pneumonia.

Physical examination revealed an underweight infant. Tonsils and cervical lymph nodes were present; he had oral and perineal candidiasis and hepatosplenomegaly. Coarse rhonchi were heard in all lung fields. A chest radiograph showed diffuse interstitial infiltrates; no thymus was visible despite the fact that a thymic silhouette was present on chest radiographs at one week and at four months of age. A lung-biopsy specimen was positive for *Pneumocystis carinii*. Serologic tests for cytomegalovirus, Epstein–Barr virus, and hepatitis B virus were negative.

The patient was persistently lymphopenic for his age and had an abnormal ratio of lymphocyte subpopulations (Table 1). Blood mononuclear cells proliferated in vitro when stimulated with phytohemagglutinin and pokeweed mitogens but gave suboptimal responses to concanavalin A. His serum showed polyclonal hyperimmunoglobulinemia, with normal agglutinin titers to human and sheep erythrocytes, but antibody to tetanus toxoid was undetectable despite two prior immunizations. Assays for erythrocyte adenosine deaminase and purine nucleoside phosphorylase were normal.

At 11 months of age panhypogammaglobulinemia developed, and the infant had a marked T-lymphocyte deficiency. Despite therapy with antibiotics and immunoglobulin infusions, his condition deteriorated, and he died at 14 months of age. At postmortem examination, the thymus was small (2 g) and dysplastic and lacked Hassall's corpuscles. The lymph nodes and spleen showed disordered architecture and lacked lymphoid follicles and periarteriolar lymphoid cells. Follicles and germinal centers were likewise absent in the gastrointestinal tract. There was no evidence of graft versus host disease or of lymphoid-cell infiltration of tissues.

Patient 2

A 1090-g white female infant remained in the Neonatal Intensive Care Unit for her first two months of life because of respiratory distress. During that time she received 25 blood transfusions.

She was readmitted to our hospital at nine months of age because of anemia. Physical examination disclosed a pale infant with cutaneous petechiae and purpura. She had generalized lymph-node enlargement, hepatosplenomegaly, and oral candidiasis. The hematocrit was 27 percent. She had thrombocytopenia (5000 to 15,000 platelets per cubic millimeter) and neutropenia (500 to 1000 neutrophils per cubic millimeter). She had no serologic evidence of Epstein–Barr viral infection, and a urine culture for cytomegalovirus was negative. A direct Coombs' test and a test for antinuclear antibody were positive. A test for platelet antibodies was positive, but a test for neutrophil antibodies was negative. She had polyclonal hyperimmunoglobulinemia (Table 1). The platelet and neutrophil counts rose with glucocorticoid therapy, which was slowly tapered over six months. When last seen, at 20 months of age, the patient was well, but the direct Coombs' test was still positive.

Patient 3

A 3100-g black female infant was stained with meconium at birth, and respiratory distress developed. During her four-week stay in the Neonatal Intensive Care Unit, she received 10 blood transfusions.

She was readmitted to our hospital at four months of age because of chronic diarrhea and weight loss. Physical examination revealed a thin infant with generalized lymph-node enlargement and hepatosplenomegaly. Serologic tests for Epstein–Barr virus, cytomegalovirus, and hepatitis B virus were negative. Immunologic studies (Table 1) showed polyclonal hyperimmunoglobulinemia and an altered ratio of T-lymphocyte subpopulations. Lymph-node enlargement, lymphocytosis, and hyperimmunoglobulinemia have persisted, but the diarrhea has abated.

EPIDEMIOLOGIC STUDIES

The three patients were in the Neonatal Intensive Care Unit at the same time, and all three received blood transfusions. We determined that the infants each received a single transfusion from a common donor. The only other patient in our hospital who received blood from this donor was an infant in the Pediatric Intensive Care Unit, in whom neutropenia developed two weeks after she had received the transfusion from the common donor. She was discharged shortly thereafter and was lost to follow-up.

We reviewed the records of 34 other infants who were in the Neonatal Intensive Care Unit at the same time as our patients. Nineteen of the 34 received blood transfusions, but none received blood from the donor in question. None of the 34 infants had subsequent illnesses similar to those observed in our patients.

With the cooperation of the American Red Cross Blood Service, we learned that the common blood donor was a healthy person, but we do not know whether the donor was a member of an AIDS risk group. Analyses of donor blood in Dr. Robert Gallo's laboratory at the National Cancer Institute disclosed an abnormal helper/suppressor T-cell ratio (0.75) and the presence of serum antibodies to HTLV-III. The retrovirus was subsequently isolated from donor blood lymphocytes, transmitted to secondary target cells, and reisolated from the secondary culture.[1] With this information, serum samples from our patients (obtained 10 to 11 months after transfusion) were analyzed in Dr. Gallo's laboratory, and all were found to be positive for antibody to HTLV-III.

DISCUSSION

Not long after AIDS was described, epidemiologic evidence indicated that the disease was probably caused by an infectious agent.[5-9] AIDS appeared to be caused by an agent that could be transmitted by a

From the Department of Pediatrics, University of Virginia Medical Center, Charlottesville, Va.

Table 1. Immunologic Findings in Three Infants with Transfusion-Associated HTLV-III.*

Patient No.	Age (Mo)	Immunoglobulins†			Lymphocytes‡					
		IgM	IgG	IgA	total	T3	T4	T8	B1	T4/T8
1	4	ND	ND	ND	7,470	ND	ND	ND	ND	ND
	9	313	984	253	1,650	61	31	27	3	1.15
	11§	7	322	9	1,480	25	0.5	9	46	0.06
2	9	390	4400	138	3,900	ND	ND	ND	ND	ND
	12¶	137	4090	82	3,600	38	16	13	46	1.23
3	4	302	2040	258	18,750	57	16	35	24	0.46
	14	71	2440	168	8,418	ND	ND	ND	ND	ND

*ND denotes not done.

†Serum immunoglobulins were measured by laser nephelometry, and the values are expressed as milligrams per deciliter. In one-year-old children the normal values for IgM, IgG, and IgA, respectively, are 41 to 149, 345 to 1213, and 16 to 84 mg per deciliter.

‡Total lymphocytes are expressed as cells per cubic millimeter of blood. The proportions of cells reactive with monoclonal antibodies against T lymphocytes (OKT3, total T cells; OKT4, helper/inducer T cells; OKT8, suppressor/cytotoxic T cells [Ortho Pharmaceuticals], and B lymphocytes [B1, Coulter Electronics] are expressed as percentages of lymphocytes.

§Immunologic studies were performed three weeks after treatment with an intravenous infusion of gamma globulin.

¶Immunologic studies were performed while the patient was receiving prednisone (1.5 mg per kilogram of body weight per day).

variety of routes, including transmission by sexual contact,[5,6] by blood products,[7] and from mothers to infants.[8,9] Seroepidemiologic studies have subsequently provided compelling evidence that HTLV-III is the etiologic agent of AIDS.[3] Although sexual transmission of HTLV-III has recently been documented,[6] other modes of transmission remain to be confirmed. The present report provides evidence that HTLV-III can be transmitted by means of blood transfusions from an infected asymptomatic donor, and that it can produce clinical disease in the recipients of such blood.

The presence of serum antibody to HTLV-III is believed to be diagnostic of AIDS or to indicate a serious risk of the disease.[3] Antibody to the virus is virtually never present in the serum of healthy adults who are not members of AIDS risk groups.[3,10] Although there are no comparable data concerning HTLV-III antibody in healthy children, there is no reason to suspect that the antibody status of normal children is different from that of normal adults.

The mothers of our patients were not tested for HTLV-III antibody, but maternal transmission was exceedingly unlikely, since none of the mothers were members of an AIDS risk group, nor did they have sexual partners at risk for AIDS. Thus, we conclude that our patients contracted HTLV-III infection through transfusion of blood from a common donor who was asymptomatically infected with HTLV-III.

Our patients had variable manifestations of HTLV-III infection. One had AIDS, one had autoimmune disease, and one had persistent lymph-node enlargement. In adults, HTLV-III infection may be asymptomatic, or it may result in a variety of clinical syndromes, including persistent lymphadenopathy, mild immune dysfunction, and AIDS.[4] Although immunodeficiency and persistent lymphadenopathy are prominent features of childhood AIDS,[8,9] autoimmune disease has received scant attention. In a report on 14 children with AIDS, Scott et al.[11] indicated that a few patients had autoimmune features. The present report documents that HTLV-III infection in infants can cause a variety of clinical syndromes, including autoimmune disease.

The determinants of the clinical features of HTLV-III infection are unknown, but the host's age and genetically determined immune responses, the mode of transmission, and other environmental factors may influence the ultimate expression of the infection. In animal models, clinical diversity is characteristic of infection with a number of retroviruses manifested by immunodeficiency and autoimmune syndromes.[12] In the case of feline leukemia virus, the pattern of disease expression is clearly linked to the maturity of the host, with immature animals more susceptible to progressive and symptomatic infection.[13]

Now that HTLV-III has been identified as the probable cause of AIDS, it is possible to confirm the modes of transmission and document the spectrum of clinical disorders caused by this agent.

We are indebted to Dr. Robert Stickley for referring Patient 1 for evaluation; to Drs. Paul Mintz and Deborah Douglas, University of Virginia Blood Bank, and Dr. Paul McCurdy, American Red Cross Blood Services, for their cooperation; to Dr. C. Ronald Scott for performing erythrocyte enzyme analyses; to Dr. John Sullivan for performing studies of Epstein–Barr viral antibody; to Dr. Robert C. Gallo and his colleagues for sharing their findings; and to Ms. Judy Smith for assistance in preparing the manuscript.

References

1. Popovic M, Sarngadharan MG, Read E, Gallo RC. Detection, isolation, and continuous production of cytopathic retroviruses (HTLV-III) from patients with AIDS and pre-AIDS. Science 1984; 224:497-500.
2. Gallo RC, Salahuddin SZ, Popovic M, et al. Frequent detection and isolation of cytopathic retroviruses (HTLV-III) from patients with AIDS and at risk for AIDS. Science 1984; 224:500-3.
3. Safai B, Sarngadharan MG, Groopman JE, et al. Seroepidemiological studies of human T-lymphotropic retrovirus type III in acquired immunodeficiency syndrome. Lancet 1984; 1:1438-40.
4. Goedert JJ, Sarngadharan MG, Biggar RJ, et al. Determinants of retrovirus (HTLV-III) antibody and immunodeficiency conditions in homosexual men. Lancet 1984; 2:711-6.
5. Harris C, Small CB, Klein RS, et al. Immunodeficiency in female sexual partners of men with the acquired immunodeficiency syndrome. N Engl J Med 1983; 308:1181-4.
6. Gazzard BG, Shanson DC, Farthing C, et al. Clinical findings and serological evidence of HTLV-III infection in homosexual contacts of patients with AIDS and persistent generalized lymphadenopathy in London. Lancet 1984; 2:480-3.
7. Curran JW, Lawrence DN, Jaffe H, et al. Acquired immunodeficiency syndrome (AIDS) associated with transfusions. N Engl J Med 1984; 310:69-75.
8. Oleske J, Minnefor A, Cooper R Jr, et al. Immune deficiency syndrome in children. JAMA 1983; 249:2345-9.
9. Cowan MJ, Hellmann D, Chudwin D, Wara DW, Chang RS, Ammann AJ. Maternal transmission of acquired immune deficiency syndrome. Pediatrics 1984; 73:382-6.
10. Cheingsong-Popov R, Weiss RA, Dalgleish A, et al. Prevalence of antibody to human T-lymphotropic virus type III in AIDS and AIDS-risk patients in Britain. Lancet 1984; 2:477-80.

11. Scott GB, Buck BE, Leterman JG, Bloom FL, Parks WP. Acquired immunodeficiency syndrome in infants. N Engl J Med 1984; 310:76-81.
12. Teich N, Wyke J, Mak T, Bernstein A, Hardy W. Pathogenesis of retrovirus-induced disease. In: Weiss R, Teich N, Varmus H, Coffin J, eds. Molecular biology of tumor viruses. RNA tumor viruses. 2nd ed. Cold Spring Harbor, N.Y.: Cold Spring Harbor Laboratory, 1982:785-998.
13. Hoover EA, Rojko JL, Olsen RG. Host-virus interactions in progressive versus regressive feline leukemia virus infection in cats. In: Essex M, Todaro G, zur Hausen H, eds. Viruses in naturally occurring cancers. Cold Spring Harbor, N.Y.: Cold Spring Harbor Laboratory, 1980:635-51.

CORRESPONDENCE

AGGRESSIVE KAPOSI'S SARCOMA IN A HETEROSEXUAL DRUG ADDICT

To the Editor: Recently described cases of aggressive lymphadenopathic and visceral Kaposi's sarcoma in the United States have occurred in homosexual men.[1-3] We have observed a similar case in a heterosexual drug addict.

A 28-year-old man was admitted for evaluation of fever and lymphadenopathy. During the preceding month he had noted progressively enlarging cervical lymph nodes, fever, drenching night sweats, a weight loss of 9 kg, and a sore throat. He had a 14-year history of addiction to cocaine and intravenous heroin, but he denied using amyl nitrate. On repeated questioning he denied having any homosexual contact, although he had had multiple heterosexual partners. The sexual history was confirmed by independent discussions with several of the patient's friends. He had no history of major infectious illnesses. On physical examination the temperature was 38.3° C. The tonsils were massively enlarged, and a shaggy exudate with rolled edges was noted on the right tonsil. There were multiple hard, matted, bilateral cervical lymph nodes, as well as enlarged axillary and inguinal nodes. There was no hepatosplenomegaly, and the remainder of the examination was unremarkable. Several days after admission oral candidiasis developed. Also, during the first week a violaceous nodule 2 cm in diameter appeared behind the right ear. At admission the white-cell count was 8900, with 54 percent neutrophils, 39 percent lymphocytes, and 7 percent monocytes. Studies of T-lymphocyte subsets of peripheral-blood lymphocytes (kindly performed by Yolene Thomas, Ph.D.) using indirect immunofluorescence and cytofluorograph analysis demonstrated an OKT4+/OKT8+ T-cell ratio of 0.37. A Monospot slide test for infectious mononucleosis and a Venereal Disease Research Laboratory test were negative. Sections of a biopsied cervical lymph node revealed a dense proliferation of spindle-shaped cells that extended irregularly in various directions, frequently lining slit-like spaces that were filled with erythrocytes. There were areas with numerous capillaries of various sizes. The stroma contained hemosiderin deposits and infiltrates of mixed lymphoplasmacytic cells. These findings were consistent with Kaposi's sarcoma. A course of combination chemotherapy and local radiotherapy was begun.

The form of Kaposi's sarcoma in this patient and in the previously described cases in homosexuals[1-3] is in marked contrast to the typical manifestations of this disease in earlier series of North American patients.[4] The explanation for the apparently increased incidence of Kaposi's sarcoma in male homosexuals is not known, although a role for an acquired immunodeficiency state has been postulated.[5] Such a condition may also be present in some heterosexual drug addicts, at least those who acquire opportunistic infections.[2] It may be relevant that our patient had an alteration in peripheral-blood T-lymphocyte subsets that was similar to that noted by Koziner et al.[6]

The development of Kaposi's sarcoma in a heterosexual drug addict suggests that factors not limited to homosexuals may be implicated in the origin of this illness and that the population at risk may be larger than was initially suspected.

Kenneth D. Gold, M.D.,
Louys Thomas, M.D.,
and T.J. Garrett, M.D.
Harlem Hospital Center
New York, NY 10037

References

1. Hymes KB, Cheung T, Greene JB, et al. Kaposi's sarcoma in homosexual men — a report of eight cases. Lancet 1981; 2:598-600.
2. Masur H, Michelis MA, Greene JB, et al. An outbreak of community-acquired Pneumocystis carinii pneumonia: initial manifestation of cellular immune dysfunction. N Engl J Med 1981; 305:1431-8.
3. Case Records of the Massachusetts General Hospital (Case 11-1982). N Engl J Med 1982; 306:657-68.
4. DiGiovanna JJ, Safai B. Kaposi's sarcoma: retrospective study of 90 cases with particular emphasis on the familial occurrence, ethnic background and prevalence of other diseases. Am J Med 1981; 71:779-83.
5. Durack DT. Opportunistic infections and Kaposi's sarcoma in homosexual men. N Engl J Med 1981; 305:1465-7.
6. Koziner B, Denny T, Myskowski PL, Kris M, Safai B. Opportunistic infections and Kaposi's sarcoma in homosexual men. N Engl J Med 1982; 306:933-4.

HTLV-III EXPOSURE DURING CARDIOPULMONARY RESUSCITATION

To the Editor: There have been no confirmed occupation-related cases of AIDS in health care workers in the United States.[1] We have been following two nurses who participated in mouth-to-mouth resuscitation of a patient with the AIDS-related complex, who was positive for human T-cell lymphotropic virus Type III/lymphadenopathy-associated virus (HTLV-III/LAV), and we here report their seronegativity nine months after exposure.

A 28-year-old man who had classic hemophilia treated with factor VIII concentrates and was known to abuse oral analgesics intravenously was diagnosed as having AIDS-related complex on the basis of viral isolation, leukopenia, weight loss, and persistent adenopathy. HTLV-III/LAV infection of his peripheral-blood lymphocytes was demonstrated by reverse transcriptase activity, immunofluorescence, and electron microscopy.[2] He had no history of fever, opportunistic infection, or persistent inversion of the T-helper/T-suppressor ratio.

Eighteen months after viral isolation, during a hospitalization for hemophilic arthropathy, the patient was found in cardiopulmonary arrest in his bathroom. Two nurses began mouth-to-mouth resuscitation, each delivering approximately 20 breaths before the patient was intubated. Resuscitation efforts were unsuccessful. Evaluation of the patient's lymph nodes at autopsy revealed a marked depletion of lymphoid elements, and pulmonary pathological studies were suggestive of the recent infusion of solubilized medications. He was positive for HTLV-III/LAV antibody by Western blot analysis[3] (performed by J.S. McDougal and M.S. Kennedy, Centers for Disease Control) at the time of his death.

These two nurses with documented mucous-membrane exposure to potentially infective saliva from a patient with AIDS-related complex have been followed prospectively for nine months. Initial samples as well as eight subsequent samples for each nurse have been negative for HTLV-III/LAV antibody. The nurses' initial physical examinations, lymphocyte counts, and T-helper/T-suppressor ratios were within normal ranges. All clinical and laboratory indexes remain stable at this writing.

Cells producing HTLV-III/LAV and cell-free viral particles have been recovered from the oral secretions of patients with AIDS-related complex,[4] suggesting that saliva may serve as a vehicle for transmission. If this mode of transmission were important, however, one might expect a higher rate of seropositivity among the spouses of patients with AIDS.[5] Although we cannot confirm that this patient with hemophilia had infectious disease at the time of resuscitation, rates of persistent viremia in persons seropositive for HTLV-III/LAV appear to be high.[6,7] This case provides further evidence that the risk of seroconversion after a point exposure to the oral secretions of an infected person is probably quite low. It should still be recommended, however, that a disposable ventilating bag and oral airway be kept at the bedside of a patient with AIDS or AIDS-related complex, to avoid mucous-membrane exposure in the event of cardiopulmonary arrest.[8]

Susan M. Saviteer, M.D., Gilbert C. White, M.D., and Myron S. Cohen, M.D.
University of North Carolina School of Medicine
Chapel Hill, NC 27514

Janine Jason, M.D.
Centers for Disease Control
Atlanta, GA 30333

References

1. McCray E, Winslow N, Solomon SL, et al. Prospective evaluation of health-care workers with parenteral or mucous membrane exposure to blood from patients with AIDS, United States: an update. Proceedings of the International Conference on AIDS. Atlanta: Department of Health and Human Resources and the World Health Organization, 1985:45.
2. Popovic M, Sarngadharan MG, Read E, Gallo RC. Detection, isolation, and continuous production of cytopathic retroviruses (HTLV-III) from patients with AIDS and pre-AIDS. Science 1984; 224:497-500.
3. Tsang VC, Peralta JM, Simons AR. Enzyme-linked immunoelectrotransfer blot techniques (EITB) for studying the specificities of antigens and antibodies separated by gel electrophoresis. Methods Enzymol 1983; 92:377-91.
4. Groopman JE, Salahuddin SZ, Sarngadharan MG, et al. HTLV-III in saliva of people with AIDS-related complex and healthy homosexual men at risk for AIDS. Science 1984; 226:447-9.
5. Redfield RR, Markham PD, Salahuddin SZ, et al. Frequent transmission of HTLV-III among spouses of patients with AIDS-related complex and AIDS. JAMA 1985; 253:1571-3.
6. Jaffe HW, Feorino PM, Darrow WW, et al. Persistent infection with human T-lymphotropic virus type III/lymphadenopathy-associated virus in apparently healthy homosexual men. Ann Intern Med 1985; 102:627-8.
7. Gomperts ED, Feorino PM, Evatt BL, et al. LAV HTLV-III presence in peripheral blood lymphocytes of seropositive young hemophiliacs. Blood (in press).
8. Advisory Committee on Infections within Hospitals — American Hospital Association. A hospitalwide approach to AIDS. Infect Control 1984; 5: 242-8.

RISK OF AIDS WITH ARTIFICIAL INSEMINATION

To the Editor: On September 14, 1984, the Privacy Committee of New South Wales advised the Department of Health in New South Wales that a moratorium should be imposed on the use of male homosexuals as sperm donors in artificial-insemination programs.

Male homosexuals were known to be donors in the programs. Also, in the light of the knowledge about the acquired immunodeficiency syndrome (AIDS) at that time, the health risk to recipients in these programs was uncertain. No screening programs for antibodies to the human T-cell lymphotropic virus Type III (HTLV-III) were then available. A moratorium was initiated in October 1984 and lifted in April 1985, when screening for antibodies to HTLV-III was introduced for sperm donors as well as for blood donors.

In July 1985, four women in an artificial-insemination program in New South Wales were found to have antibodies to HTLV-III, and lymphadenopathy developed in one of them. The source of their exposure was identified as a semen donor who had participated in the program before the moratorium. It is reassuring that other programs for artificial insemination are now introducing the screening of semen donors for antibodies to HTLV-III (June 20 issue).*

The Privacy Committee is an independent statutory committee that acts as ombudsman for privacy and investigates and advises on issues concerning privacy. The committee has given advice on confidentiality and privacy in relation to AIDS, including such issues as testing for antibodies, blood donation, semen donation, and research.

Jacqueline Morgan, M.B.,B.S., M.Sc.Soc., and Jim Nolan, B.A., B.Leg.S.
Box 6, G.P.O.
Sydney, New South Wales 2001, Australia

*Schiff I, Correia B, Ravnikar VA, Schur PH. HTLV-III antibody testing in sperm donors. N Engl J Med 1985; 312:1638.

Clinical Studies

Experimental Treatment and General Follow-Up

MEDICAL INTELLIGENCE

PRELIMINARY OBSERVATIONS ON THE EFFECT OF RECOMBINANT LEUKOCYTE A INTERFERON IN HOMOSEXUAL MEN WITH KAPOSI'S SARCOMA

Susan E. Krown, M.D., Francisco X. Real, M.D., Susanna Cunningham-Rundles, Ph.D., Patricia L. Myskowski, M.D., Benjamin Koziner, M.D., Seymour Fein, M.D., Abraham Mittelman, M.D., Herbert F. Oettgen, M.D., and Bijan Safai, M.D.

PRELIMINARY clinical trials have shown that both natural and recombinant-DNA-produced human interferons are occasionally capable of inhibiting the growth of some tumors.[1-4] Although the tumors responding to interferon have most often been those without evidence for a viral association, case reports have appeared of therapeutic effects in patients with nasopharyngeal carcinoma,[5] for which there is strong serologic evidence supporting a viral association, and in patients with laryngeal papilloma,[6] for which the available evidence supports a viral pathogenesis. Interferons have also been shown to modify the course of chronic viral infections in human beings, including infections induced by hepatitis B virus[7] and by cytomegalovirus.[8]

Recently, a syndrome of cellular immunodeficiency, susceptibility to opportunistic infection, and the development of Kaposi's sarcoma has been described,[9-11] which primarily afflicts young homosexual men. Although the reasons for this outbreak are unclear, persistent cytomegalovirus infection has been considered as a possible cause of both the immunodeficiency and the sarcoma in these patients.[12,13] This preliminary report describes the effects of recombinant leukocyte A interferon (IFLrA), a purified human interferon produced by recombinant-DNA techniques, on tumor growth and immune function in 13 patients treated during the course of a Phase I trial of this agent. Of 12 evaluable patients, 5 had major objective responses (3 complete and 2 partial), and 3 others had minor temporary responses. Our data suggest that interferon may prove to be useful in the treatment of Kaposi's sarcoma in immunosuppressed patients.

Methods

IFLrA (supplied by Hoffmann–La Roche) was prepared from *Escherichia coli* as previously described.[14,15] The molecular weight of IFLrA was estimated to be 19,241 daltons[15]; the specific activity was 2×10^8 to 4×10^8 U per milligram of protein.

All patients had measurable, biopsy-confirmed Kaposi's sarcoma. Patients were evaluated by means of a physical examination; upper and lower gastrointestinal endoscopy with estimation of the number of gastrointestinal lesions; chest x-ray films; complete blood count; studies of blood urea nitrogen, creatinine, serum calcium, phosphorus, uric acid, total protein, albumin, total bilirubin, serum aspartate aminotransferase, alkaline phosphatase, and lactic dehydrogenase; determination of the prothrombin time; and urinalysis. Serum samples were obtained periodically for measurement of antibodies to herpes simplex virus, cytomegalovirus, and Epstein–Barr viral capsid antigen and for hepatitis B surface antigen and antibody.

Immunocompetence was assessed in vivo by means of skin tests with dermatophytin-O, mumps, tuberculin, and streptokinase–streptodornase antigens, and sensitization and challenge with 2,4-dinitrochlorobenzene as previously described.[16] For in vitro evaluation of immune function, mononuclear cells were separated from heparinized venous blood by centrifugation on Ficoll–Isopaque. T cells were counted by rosette formation with sheep erythrocytes after incubation at 4°C for one hour. The percentage of mononuclear cells binding mouse monoclonal antibodies OKT4 and OKT8 (Ortho Pharmaceutical, Raritan, N.J.) was determined by indirect-immunofluorescence analysis on a cytofluorograph system 30L (Ortho Instruments). Lymphocyte proliferation was measured by incorporation of [^{14}C]thymidine in response to stimulation with phytohemagglutinin.[17] The natural cytotoxicity of peripheral-blood mononuclear cells against K562 target cells was determined with a four-hour ^{51}Cr-release assay.[18] In some patients, the ability of IFLrA to augment natural cytotoxicity before treatment was tested in vitro by addition of 800 units of IFLrA to 10^6 mononuclear cells in 0.225-ml cultures.

Serum interferon titers were measured by means of a modified bioassay with MDBK cells (a bovine kidney-cell line) as targets and with vesicular stomatitis virus.[19] A modification of the bioassay was used to test for the development of neutralizing antibodies to IFLrA.[4]

After the patients had given written informed consent, they were treated with daily intramuscular injections of IFLrA for 28 days. The daily dose of IFLrA was either 36×10^6 U (nine patients) or 54×10^6 U (four patients). Patients with evidence of tumor regression or stable disease at the end of the first 28 days continued to receive treatment with IFLrA at the same dose three days a week.

A complete response was defined as complete disappearance of all signs and symptoms of disease for at least one month, confirmed by biopsy of skin and node lesions and, when appropriate, by endoscopy. A partial response was defined as at least a 50 percent decrease in the totals of the sizes of all measurable skin, nodal, and oral mucosal lesions, lasting for at least one month, without progression of gastrointestinal disease and without the appearance of new lesions or an increase in the size of any lesion. The size of each lesion was taken to be the product of the longest dimension and the maximum dimension perpendicular to it. A minor response was defined as at least a 25 percent (but less than 50 percent) decrease in the totals of the sizes of all measurable skin, nodal, and oral mucosal lesions, lasting for at least one month, or as a greater regression of disease that persisted for less than one month. (The only patient with a minor response who had gastrointestinal involvement had progression of disease before his gastrointestinal tract was reevaluated.) Progression was defined as at least a 25 percent increase in the size of any lesion or the appearance of any new lesions. Patients were considered evaluable for response if they completed four weeks of treatment. Complete and partial responses were considered major objective responses.

From the Clinical Immunology, Dermatology, and Hematology/Lymphoma Services, Department of Medicine, Memorial Sloan–Kettering Cancer Center, New York, and the Department of Medical Oncology and Immunology, Hoffmann–La Roche, Nutley, N.J.

Supported in part by a grant (CA-08748) from the National Cancer Institute. Dr. Real is a fellow of the Spanish Ministry of Culture.

Table 1. Extent of Kaposi's Sarcoma, Tumor Burden, Duration of Treatment, and Response to IFLrA.

Patient No.	Organs Involved*				Estimated Tumor Burden†	Duration of Treatment	Time Since Last Dose of IFLrA	Status at Last Follow-up	Therapeutic Response
	Skin	Lymph Nodes	Oral Mucosa	Gastrointestinal Tract					
1	+	+	+	+	Moderate	6 mo	10 mo‡	Alive, no evidence of disease	Complete
2	+	−	−	−	Minimal	4 mo	7 mo‡	Alive, no evidence of disease	Complete
3	+	+	+	−	Moderate	10 mo	6 wk‡	Alive, no evidence of disease	Complete
4	+	+	−	−	Moderate	4 mo	5 mo†	Dead	Partial
5	+	+	+	+	Large	12 mo	On treatment‡	Alive, residual disease	Partial
6	+	+	−	−	Moderate	3 mo	9 mo‡	Alive, residual disease	Minor
7	+	+	+	+	Large	11 wk	9 mo‡	Alive, residual disease	Minor
8	+	+	−	−	Moderate	8 wk	6 mo†	Dead	Minor
9	+	+	+	+	Large	3 mo	5 mo†	Dead	Progression
10	+	+	−	+	Moderate	9 wk	11 mo‡	Alive, residual disease	Progression
11	+	+	−	−	Large	7 wk	5 mo†	Dead	Progression
12	+	−	−	+	Moderate	8 wk	5 mo†	Dead	Progression
13	+	+	−	−	Moderate	9 days	6 wk†	Dead	Not evaluable

*+ denotes organ involved, and − organ not involved.

†Minimal denotes ≤20 skin lesions, without lymph-node, oral mucosal, or gastrointestinal involvement; moderate >20 but ≤50 skin lesions or ≤20 gastrointestinal lesions (or both), with or without lymph-node or oral mucosal involvement (or both); and large >50 skin lesions or >20 gastrointestinal lesions (or both), with or without lymph-node or oral mucosal involvement (or both).

‡Patient alive at last follow-up.

Results

The patients were all homosexual or bisexual men who were 32 to 50 years old. The extent of disease, estimation of tumor burden, duration of treatment, and response are summarized in Table 1. All patients had measurable skin lesions and enlarged lymph nodes, and some had evaluable lesions involving the oral mucosa (five patients), the stomach (four patients), or both the stomach and colon (two patients). A lymph-node biopsy showed Kaposi's sarcoma in 11 patients, and lymphoid hyperplasia without characteristic lesions of the sarcoma in 2.

Two patients had been treated previously for Kaposi's sarcoma, without response. One had been treated with a partially purified human alpha interferon six months before the trial. He then received 400 rad of total-skin electron-beam radiation and an investigational antiviral agent, 2′fluoro,5-iodo-ara-cytosine. The other patient had also been treated previously with this agent.

One patient, who had been treated for only nine days, was not considered evaluable for therapeutic response. He was febrile before and during treatment, and was subsequently found to have cerebral toxoplasmosis. Of the 12 evaluable patients, 5 had a major objective response (3 had a complete response, and 2 a partial response), 3 had a minor response, and 4 had disease progression. A complete response occurred in one patient with lesions confined to the skin; in another with involvement of the skin, lymph nodes, oral mucosa, and stomach; and in a third with skin, oral mucosal, and node lesions. The first two of these three patients were treated for 4 and 6 months, respectively, and remained free of disease 7 and 10 months after the end of treatment. The third had a complete response that was confirmed after 9 months, stopped treatment after 10 months, and remained disease-free 6 weeks later. Partial responses were observed in one patient with hundreds of skin lesions, as well as lymph-node, oral mucosal, gastric, and colonic involvement, and in another with skin and lymph-node disease only. In the first of these two patients a partial response (including over 90 percent regression of skin lesions and complete regression of gastric lesions) continued during maintenance therapy for 12 months after initiation of treatment. In the second patient interferon treatment was discontinued because of bacterial pneumonia and exacerbations of preexisting renal tubular acidosis. After treatment was stopped new lesions from the sarcoma developed on the skin, and primary lymphoma subsequently developed in the brain, which led to death 10 months after the start of treatment. At autopsy, Kaposi's sarcoma was confined to the skin.

Minor responses were observed in three patients during the first month of treatment. However, when the dosage schedule was changed in the second month from seven to three times a week, new lesions appeared. In the four remaining patients the disease was stable during the first month of daily treatment, but new skin lesions developed during the second month. Biopsy of regressing skin lesions showed a variable degree of perivascular lymphocytic infiltration in all patients.

Side effects, similar to those reported previously with both partially purified and recombinant-DNA-produced interferons,[1-4] included fever, chills, weakness, fatigue, anorexia, headache, myalgias, and joint pain. Hair loss and paresthesias occurred infrequent-

Table 2. Results of Pretreatment Immunologic Evaluation.*

Patient No.	Skin Tests		Serum Immunoglobulins				Sheep Erythrocyte Rosettes	OKT4/OKT8 Ratio	Natural Killer-Cell Activity	Response to PHA	Therapeutic Response
	DNCB	Antigens	IgG	IgA	IgM	IgE					
		positive tests/ total tests	*mg/dl*	*mg/dl*	*mg/dl*	*IU/ml*	*%*		*% specific ^{51}Cr release*	*cpm*	
1	−	0/4	1262	242	238	27	81	1.37	14.3	15,130	Complete
2	+	1/4	1137	154	150	44	65	0.87	14.7	17,998	Complete
3	+	1/3†	1118	113	129	217	83	0.82	19.2	5,543	Complete
4	+	0/4	1555	351	200	94	61	0	19.2	5,917	Partial
5	−	0/4	1882	152	140	205	80	1.54	14.0	10,828	Partial
6	−	0/4	ND	ND	ND	ND	80	1.61	21.5	18,788	Minor
7	−	0/4	2777	822	162	ND	73	ND	14.0	4,044	Minor
8	−	1/4	2483	872	184	22	70	0.76	29.3	9,958	Minor
9	−	0/4	1335	380	151	ND	84	0	14.0	854	Progression
10	+	0/4	2757	215	125	16	73	0.35	21.3	9,094	Progression
11	ND	ND	1900	365	85	ND	68	0.56	2.0	13,736	Progression
12	ND	ND	1466	264	272	53	86	0.38	14.5	7,181	Progression
13	ND	ND	1518	503	461	12	82	0	11.0	1,129	Not evaluable
Normal values‡	+	3–4/4	800–1800	90–450	60–250	10–400	72±11	1.83 ±0.27	>14.7	>17,000	

*DNCB denotes dinitrochlorobenzene, PHA phytohemagglutinin, and ND not done.

†Mumps skin test not done.

‡*Serum immunoglobulins* — historical controls, with use of commercial radial-immunodiffusion plates (Behring Diagnostics); *sheep erythrocyte rosettes* — mean ±SD for 180 normal, adult, blood-bank donors; *OKT4/OKT8 ratio* — mean ±SD for 45 normal blood donors and hospital personnel (not matched for age or sex) studied during the same time period; *natural killer-cell activity* — lowest level observed among 59 healthy controls.[18] Among 42 age-matched and sex-matched healthy hospital personnel studied in parallel with this patient group, the range of activity was 15.1 to 76.3 percent; *response to PHA* — mean −2 SD for 36 normal controls.[17] Among 42 age-matched and sex-matched healthy hospital personnel studied in parallel with this patient group, the range of response was 16,798 to 28,450 cpm.

ly. Orthostatic hypotension was observed in several patients. The mean nadir for the white-cell count was 2200 per cubic millimeter (range, 1300 to 4900); in 10 patients the lowest granulocyte count was under 1000 cells per cubic millimeter. However, after an initial decrease, blood counts often stabilized or increased despite continued treatment. Reversible increases in aspartate aminotransferase were observed in 8 of 12 patients. Two patients required dose reduction because of toxicity: one because of symptomatic hypotension and weakness, and the other because of severe fatigue and neutropenia.

Major episodes of infection were infrequent during treatment. All patients tested had serologic evidence of prior infection with cytomegalovirus, herpes simplex virus, and Epstein–Barr virus. In general, marked changes in serum titers of antibodies to viral antigens were not observed. The single patient who was positive for hepatitis B surface antigen remained so after treatment.

The results of tests of immune function before interferon treatment are summarized in Table 2. Skin-test reactivity to dinitrochlorobenzene and microbial antigens was diminished, and no appreciable changes occurred during treatment. Normal or elevated levels of serum immunoglobulins were observed in all patients tested.

The percentage of sheep erythrocyte-rosetting lymphocytes was within the normal range in all patients. However, the percentage of $OKT4^+$ cells and the $OKT4^+/OKT8^+$ ratio were markedly lower than normal. After three weeks of daily treatment the mean $OKT4^+/OKT8^+$ ratio increased from 0.63 to 0.96. No relation between the pretreatment $OKT4^+/OKT8^+$ ratio, or changes induced by therapy, and the subsequent therapeutic response was observed.

Eight of thirteen patients lacked natural killer-cell activity (≤14.7 percent specific ^{51}Cr release; see Methods and ref. 18) before treatment. Augmentation of natural killer-cell activity in vitro by IFLrA, studied in nine patients (Table 3), occurred in five. In seven patients natural killer-cell activity increased markedly during treatment with IFLrA, ranging from 57 to 182 percent above the pretreatment value (Table 3). Changes in activity, either in vitro or during treatment, did not correlate with therapeutic response.

Before treatment with IFLrA the lymphocyte proliferative response to phytohemagglutinin was markedly depressed in 10 of 12 evaluable patients (Tables 2 and 3). The response to phytohemagglutinin increased to normal in six patients during treatment. Of the eight patients with a normal response before or during treatment, five had major objective responses, whereas none of the four who had a persistently low response to phytohemagglutinin had a major objective response. The correlation between the response to phytohemagglutinin and the therapeutic response was not significant ($P = 0.075$, Fisher's exact test, two-sided).

Before treatment, six patients had measurable serum levels of interferon (5 to 84 units per milliliter) (Table 3). Except for the single patient who could not be evaluated, none of the patients with circulating interferon activity had clinically evident infection. A partial response was seen in one of five evaluable patients with circulating interferon; four of seven without interferon activity before treatment had major objective responses ($P = 0.293$, Fisher's exact test, two-sided). The presence of circulating interferon activity before treatment was not correlated with pretreatment blood counts or measures of immune function. Serum interferon concentrations and the time of the maxi-

Table 3. Changes in Immune Reactivity, Serum Interferon, and Therapeutic Response to IFLrA.*

Therapeutic Response; Patient No.	Natural Killer-Cell Activity			PHA Response		Serum Interferon Titers†			IFLrA Dose
	Before IFLrA	Increase in vitro	Increase during treatment (% increase)	Before IFLrA	During treatment	Before IFLrA	Maximum on Day 1	Time of maximum	
						U/ml	*U/ml*	*hr*	$U \times 10^{-6}$
Complete									
1	↓	ND	+ (185)	↓	N	—	228	2	36
2	↓	+	–	N	N	—	108	6	36
3	N	+	+ (79)	↓	N	—	240	4	36
Partial									
4	N	–	–	↓	N	84	392	4	54
5	↓	ND	+ (71)	↓	N	—	160	3	36
Minor									
6	N	ND	–	N	N	5	216	3	36
7	↓	+	+ (79)	↓	↓	30	1000	3	36
8	N	+	+ (57)	↓	N	20	160	2	36
Progression									
9	↓	–	+ (75)	↓	↓	18	192	6	36
10	N	ND	–	↓	N	—	252	6	54
11	↓	–	–	↓	↓	—	476	12	54
12	↓	–	–	↓	↓	—	80	6	36
Inevaluable									
13	↓	+	+ (182)	↓	↓	70	120	24	54

*PHA denotes phytohemagglutinin, ↓ decreased response, ND not done, + increased response, N normal response, and – no increase.

†Dash indicates no detectable serum interferon activity.

mum serum drug concentrations were similar to those reported previously for IFLrA.[2,3]

Neutralizing antibody to IFLrA developed in one patient. He had been treated with IFLrA for four months, had antibody titers below 1:5 before treatment and on Day 35, and had a complete response. A serum sample obtained four days after his last dose of IFLrA showed an antibody titer of 1:15.

Discussion

Our initial experience indicates that IFLrA, a highly purified human alpha interferon produced by recombinant-DNA technology, is capable of inducing tumor regression in patients presenting with an apparently new form of Kaposi's sarcoma. Of 12 evaluable patients, five had major objective responses, and three others had minor responses initially, followed by disease progression during the second month of treatment. Responses were observed in patients with a moderate to large tumor mass and were not confined to patients with a minimal tumor burden (of which there was only one). Treatment was well tolerated, and the patients had few of the major infectious complications to which such patients are susceptible. Although reports of interferon-induced tumor regression have appeared previously,[1,5,6] these studies used partially purified multispecies material in which the relative contributions of different interferon species and noninterferon proteins to the observed responses could not be assessed. Objective evidence for tumor regression has been reported by others[2-4] in patients with various tumors treated with various doses and schedules of IFLrA in Phase I trials; we used a pure, single species of alpha interferon against a specific tumor.

Although no data have been published concerning response rates to chemotherapy, there is no reason to expect that Kaposi's sarcoma in homosexual men would show a drug sensitivity substantially different from that shown by classical Kaposi's sarcoma, in which chemotherapeutic agents have induced high response rates.[20,21] To our knowledge there has been no experience with interferon in classical Kaposi's sarcoma. Nevertheless, our decision to explore the role of interferon in the treatment of this disorder was based on the following evidence: this tumor, which by itself does not often lead to severe morbidity and mortality,[10,11,22] is associated with profound immunodeficiency; Kaposi's sarcoma occurring in the setting of transplant-related immunosuppression may regress "spontaneously" when immunosuppression is relaxed, suggesting that an intact immune system may contribute to tumor control[23]; and viral infection may be related to the development of both the neoplasm and the immunodeficiency.[12,13] Interferon, which has been demonstrated to have stimulatory effects on the activities of human natural killer cells, cytotoxic T cells, and macrophages,[24] in addition to its antitumor and antiviral effects, appears to combine in a single agent a number of properties of particular relevance to the spectrum of abnormalities encountered in patients with Kaposi's sarcoma, while lacking the immunosuppressive effects of cytotoxic chemotherapy.

As previously reported,[22] the normal ratio of T cells bearing OKT4 and OKT8 antigens was reversed in our patients; most had decreased or absent OKT4-positive cells. Although the majority of patients continued to have abnormal $OKT4^{+}/OKT8^{+}$ ratios, there was a modest increase in the mean ratio after three weeks of treatment. Our findings differ from those of Horning et al.,[3] who found a proportional decrease in both helper and suppressor T cells in patients receiving high doses of IFLrA on a schedule of intermittent escalating doses. Since their patients did not have Kaposi's sarcoma or abnormal ratios of T-cell subsets before treatment, one can speculate that tumor type, dose and schedule of interferon administration, and pretreatment immune status may all affect changes induced by treatment.

Interferon has been widely recognized as a stimulator of natural killer-cell activity in vivo[25] and would be expected to be effective pharmacologically in patients with a suitable pool of target precursor natural killer cells. Although 8 of 13 patients had an increase in natural killer-cell activity (after in vitro incubation with IFLrA or in vivo treatment with IFLrA, or both), there was no clear correlation between augmented natural killer-cell activity and therapeutic response. In fact, some patients without an increase in natural killer-cell activity had objective tumor regression, suggesting that the natural killer system had been previously activated (perhaps in relation to preexisting levels of circulating interferon) and had thus become refractory to further activation. It is also possible that in some patients in whom in vitro augmentation cannot be achieved, IFLrA may be of benefit in vivo by maintaining endogenous cytotoxicity, which might otherwise decline, or by enhancing the kinetics of tumor target lysis. The latter possibility is suggested by the observation of restored in vitro induction of natural killer-cell activity by IFLrA after therapy, without an increase in endogenous cytotoxicity, in the only patient tested for this.

A normal T-lymphocyte proliferative response to phytohemagglutinin before therapy or improvement of T-lymphocyte function during treatment appeared to be associated with a clinical response, although the association was not statistically significant in this small sample. T-lymphocyte function did not decrease during therapy in any patient, in contrast to the findings in other trials of interferons, in which decreased lymphoproliferative responses to T-cell mitogens were regularly observed[26] or in which both increased and decreased mitogen responses were observed in different patients.[1]

Our findings, although preliminary, suggest that IFLrA is a useful agent in the treatment of Kaposi's sarcoma in immunosuppressed patients, and that it is capable of restoring at least some aspects of cell-mediated immune function. The study provides no evidence in support of or against either a viral origin for the sarcoma or an antiviral mechanism for the antitumor activity of interferon in this disease. As previously reported,[2] neutralizing antibodies to IFLrA developed in one patient. The importance of such antibodies is unknown, but their development did not preclude a therapeutic response in this case. Continued study will be required to characterize and assess the possible importance (regarding the cause or prognosis of disease) of the high levels of circulating interferon found in some patients before treatment. This interferon can be classified as the alpha type by virtue of its antiviral activity on bovine MDBK cells,[27] and although it has not been specifically tested, it probably represents the same type of acid-labile alpha interferon that was recently reported in the serum of some patients with autoimmune diseases[28] and acquired immunodeficiency.[29] It will also be important to investigate other aspects of interferon's action on cell functions, which may be related more closely to its therapeutic activity in this disease. Although it is premature to make firm recommendations, it may be worthwhile to consider the addition of IFLrA to other cytoreductive or immunomodulatory agents in the treatment of Kaposi's sarcoma.

We are indebted to Anne Golden for excellent assistance in the conduct and analysis of this study, to the Clinical Immunology Research nursing staff for their care of the patients, to Dr. Robert E. Wittes for helpful contributions to the discussion, to Dr. Nancy Geller for statistical analysis, to Pat Anderson, Soonie Chang, Agnes Chu, Thomas Denny, David Gebhard, Lia Kirsch, and Dorothy Yao for excellent technical assistance, and to Sonia Dawkins for preparing the manuscript.

References

1. Gutterman JU, Blumenschein GR, Alexanian R, et al. Leukocyte interferon-induced tumor regression in human metastatic breast cancer, multiple myeloma, and malignant lymphoma. Ann Intern Med 1980; 93:399-406.
2. Gutterman JU, Fine S, Quesada J, et al. Recombinant leukocyte A interferon: pharmacokinetics, single-dose tolerance, and biologic effects in cancer patients. Ann Intern Med 1982; 96:549-56.
3. Horning SJ, Levine JF, Miller RA, Rosenberg SA, Merigan TC. Clinical and immunologic effects of recombinant leukocyte A interferon in eight patients with advanced cancer. JAMA 1982; 247:1718-22.
4. Sherwin S, Knost J, Fein S, et al. A multiple dose phase I trial of recombinant leukocyte A interferon using a 3 × weekly schedule. Proc Am Soc Clin Oncol 1982; 1:35. abstract.
5. Treuner J, Neithammer D, Dannecker G, Hagmann R, Neef V, Hofschneider PH. Successful treatment of nasopharyngeal carcinoma with interferon. Lancet 1980; 1:817-8.
6. Haglund S, Lundquist P-G, Cantell K, Strander H. Interferon therapy in juvenile laryngeal papillomatosis. Arch Otolaryngol 1981; 107:327-32.
7. Greenberg HB, Pollard RB, Lutwick LI, Gregory PB, Robinson WS, Merigan TC. Effects of human leukocyte interferon on hepatitis B virus infection in patients with chronic active hepatitis. N Engl J Med 1976; 295:517-22.
8. Cheeseman SH, Rubin RH, Stewart JA, et al. Controlled clinical trial of prophylactic human-leukocyte interferon in renal transplantation: effects on cytomegalovirus and herpes simplex virus infections. N Engl J Med 1979; 300:1345-9.
9. Hymes KB, Cheung T, Greene JB, et al. Kaposi's sarcoma in homosexual men — a report of eight cases. Lancet 1981; 2:598-600.
10. Urmacher C, Myskowski P, Ochoa M Jr, Kris M, Safai B. Outbreak of Kaposi's sarcoma with cytomegalovirus infection in young homosexual men. Am J Med 1982; 72:569-75.
11. Masur H, Michelis MA, Greene JB, et al. An outbreak of community-acquired *Pneumocystis carinii* pneumonia: initial manifestation of cellular immune dysfunction. N Engl J Med 1981; 305:1431-8.
12. Safai B, Miké V, Giraldo G, Beth E, Good RA. Association of Kaposi's sarcoma with second primary malignancies: possible etiopathogenic implications. Cancer 1980; 45:1472-9.
13. Giraldo G, Beth E, eds. The role of viruses in human cancer. Vol. 1. New York: Elsevier/North-Holland, 1980:57-73.
14. Staehlin T, Hobbs DS, Kung H-f, Lai C-Y, Pestka S. Purification and characterization of recombinant human leukocyte interferon (IFLrA) with monoclonal antibodies. J Biol Chem 1981; 256:9750-4.
15. Pestka S, Maeda S, Chiang T-R, et al. Cloning and expression of human interferons in microorganisms. Tex Rep Biol Med 1982; 41:198-208.
16. Pinsky CM. Skin tests. In: Herberman RB, McIntire KR, eds. Immunodiagnosis of cancer. New York: Marcel Dekker, 1979:722-38.
17. Cunningham-Rundles S, Hansen JA, Dupont B. Lymphocyte transformation *in vitro* in response to mitogens and antigens. In: Bach F, Good RA, eds. Clinical immunobiology. Vol. 3. New York: Academic Press, 1976: 151-94.
18. Cunningham-Rundles S, Filippa DA, Braun DW Jr, Antonelli P, Ashikari

H. Natural cytotoxicity of peripheral blood lymphocytes and regional lymph node cells in breast cancer in women. J Natl Cancer Inst 1981; 67:585-90.
19. Rubinstein S, Familletti PC, Pestka S. Convenient assay for interferons. J Virol 1981; 37:755-8.
20. Vogel CL. Management of Kaposi's sarcoma: chemotherapy I. Antibiot Chemother 1981; 29:82-7.
21. Olweny CLM, Toya T, Katongole-Mbidde E, et al. Treatment of Kaposi's sarcoma by combination of actinomycin-D, vincristine and imidazole carboxamide (NSC-45388): results of a randomized clinical trial. Int J Cancer 1974; 14:649-56.
22. Gottlieb MS, Schroff R, Schanker HM, et al. *Pneumocystis carinii* pneumonia and mucosal candidiasis in previously healthy homosexual men: evidence of a new acquired cellular immunodeficiency. N Engl J Med 1981; 305:1425-31.
23. Harwood AR, Osoba D, Hofstader SL, et al. Kaposi's sarcoma in recipients of renal transplants. Am J Med 1979; 67:759-65.
24. Borden EC, Ball LA. Interferons: biochemical, cell growth inhibitory, and immunological effects. Prog Hematol 1981; 12:299-339.
25. Herberman RR, Ortaldo JR, Bonnard GD. Augmentation by interferon of human natural and antibody-dependent cell-mediated cytotoxicity. Nature 1979; 277:221-3.
26. Krown SE, Stoopler MB, Gralla RJ, et al. Phase II trial of human leukocyte interferon in non-small cell lung cancer: preliminary results. In: Terry WD, Rosenberg SA, eds. Immunotherapy of human cancer. New York: Excerpta Medica, 1982:397-405.
27. Gresser I, Bandu M-T, Brouty-Boye D, Tovey M. Pronounced antiviral activity of human interferon on bovine and porcine cells. Nature 1974; 251:543-5.
28. Preble OT, Black RJ, Friedman RM, Klippel JH, Vilcek J. Systemic lupus erythematosus: presence in human serum of an unusual acid-labile leukocyte interferon. Science 1982; 216:429-31.
29. Preble OT, Johnston MI, Jacobsen H, Friedman RM, Klippel JH. Acid-labile leukocyte interferon in patients with autoimmune diseases. Presented at the third International Congress for Interferon Research, Miami, Fla., November 1-3, 1982.

ORIGINAL ARTICLE

INTRA-BLOOD–BRAIN-BARRIER SYNTHESIS OF HTLV-III-SPECIFIC IgG IN PATIENTS WITH NEUROLOGIC SYMPTOMS ASSOCIATED WITH AIDS OR AIDS-RELATED COMPLEX

LIONEL RESNICK, M.D., FULVIA DIMARZO-VERONESE, PH.D., JÖRG SCHÜPBACH, M.D., WALLACE W. TOURTELLOTTE, M.D., PH.D., DAVID D. HO, M.D., FRANCO MÜLLER, PH.D., PAUL SHAPSHAK, PH.D., MARKUS VOGT, M.D., JEROME E. GROOPMAN, M.D., PHILLIP D. MARKHAM, PH.D., AND ROBERT C. GALLO, M.D.

Abstract Intra-blood–brain-barrier production of virus-specific antibody is good evidence of infection within the blood–brain barrier. Patients with the acquired immunodeficiency syndrome (AIDS) have an increased incidence of neurologic abnormalities — i.e., unexplained, diffuse encephalopathy manifested clinically as chronic progressive dementia. To define the role of human T-cell lymphotropic virus Type III (HTLV-III), the etiologic agent of AIDS, in the pathogenesis of neurologic dysfunction, we compared cerebrospinal fluid and serum from patients with neurologic symptoms associated with AIDS and the AIDS-related complex for the presence of antibodies directed against HTLV-III. Antibodies directed against HTLV-III antigens were detected by four immunologic tests: a fixed-cell immunofluorescence assay, an enzyme-linked immunosorbent assay, immunoblots of viral lysates, and immunoprecipitation of cellular lysates. All patients were seropositive, and 22 of 23 (96 percent) had HTLV-III-specific antibodies in their cerebrospinal fluid. Unique oligoclonal IgG bands were detected in the cerebrospinal fluid, and the rate of IgG synthesis within the blood–brain barrier was elevated. In eight of nine patients tested, the enzyme-linked immunosorbent assay showed that the percentage of HTLV-III-specific IgG in cerebrospinal fluid was higher than in serum, suggesting that HTLV-III infection of neurologic tissue occurs in the majority of patients with neurologic disease associated with AIDS or its related complex.

HUMAN T-cell leukemia (T-lymphotropic) virus Type III (HTLV-III) is the etiologic agent of the acquired immunodeficiency syndrome (AIDS) and the AIDS-related complex.[1-7] In addition to the variety of complications resulting from the underlying immune dysfunction caused by the virus, central nervous system dysfunction occurs frequently in patients with AIDS.[8] Neurologic symptoms are commonly observed, and neuropathologic abnormalities are demonstrated in the majority of patients at postmortem examination.[9] Spinal-cord disease with signs and symptoms of paraparesis and ataxia, pathologically representing a vacuolar myelopathy, afflicts approximately 20 percent of patients with AIDS.[10] In some patients, well-defined focal lesions in the brain are the result of opportunistic infections, such as toxoplasmosis, or neoplasms, such as central nervous system lymphoma. However, more common than these focal disturbances is the development of an unexplained diffuse encephalopathy in which progressive dementia is the dominant feature.[9] Histopathologically, the encephalopathy is associated with gross cerebral atrophy and microglial nodules.[11] The discovery of HTLV-III sequences in the brain tissue of patients with AIDS encephalopathy indicates the potential neurotropism of this virus and suggests that HTLV-III may have a role in the pathogenesis of AIDS encephalopathy.[12] In addition, HTLV-III has been isolated from the cerebrospinal fluid and neurologic tissues of patients with AIDS-related neurologic dysfunction.[3,13-15]

Serum antibodies against HTLV-III, indicating prior infection, have been found in nearly 100 percent of cases of AIDS and in approximately 90 percent of cases of AIDS-related complex.[6] In an effort to define the role of HTLV-III in the pathogenesis of central nervous system dysfunction, we conducted a seroepidemiologic study comparing cerebrospinal fluid and serum for the presence of antibody directed against HTLV-III. The majority of the patients with AIDS and AIDS-related complex who were selected for this study had clinical neurologic abnormalities.

Antibodies directed against HTLV-III antigens were detected by four different immunologic tests: a fixed-cell indirect-immunofluorescence assay, an enzyme-linked immunosorbent assay, immunoblot analysis of viral lysates, and radioimmunoprecipitation of cellular lysates. Both serum and cerebrospinal fluid of patients with AIDS or AIDS-related complex were found to contain specific antibodies directed against HTLV-III antigens. Unique oligoclonal IgG bands were detected in the cerebrospinal fluid, and measurement of the IgG synthesis rate within the blood–brain barrier gave evidence of elevated IgG synthesis in patients with AIDS or its complex. In the majority of patients tested, a higher percentage of HTLV-III-specific IgG was found in cerebrospinal fluid than in serum, suggesting that IgG synthesis against HTLV-

From the Laboratory of Tumor Cell Biology, National Institutes of Health, Bethesda, Md.; the Department of Cell Biology, Litton Bionetics, Inc., Kensington, Md.; the Neurology Service, Veterans Administration Wadsworth Medical Center, Los Angeles; the Infectious Disease Unit, Massachusetts General Hospital, Boston; the Department of Medicine, New England Deaconess Hospital, Boston; the Department of Medicine and Institute for Medical Microbiology, University Hospital, Zurich; and the Departments of Medicine and Dermatology, Mount Sinai Hospital–Medical Center, Miami Beach, Fla.

Supported in part by Merit Review Funds from the Veterans Administration, a grant (1 RD1-NS-116776-001) from the National Institute of Neurological and Communicative Disorders and Stroke, and by the Key Pharmaceuticals Medical Research and Education Foundation.

III antigens was selective. The finding of intra-blood–brain-barrier synthesis of HTLV-III-specific IgG, irrespective of clinical symptoms, suggests that HTLV-III infection of neurologic tissue occurs in the majority of patients with neurologic abnormalities associated with AIDS or AIDS-related complex.

Methods

Selection of Patients

Patients with AIDS were identified clinically as persons presenting with opportunistic infection, Kaposi's sarcoma, or both, in accordance with the definition of the Centers for Disease Control.[16] Patients with AIDS-related complex were defined as having unexplained lymphadenopathy in two or more extrainguinal sites, with or without constitutional symptoms but with a persistent decrease in Leu3+/OKT4+ cells that lasted for more than three months.[17] The majority of patients selected had neurologic disease, although two had no neurologic signs or symptoms and one presented with acute unexplained meningitis followed by the development of AIDS-related complex.

Serum and Cerebrospinal Fluid Samples

Serum and cerebrospinal fluid samples were collected under sterile conditions and stored at −70°C. Some of the samples had already been used in other tests and had undergone repeated freezing and thawing. Cerebrospinal fluid samples from normal controls and other patients with neurologic diseases were obtained from the neurology department at the National Institutes of Health and the National Neurologic Research Bank. The serologic studies were done under code, with use of the fixed-cell indirect immunofluorescence assay, an enzyme-linked immunosorbent assay, Western blot technique, and a metabolic labeling radioimmunoprecipitation technique described below. The formula determining IgG-synthesis rate in the blood–brain area, detection of oligoclonal IgG bands in cerebrospinal fluid, and quantitation of HTLV-III-specific IgG in cerebrospinal fluid were applied to cases in which serum and cerebrospinal fluid samples were obtained simultaneously.

Immunologic Procedures for Detection of HTLV-III Antibodies

Fixed-cell indirect immunofluorescence assays were performed as previously described.[18] A result was scored as positive if more than 10 percent of the cells exhibited fluorescence as compared with a negative control.

The enzyme-linked immunosorbent assay was performed as described by Sarngadharan et al.[4] Assays were performed in duplicate, and the serum absorbance readings were scored as follows: more than twice the average of four normal negative controls, score +; more than three times the normal average, score ++ (clearly positive); more than five times the normal average, score +++; and more than six times the normal average, score ++++. The cerebrospinal fluid absorbance reading was scored + if it was more than X_0 +2 SD (X_0 is the average absorption of 12 normal negative cerebrospinal fluid controls).

Western blot analysis of donor cerebrospinal fluid or serum for the presence of antibodies reacting with HTLV-III structural proteins was performed as previously described.[19] The results of specific antigen–antibody reactions were assessed visually: − denoted no reaction, and + a detectable reaction.

Metabolic labeling and radioimmunoprecipitation were performed as follows. Tissue culture (3×10^7) H9 cells infected with HTLV-III were radioactively labeled by overnight incubation in medium containing [^{3}H]leucine (100 μCi per milliliter). Labeled cells were washed twice in phosphate-buffered saline containing 0.1 percent cold leucine and disrupted at 4°C by repeated aspiration through a 21-gauge needle in 5 ml of 10 mM sodium phosphate (pH 7.2), 0.9 percent sodium chloride, 1 percent Triton X, 0.5 percent sodium deoxycholate, and 0.1 percent sodium dodecyl sulfate. The extract was absorbed for four hours at room temperature with 5 ml of a 10 percent suspension of protein A–Sepharose and 100 μl of normal human serum. The lysate was then clarified by centrifugation at $100{,}000\times g$ for 60 minutes. Immunoprecipitation analysis was performed by adding either 10 μl of serum or 50 μl of cerebrospinal fluid and 200 μl of a 10 percent suspension of protein A–Sepharose to 1 ml of labeled extract and incubating the solution for 18 hours at 4°C. Immunoprecipitates were collected by centrifugation at $2000\times g$ for 10 minutes, washed extensively in phosphate-buffered saline and resuspended in 50 μl of 0.65 M TRIS-hydrochloride (pH 6.7), 1 percent sodium dodecyl sulfate, 10 percent glycerol, 2.5 percent 2-mercaptoethanol, and 0.1 percent bromophenol blue, heated for 3 minutes at 90°C, and analyzed by sodium dodecyl sulfate–polyacrylamide gel electrophoresis.

Intra-Blood–Brain-Barrier IgG Synthesis

IgG and albumin concentrations were quantified by electroimmunodiffusion,[20] and the intra-blood–brain-barrier IgG synthesis rate (milligrams per day) was calculated[21] as

$$\left[\left(\mathrm{IgG_{CSF}} - \frac{\text{IgG serum}}{369}\right) - \left(\mathrm{ALB_{CSF}} - \frac{\text{ALB serum}}{230}\right) \times \left(\frac{\text{IgG serum}}{\text{ALB serum}}\right)(0.43)\right] \times 5,$$

where concentrations are in milligrams per deciliter, ALB denotes albumin, CSF cerebrospinal fluid, 369 and 230 the average normal serum/cerebrospinal fluid ratios for IgG and albumin, respectively, 0.43 the molecular-weight ratio of albumin/IgG, and 5 the daily production of cerebrospinal fluid in deciliters.

Oligoclonal-IgG-Band Determination

Oligoclonal IgG bands were detected by isoelectric focusing electrophoresis, IgG-specific immunofixation, and silver nitrate staining as described.[22] Oligoclonal IgG bands are defined as IgG bands that are found exclusively in cerebrospinal fluid or that are more intense in cerebrospinal fluid than in autologous serum.

Quantitation of HTLV-III-Specific IgG in Cerebrospinal Fluid and Serum

HTLV-III-specific IgG antibodies in human cerebrospinal fluid and serum samples were quantitated by an enzyme-linked immunosorbent assay in which a known quantity of affinity-purified human HTLV-III-specific antibodies was used as a reference. The purification of these antibodies involved the following steps. Density-banded HTLV-IIIB was coupled to activated CH-Sepharose according to the manufacturer's instructions (Pharmacia). A serum sample with high titers of antibodies to HTLV-III was diluted with an equal volume of phosphate-buffered saline and incubated with the HTLV-III-coated CH-Sepharose overnight at 4°C. The beads were washed with a 20-fold volume of phosphate-buffered saline. The bound antibodies were eluted with a buffer consisting of 0.2 M glycine (pH 2.5) containing 4 M magnesium chloride. The eluate was dialyzed against phosphate-buffered saline, and the protein concentration was determined. The affinity-purified antibodies were serially diluted in HTLV-III-antibody-negative cerebrospinal fluid or serum and served as standards on the assay plates on which the cerebrospinal fluid or serum was tested.

Results

The majority of patients with AIDS or AIDS-related complex who were tested for the presence of antibodies to HTLV-III had neurologic manifestations whose cause had not been diagnosed. Table 1 summarizes the clinical and systemic findings in the 23 patients in this study. The most common diagnosis was diffuse encephalopathy manifested clinically as progressive dementia. Two patients had no neurologic manifestations. Seven patients had confirmed active neurologic disorders, including central

Table 1. Clinical Features and Systemic Findings in 23 Patients with AIDS or AIDS-Related Complex.

Patient No.	Age/Sex	Risk Factors	Systemic Diagnoses*	Neurologic Findings
1	30/M	Homosexual	Kaposi's sarcoma	Chronic headaches, dementia
2	29/M	Homosexual	*P. carinii* pneumonia	Dementia
3	34/M	Intravenous drug addict	*P. carinii* pneumonia	Dementia, seizures, ataxia
4	40/M	Homosexual	Esophageal candidiasis, persistent lymphadenopathy, cerebral toxoplasmosis	Hemiparesis
5	42/M	Homosexual	CMV pneumonia, dissem. *M. avium-intracellulare*	Mental status altered by cycloserine
6	30/F	Intravenous drug addict	*P. carinii* pneumonia	None
7	27/M	Homosexual	Kaposi's sarcoma	None
8	25/F	Intravenous drug addict, sexual partner with AIDS-related complex	Esophageal candidiasis, persistent lymphadenopathy	Dementia, incontinence
9	24/F	Sexual partner with AIDS-related complex	Esophageal candidiasis, persistent lymphadenopathy	Ataxia, paraparesis
10	23/M	Homosexual	Persistent lymphadenopathy	Acute meningitis
11	36/M	Homosexual	*P. carinii* pneumonia	Dementia
12	29/M	Homosexual	Kaposi's sarcoma, cerebral non-Hodgkin lymphoma	Dementia
13	36/M	Homosexual	*P. carinii* pneumonia	Dementia
14	28/M	Homosexual	Esophageal candidiasis, persistent lymphadenopathy	Acute psychosis
15	28/M	Homosexual	*P. carinii* pneumonia, cerebral toxoplasmosis, cerebral non-Hodgkin lymphoma, dissem. *M. avium-intracellulare*, intestinal cryptosporidiosis CMV retinitis	Paraparesis, ataxia, seizures, incontinence, psychomotor retardation
16	61/M	Transfusion recipient	*P. carinii* pneumonia	Dementia
17	19/M	Haitian	Dissem. CMV, dissem. *M. avium-intracellulare*	Psychomotor retardation
18	31/M	Homosexual	*P. carinii* pneumonia	Personality change
19	31/M	Homosexual	*P. carinii* pneumonia, dissem. *M. avium-intracellulare*, cerebral non-Hodgkin lymphoma	Ataxia, psychomotor retardation
20	4/M	Transfusion recipient	Cerebral cryptococcosis	Loss of developmental milestones
21	42/M	Homosexual	Kaposi's sarcoma	Chronic headaches
22	26/M	Homosexual	*P. carinii* pneumonia, cerebral toxoplasmosis	Hemiparesis
23	31/M	Homosexual	Esophageal candidiasis, persistent lymphadenopathy	Dementia

*CMV denotes cytomegalovirus infection; and dissem., disseminated.

nervous system lymphoma, cryptococcal meningitis, a drug-induced change in mental status, and cerebral toxoplasmosis. One patient presented with an acute self-limiting illness with fever, meningitis, and skin eruption, followed by the development of AIDS-related complex.

All patients tested had positive serum for HTLV-III according to enzyme-linked immunosorbent assay and Western blot techniques, and all except Patient 10 had positive cerebrospinal fluid according to the Western blot procedure (Table 2 and Fig. 1). The cerebrospinal fluid of Patient 10 was also negative according to immunoprecipitation of [^{3}H]leucine-labeled H9 cells infected with HTLV-III. The enzyme-linked immunosorbent assay failed to identify as positive two cerebrospinal fluid samples that were positive by Western blot technique. The immunofluorescence assay failed to identify 8 of 10 cerebrospinal fluid samples that were positive by Western blot. By comparison, serum and cerebrospinal fluid samples from pooled normal controls and from 30 patients with multiple neurologic diseases — e.g., multiple sclerosis, Parkinson's disease, amyotrophic lateral sclerosis, systemic lupus erythematosus, brain tumors, Guillain–Barré syndrome, progressive supranuclear palsy, and Alzheimer's disease — were negative by enzyme-linked immunosorbent assay and Western blot. The most marked reactions in the Western blot assay were directed against the antigens gp41, which represents the transmembrane portion of the envelope of HTLV-III,[23] and p24, the major viral core protein coded for by the *gag* gene of HTLV-III. All serum samples tested had reactivity against gp41 by either the Western blot or immunoprecipitation assay. According to the Western blot technique, only serum from Patient 10 contained no evidence of antibodies against gp41. However, with use of the immunoprecipitation assay, serum antibodies to gp41 were also detected. All positive cerebrospinal fluid samples exhibited evidence of reactivity against gp41. Anti-

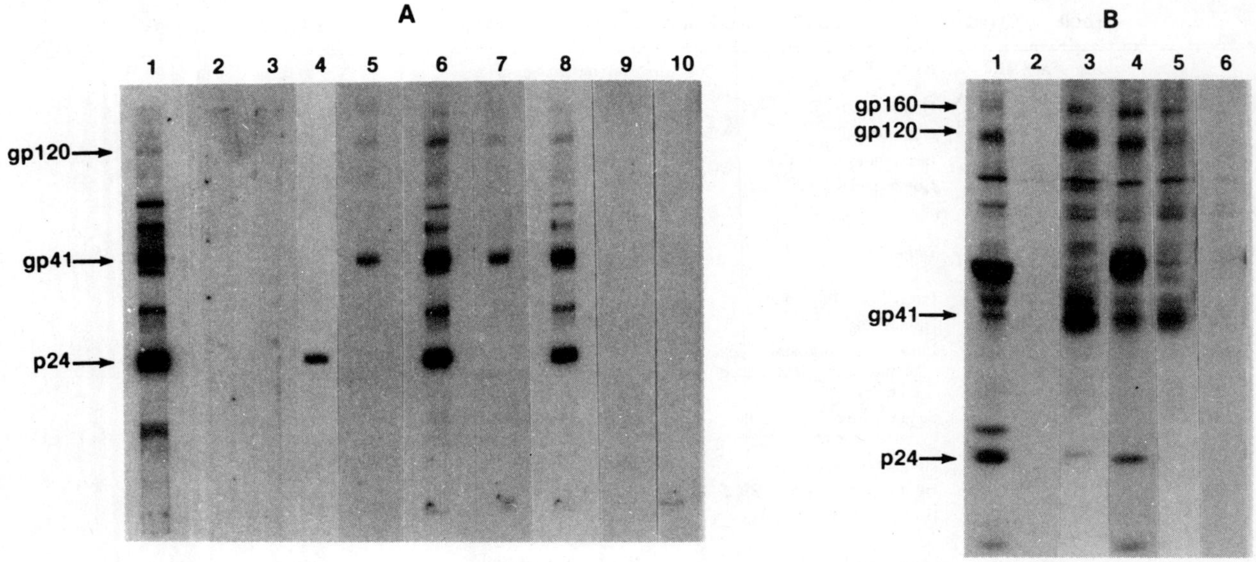

Figure 1. Results of Western Blot Assay (A) and Immunoprecipitation of Metabolically Labeled HTLV-III Proteins (B) in Representative Serum and Cerebrospinal Fluid of Patients with AIDS or AIDS-Related Complex.

Tests were performed as described in the Methods section. In Panel A, Lanes 1 through 6 represent serum samples, and Lanes 7 through 10 cerebrospinal fluid samples. Lane 1 represents a patient with AIDS (control); Lanes 2 and 9, a healthy control; Lanes 3 and 10, a patient with multiple sclerosis; Lane 4, a patient with AIDS-related complex (Patient 10); Lanes 5 and 7, a patient with AIDS (Patient 5); and Lanes 6 and 8, another patient with AIDS (Patient 1).

In Panel B, Lanes 1 through 3 represent serum samples, and Lanes 4 through 6 cerebrospinal fluid samples. Lane 1 represents a patient with AIDS (control); Lane 2, a healthy control; Lanes 3 and 6, a patient with AIDS-related complex (Patient 10); Lane 4, a patient with AIDS (Patient 1); and Lane 5, another patient with AIDS (Patient 5).

bodies against p24 were present in about 40 percent of the serum and cerebrospinal fluid samples analyzed. In the majority of cases, if antibody against p24 was present in the serum, it was also present in the cerebrospinal fluid.

As shown in Table 3, total intra-blood–brain-barrier IgG synthesis was elevated in six of nine patients tested and in the normal range in three. In addition, four of the nine patients had elevated cerebrospinal fluid albumin concentrations. The patients in whom the total intra-blood–brain-barrier IgG-synthesis rate was elevated had antibody directed against p24 and gp41 in cerebrospinal fluid and serum and, in addition, had unique oligoclonal IgG bands in the cerebrospinal fluid that were detected by isoelectric focusing electrophoresis. A quantitative enzyme-linked immunosorbent assay demonstrated that 0.2 to 2.8 percent of the cerebrospinal fluid IgG was specifically directed against HTLV-III antigens in patients with AIDS or AIDS-related complex. In eight of nine patients tested, regardless of clinical symptoms or the duration of disease, the percentage of HTLV-III-specific IgG in the cerebrospinal fluid was higher than in serum.

Discussion

This report describes the presence and quantitation of cerebrospinal fluid antibodies directed against HTLV-III antigens in patients with neurologic symptoms associated with AIDS or AIDS-related complex. The high prevalence of serum antibodies directed against HTLV-III antigens in these patients is consistent with previous reports.[4,6,16] All serum samples tested were positive by enzyme-linked immunosorbent assay, Western blot technique, or immunoprecipitation; the latter two tests were more sensitive and specific. The enzyme-linked immunosorbent assay identified all positive serum samples but missed two cerebrospinal fluid samples identified as positive by Western blot. The immunofluorescence assay lacked sensitivity, identifying only 2 of 10 positive cerebrospinal fluid samples identified by Western blot. These findings should be taken into consideration when the immunofluorescence assay is being evaluated as a confirmatory test in conjunction with screening by enzyme-linked immunosorbent assay.

In general, Western blot analysis indicated that the antibodies were either directed against p24 and gp41, or against gp41 but not p24. All serum and cerebrospinal fluid samples that were positive against HTLV-III had evidence of reactivity against gp41. The immunoprecipitation assay helped to identify antibodies directed against HTLV-III envelope glycoproteins in one patient that were not detected by Western blot. These included the envelope precursor, gp160, and the two cleavage products, gp120 and gp41.[23,24] The immunoprecipitation assay, however, did not identify antibodies to p24 in patients whose samples did not exhibit reactivity to Western blot testing.

Table 2. Presence or Absence of Antibodies Directed against HTLV-III Antigens in Cerebrospinal Fluid and Serum of Patients with AIDS or AIDS-Related Complex.*

Patient No.	Cerebrospinal Fluid ELISA	Cerebrospinal Fluid WB (RIP) p24	Cerebrospinal Fluid WB (RIP) gp41	Serum ELISA	Serum WB (RIP) p24	Serum WB (RIP) gp41
1	+	+(+)	+(+)	++++	+	+
2	+	+	+	+++	+	+
3	+	+	+	+++	+	+
4	+	−	+	+++	−	+
5	+	−(−)	+(+)	++	−	+
6	+	+	+	++	+	+
7	+	+	+	+	+	+
8	+	+	+	++	+	+
9	+	−	+	++	−	+
10	−	−(−)	−(−)	+	+(+)	−(+)
11	+	−	+	+++	−	+
12	+	+	+	++	+	+
13	+	−	+	++	−	+
14	−	−	+	+++	+	+
15	−	−	+	++	−	+
16	+	−	+	++	−	+
17	+	+	+	++++	+	+
18	+	−	+	ND	ND	ND
19	+	+	+	ND	ND	ND
20	+	−	+	ND	ND	ND
21	+	−	+	ND	ND	ND
22	+	−	+	ND	ND	ND
23	+	−	+	ND	ND	ND

*See Methods section for explanation of performance of tests and scoring of results. ELISA denotes enzyme-linked immunosorbent assay, WB Western blot analysis, RIP radioimmunoprecipitation, and ND not done. The indirect immunofluorescence assay was positive in 2 of 10 cerebrospinal fluid samples positive by Western blot analysis.

Altogether, 22 of 23 (96 percent) cerebrospinal fluid samples from patients with AIDS or AIDS-related complex contained HTLV-III-specific antibodies. The only negative cerebrospinal fluid sample was from Patient 10, in whom acute meningitis was evident at presentation and AIDS-related complex subsequently developed. This patient was in the process of acute seroconversion, since antibodies against HTLV-III were developing in his serum but not yet in his cerebrospinal fluid during his presentation.

Natural leakage of IgG from blood to cerebrospinal fluid is a function of the serum concentration of IgG and the permeability of the blood–brain barrier (i.e., the cerebrospinal fluid/serum ratio).[25] The formula for the intra-blood–brain-barrier IgG-synthesis rate has been reliably determined in asymptomatic normal subjects and in patients with multiple sclerosis and other neurologic conditions with a modest range of blood–brain-barrier abnormalities, by means of isotopic-tracer techniques.[26] Patients with multiple sclerosis and subacute sclerosing panencephalitis have evidence of de novo intra-blood–brain-barrier IgG synthesis, in that the synthesis rate is elevated (>3 mg per day) and unique IgG oligoclonal bands are present in cerebrospinal fluid.[27] Also, elevated cerebrospinal fluid/antibody ratios against viruses such as visna have been interpreted as indicating intra-blood–brain-barrier synthesis of virus-specific IgG.[28] In acute human central nervous system infections with herpes simplex virus, varicella–zoster virus, and mumps virus, as well as in chronic measles and rubella panencephalitis, antibodies to the virus are formed in the blood–brain barrier and correlate temporally with central nervous system infection.[29-32] Therefore, these findings, when applied to the study of cerebrospinal fluid from patients with HTLV-III infection, provide evidence for the de novo synthesis of intra-blood–brain-barrier IgG, a signal of HTLV-III infection within the blood–brain barrier. Using the formula for intra-blood–brain-barrier IgG synthesis and isoelectric focusing to detect oligoclonal IgG bands in cerebrospinal fluid, we identified a group of patients with AIDS or its related complex who had elevated total intra-blood–brain barrier IgG synthesis and oligoclonal IgG bands.

Table 3. Intra-Blood–Brain-Barrier Total and HTLV-III-Specific IgG Synthesis in Nine Patients.

Patient No.	Cerebrospinal Fluid				Blood–Brain-Barrier IgG Synthesis		Oligoclonal IgG Bands*	Serum			
	HTLV-III-specific IgG		Total IgG†	Albumin‡	Total§	HTLV-III specific‖		HTLV-III-specific IgG		Total IgG¶	Albumin**
	% of total IgG	mg/dl	mg/dl	mg/dl	mg/day		no.	% of total IgG	mg/dl	mg/dl	mg/dl
1	2.7	0.61	22.8	41.0	69	+	12	2.5	57.0	2291	5688
2	0.8	0.21	27.2	34.6	36	+	3	0.4	13.8	3739	3276
3	0.9	0.18	21.0	73.6	15	+	2	0.5	11.3	2412	4784
4	0.2	0.02	12.4	42.4	2	?	0	0.2	4.8	2432	4482
5	0.4	0.02	6.4	19.4	−11	+	0	0.1	4.1	3015	4121
6	2.8	0.58	20.9	21.9	41	+	ND	0.4	10.3	2613	2349
7	2.0	0.42	20.9	17.5	57	+	ND	0.2	1.5	2549	2618
8	2.5	0.20	7.8	28.8	10	+	ND	0.6	9.4	1614	4500
9	2.8	0.10	3.4	13.3	1	+	ND	0.6	7.0	1153	2917

*IgG bands found exclusively in cerebrospinal fluid or found to be more intense in cerebrospinal fluid than in autologous serum. ND denotes not done.

†Normal range, 0.9 to 8.2 mg per deciliter.

‡Normal range, 5.5 to 34.3 mg per deciliter.

§Normal <3 mg per day.

¶Normal range, 900 to 1800 mg per deciliter.

‖+denotes that the percentage of HTLV-III-specific IgG — i.e., the cerebrospinal fluid/serum ratio — is more than 1, and ? that a definitive assessment could not be made.

**Normal range, 3600 to 5600 mg per deciliter.

Patients with antibodies directed against a wide variety of HTLV-III antigens were also found to have multiple unique oligoclonal IgG bands in the cerebrospinal fluid. The finding of higher percentages of HTLV-III-specific antibodies in cerebrospinal fluid than in serum in the majority of patients is compatible with local infection and active viral replication within the cerebrospinal fluid. Leakage of HTLV-III-specific antibodies from the serum to the cerebrospinal fluid, secondary to changes in blood–brain-barrier permeability, would not be expected to give rise to higher percentages of HTLV-III-specific antibodies in cerebrospinal fluid than in serum. However, only 0.2 to 2.8 percent of the total cerebrospinal fluid IgG was specifically directed against HTLV-III antigens, suggesting polyclonal activation of the immune system locally within the cerebrospinal fluid. The identification of the antigens recognized by the vast majority of antibodies in the cerebrospinal fluid remains to be determined. As a result of the immunosuppressive action of HTLV-III, these antibodies may be directed against other infectious agents or, alternatively, if autoimmune phenomena are involved, quite possibly against neurologic tissue.

The finding of intra-blood–brain-barrier HTLV-III-specific IgG may be of prognostic importance. Two patients with AIDS and no apparent neurologic symptoms had evidence of intra-blood–brain-barrier HTLV-III-specific synthesis of antibodies directed against multiple HTLV-III antigens detected by Western blot. HTLV-III may infect neurologic tissue at an early point, with subsequent blood–brain-barrier synthesis of antibodies specifically directed against HTLV-III, leading ultimately to chronic neurologic disease. Manifestation of neurologic disease may be dependent on multiple factors, such as the duration of HTLV-III infection of the central nervous system, concomitant infections with other agents, or the development of autoimmune phenomena. The patients with HTLV-III infection but no neurologic disease should be followed closely to determine which factors may be of importance if neurologic manifestations develop.

It remains to be established whether HTLV-III has a direct role in the unexplained neurologic syndromes — i.e., dementia — associated with AIDS or AIDS-related complex. The discovery of HTLV-III sequences in the brain, isolation of HTLV-III in the cerebrospinal fluid and neurologic tissue,[3,14,15] and the production of intra-blood–brain-barrier HTLV-III-specific IgG are consistent with a direct etiologic role of HTLV-III in unexplained, chronic neurologic disease associated with AIDS or AIDS-related complex. Moreover, HTLV-III is morphologically and genetically related to visna, a retrovirus directly responsible for a chronic degenerative neurologic disease of sheep.[33] If HTLV-III does play a part in these neurologic conditions, the contribution of HTLV-III to the neurologic disease process may be measured by determining the amount of cerebrospinal fluid IgG specific for HTLV-III. It is of interest that the two patients with known neurologic disease had markedly lower quantities of cerebrospinal fluid HTLV-III-specific IgG in comparison to the patients with neurologic disease of unknown cause or those without neurologic disease. Quantitative analysis of HTLV-III-specific IgG in the cerebrospinal fluid may become the basis of a diagnostic test for HTLV-III infection of neurologic tissue, and the modulation of HTLV-III-specific IgG may also become a quantifiable aspect in the evaluation of potential therapies for HTLV-III-induced neurologic diseases.

Note added in proof: Since submission of this article, we have obtained the following percentages for HTLV-III-specific IgG synthesis in the cerebrospinal fluid: Patient 1, 3 percent; Patient 2, 2 percent; Patient 3, 3 percent; Patient 4, 0; Patient 5, 0; Patient 6, 6 percent; Patient 7, 4 percent; Patient 8, 8 percent; and Patient 9, 0.

We are indebted to M. Sarngadharan for helpful discussions and critical review of the manuscript, to F. Clara, M. Hirsch, M. Kaplan, D. McFarlin, and R. Lüthy for providing valuable specimens, and to M. Lee, M. Osborne, M. Walsh, P. Schmid, A. Devico, and D. Stokes for technical assistance.

References

1. Gallo RC, Salahuddin SZ, Popovic M, et al. Frequent detection and isolation of cytopathic retroviruses (HTLV-III) from patients with AIDS and at risk for AIDS. Science 1984; 224:500-3.
2. Popovic M, Sarngadharan MG, Read E, Gallo RC. Detection, isolation, and continuous production of cytopathic retroviruses (HTLV-III) from patients with AIDS and pre-AIDS. Science 1984; 224:497-500.
3. Salahuddin SZ, Markham PD, Popovic M, et al. Isolation of infectious human T-cell leukemia/lymphotropic virus type III (HTLV-III) from patients with acquired immunodeficiency syndrome (AIDS) or AIDS-related complex (ARC) and from healthy carriers: a study of risk groups and tissue sources. Proc Natl Acad Sci USA 1985; 82:5530-4.
4. Sarngadharan MG, Popovic M, Bruch L, Schüpbach J, Gallo RC. Antibodies reactive with human T-lymphotropic retroviruses (HTLV-III) in the serum of patients with AIDS. Science 1984; 224:506-8.
5. Broder S, Gallo RC. A pathogenic retrovirus (HTLV-III) linked to AIDS. N Engl J Med 1984; 311:1292-7.
6. Safai B, Sarngadharan MG, Groopman JE, et al. Seroepidemiological studies of human T-lymphotropic retrovirus type III in acquired immunodeficiency syndrome. Lancet 1984; 1:1438-40.
7. Biggar RJ, Bouvet E, Effesen P, et al. AIDS in Europe, status quo 1983 — recommendations: report of a meeting co-sponsored by the Danish Cancer Society, the World Health Organization and the European Organizations for Cooperation in Cancer Prevention Studies, Aarhus, Denmark, October, 1983. Eur J Cancer Clin Oncol 1984; 20:169-73.
8. Jordan BD, Navia B, Petito C, Cho E, Price R. Neurological syndromes complicating AIDS. Front Radiat Ther Oncol 1985; 19:82-7.
9. Snider WD, Simpson DM, Nielsen S, Gold JWM, Metroka C, Posner JB. Neurological complications of acquired immune deficiency syndrome: analysis of 50 patients. Ann Neurol 1983; 14:403-18.
10. Petito CK, Navia BA, Cho E-S, Jordan BD, George DC, Price RW. Vacuolar myelopathy pathologically resembling subacute combined degeneration in patients with the acquired immunodeficiency syndrome. N Engl J Med 1985; 312:874-9.
11. Nielsen S, Petito CK, Urmacher CD, Posner JB. Subacute encephalitis in acquired immune deficiency syndrome: a postmortem study. Am J Clin Pathol 1984; 82:678-82.
12. Shaw GM, Harper ME, Hahn BH, et al. HTLV-III infection in brains of children and adults with AIDS encephalopathy. Science 1985; 227: 177-82.
13. Gajdusek DC, Amyx HL, Gibbs CJ Jr, et al. Infection of chimpanzees by human T-lymphotropic retroviruses in brain and other tissues from AIDS patients. Lancet 1985; 1:55-6.
14. Ho DD, Rota TR, Schooley RT, et al. Isolation of HTLV-III from cerebrospinal fluid and neural tissues of patients with neurologic syndromes related to the acquired immunodeficiency syndrome. N Engl J Med 1985; 313:1493-7.
15. Levy JA, Shimabukuro J, Hollander H, Mills J, Kaminsky L. Isolation of AIDS-associated retroviruses from cerebrospinal fluid and brain of patients with neurological symptoms. Lancet 1985; 2:586-8.

16. Fauci AS, Macher AM, Longo DL, et al. Acquired immunodeficiency syndrome: epidemiologic, clinical, immunologic, and therapeutic considerations. Ann Intern Med 1984; 100:92-106.
17. Persistent, generalized lymphadenopathy among homosexual males. MMWR 1982; 31:249-51.
18. Ho DD, Schooley RT, Rota TR, et al. HTLV-III in the semen and blood of a healthy homosexual man. Science 1984; 226:451-3.
19. Schüpbach J, Haller O, Vogt M, et al. Antibodies to HTLV-III in Swiss patients with AIDS and pre-AIDS and in groups at risk for AIDS. N Engl J Med 1985; 312:265-70.
20. Tourtellotte WW, Tavolato B, Parker JA, Comiso P. Cerebrospinal fluid electroimmunodiffusion: an easy, rapid, sensitive, reliable, and valid method for the simultaneous determination of immunoglobulin-G and albumin. Arch Neurol 1971; 25:345-50.
21. Tourtellotte W, Potvin AR, Fleming JO, et al. Multiple sclerosis: measurement and validation of central nervous system IgG synthesis rate. Neurology (Minneap) 1980; 30:240-4.
22. Staugaitis SM, Shapshak P, Tourtellotte WW, Lee MM, Reiber H-OO. Isoelectric focusing of unconcentrated cerebrospinal fluid: applications to ultrasensitive analysis of oligoclonal immunoglobulin G. Electrophoresis 1985; 6:287-91.
23. diMarzo Veronese F, DeVico AL, Copeland TD, Oroszlan S, Gallo RC, Sarngadharan MG. Characterization of gp41 as the transmembrane protein coded by the HTLV-III/LAV envelope gene. Science 1985; 229:1402-5.
24. Allan JS, Coligan JE, Barin F, et al. Major glycoprotein antigens that induce antibodies in AIDS patients are encoded by HTLV-III. Science 1985; 228:1091-4.
25. Tourtellotte WW, Ma BI. Multiple sclerosis: the blood-brain-barrier and the measurement of de novo central nervous system IgG synthesis. Neurology (Minneap) 1978; 28:76-83.
26. Tourtellotte WW, Staugaitis SM, Walsh MJ, et al. The basis of intra-blood-brain-barrier IgG synthesis. Ann Neurol 1985; 17:21-7.
27. Vandvik B, Norrby E, Nordal HJ, Degre M. Oligoclonal measles virus-specific IgG antibodies isolated from cerebrospinal fluids, brain extracts, and sera from patients with subacute sclerosing panencephalitis and multiple sclerosis. Scand J Immunol 1976; 5:979-92.
28. Griffin DE, Narayan O, Bukowski JF, Adams RJ, Cohen SR. The cerebrospinal fluid in visna, a slow viral disease of sheep. Ann Neurol 1978; 4:212-8.
29. Vandvik B, Sköldenberg B, Forsgren M, Stiernstedt G, Jeansson S, Norrby E. Long-term persistence of intrathecal virus-specific antibody responses after herpes simplex virus encephalitis. J Neurol 1985; 231:307-12.
30. Vartdal F, Vandvik B, Norrby E. Intrathecal synthesis of virus-specific oligoclonal IgG, IgA and IgM antibodies in a case of varicella-zoster meningoencephalitis. J Neurol Sci 1982; 57:121-32.
31. Vandvik B, Nilsen RE, Vartdal F, Norrby E. Mumps meningitis: specific and non-specific antibody responses in the central nervous system. Acta Neurol Scand 1982; 65:468-87.
32. Wolinsky JS, Waxham MN, Hess JL, Townsend JJ, Baringer JR. Immunochemical features of a case of progressive rubella panencephalitis. Clin Exp Immunol 1982; 48:359-66.
33. Gonda MA, Wong-Staal F, Gallo RC, Clements JE, Narayan O, Gilden RV. Sequence homology and morphological similarity of HTLV-III and visna virus, a pathogenic lentivirus. Science 1985; 227:173-7.

ORIGINAL ARTICLE

ISOLATION OF HTLV-III FROM CEREBROSPINAL FLUID AND NEURAL TISSUES OF PATIENTS WITH NEUROLOGIC SYNDROMES RELATED TO THE ACQUIRED IMMUNODEFICIENCY SYNDROME

David D. Ho, M.D., Teresa R. Rota, M.A., Robert T. Schooley, M.D., Joan C. Kaplan, Ph.D., J. Davis Allan, M.D., Jerome E. Groopman, M.D., Lionel Resnick, M.D, Donna Felsenstein, M.D., Charla A. Andrews, M.S., and Martin S. Hirsch, M.D.

Abstract We conducted virus-isolation studies on 56 specimens from the nervous system of 45 patients in order to determine whether human T-cell lymphotropic virus Type III (HTLV-III) is directly involved in the pathogenesis of the neurologic disorders frequently encountered in the acquired immunodeficiency syndrome (AIDS) and the AIDS-related complex. We recovered HTLV-III from at least one specimen from 24 of 33 patients with AIDS-related neurologic syndromes. In one patient, HTLV-III was isolated from the cerebrospinal fluid during acute aseptic meningitis associated with HTLV-III seroconversion. HTLV-III was also isolated from cerebrospinal fluid from six of seven patients with AIDS or its related complex and unexplained chronic meningitis. In addition, of 16 patients with AIDS-related dementia, 10 had positive cultures for HTLV-III in cerebrospinal fluid, brain tissue, or both. Furthermore, we cultured HTLV-III from the spinal cord of a patient with myelopathy and from the sural nerve of a patient with peripheral neuropathy. These findings suggest that HTLV-III is neurotropic, is capable of causing acute meningitis, is responsible for AIDS-related chronic meningitis and dementia, and may be the cause of the spinal-cord degeneration and peripheral neuropathy in AIDS and AIDS-related complex.

INFECTIONS and neoplasms of the central nervous system are frequent complications of the acquired immunodeficiency syndrome (AIDS).[1] Recently, several distinct neurologic syndromes have also been reported. Subacute encephalitis, a progressive dementing illness characterized by brain atrophy, occurs in about one third of patients with AIDS.[2] In addition, approximately one fifth of patients with AIDS have vacuolar degeneration of the spinal cord that results in paraparesis, ataxia, and incontinence.[3] Furthermore, many have unexplained chronic meningitis or peripheral neuropathy.[1,4] Several reports suggest that human T-cell lymphotropic virus Type III (HTLV-III), the etiologic agent of AIDS,[5-8] may be directly involved in these processes. Shaw et al. have detected HTLV-III sequences in the brains of 5 of 15 patients with AIDS and encephalopathy.[9] In addition, HTLV-III infection has been established in chimpanzees by inoculation with brain tissues from AIDS patients.[10] HTLV-III is also morphologically, genomically, and taxonomically related to visna, a nononcogenic retrovirus (lentivirus) responsible for a slowly degenerative neurologic disease of sheep.[11,12] The above considerations prompted us to conduct studies to isolate HTLV-III from cerebrospinal fluid, brain, spinal cord, and peripheral nerve obtained from patients with AIDS or AIDS-related complex.

Methods

Forty-five patients from Massachusetts General Hospital and New England Deaconess Hospital were included in this study. Many were selected because they had neurologic diseases. Autopsy or biopsy specimens (approximately 0.2 cm^3) of brain, spinal cord, and peripheral nerve were each homogenized in 2 ml of RPMI-1640 medium and passed through a filter with a pore size of 0.45 μm (Nalgene). Approximately 1 ml of each filtered tissue homogenate or 0.25 to 0.75 ml of cerebrospinal fluid (five samples were prefiltered; see below) was cultured with 5×10^6 normal peripheral-blood mononuclear cells pretreated with phytohemagglutinin (Sigma, 10 μg per milliliter) and hexadimethrine bromide (Polybrene; Sigma, 2 μg per milliliter). Individual cultures were maintained in 5 ml of RPMI-1640 medium supplemented with HEPES buffer (10 mM), L-glutamine (2 mM), penicillin (250 units per milliliter), streptomycin (250 μg per milliliter), fetal-calf serum (20 percent), and interleukin-2 (Electronucleonics, 10 percent). Thereafter, supernatant fluids were assayed for reverse transcriptase activity twice weekly, according to a method previously described.[13,14] Cultures positive for reverse transcriptase were subsequently tested for expression of HTLV-III antigen by indirect immunofluorescence,[13] by means of a human immune serum and a murine monoclonal antibody (provided by M.G. Sarngadharan) specific for the p41 antigen of HTLV-III. Cultures demonstrating both reverse transcriptase activity (>10^4 cpm per milliliter on at least two determinations) and HTLV-III-specific immunofluorescence were considered positive for HTLV-III. Cultures negative for reverse transcriptase were discarded after four weeks. Serologic status with respect to HTLV-III was assessed by fixed-cell indirect immunofluorescence[13] and by immunoblot (Western) techniques.[8]

Specimens were also cultured for other viruses on human embryonic lung, human embryonic kidney, and monkey kidney cells. These cell cultures are designed to detect pathogenic central nervous system viruses, including herpes simplex virus, cytomegalovirus, and most enteroviruses, myxoviruses, and paramyxoviruses.

Results

A total of 56 specimens of the central nervous system (37 samples of cerebrospinal fluid, 15 of brain tissue, 2 of spinal cord, and 2 of peripheral nerve) from 45 patients (29 with AIDS, 7 with AIDS-related complex, and 9 previously healthy men) were obtained for HTLV-III culture. Forty-one patients were seropositive for HTLV-III when first evaluated, 2 had seroconversion during acute meningitis, 1 remained seronegative, and 1 did not undergo serologic testing.

From the Infectious Disease Unit, Massachusetts General Hospital and Harvard Medical School, Boston; the Department of Medicine, New England Deaconess Hospital and Harvard Medical School, Boston; and the Department of Dermatology, Mount Sinai Medical Center, Miami Beach, Fla.

Supported in part by grants (CA 12464, CA 35020, and CA 37461) from the National Institutes of Health and by the Mashud A. Mezerhane B. Fund. Dr. Ho is a recipient of the Clinical Investigator Award from the National Institutes of Health.

Table 1. Isolation of HTLV-III from the Central Nervous System of 45 Patients with AIDS or AIDS-Related Complex, According to Neurologic Complication.

Complication	No. of Patients*	No. with HTLV-III
Meningitis	9	7
Dementia	16	10
Myelopathy	4	4
Peripheral neuropathy	3	3
Others†	6	5
Unrelated‡	3	0
None	9	0

*Some patients are listed in more than one category.
†Patients 28 through 33 of Table 2.
‡Patients 34 through 36 of Table 2.

Thirty-three patients had AIDS-related neurologic disorders, including unexplained dementia, myelopathy, meningitis, peripheral neuropathy, and other disorders (meningoencephalitis, parietal mass lesion, psychosis, central nervous system lymphoma, tuberculous cerebellar abscess, and central nervous system toxoplasmosis). Twenty-four of these 33 were positive for HTLV-III in specimens from at least one central nervous system site. In contrast, none of 12 patients with unrelated neurologic deficits or no deficits had HTLV-III in cerebrospinal fluid or brain (see below). These results are summarized in Table 1 and tabulated with a clinical description of each patient in Table 2. The cases of four patients are described below.

Patient 1

A previously healthy 23-year-old homosexual man had had a single sexual partner in the past year. Their sexual contacts were infrequent, and the last occurred in January 1985. Approximately six weeks later, fevers (temperatures to 39.4°C), severe headache, neck stiffness, photophobia, arthralgias, and a truncal maculopapular rash abruptly developed. The results of an evaluation in the emergency ward on February 18, 1985, including an examination of cerebrospinal fluid, were within normal limits. Treatment was symptomatic, with acetaminophen for presumed viral infection of unclear origin. Over the ensuing eight days, these symptoms gradually resolved but diffuse urticaria appeared and was managed with diphenhydramine. Eight days later, fever, headache, neck stiffness, and photophobia recurred. Repeat evaluation showed leukocytosis and cerebrospinal fluid lymphocytic pleocytosis (28 cells per cubic millimeter). The patient was again treated symptomatically for presumed viral meningitis, and the symptoms resolved in a week. The patient has remained well, but has since had prominent generalized lymphadenopathy.

During the acute, self-limited meningitis, HTLV-III seroconversion was demonstrated by both the indirect immunofluorescence technique (titer increased from 0 to 1:32, then to 1:128) and Western blot analysis. In addition, cerebrospinal fluid obtained during the second phase of illness yielded HTLV-III on culture, though a blood culture was negative for the virus. Multiple additional studies were conducted to exclude other possible causes of the meningitis. Cerebrospinal fluid cultures were negative for bacteria, mycobacteria, and fungi. In addition, cerebrospinal fluid viral cultures on human embryonic lung, human embryonic kidney, and monkey kidney cells were negative.

Table 2. Systemic Diagnoses, Neurologic Complications, and HTLV-III Isolation in 45 Patients.

Patient No.	Diagnoses*	Complications	HTLV-III Isolation†	
1	AIDS-related complex	Acute meningitis	CSF	+
			Blood	−
2	‡	Acute meningitis	CSF	−
			Blood	+
3	AIDS, cryptococcosis	Chronic meningitis	CSF — filtered	+
4	AIDS, *P. carinii* pneumonia, tuberculosis	Chronic meningitis	CSF — filtered	+
5	AIDS-related complex	Chronic meningitis	CSF	+
6	AIDS, Kaposi's sarcoma, *P. carinii* pneumonia	Chronic meningitis	CSF	+
7	AIDS, esophageal candidiasis	Chronic meningitis	CSF	+
8	AIDS-related complex	Chronic meningitis	CSF	+
9	AIDS, Kaposi's sarcoma	Chronic meningitis	CSF	−
10	AIDS, *P. carinii* pneumonia, dissem. *M. avium-intracellulare*, toxoplasmosis, cryptosporidiosis	Dementia, myelopathy, peripheral neuropathy	CSF	+
			Brain	+
			Lumbar cord	+
			Cervical cord	−
			Sural nerve	−
			Blood	−
			Heart	−
			Lung	−
11	AIDS, Kaposi's sarcoma	Chronic meningitis, myelopathy, dementia	Brain	+
			Liver	−
			Thyroid	−
12	AIDS, *P. carinii* pneumonia	Myelopathy, dementia	CSF — filtered	+
13	AIDS, *P. carinii* pneumonia, esophageal candidiasis	Dementia, myelopathy	CSF	+
14	AIDS, toxoplasmosis	Dementia	Brain	+
15	AIDS, Kaposi's sarcoma, lymphoma	Dementia	Brain	+
			Kidney	−
			Lung	−
16	AIDS, *P. carinii* pneumonia	Dementia	Brain — temporal	+
			Brain — frontal	−
			Brain — occipital	−
17	AIDS, lymphoma	Dementia	Brain — area 1	−
			Brain — area 2	+
18	AIDS, Kaposi's sarcoma, lymphoma	Dementia	CSF — filtered	+
19	AIDS, Kaposi's sarcoma, *P. carinii* pneumonia	Dementia	CSF	+
20	AIDS-related complex	Dementia	CSF	−
21	AIDS-related complex	Dementia	CSF	−
22	AIDS-related complex	Dementia	CSF	−
23	AIDS, Kaposi's sarcoma	Dementia	CSF	−

Tests of acute-phase and convalescent-phase serum ruled out acute infection with cytomegalovirus, herpes simplex Types I and II, influenza, mumps, measles, lymphocytic choriomeningitis virus, and *Toxoplasma gondii*. Because the patient's illness occurred in the winter, an enteroviral agent was considered less likely, and thus stool culture for enterovirus was not performed. Specific serologic testing for the large number of enteroviruses was not feasible; however, culture of cerebrospinal fluid for enteroviruses was negative. A serologic test for syphilis and a test for heterophil antibodies were negative on two determinations. Liver-function tests were normal; the serum contained antibody to hepatitis B surface antigen. Arthropod-borne diseases were considered highly unlikely because of seasonal and geographic considerations.

Patient 10

A 28-year-old homosexual man contracted *Pneumocystis carinii* pneumonia in 1982. Subsequently, his clinical course was complicated by recurrent perianal herpes simplex infection, central nervous system toxoplasmosis, and disseminated *Mycobacterium avium-intracellulare* and cytomegalovirus infections. He also had intestinal cryptosporidiosis with resultant vitamin B_{12} deficiency. Despite monthly parenteral vitamin B_{12} supplementation, gradual onset of a gait disturbance occurred in October 1984. This progressed to paraplegia, with urinary and fecal incontinence over the next three months. In January 1985 the patient was hospitalized for these problems. Physical examination was notable for severe lower-extremity weakness, abnormal vibratory and position sense in the toes, and dementia. A cranial CT scan demonstrated marked cerebral atrophy and hydrocephalus; a myelogram showed no evidence of cord compression. Examination of the cerebrospinal fluid was unremarkable, and cultures for bacteria, fungi, and viruses for which cultures are routinely performed were negative. However, a culture of cerebrospinal fluid was positive for HTLV-III (Table 2). The patient's course deteriorated, and he died in March 1985. Histopathologic examination of the nervous system showed microglial nodule formation, gliosis, and demyelination in the cerebrum. In addition, a lymphoma was found in the left occipital region. There was no evidence of spinal-cord compression, but vacuolar degeneration of the lumbar cord was noted, particularly in the dorsal columns and lateral horns. Postmortem specimens obtained from the frontal lobe of the brain and lumbar spinal cord 24 hours after death also yielded HTLV-III on culture (Table 2).

Table 2 *(continued)*.

Patient No.	Diagnoses*	Complications	HTLV-III Isolation†	
24	AIDS, *P. carinii* pneumonia, dissem. *M. avium-intracellulare*, dissem. CMV	Dementia	CSF	–
25	AIDS, *P. carinii* pneumonia, tuberculosis	Dementia	CSF — filtered	–
26	AIDS-related complex	Peripheral neuropathy	CSF Sural nerve	+ +
27	AIDS-related complex	Peripheral neuropathy	CSF	+
28	‡	Meningoencephalitis, cerebral vasculitis	CSF Brain Blood	+ + –
29	‡	Parietal mass lesion	CSF Brain	+ +
30	§	Dementia, psychosis	CSF	+
31	AIDS	Central nervous system lymphoma	CSF	+
32	AIDS, Kaposi's sarcoma	Tuberculous cerebellar abscess	CSF Brain — cerebellum	+ +
33	AIDS	Central nervous system toxoplasmosis	CSF	–
34	‡	Neurosyphilis	CSF	–
35	‡	Astrocytoma	Brain tumor	–
36	AIDS, *P. carinii* pneumonia	Cerebral vascular accident	CSF	–
37	AIDS, dissem. CMV, dissem. *M. avium-intracellulare*, cryptosporidiosis	None	CSF	–
38	AIDS, *P. carinii* pneumonia, dissem. CMV, esophageal candidiasis	None	CSF	–
39	AIDS, Kaposi's sarcoma, *P. carinii* pneumonia, dissem. *M. avium-intracellulare*	None	Brain	–
40	‖	None	Brain	–
41	AIDS, cryptococcosis	None	CSF	–
42	AIDS, *P. carinii* pneumonia, Kaposi's sarcoma	None	CSF	–
43	‡	None	CSF	–
44	AIDS, *P. carinii* pneumonia, dissem. CMV	None	CSF	–
45	AIDS, *P. carinii* pneumonia	None	CSF	–

*CMV denotes cytomegalovirus infection; and dissem., disseminated.

†CSF denotes cerebrospinal fluid, and CSF — filtered denotes pre-filtered (pore size, 45 μm) cerebrospinal fluid.

‡Previously healthy homosexual man.

§Previously healthy Haitian.

‖Previously healthy homosexual man who had received a liver transplant.

Patient 11

A 39-year-old homosexual man was in good health until June 1984, when he began to have marked fatigue. In August he was hospitalized because of a urinary tract infection and also underwent evaluation of chronic frontal headaches and fevers. A neurologic examination was normal, as was a cranial CT scan. However, the cerebrospinal fluid contained 24 mononuclear cells per cubic millimeter, with normal glucose and protein concentrations. A serologic test for syphilis and cerebrospinal fluid cultures for bacteria, mycobacteria, fungi, and routinely cultured viruses were negative. Serum antibody to HTLV-III was detected by the immunofluorescence technique. The patient was discharged without a specific diagnosis and given symptomatic treatment.

The headaches, fatigue, and intermittent fevers continued. Subsequent examinations of cerebrospinal fluid showed persistent mononuclear pleocytosis, a normal glucose concentration, and a progressive increase in protein level (maximum, 128 mg per 100 ml [1.3 g per liter]). In October 1984, biopsy of a new skin lesion revealed Kaposi's sarcoma. At the same time, mild changes in affect, orthostatic hypotension, and a neurogenic bladder developed. A myelogram was normal, but a cranial CT scan showed mild ventricular dilatation. By November, the occurrence of memory loss, weakness of both lower extremities and the right upper extremity, and hyperesthesia of the right leg necessitated hospitalization. A CT scan demonstrated increasing ventricular dilatation, particularly of the left lateral horn. No mass lesions were noted. The cerebrospinal fluid had 6 mononuclear cells per cubic millimeter, the glucose level was 57 mg per 100 ml (3.2 mmol per liter), and the protein level 69 mg per 100 ml (0.7 g per liter). Repeat cultures of cerebrospinal fluid for bacteria, mycobacteria, fungi, and routinely cultured viruses were negative, as were serologic studies for syphilis and cryptococci. Subsequently, the patient had progressive deterioration marked by paraplegia and dementia; he died in December 1984. Postmortem findings confirmed the clinical diagnosis of AIDS-related subacute encephalitis and spinal-cord degeneration. Cultures of brain tissue (frontal lobe) were negative for bacteria, mycobacteria, fungi, and routinely cultured viruses. However, the same specimen was positive for HTLV-III after only five days of culture.

Patient 26

A 45-year-old homosexual man had generalized lymphadenopathy that had begun in early 1984. Beginning in October 1984, severe numbness and tingling in a glove-and-stocking distribution involved both hands and both feet. The patient also had mild weakness of the upper extremities and severe weakness of the lower extremities, resulting in an unsteady gait. Diagnostic evaluations demonstrated normal vitamin B_{12} and folate levels, negative testing for syphilis and screening for toxins, normal fasting glucose and blood chemistries, and an unremarkable cranial CT scan. Electromyographic and nerve-conduction studies showed slowed conduction velocity, fibrillations, and fasciculations. The cerebrospinal fluid was abnormal, with 15 lymphocytes per cubic millimeter, a protein level of 210 mg per 100 ml (2.1 g per liter), and a glucose level of 43 mg per 100 ml (2.4 mmol per liter). Subsequently, biopsy of the sural nerve showed demyelination and chronic inflammation. Cultures of both the cerebrospinal fluid and sural nerve were negative for bacteria, mycobacteria, fungi, and routinely cultured viruses. However, both specimens were positive for HTLV-III.

Discussion

We have demonstrated the recovery of HTLV-III from cerebrospinal fluid, brain, spinal cord, and peripheral nerve of patients with AIDS-related neurologic complications. The isolation of virus from cerebrospinal fluid cannot be solely due to the presence of leukocytes, since many samples were either free of cells (especially samples from patients with dementia) or prefiltered (see Table 2). It is also unlikely that small amounts of blood in the neural tissues could have accounted for the isolations of HTLV-III, since multiple vascular tissues or blood (or both) from some of the same patients were virus-negative. However, it is unknown which cell type in the neural tissues harbors the virus. All cerebrospinal fluid and brain cultures for HTLV-III were negative for the 12 patients who did not have AIDS-related neurologic problems (Patients 34 through 45). Therefore, our current findings extend the results of previous studies,[9,10] which suggest that HTLV-III is not strictly lymphotropic but is also neurotropic. This in turn raises the possibility that the central nervous system may serve as a sanctuary for the virus and that any effective antiviral treatment must penetrate the blood–brain barrier for successful eradication.

HTLV-III appears to be capable of inducing both acute self-limited aseptic meningitis and chronic neurologic diseases in infected persons. In Patient 1, the isolation of HTLV-III from cerebrospinal fluid, the documented HTLV-III seroconversion and subsequent rise in antibody titer, and the systematic exclusion of other potential causes all support the diagnosis of acute HTLV-III meningitis. The course and some of the clinical features in this patient were also similar to those observed in 12 patients with acute (primary) AIDS retrovirus infection who were recently described by Cooper et al.[15] Patient 2 also had a similar illness, with acute, self-limited meningitis. Although HTLV-III was not recovered from his cerebrospinal fluid, the documented seroconversion in addition to the isolation of the virus from his blood suggest that he too had HTLV-III-induced meningitis. Furthermore, HTLV-III has been isolated from cerebrospinal fluid of six of seven patients with chronic meningitis, which remained unexplained after thorough evaluations. On the basis of the above results, we believe that HTLV-III must be added to the list of viruses capable of causing aseptic meningitis, particularly in persons at high risk for AIDS.

In the patients with dementia (Patients 10 through 25), all cerebrospinal fluid and brain cultures for bacteria, mycobacteria, fungi, and routinely cultured viruses were negative. In particular, cultures were negative for cytomegalovirus, which has been proposed as an agent of subacute encephalitis.[1,2] In contrast, HTLV-III was isolated from at least one central nervous system specimen from 10 of the 16 patients mentioned above. Virus was recovered in 6 of 9 samples of brain tissue and 5 of 11 samples of cerebrospinal fluid. Five of the brain samples grew HTLV-III rapidly, within one week of inoculation, suggesting that HTLV-III was present in high titers. Indeed, molecular hybridization studies have shown that brain is the most heavily infected tissue, as compared with spleen, lymph node, liver, and lung.[9] We believe that HTLV-III is directly involved in the pathogenesis of subacute encephalitis associated with AIDS and AIDS-related complex, on the basis of our isolation of the virus as described above; the detection of HTLV-III sequences in brain cells in AIDS-related subacute encephalitis, as shown by in situ hybridization[9]; and the similarity of HTLV-III to visna virus.[11,12] Our hypothesis is also supported by recent quantitative serologic studies demonstrating synthesis of HTLV-III-specific immunoglobulins within the blood–brain barrier of patients with neurologic complications of AIDS or AIDS-related complex.[16]

The syndromes of vacuolar myelopathy and peripheral neuropathy in the setting of AIDS or its related complex have been reported only recently.[3,4] The pathogenesis of these disorders is unknown at present. The 100 percent isolation rate for HTLV-III in our patients with these two disorders (Table 1) and the direct recovery of virus from spinal cord (Patient 10) and sural nerve (Patient 26) suggest that the myelopathy and peripheral neuropathy may be other direct neurologic sequelae of HTLV-III infection.

Several patients (Patients 2 and 28 through 30) did not have clinical manifestations of immunodeficiency but did have neurologic problems in association with HTLV-III isolation from the central nervous system. These cases suggest that HTLV-III-related neurologic disease may occur before or in the absence of HTLV-III-related immunodeficiency. Furthermore, the patients' atypical neurologic presentations serve to remind us that HTLV-III may cause central nervous system syndromes yet undefined. As the number of cases of AIDS and HTLV-III infection continues to rise, a considerable increase in neurologic complications in patients with or at risk for AIDS should be anticipated.

Note added in proof: Since acceptance of this paper, a report describing isolation of AIDS-associated retrovirus from 13 cerebrospinal fluid specimens and 1 brain specimen has appeared.[17]

We are indebted to R. Byington, T. Flynn, E. Keller, J. Steele, D. Gabuzda, and our colleagues in the Departments of Medicine, Neurology, and Neuropathology of Massachusetts General Hospital for valuable assistance.

References

1. Snider WD, Simpson DM, Nielsen S, Gold JWM, Metroka CE, Posner JB. Neurological complications of acquired immune deficiency syndrome: analysis of 50 patients. Ann Neurol 1983; 14:403-18.
2. Nielsen S, Petito CK, Urmacher CD, Posner JB. Subacute encephalitis in acquired immune deficiency syndrome: a postmortem study. Am J Clin Pathol 1984; 82:678-82.
3. Petito CK, Navia BA, Cho E-S, Jordan BD, George DC, Price RW. Vacuolar myelopathy pathologically resembling subacute combined degeneration in patients with the acquired immunodeficiency syndrome. N Engl J Med 1985; 312:874-9.
4. Levy RM, Bredesen DE, Rosenblum ML. Neurological manifestations of the acquired immunodeficiency syndrome (AIDS): experience at UCSF and review of the literature. J Neurosurg 1985; 62:475-95.
5. Popovic M, Sarngadharan MG, Read E, Gallo RC. Detection, isolation, and continuous production of cytopathic retroviruses (HTLV-III) from patients with AIDS and pre-AIDS. Science 1984; 224:497-500.
6. Gallo RC, Salahuddin SZ, Popovic M, et al. Frequent detection and isolation of cytopathic retroviruses (HTLV-III) from patients with AIDS and at risk for AIDS. Science 1984; 224:500-3.
7. Schüpbach J, Popovic M, Gilden RV, Gonda MA, Sarngadharan MG, Gallo RC. Serological analysis of a subgroup of human T-lymphotropic retroviruses (HTLV-III) associated with AIDS. Science 1984; 224:503-5.
8. Sarngadharan MG, Popovic M, Bruch L, Schüpbach J, Gallo RC. Antibodies reactive with human T-lymphotropic retroviruses (HTLV-III) in the serum of patients with AIDS. Science 1984; 224:506-8.
9. Shaw GM, Harper ME, Hahn BH, et al. HTLV-III infection in brains of children and adults with AIDS encephalopathy. Science 1985; 227:177-82.
10. Gajdusek DC, Amyx HL, Gibbs CJ, et al. Infection of chimpanzees by human T-lymphotropic retroviruses in brain and other tissues from AIDS patients. Lancet 1985; 1:55-6.
11. Gonda MA, Wong-Staal F, Gallo RC, Clements JE, Narayan O, Gilden RV. Sequence homology and morphologic similarity of HTLV-III and visna virus, a pathogenic lentivirus. Science 1985; 227:173-7.
12. Sonigo P, Alizon M, Staskus K, et al. Nucleotide sequence of the visna lentivirus: relationship to the AIDS virus. Cell 1985; 42:369-82.
13. Ho DD, Schooley RT, Rota TR, et al. HTLV-III in the semen and blood of a healthy homosexual man. Science 1984; 226:451-3.
14. Ho DD, Rota TR, Hirsch MS. Infection of human endothelial cells by human T-lymphotropic virus type I. Proc Natl Acad Sci USA 1984; 81:7588-90.
15. Cooper DA, Gold J, Maclean P, et al. Acute AIDS retrovirus infection: definition of a clinical illness associated with seroconversion. Lancet 1985; 1:537-40.
16. Resnick L, diMarzo-Veronese F, Schüpbach J, et al. Intra-blood–brain-barrier synthesis of HTLV-III-specific IgG in patients with neurologic symptoms associated with AIDS or AIDS-related complex. N Engl J Med 1985; 313:1498-504.
17. Levy JA, Shimabukuro J, Hollander H, Mills J, Kaminsky L. Isolation of AIDS-associated retroviruses from cerebrospinal fluid and brain of patients with neurological symptoms. Lancet 1985; 2:586-8.

SPECIAL REPORT

DEVELOPMENT OF ANTIRETROVIRAL THERAPY FOR THE ACQUIRED IMMUNODEFICIENCY SYNDROME AND RELATED DISORDERS

A Progress Report

ROBERT YARCHOAN, M.D. AND SAMUEL BRODER, M.D.

Abstract We review the rationale for, and progress in, the development of antiviral therapy for the acquired immunodeficiency syndrome (AIDS). A consideration of the replicative cycle of the human immunodeficiency virus (HIV) can lead to the identification of several steps that represent potential targets for antiretroviral therapy, and several substances that can inhibit the replication of HIV in vitro have already been identified. The 2′,3′-dideoxynucleosides are a class of nucleoside analogues in which the 3′-hydroxy group is modified so that it cannot form phosphodiester linkages for nucleic acid chains. Some are potent in vitro inhibitors of HIV replication, possibly acting as chain terminators of viral DNA during reverse transcription. One of these dideoxynucleoside analogues, 3′-azido-2′,3′-dideoxythymidine (AZT), has now been administered for up to 18 months to patients with AIDS. The drug has been shown to improve immunologic function, to reverse, at least partially, HIV-induced neurologic dysfunction in some patients, and to improve certain other clinical abnormalities associated with AIDS. The principal toxic effect associated with AZT is dose-dependent suppression of bone marrow, resulting particularly in anemia and leukopenia; however, most patients in whom this toxic effect occurs can subsequently tolerate a lower dose of the drug. The demonstration that AZT can be beneficial in patients with AIDS has removed some of the uncertainty about the rationale for an antiretroviral intervention in HIV infection.

THE acquired immunodeficiency syndrome (AIDS) is a lethal multisystem disease that has become a major public health problem since its recognition in 1981.[1-3] AIDS is caused by the third known human T-lymphotropic virus (HTLV-III),[4] which can replicate within critical cells of the immune system (particularly T cells and macrophages), leading to loss of CD4+ (T4+, or helper–inducer) T cells and profound immunosuppression.[5-8] The virus has several other names, including lymphadenopathy-associated virus (LAV)[9] and AIDS-related virus (ARV).[10] It has recently been proposed by the subcommittee on human retroviruses of the International Committee on the Taxonomy of Viruses that the virus that causes AIDS be called human immunodeficiency virus (HIV),[11] and this may become the general designation for this category of retrovirus.

More than 30,000 cases of AIDS have been reported in the United States, and the disease is seen with increasing frequency throughout the world. There may be a long prodromal period before the development of frank AIDS[12,13]; it is estimated that more than 1 million people in this country are now infected with HIV, and this number is likely to increase. In perhaps 30 percent of infected persons or more, AIDS may develop in a three- to five-year period,[14] so that even if the spread of HIV infection slows, the number of cases of AIDS will continue to increase. It is worth stressing that the full natural history of this infection is not known, and unexpected long-term consequences may accompany infection with this pathogen.

The principal investigators conducting the randomized, placebo-controlled AZT trial were D. Durack, *Duke University Medical Center*, Durham, N.C.; M. Fischl, *University of Miami*, Miami, Fla.; M. Gottlieb, *University of California, Los Angeles;* M. Grieco, *St. Luke's–Roosevelt Hospital*, N.Y.; J. Groopman, *New England Deaconess Hospital*, Boston; M. Hirsch, *Massachusetts General Hospital*, Boston; G.G. Jackson, *University of Illinois*, Chicago; O. Laskin, *Cornell Medical Center*, N.Y.; J. Leedom, *University of Southern California, Los Angeles;* D. Mildvan, *Beth Israel Medical Center*, N.Y.; D. Richman, *University of California, San Diego;* and P. Volberding, *University of California, San Francisco.*

RATIONALE FOR THE USE OF ANTIVIRAL THERAPY IN AIDS

The demonstration that HIV is the causative agent of AIDS,[4] accompanied by the availability of purified virus on a large scale, made it possible to develop treatments aimed at inhibiting the replication of the retrovirus. Consideration of antiretroviral therapy for the treatment of AIDS is based on the assumption that continued retroviral replication is involved in both the pathogenesis and progression of the disease. In regard to the immunodeficiency, the characteristic depletion of CD4+ T cells can be mediated directly by HIV infection of these cells,[5,15] although it is possible that indirect mechanisms may also have a role.[16] If the immune system of patients with AIDS retains some regenerative potential (either alone or with immunoreconstitutive therapy[17]), then inhibition of HIV replication may permit some restoration of immunity or at least prevent further clinical deterioration, thereby prolonging survival. Some clinical investigators, however, have considered retroviruses to be inherently untreatable once established in vivo, and these rationales for attempting to develop antiretroviral drugs remain somewhat controversial. Nevertheless, as we will discuss later, certain recent clinical results support the basic assumptions underlying intervention against established retroviral infections.

Antiretroviral therapy may also address other disease manifestations of HIV infection. Since the first observation that the brain is an important site of HIV replication,[18] there has been a growing recognition that serious neurologic dysfunction, ranging from peripheral neuropathy to profound dementia, may be caused by the virus.[19-21] Although it is still not known precisely how HIV enters the nervous system (one possibility is that it is transported there by infected macrophages[7]) or how it induces neurologic damage, it is clear that successful therapeutic strategies must deal with the fact of viral replication within the nervous system.

Stages in the Life Cycle of HIV That May Be Targets for Antiviral Agents

Before we turn our attention to a discussion of certain recent practical clinical developments in the antiretroviral therapy of AIDS, it may be worthwhile to review briefly the replicative cycle of HIV and consider how specific stages of viral replication might be targets for therapeutic strategies (Table 1).

HIV belongs to a family of RNA viruses known as retroviruses, which by definition must replicate through a DNA intermediary (i.e., at one step in their cycle of replication genetic information flows from RNA to DNA in a "retro" direction).[23,24] Many members of this family of viruses can induce neoplastic transformation in infected cells, and the terms "RNA tumor virus" and "leukemia virus" have been used to describe these viruses. HIV, however, has not been shown to be a transforming agent itself, although it is linked to the causation of certain cancers through its ability to induce immunosuppression, thus providing a vivid reminder of the relation between abnormalities in the immune system and the development of neoplasms.[25]

The first step in the infection of a target cell by HIV is its binding to CD4 antigen (and possibly other receptors) on the cell surface.[26,27] There is evidence that this binding between the viral envelope glycoprotein and the CD4 antigen may play a leading part in T-cell lysis through syncytia formation.[28,29] This binding could be blocked by antibodies to either the viral envelope glycoprotein or the CD4 antigen; alternatively, synthetic ligands could be used to block viral attachment.[30] Although there is substantial variation in the envelope of different isolates of HIV,[31,32] the envelope glycoprotein is constrained by its need to bind to CD4, and it is likely that a relatively invariant region of the envelope will be shown to be crucial for viral infection.

After attachment, HIV enters a target cell by an incompletely defined mechanism that may involve a fusion process. It then loses its envelope coat, and viral RNA (along with reverse transcriptase) is released into the cytoplasm. Compounds that block these steps in other viruses have been identified (e.g., amantadine is believed to block the uncoating of influenza A virus[33]), and similar agents may be developed for HIV.

At this point, the HIV *pol* product, reverse transcriptase, makes a complementary-strand (first-strand) DNA copy of the RNA genome and then catalyzes the production of a positive-strand DNA copy so that the genetic information is eventually encoded in a double-stranded DNA form.[31,34] Reverse-transcriptase activity is essential for viral replication and can for all practical purposes be considered a unique viral function. It is thought that an inherent RNase H activity of the reverse transcriptase eliminates the viral genomic RNA strand, making it possible for the reverse transcriptase to generate the second DNA strand.[35] If a DNA copy of the uncoated viral RNA is not made promptly, the RNA is susceptible to degradation by cellular enzymes. For these reasons, reverse transcriptase has been a major target for antiviral therapy in AIDS, and indeed, as we will discuss below, most of the agents now being investigated, including 3′-azido-2′,3′-dideoxythymidine (AZT), act at this step.[36-41] It should be noted that the progress in this area has been possible partly because of pioneering research directed at finding agents that inhibit the reverse transcriptase of murine and avian retroviruses.[42-47]

The DNA copy of retroviral genetic material may either remain in an unintegrated form or become integrated into the genome of the host cell through a viral "integrase" (thought to be a *pol* gene product).[48] At some later point, the DNA is transcribed to mRNA and to viral genomic RNA with use of host RNA polymerases, and the mRNA is translated to form viral proteins, again with use of the biochemical apparatus of the host cell. The guanosine analogue ribavirin is believed to interfere with what is called the 5′-capping of mRNA in other viral systems, and it may have a related activity against HIV.[33,49]

The production of HIV proteins is under the regulatory control of at least two unique viral genes — *tat*-III and *art* (or *trs*).[50-52] The products of these genes are required for efficient replication of HIV, and they may be future targets for antiviral therapy. The *tat*-III gene product, for example, is believed to increase production of viral proteins markedly after binding to a region on what is called the 5′-long termi-

Table 1. Stages of HIV Replication That May Be Targets for Therapeutic Intervention.

Stage	Possible Intervention
Binding to target cell	Antibodies to virus or cellular receptor
Entry into target cell and uncoating of RNA	Drugs (by analogy with calmodulin antagonists for Epstein–Barr infection[22] or amantadine for type A influenza virus infection)
Transcription of RNA to DNA by reverse transcriptase	Reverse transcriptase inhibitors
Degradation of RNA by RNase activity (encoded by viral *pol* gene)	RNase H inhibitors
Integration of DNA into host genome	Agents that inhibit *pol*-encoded integrase function may be found
Transcription of DNA to RNA	Inhibitors proved to be specific for the retrovirus at this step are not available
Translation of RNA	Inhibitors of *tat*-III or *art*–*trs*; "anti-sense" constructs
Viral component production and assembly	Myristylation, glycosylation, or protease inhibitors or modifiers
Viral budding	Interferons; antibodies to a viral antigen

nal repeat of the viral mRNA.[53] Drugs might be developed (perhaps designed on the basis of x-ray diffraction studies and computer-generated models of the protein[53-55]) with the goal of binding to and inhibiting the function of *tat*-III.

Another approach that may serve to inhibit the production of viral proteins is the use of "anti-sense" oligodeoxynucleotides.[56,57] These are short sequences of DNA (or DNA that has been chemically modified) with base pairs that are complementary to a segment of the viral genome. Such oligonucleotides could theoretically block expression of viral proteins through a hybridization arrest of mRNA[57,58] or by interference with the binding of a regulatory protein (e.g., *tat*-III).

The final steps of viral replication involve secondary processing of certain viral proteins by proteases (which is thought to be a function of one of the viral *pol* gene products[34]) and myristylating and glycosylating enzymes in the host[59,60]; these steps could theoretically be affected by specific inhibitors. Finally, the virus is released by budding. Alpha-interferon, which has been shown to inhibit HIV replication,[61] is thought possibly to act at this step.

It has become evident that macrophages,[6,7] B cells infected with the Epstein–Barr virus[62] (which are increased in patients with AIDS[63,64]), and even certain T cells[65,66] may be chronically infected with HIV without being destroyed. Agents that act at the later steps of viral replication (after reverse transcription) may block viral production by these chronically infected cells, whereas agents that act at reverse transcription or earlier steps may serve to protect uninfected cells from HIV infection. A combination of early- and late-acting agents may therefore be more effective than either alone and may also reduce the chance that the virus will develop resistance to any single agent.

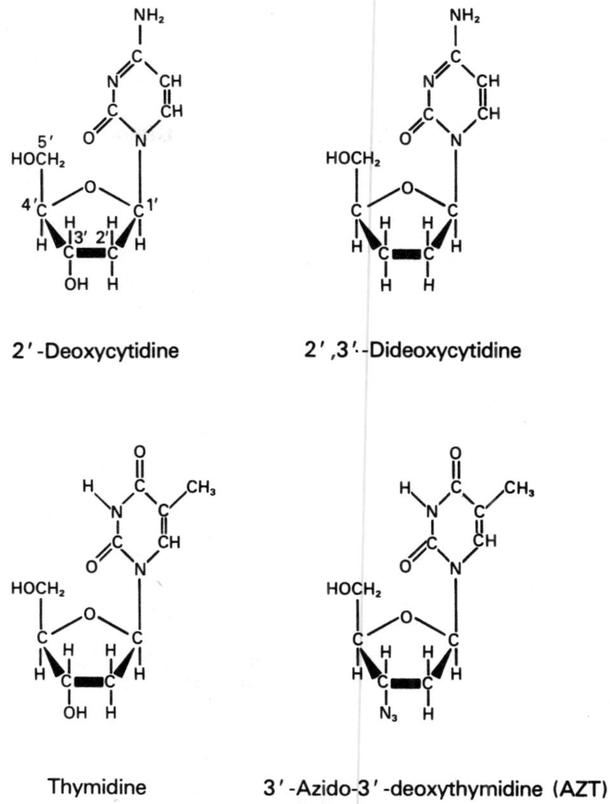

Figure 1. Structure of Two Dideoxynucleosides (Right) as Compared with Their Normal Deoxynucleoside Counterparts (Left).
2'-3'-Dideoxycytidine and the 3'-azido analogue of 2',3'-dideoxythymidine (AZT), two dideoxynucleosides with potent in vitro activity against HIV, differ from their normal 2'-deoxynucleoside counterparts, 2'-deoxycytidine and thymidine (2'-deoxythymidine), in that the 3'-hydroxy (–OH) group is modified so that it cannot form 3'-phosphodiester linkages.

Dideoxynucleoside Analogues as Inhibitors of HIV Infection

We will now discuss a group of compounds — the 2',3'-dideoxynucleoside analogues — that can be metabolized in mammalian cells to become potent inhibitors of HIV replication. Dideoxynucleosides have previously been studied in the pioneering laboratories of Horwitz, Robins, Cohen, and Prusoff,[67-69] and indeed, as phosphorylated products, they are familiar to molecular biologists as reagents in the Sanger sequencing reaction.[70] Some of these compounds block the infection of target cells by HIV at concentrations that are 10- to 20-fold lower than those at which they inhibit the proliferation and survival of the cells, even under conditions of high multiplicity of infection (many infectious virions per cell).[40,41] As will be discussed later, one drug, the 3'-azido derivative of 2',3'-dideoxythymidine, or AZT, has recently been shown to induce immunologic improvements[71] and to confer a survival advantage in certain patients with AIDS.[72,73]

The dideoxynucleosides that have been shown to inhibit the replication of HIV differ from the normal substrates for nucleic acid synthesis (2'-deoxynucleosides) in that the 3'-hydroxy group is replaced by hydrogen or another group that cannot form phosphodiester linkages (Fig. 1). Some but not all of these compounds can be metabolized by mammalian kinases to 5'-triphosphate forms (Fig. 2).[45,74,75] There is evidence that these phosphorylated nucleosides inhibit HIV replication by acting as chain terminators[68,70,76]; because of the 3' modification, once viral reverse transcriptase is fooled into adding the nucleosides to the end of a growing chain of DNA, no subsequent 5'→3' phosphodiester linkages can be made (Fig. 3). The DNA polymerase of HIV (reverse transcriptase) and other retroviruses is much more susceptible to the inhibitory effects of phosphorylated nucleosides (as triphosphates) than is mammalian DNA polymerase alpha,[45,74,76] and this is probably one reason for the selective antiretroviral activity of these compounds.

As noted above, dideoxynucleosides must be phosphorylated to an active 5'-triphosphate moiety by cellular kinases in the host. Different species of animals (or even different cell types within one species) differ in the efficiency with which they phosphorylate these

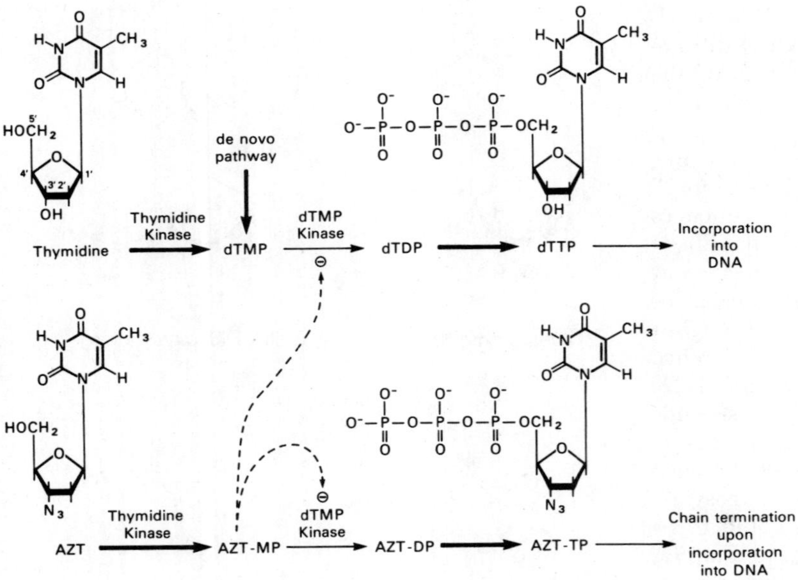

Figure 2. Intracellular Metabolism of AZT and Thymidine.
Thymidine (2′-deoxythymidine), whose structure is shown at top left, is phosphorylated at the 5′ position by cellular thymidine kinase to form thymidine-5′-monophosphate (dTMP). dTMP can also be produced through the de novo pathway by methylation of deoxyuridine-5′-monophosphate. dTMP is then further phosphorylated to thymidine-5′-diphosphate (dTDP) by dTMP kinase (thymidylate kinase), and dTDP is again phosphorylated at the 5′ position by nucleoside diphosphate kinase to form thymidine-5′-triphosphate (dTTP) (structure shown at top right). The latter compound can be a substrate for incorporation into a growing chain of DNA. AZT (structure shown at bottom left) is phosphorylated by the same series of cellular enzymes to form (in succession) AZT-5′-monophosphate (AZT-MP), AZT-5′-diphosphate (AZT-DP), and AZT-5′-triphosphate (AZT-TP) (structure shown at bottom right).[74] When AZT-TP is incorporated into a growing chain of DNA, no 5′→3′ diester linkages can be added because of the 3′-azido ($-N_3$) substitution, and it is believed that the growing chain of DNA is terminated (see Fig. 3). It is thought that viral reverse transcriptase is more easily fooled into binding and incorporating the AZT congener than is cellular DNA polymerase alpha. AZT-MP is phosphorylated very slowly by dTMP kinase (relative maximum velocity = 0.3 percent as compared with dTMP; K_m = 8.6 μM), and the phosphorylation of AZT-MP to AZT-TP is limited in human cells.[74] In addition, AZT-MP interferes with the phosphorylation of dTMP by competitive substrate inhibition (K_{is} = 8.6 μM).[74] Cells exposed to AZT may have high levels of dTMP and decreased levels of dTTP,[71,74] and this may be one factor that contributes to the toxicity of the drug. Patients with folate or vitamin B_{12} deficiency may have decreased production of dTMP by the de novo pathway and may therefore be particularly sensitive to AZT-induced dTTP depletion unless they receive vitamin replacement therapy.[80]

drugs,[45,74,75] and for this reason, extreme caution must be used in extrapolating from experimental results obtained in one species (or in one cell type within a species) to another. For example, 2′,3′-dideoxythymidine is poorly phosphorylated in human cells and is the least potent of any 2′,3′-dideoxynucleoside tested.[41] Substitution of the 3′-hydrogen by an azido group, however, produces AZT (Fig. 1), an excellent substrate for human thymidine kinase (K_m = 3.0 μM)[74] that is many times more efficient at inhibiting HIV replication.[40,41]

Another pyrimidine analogue, 2′,3′-dideoxycytidine, is even more potent than AZT on a molar basis; essentially complete in vitro inhibition of HIV is obtained at a concentration of 0.5 μM, even under conditions of substantial viral excess, and the virus-inhibiting effect remains for prolonged culture periods.[41,76] At low viral doses, substantial antiretroviral activity can be seen, even at 10-nM concentrations. Additional testing has demonstrated that 2′,3′-dideoxycytidine has other properties desirable in a potential therapeutic agent for HIV infection. It is relatively resistant to cytidine deaminase (a major catabolic enzyme for cytidine analogues),[75] it is well absorbed when administered orally in animals, it has straightforward pharmacokinetic clearance by the kidney, and it produces comparatively few toxic effects in laboratory animals.[77] A Phase I (feasibility and toxicity) study of 2′,3′-dideoxycytidine in patients with AIDS is currently being conducted as the next step in the development of the drug. A comparable study of a purine analogue, 2′,3′-dideoxyadenosine, is planned.

AZT was synthesized 20 years ago by Horwitz et al.[67] and was shown by Ostertag et al. over 12 years ago to inhibit in vitro replication of C-type murine retrovirus.[46] Early in 1985, it was observed that AZT at concentrations of 1 to 3 μM inhibited HIV replication, even under test conditions with a high multiplicity of infection.[40] (Under less stringent test conditions, substantially lower concentrations of AZT have been shown to be inhibitory.) Five months later, a Phase I trial of AZT in patients with AIDS and related conditions was begun.[71] One of the purposes of this trial was to study the pharmacokinetics of AZT. The drug was found to be well absorbed when given orally (its bioavailability was approximately 60 percent), and levels that inhibited the replication of HIV were shown to be achievable in patients (Fig. 4).[71,78] The half-life of AZT was found to be approximately one hour, with much of the drug clearance occurring by means of glucuronidation.[71,78,79] (At least one drug that is known to interfere with glucuronidation, probenecid, increases the half-life of AZT,[79] and it is possible that other inhibitors of glucuronidation, such as acetaminophen, morphine, and sulfonamides, could have similar effects.) Finally, AZT was found to have excellent penetration across the blood–brain barrier (Fig. 4).[71,78]

In this trial, it was also observed that patients who were given intermediate oral doses of AZT (15 to 30

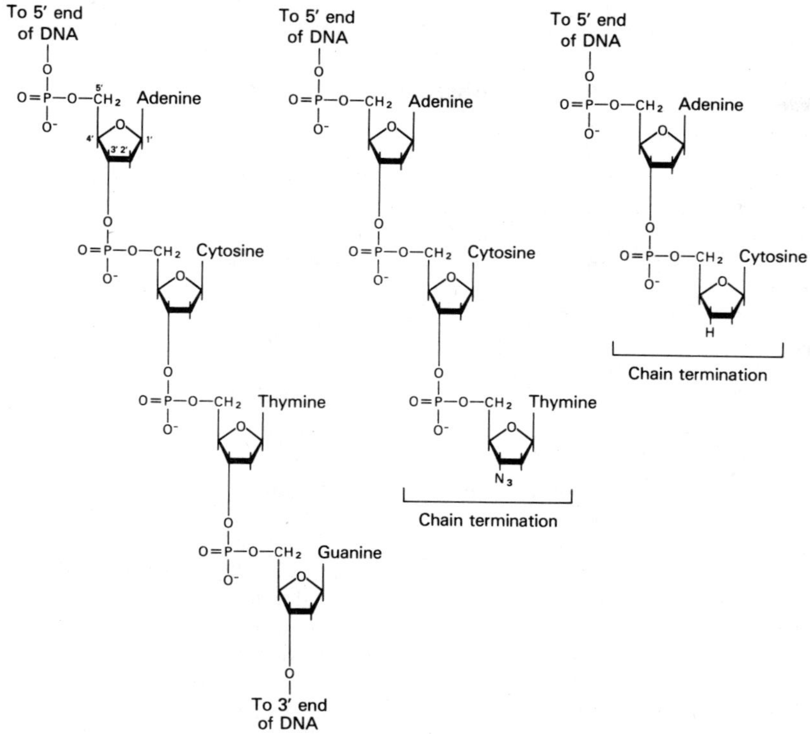

Figure 3. One Postulated Mechanism of Action of Dideoxynucleoside Triphosphates in Inhibiting HIV Replication.

Shown at left is a normal DNA chain. When AZT-TP (center) or 2′,3′-dideoxycytidine-5′-triphosphate (right) is bound by a DNA polymerase and incorporated onto the growing 3′ end of a DNA chain, it is not possible to form subsequent 5′→3′ phosphodiester linkages, which are necessary to add other nucleosides, and chain termination occurs. HIV reverse transcriptase is much more sensitive to the inhibitory effects of 2′,3′-dideoxynucleosides than is mammalian DNA polymerase alpha, an important enzyme in DNA synthesis and repair (see text).

mg per kilogram of body weight per day) over a six-week period had partial restoration of immune function, including twofold to threefold increases in the absolute number of helper–inducer (CD4+) T cells and the development of cutaneous delayed-type hypersensitivity reactions in previously anergic persons; these changes were often detectable after the second week of therapy.[71] Finally, the majority of patients given AZT gained weight and reported less fatigue, and some had improvements in other clinical abnormalities associated with AIDS.[71,80]

Toxic effects on bone marrow (particularly those resulting in anemia and leukopenia and, at times, in reductions in the number of CD4+ lymphocytes) are observed in most patients receiving high doses of oral AZT (90 mg per kilogram per day) for four to six weeks and in some patients receiving lower doses (25 to 30 mg per kilogram per day) for more than eight weeks.[71,80] An increase in the red-cell mean corpuscular volume (reflecting megaloblastic changes) is often an early sign of these toxic effects.[80] In most cases in which anemia or neutropenia represents the dose-limiting toxic effect, however, the patients can subsequently tolerate reduced doses of the drug (6 to 15 mg per kilogram per day orally). (There is little experience at this time, however, with the combined administration of AZT and other hematotoxic drugs, and such combinations might cause unacceptable toxic effects on bone marrow.) It is likely that an AZT-induced deficiency of thymidine triphosphate[71,74] contributes to the hematologic toxic effects (Fig. 2). Interestingly, thrombocytopenia is less common, and some patients even have increases in the number of platelets during short courses of AZT.[71] Approximately half the patients receiving AZT have reported mild headaches, and three patients receiving high doses (90 mg per kilogram per day orally) or concurrent antibiotic therapy have had transient agitation.[71,81] In addition, some patients had nausea and vomiting.[82] Otherwise, nonhematologic toxicity has rarely been observed.

We have now administered AZT to patients with AIDS for as long as 18 months, and they generally appear to tolerate the drug for this period.[81] Some patients with AIDS-related complex or Kaposi's sarcoma and relatively normal immunologic and bone marrow function at the start of therapy have had sustained increases in the number of CD4+ T cells.[80,81] However, some patients with AIDS have had late decreases in the number of CD4+ T cells and secondary infections with *Pneumocystis carinii* pneumonia.[80,81] It is unclear at this time whether these declines represent disease progression[83] or cumulative AZT toxicity, and this issue is a subject for future research. Overall, patients receiving AZT have fared well, and as a group, they appear to live longer than historical controls.[81,84] Drawing definite conclusions about survival in an open trial, however, can be misleading, particularly with a disease such as AIDS, in which substantial differences in survival can result from subtle base-line differences in the patient populations.

To address this point specifically and to determine whether some of the improvements observed in the AZT Phase I trial may have been due to a placebo effect, a multicenter randomized, double-blind, placebo-controlled trial was conducted in patients with AIDS who had recently recovered from *P. carinii* pneumonia and in patients with AIDS-related complex. In such a trial, a true drug effect can be distinguished from artifacts resulting from differences in supportive care, biases in reporting, or placebo effects. This study included 282 patients; nearly equal numbers were enrolled in each arm.[72,73] The investigation demonstrat-

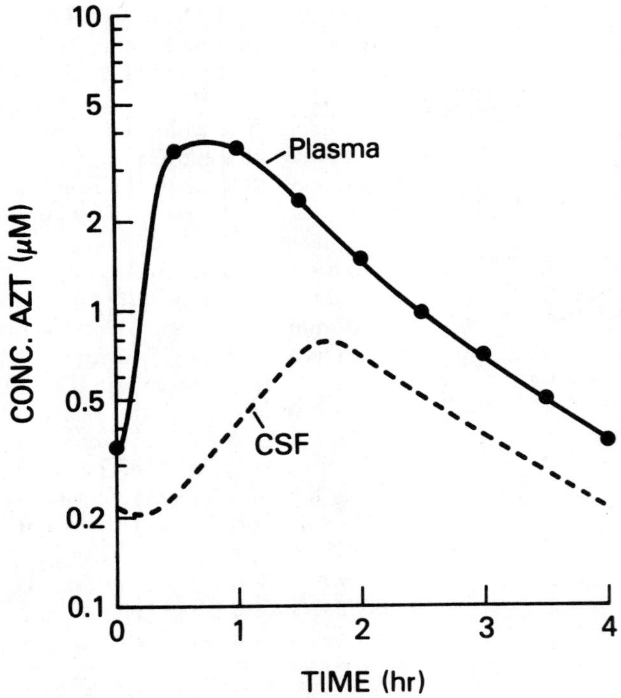

Figure 4. Model of AZT Pharmacokinetics.
Idealized plasma and cerebrospinal fluid (CSF) concentrations of AZT in a typical (70-kg) patient receiving 200 mg (3.57 mg per kilogram of body weight) of oral AZT every four hours.

ed that over a period of six months, there was a substantially decreased mortality rate in the patients receiving AZT (19 deaths in the placebo arm and only 1 death in the drug arm by September 1986).[72,73] As of this writing, AZT is being made widely available on an investigational basis to patients with AIDS who have had *P. carinii* pneumonia and who satisfy certain other criteria. This experience serves as a reminder that placebo-controlled trials in certain settings can greatly accelerate the pace of drug development.

As noted above, AZT has excellent penetration across the blood–brain barrier; four hours after a dose is taken, the levels in the cerebrospinal fluid average 50 to 60 percent of simultaneously measured plasma levels.[71,78,82] This finding suggested that AZT might benefit patients with HIV-associated neurologic dysfunction. As a first step in testing this hypothesis, we administered AZT to seven such patients. Each of the six patients with HIV-associated dementia, peripheral neuropathy, or both has had some improvement of symptoms as assessed by clinical examinations, neuropsychometric testing, nerve-conduction studies, or positron emission tomography (in one patient, however, the drug subsequently had to be stopped because of neutropenia). The seventh patient, who had a T10 paraplegia, had no demonstrable response.[81,82] These results suggest that AZT can at least transiently induce improvements in cognitive function, coordination, and peripheral-nerve function in a subset of patients with HIV-associated neurologic disease. However, only a limited number of such patients have been studied so far, and we do not know how long the effects will last; further therapeutic studies with AZT (and other antiviral agents) are needed in this population.

The clinical experience with AZT is limited at this time, and the long-term sequelae of drug administration are not known. The optimal dose for therapy is still being explored, and it may vary in different groups of patients; for example, one may be willing to tolerate relatively more toxicity in patients with HIV-associated dementia. We also need to learn the best schedule of administration and whether the development of AIDS may be slowed or prevented by administering AZT early in the course of an HIV infection. Strategies that may permit more antiviral activity without a concomitant increase in bone marrow toxicity should now be investigated. In this regard, it has recently been observed that acyclovir (a guanosine analogue with potent activity against herpesviruses but little or no antiretroviral activity by itself) can potentiate the antiretroviral effect of AZT in vitro through an unknown mechanism.[76] Acyclovir does not characteristically cause bone marrow suppression, and it is possible that the combination of this agent and AZT may be of benefit. A clinical trial to test this hypothesis is currently under way.

It is hoped that further research may permit us to use AZT more effectively in patients with AIDS or identify other agents that are even more effective. The use of AZT is only a first step. Even at this point, however, the demonstration that one dideoxynucleoside analogue has clinical efficacy in some patients with AIDS and that even the neurologic dysfunction caused by the disease may be partly reversible in some cases has removed some of the uncertainty about the rationale for an antiretroviral intervention in established AIDS. It may also help to dispel the prevailing sense of hopelessness about the disease.

References

1. Gottlieb MS, Schroff R, Schanker HM, et al. *Pneumocystis carinii* pneumonia and mucosal candidiasis in previously healthy homosexual men: evidence of a new acquired cellular immunodeficiency. N Engl J Med 1981; 305:1425-31.
2. Masur H, Michelis MA, Greene JB, et al. An outbreak of community-acquired *Pneumocystis carinii* pneumonia: initial manifestation of cellular immune dysfunction. N Engl J Med 1981; 305:1431-8.
3. Siegal FP, Lopez C, Hammer GS, et al. Severe acquired immunodeficiency in male homosexuals, manifested by chronic perianal ulcerative herpes simplex lesions. N Engl J Med 1981; 305:1439-44.
4. Gallo RC, Salahuddin SZ, Popovic M, et al. Frequent detection and isolation of cytopathic retroviruses (HTLV-III) from patients with AIDS and at risk for AIDS. Science 1984; 224:500-3.
5. Popovic M, Sarngadharan MG, Read E, Gallo RC. Detection, isolation, and continuous production of cytopathic retroviruses (HTLV-III) from patients with AIDS and pre-AIDS. Science 1984; 224:497-500.
6. Ho DD, Rota TR, Hirsch MS. Infection of monocyte/macrophages by human T lymphotropic virus type III. J Clin Invest 1986; 77:1712-5.
7. Gartner S, Markovits P, Markovitz DM, Kaplan MH, Gallo RC, Popovic M. The role of mononuclear phagocytes in HTLV-III/LAV infection. Science 1986; 233:215-9.
8. Fahey JL, Prince H, Weaver M, et al. Quantitative changes in T helper or T suppressor/cytotoxic lymphocyte subsets that distinguish acquired immune deficiency syndrome from other immune disorders. Am J Med 1984; 76:95-100.

9. Barré-Sinoussi F, Chermann JC, Rey F, et al. Isolation of a T-lymphotropic retrovirus from a patient at risk for acquired immune deficiency syndrome (AIDS). Science 1983; 220:868-71.
10. Levy JA, Hoffman AD, Kramer SM, Landis JA, Shimabukuro JM, Oshiro JS. Isolation of lymphocytopathic retroviruses from San Francisco patients with AIDS. Science 1984; 225:840-2.
11. Coffin J, Haase A, Levy JA, et al. Human immunodeficiency viruses. Science 1986; 232:697.
12. Groopman JE, Salahuddin SZ, Sarngadharan MG, et al. HTLV-III in saliva of people with AIDS-related complex and healthy homosexual men at risk for AIDS. Science 1984; 226:447-9.
13. Ho DD, Schooley RT, Rota TR, et al. HTLV-III in the semen and blood of a healthy homosexual man. Science 1984; 226:451-3.
14. Goedert JJ, Biggar RJ, Weiss SH, et al. Three-year incidence of AIDS in five cohorts of HTLV-III–infected risk group members. Science 1986; 231:992-5.
15. Klatzmann D, Barré-Sinoussi F, Nugeyre MT, et al. Selective tropism of lymphadenopathy associated virus (LAV) for helper-inducer T lymphocytes. Science 1984; 225:59-63.
16. Laurence J, Gottlieb AB, Kunkel HG. Soluble suppressor factors in patients with acquired immune deficiency syndrome and its prodrome: elaboration in vitro by T lymphocyte-adherent cell interactions. J Clin Invest 1983; 72:2072-81.
17. Lane HC, Masur H, Longo DL, et al. Partial immune reconstitution in a patient with the acquired immunodeficiency syndrome. N Engl J Med 1984; 311:1099-103.
18. Shaw GM, Harper ME, Hahn BH, et al. HTLV-III infection in brains of children and adults with AIDS encephalopathy. Science 1985; 227:177-82.
19. Ho DD, Rota TR, Schooley RT, et al. Isolation of HTLV-III from cerebrospinal fluid and neural tissues of patients with neurologic syndromes related to the acquired immunodeficiency syndrome. N Engl J Med 1985; 313:1493-7.
20. Resnick L, diMarzo-Veronese F, Schüpbach J, et al. Intra-blood–brain-barrier synthesis of HTLV-III-specific IgG in patients with neurologic symptoms associated with AIDS or AIDS-related complex. N Engl J Med 1985; 313:1498-504.
21. Navia BA, Jordan BD, Price RW. The AIDS dementia complex. I. Clinical features. Ann Neurol 1986; 19:517-24.
22. Nemerow GR, Cooper NR. Infection of B lymphocytes by a human herpesvirus, Epstein–Barr virus, is blocked by calmodulin antagonists. Proc Natl Acad Sci USA 1984; 81:4955-9.
23. Baltimore D. RNA-dependent DNA polymerase in virions of RNA tumour viruses. Nature 1970; 226:1209-11.
24. Temin HM, Mizutani S. RNA-dependent DNA polymerase in virions in Rous sarcoma virus. Nature 1970; 226:1211-3.
25. Klein G. Immune and non-immune control of neoplastic development: contrasting effects of host and tumor evolution. Cancer 1980; 45:2486-99.
26. Dalgleish AG, Beverley PCL, Clapham PR, Crawford DH, Greaves MF, Weiss RA. The CD4 (T4) antigen is an essential component of the receptor for the AIDS retrovirus. Nature 1984; 312:763-7.
27. Klatzmann D, Champagne E, Chamaret S, et al. T-lymphocyte T4 molecule behaves as the receptor for human retrovirus LAV. Nature 1984; 312:767-8.
28. Sodroski J, Goh WC, Rosen C, Campbell K, Haseltine WA. Role of the HTLV-III/LAV envelope in syncytium formation and cytopathicity. Nature 1986; 322:470-4.
29. Lifson JD, Feinberg MB, Reyes GR, et al. Induction of CD4-dependent cell fusion by the HTLV-III/LAV envelope glycoprotein. Nature 1986; 323:725-8.
30. Pert CB, Hill JM, Ruff MR, et al. Octapeptides deduced from the neuropeptide receptor-like pattern of antigen T4 in brain potently inhibit human immunodeficiency virus receptor binding and T-cell infectivity. Proc Natl Acad Sci USA 1986; 83:9254-8.
31. Wong-Staal F, Gallo RC. Human T-lymphotropic retroviruses. Nature 1985; 317:395-403.
32. Hahn BH, Shaw GM, Taylor ME, et al. Genetic variation in HTLV-III/LAV over time in patients with AIDS or at risk for AIDS. Science 1986; 232:1548-53.
33. Dolin R. Antiviral chemotherapy and chemoprophylaxis. Science 1985; 227:1296-303.
34. Tanese N, Sodroski J, Haseltine WA, Goff SP. Expression of reverse transcriptase activity of human T-lymphotropic virus type III (HTLV-III/LAV) in *Escherichia coli*. J Virol 1986; 59:743-5.
35. Johnson MS, McClure MA, Feng D-F, Gray J, Doolittle RF. Computer analysis of retroviral *pol* genes: assignment of enzymatic functions to specific sequences and homologies with nonviral enzymes. Proc Natl Acad Sci USA 1986; 83:7648-52.
36. Mitsuya H, Popovic M, Yarchoan R, Matsushita S, Gallo RC, Broder S. Suramin protection of T cells in vitro against infectivity and cytopathic effect of HTLV-III. Science 1984; 226:172-4.
37. Rozenbaum W, Dormont D, Spire B, et al. Antimoniotungstate (HPA 23) treatment of three patients with AIDS and one with prodrome. Lancet 1985; 1:450-1.
38. Sandstrom EG, Kaplan JC, Byington RE, Hirsch MS. Inhibition of human T-cell lymphotropic virus type III in vitro by phosphonoformate. Lancet 1985; 1:1480-2.
39. Anand R, Moore J, Feorino P, Curran J, Srinivasan A. Rifabutine inhibits HTLV-III. Lancet 1986; 1:97-8.
40. Mitsuya H, Weinhold KJ, Furman PA, et al. 3′-Azido-3′-deoxythymidine (BW A509U): an antiviral agent that inhibits the infectivity and cytopathic effect of human T-lymphotropic virus type III/lymphadenopathy-associated virus *in vitro*. Proc Natl Acad Sci USA 1985; 82:7096-100.
41. Mitsuya H, Broder H. Inhibition of the *in vitro* infectivity and cytopathic effect of human T-lymphotropic virus type III/lymphadenopathy-associated virus (HTLV-III/LAV) by 2′,3′-dideoxynucleosides. Proc Natl Acad Sci USA 1986; 83:1911-5.
42. Ting RC, Yang SS, Gallo RC. Reverse transcriptase, RNA tumour virus transformation and derivatives of rifamycin SV. Nature [New Biol] 1972; 236:163-6.
43. Furmanski P, Bourguignon GJ, Bolles CS, Corombos JD, Das MR. Inhibition by 2′,3′-dideoxythymidine of retroviral infection of mouse and human cells. Cancer Lett 1980; 8:307-15.
44. De Clercq E. Suramin: a potent inhibitor of the reverse transcriptase of RNA tumor viruses. Cancer Lett 1979; 8:9-22.
45. Waqar MA, Evans MJ, Manly KF, Hughes RG, Huberman JA. Effects of 2′,3′-dideoxynucleosides on mammalian cells and viruses. J Cell Physiol 1984; 121:402-8.
46. Ostertag W, Roesler G, Krieg CJ, et al. Induction of endogenous virus and of thymidine kinase by bromodeoxyuridine in cell cultures transformed by Friend virus. Proc Natl Acad Sci USA 1974; 71:4980-5.
47. Chandra P, Demirhan I, De Clercq E. A study of antitemplate inhibition of mammalian, bacterial and viral DNA polymerases by 2- and 2′-substituted derivatives of polyadenylic acid. Cancer Lett 1981; 12:181-93.
48. Shaw GM, Hahn BH, Arya SK, Groopman JE, Gallo RC, Wong-Staal F. Molecular characterization of human T-cell leukemia (lymphotropic) virus type III in the acquired immune deficiency syndrome. Science 1984; 226:1165-71.
49. McCormick JB, Getchell JP, Mitchell SW, Hicks DR. Ribavirin suppresses replication of lymphadenopathy-associated virus in cultures of human adult T lymphocytes. Lancet 1984; 2:1367-9.
50. Sodroski J, Rosen C, Wong-Staal F, et al. *Trans*-acting transcriptional regulation of human T-cell leukemia virus type III long terminal repeat. Science 1985; 227:171-3.
51. Sodroski J, Goh WC, Rosen C, Dayton A, Terwilliger E, Haseltine W. A second post-transcriptional *trans*-activator gene required for HTLV-III replication. Nature 1986; 321:412-7.
52. Feinberg MB, Jarrett RF, Aldovini A, Gallo RC, Wong-Staal F. HTLV-III expression and production involve complex regulation at the levels of splicing and translation of viral RNA. Cell 1986; 46:807-17.
53. Fisher AG, Feinberg MB, Josephs SF, et al. The *trans*-activator gene of HTLV-III is essential for virus replication. Nature 1986; 320:367-71.
54. Rosen CA, Sodroski JG, Goh WC, Dayton AI, Lippke J, Haseltine WA. Post-transcriptional regulation accounts for the *trans*-activation of the human T-lymphotropic virus type III. Nature 1986; 319:555-9.
55. Smith TJ, Kremer MJ, Luo M, et al. The site of attachment of human rhinovirus 14 for antiviral agents that inhibit uncoating. Science 1986; 233:1286-93.
56. Izant JG, Weintraub H. Inhibition of thymidine kinase gene expression by anti-sense RNA: a molecular approach to genetic analysis. Cell 1984; 36:1007-15.
57. Pestka S, Daugherty BL, Jung V, Hotta K, Pestka RK. Anti-mRNA: specific inhibition of translation of single mRNA molecules. Proc Natl Acad Sci USA 1984; 81:7525-8.
58. Zamecnik PC, Goodchild J, Taguchi Y, Sarin PS. Inhibition of replication and expression of human T-cell lymphotropic virus type III in cultured cells by exogenous synthetic oligonucleotides complementary to viral RNA. Proc Natl Acad Sci USA 1986; 83:4143-6.
59. Schultz AM, Oroszlan S. In vivo modification of retroviral *gag* gene-encoded polyproteins by myristic acid. J Virol 1983; 46:355-61.
60. Henderson LE, Krutzsch HC, Oroszlan S. Myristyl amino-terminal acylation of murine retrovirus proteins: an unusual post-translational proteins modification. Proc Natl Acad Sci USA 1983; 80:339-43.
61. Ho DD, Hartshorn KL, Rota TR, et al. Recombinant human interferon alfa-A suppresses HTLV-III replication in vitro. Lancet 1985; 1:602-4.
62. Montagnier L, Gruest J, Chamaret S, et al. Adaptation of lymphadenopathy associated virus (LAV) to replication in EBV-transformed B lymphoblastoid cell lines. Science 1984; 225:63-6.
63. Birx DL, Redfield RR, Tosato G. Defective regulation of Epstein–Barr virus infection in patients with acquired immunodeficiency syndrome (AIDS) or AIDS-related disorders. N Engl J Med 1986; 314:874-9.
64. Yarchoan R, Redfield RR, Broder S. Mechanisms of B cell activation in

patients with acquired immunodeficiency syndrome and related disorders: contribution of antibody-producing B cells, of Epstein–Barr virus-infected B cells, and of immunoglobulin production induced by human T cell lymphotropic virus, type III/lymphadenopathy-associated virus. J Clin Invest 1986; 78:439-47.
65. Hoxie JA, Haggarty BS, Rackowski JL, Pillsbury N, Levy JA. Persistent noncytopathic infection of normal human T lymphocytes with AIDS-associated retrovirus. Science 1985; 229:1400-2.
66. Folks T, Powell DM, Lightfoote MM, Benn S, Martin MA, Fauci AS. Induction of HTLV-III/LAV from a nonvirus-producing T-cell line: implications for latency. Science 1986; 231:600-2.
67. Horwitz JP, Chua J, Noel M. Nucleosides. V. The monomesylates of 1-(2′-deoxy-β-D-lyxofuranosyl)thymine. J Org Chem 1964; 29:2076-8.
68. Toji L, Cohen SS. The enzymatic termination of polydeoxynucleotides by 2′,3′-dideoxyadenosine triphosphate. Proc Natl Acad Sci USA 1969; 63:871-7.
69. Lin T-S, Prusoff WH. Synthesis and biological activity of several amino analogues of thymidine. J Med Chem 1978; 21:109-12.
70. Sanger F, Nicklen S, Coulson AR. DNA sequencing with chain-terminating inhibitors. Proc Natl Acad Sci USA 1977; 74:5463-7.
71. Yarchoan R, Klecker RW, Weinhold KJ, et al. Administration of 3′-azido-3′-deoxythymidine, an inhibitor of HTLV-III/LAV replication, to patients with AIDS or AIDS-related complex. Lancet 1986; 1:575-80.
72. Barnes DM. Promising results halt trial of anti-AIDS drug. Science 1986; 234:15-6.
73. Wright K. First tentative signs of therapeutic promise. Nature 1986; 323:283.
74. Furman PA, Fyfe JS, St. Clair MH, et al. Phosphorylation of 3′-azido-3′-deoxythymidine and selective interaction of the 5′-triphosphate with human immunodeficiency virus reverse transcriptase. Proc Natl Acad Sci USA 1986; 83:8333-7.
75. Cooney DA, Dalal M, Mitsuya H, et al. Initial studies on the cellular pharmacology of 2′,3′-dideoxycytidine, an inhibitor of HTLV-III infectivity. Biochem Pharmacol 1986; 35:2065-8.
76. Mitsuya H, Matsukura M, Broder S. Rapid *in vitro* systems for assessing activity of agents against HTLV-III/LAV. In: Broder S, ed. AIDS: modern concepts and therapeutic challenges. New York: Marcel Dekker, 1987:303-33.
77. Kelly JA, Litterst CL, Roth JS, et al. The disposition and metabolism of 2′,3′-dideoxycytidine, an *in vitro* inhibitor of HTLV-III infectivity, in mice and monkeys. Drug Metab Dispos (in press).
78. Klecker RW, Collins JM, Yarchoan R, et al. Plasma and cerebrospinal fluid pharmacokinetics of 3′-azido-3′-deoxythymidine: a novel pyrimidine analog with potential application for the treatment of AIDS and related disorders. Clin Pharmacol Ther (in press).
79. de Miranda P, Good SS, Blum MR, Thomas RV, Yarchoan R, Broder S. The effect of probenecid on the pharmacokinetic disposition of azidothymidine (AZT). Presented at the International Conference on Acquired Immunodeficiency Syndrome (AIDS), Paris, June 23-25, 1986.
80. Yarchoan R, Broder S. Strategies for the pharmacologic intervention against HTLV-III/LAV. In: Broder S, ed. AIDS: modern concepts and therapeutic challenges. New York: Marcel Dekker, 1987:335-60.
81. *Idem.* Preliminary results on the use of dideoxynucleosides in the therapy of AIDS. In: Chanock RM, Lerner RA, Brown F, Ginsberg HS, eds. Vaccine 87. Cold Spring Harbor, N.Y.: Cold Spring Harbor Press (in press).
82. Yarchoan R, Berg G, Brouwers P, et al. Response of human-immunodeficiency-virus-associated neurological disease to 3′-azido-3′-deoxythymidine. Lancet 1987; 1:132-5.
83. Broder S, Gallo RC. A pathogenic retrovirus (HTLV-III) linked to AIDS. N Engl J Med 1984; 311:1292-7.
84. Rivin BE, Monroe JM, Hubschman BP, Thomas PA. AIDS outcome: a first follow-up. N Engl J Med 1984; 311:857.

SPECIAL ARTICLE

THE PROSPECTS FOR AND PATHWAYS TOWARD A VACCINE FOR AIDS

Donald P. Francis, M.D., D.Sc., and John C. Petricciani, M.D.

Acquired immunodeficiency syndrome (AIDS) is a severe disease of the immune system caused by a horizontally transmitted retrovirus. Although this virus has been given several names, including lymphadenopathy-associated virus (LAV),[1,2] immunodeficiency-associated virus (IDAV),[3] human T-cell lymphotropic virus Type III (HTLV-III),[4] and AIDS-associated retrovirus (ARV),[5] it is referred to as HTLV-III/LAV in this discussion. This virus preferentially infects lymphocytes of the T helper subset and destroys them, leaving the host unable to cope with a variety of infectious and neoplastic diseases.[6] The clinical syndrome AIDS is the most severe clinical manifestation of HTLV-III/LAV infection, but there appears to be a wide range of milder conditions, including a transient mononucleosis-like syndrome, persistent generalized lymphadenopathy, and various hematologic conditions that may be part of a wider clinical spectrum associated with this infection. Studies of the natural history of HTLV-III/LAV infection among homosexual men followed for several years have shown that generalized lymphadenopathy has developed in about 25 percent of infected men and AIDS in 7 to 15 percent.[7-9]

HTLV-III/LAV was presumably introduced into the United States in the 1970s, and although it is difficult to transmit as compared with many other infectious agents, it has spread effectively in situations in which personal behavior or prescribed medical therapies have exposed people to the virus.[10,11] Several practical recommendations have been made to decrease the transmission of this virus in the United States.[12,13] Some are directed toward the modification of sexual behavior — specifically, the avoidance of sexual contact with persons with clinical, laboratory, or epidemiologic evidence of infection. Others have been directed toward protecting blood and blood products from infection with this virus; specifically, members of groups at risk for AIDS were asked in March 1983 to refrain voluntarily from donating plasma or blood. Later, heat treatment of factor VIII concentrates was instituted, and more recently, serologic screening tests for antibody to HTLV-III/LAV were approved, and all donors are now being tested.

But these control measures are unlikely to eliminate transmission completely because AIDS is transmitted primarily through sexual contact. The only certain barrier to further spread of the disease is a vaccine.[14]

The production of an effective vaccine for AIDS depends on the ability to manufacture large quantities of a safe antigen that stimulates protective immunity when it is injected into human beings. The recent licensure of a vaccine for feline leukemia virus, a retrovirus causing an AIDS-like disease in cats, brings home the scientific possibility that a successful retrovirus vaccine for human beings might work. However, although they are related, HTLV-III/LAV and feline leukemia virus are different viruses, and many difficult scientific problems must be solved before an AIDS vaccine can be developed. Moreover, there are several nonscientific issues that may inhibit the development of an AIDS vaccine. The most important one relates to the interest of the private sector in investing in an AIDS-vaccine project. It is expensive to develop a new vaccine and bring it to the public, and companies capable of it may be reluctant to invest large sums of money for an uncertain return. The uncertainties of an AIDS-vaccine market center on (1) how big the market is (i.e., how large the population is for which the vaccine will be recommended [both nationally and internationally]); (2) who will pay for the vaccine (the individual, third-party insurers, the government); and (3) what the liability risks are.

We here outline a suggested pathway toward the development of an AIDS vaccine, encourage collaborative studies to speed the development process, and present options for the use of such a vaccine once it is developed.

The Causative Virus

Although AIDS is clinically unique, its causative virus shares many features with other well-studied retroviruses. Its genome codes for a small number of proteins, including several structural proteins, an enzyme essential for its replication, and one or two peptides of unknown function. Specifically, the HTLV-III/LAV genome contains genes that have been termed "gag," "pol," and "env."[15-18] The gag gene codes for proteins that make up the core of the virus — one with a molecular weight of about 18,000 and the other with a molecular weight of about 24,000 (p24). A third gag-encoded protein, with a molecular weight of about 15,000, is most likely the ribonucleoprotein. The pol gene codes for the replication enzyme reverse transcriptase, and the env gene codes for the proteins (presumably two) that make up the outer coat, or envelope, of the virus. One, the major envelope protein, appears to be large (molecular weight, 110,000 to 120,000 [gp120]) and extensively glycosylated.[15-19] The other, with a molecular weight of about 41,000 (gp41), is presumably the transmembrane protein, which joins the envelope to the virus core. Antibodies

From the Division of Viral Diseases, Center for Infectious Diseases, Centers for Disease Control, Atlanta; and the Division of Blood and Blood Products, Center for Drugs and Biologics, Food and Drug Administration, Bethesda, Md.

in the serum of infected people commonly react to most if not all of the major structural proteins, both core and envelope.[17,19-21]

The role of antibodies in host defense against infection is unknown, however. Some of these antibodies may be protective, as evidenced by the finding that serum from some infected persons can neutralize HTLV-III/LAV in vitro.[22,23] The prevalence of these antibodies, at least at high titer as determined by currently available techniques, appears to be low. Moreover, antibody testing has so far not been able to classify infected persons as protected or unprotected. This contrasts markedly with the situation in feline leukemia virus infections, in which the presence of neutralizing antibody is highly correlated with protection from severe disease.[24] But the rarity of neutralizing antibody in persons infected with HTLV-III/LAV does not by itself preclude the possibility that people can be protected with an AIDS vaccine, because antibodies induced by a vaccine may be functionally quite different from those induced in the presence of persistent infection.

The biologic and genetic stability of the viral antigens is critical to the effectiveness of an AIDS vaccine. If the frequency of genetic mutations is so high that it effectively allows the virus to escape from a vaccine-induced host immune response, then a vaccine may not be effective. On the other hand, if the frequency of mutations is low or if there are highly conserved regions against which protective antibodies can be produced, then a vaccine becomes a much more viable prospect. HTLV-III/LAV appears to have several subtype variations, some or all of which may need to be considered in vaccine development. Nucleic acid variations from one isolate to another include those in the env region, whose ultimate protein product is likely to be the target of protective immunity.[15-18] Indeed, the variations in the env region include sites of potential glycosylation. These glycosylation sites, along with other sites of variation, could be important in terms of vaccination, because they could substantially affect both the tertiary structure of a protein and its immunogenicity. Understanding the extent of marked subtype variation will be extremely important for vaccine planning.

Vaccines against Other Naturally Occurring Retroviruses

If it is found that the genetic variation of HTLV-III/LAV is limited and predictable, vaccine-induced antibodies directed toward its structural proteins, especially envelope proteins, could protect against subsequent infection. In this regard, two vaccines against retrovirus infection in other animal species may serve as useful models. The best example is infection of cats with feline leukemia virus. This is a common worldwide infection of pet cats, which causes diseases quite similar to AIDS in human beings.[24] Feline leukemia virus does have subtype variations, but the antigenic sites that are conserved in all known isolates have been identified and incorporated in the vaccine. Vaccination against feline leukemia virus with early vaccine preparations was initially ineffective and may have actually worsened the outcome of subsequent infection.[25] However, the later use of an inactivated vaccine purified from the supernatant fluid of cultured cells has been effective, and the vaccine was recently licensed in the United States ("Leukocell," Norden Laboratories, Lincoln, Nebr.). Although the exact manufacturing process of the commercial vaccine is a trade secret, prototype vaccines from which it was modeled were made by simply concentrating whole virus and virus subunits from high-titer supernatant fluid of FL 74 cells in a manner that preserved envelope glycoprotein.[26] The inactivated product, combined with adjuvant, was then used as a vaccine. Both prototype and commercial products have induced measurable antibodies and protection after both laboratory challenge and natural exposure.[26,27] The feline leukemia virus vaccine model is important for the development of retroviral vaccines in a general sense. Yet, because the pathogenic process of feline leukemia virus appears to be quite different from that of HTLV-III/LAV and because the safety requirements for animal vaccines are quite different from those for human vaccines, the development of an AIDS vaccine offers considerably more challenge.

Vaccines for another animal retrovirus disease, bovine leukosis/leukemia — a rare complication of a common infection of cattle by bovine leukemia virus — are at a more basic developmental stage. Attempts to prevent this infection with vaccine have had mixed results, much like those of the early attempts against feline leukemia virus. Trials in this country with purified virus preparations have failed,[28] but there are reports from abroad of a preparation that shows a relatively high efficacy.[29]

Options for Antigen Production

There are several ways a human retrovirus vaccine could be made. Current viral vaccines for human beings use both live and killed virus to induce protective antibodies, and among the killed-virus vaccines there are examples of both whole-virus and subunit preparations. Because retroviruses have a predilection for recombination and because they have been associated with malignant diseases, it is highly unlikely that a live attenuated retrovirus vaccine would be acceptable for human beings.

A killed-virus vaccine, on the other hand, should be much more acceptable. Problems arise here, however, in selecting a cell line for producing the virus, choosing methods for purifying the viral antigens, and freeing them from viral nucleic acid. HTLV-III/LAV has limited cell tropism, and cells derived from human tumors may be the only ones that will support the large-scale production of immunogenic antigens. Although the use of such abnormal cells raises additional safety issues in connection with the vaccine, there appears to be a consensus that under certain conditions, some tumor-derived cells could be acceptable.[30] For example, the Food and Drug Administration has already accepted Chinese hamster ovary cells for use in the production of an investigational recombinant vaccine against hepatitis B virus. An additional problem with whole or subunit vaccines is that the extensive processing required to produce a safe vaccine from retrovirus cell cultures may potentially cause the loss of a sizable proportion of some structural antigens, especially envelope glycoproteins, which may be important in inducing protective immunity. In the future, the direct biochemical synthesis of antigenic peptides may be an alternative to cell culture. These peptides, chosen by computer prediction models that target hydrophilic subregions of viral proteins, may prove to be an inexpensive source of antigenic material.

Perhaps the best option at this time is recombinant DNA technology. Already several groups have been able to incorporate HTLV-III/LAV genes into bacteria, yeast, and mammalian cells, all of which have produced virus-specific proteins. The advantages of these antigen-production systems are that the infective virus cannot be produced, because only a small portion of the viral genome is incorporated, and that high-yield production systems can be designed that, when combined with other modern biochemical techniques, can ensure large quantities of safe and economical immunogens. On the other hand, the theoretical disadvantages of these systems are (1) that the immunity-inducing epitopes may be inadequately represented on the expressed proteins; (2) that the post-translational processing of the expressed proteins may make them different from the natural product; and (3) that the relative amounts of the immunologically important proteins may be different and therefore less immunogenic in the expressed antigens as compared with the natural ones.

The choice of which recombinant system (bacterial, yeast, or mammalian cells) to use may have to take into consideration the fact that bacterial and yeast cells do not effectively glycosylate their expressed proteins. Since the envelope glycoprotein of HTLV-III/LAV is heavily glycosylated, it may be essential to use mammalian cells to duplicate the natural antigen accurately. Although the immunogenic importance of glycosylation has not been determined for the AIDS agent, mammalian cell systems should probably be given high priority as expression vectors. Other possibilities, such as vaccinia-vector vaccines, are still in early research and developmental stages, and they will probably require much more time before they are ready for clinical trials.

Regardless of which recombinant production system is used, a decision must be made about which antigen or antigens should be incorporated into an AIDS vaccine. Simplicity would seem to override complexity in this matter, and at least at the beginning, the best choice would appear to be a vaccine containing only the major envelope glycoprotein, gp 120. Should this fail to induce protective antibodies, continued trials of different subunits of the same protein, different proteins alone, or different proteins in combination with the envelope protein could be instituted. How much effort should be devoted to trying (or adding) the transmembrane protein (gp41) or any gag-encoded proteins in advance of knowing the results of a prototype envelope vaccine remains an open question. It should be remembered, however, that in the feline system one of these other proteins (the transmembrane protein, p15E) is immunosuppressive.[31]

Another question arises regarding adjuvants. Should vaccine developers use alum, which is accepted as a safe adjuvant, or should they try others that may be more effective? In the interests of both speed and simplicity, logic would lead one to explore the use of alum as the adjuvant for prototype vaccines, while leaving the door open for the exploration of others if alum proves unsatisfactory.

Pathway for Evaluation

Assuming that expressed envelope proteins will soon be available in adequate quantity and purity for testing, an evaluation pathway that will document safety and efficacy while minimizing the time for approval needs to be established. The specifics of this pathway will be finally determined during formal interaction with the Food and Drug Administration as clinical trials progress, but a reasonable approach is suggested here.

A first step in evaluation is to test the ability of the vaccine to induce antibodies in animals and test the effect of these antibodies on viral replication. If a prototype vaccine induces antibodies in small laboratory animals and the antibodies neutralize the virus in an in vitro assay, the vaccine could then be advanced to the next step — experiments with primate challenge. For this purpose, the chimpanzee model has been developed.[32-34] Possibly, a less expensive and more readily available susceptible animal will eventually be found, but until that time the chimpanzee remains the best model, since it is readily infected with HTLV-III/LAV and has a quite predictable response to infection. After intravenous inoculation of chimpanzees with 10^3 to 10^4 times the $TCID_{50}$, virus can be isolated from peripheral-blood lymphocytes within a few weeks, and antibody can be detected soon thereafter. A prototype vaccine's ability to protect could be tested by immunizing chimpanzees with the vaccine and subsequently challenging the animals with a dose of HTLV-III/LAV known to be infectious. After challenge, the animals could be monitored for infection by both viral isolation and antibody testing. For example, weekly cultures of peripheral-blood lymphocytes would provide data on whether viral replication is detectable, and weekly testing for antibody to antigens not in the vaccine (e.g., p24) could be used to determine whether viral replication, undetectable by lymphocyte culture, had occurred. The length of follow-up in the chimpanzees would probably not need to exceed a few months. How many animals to use per prototype vaccine would depend on the availability of adequately housed chimpanzees and the safety concerns of each prototype vaccine. However, it should be recognized early in any vaccine-development program that there are serious limitations on the number of chimpanzees available for research generally and that it will be possible to develop only a moderate amount of safety and efficacy data from work with them before moving on to clinical trials in human beings.

Human Trials

Once a candidate vaccine has been shown to protect chimpanzees (or another equally susceptible animal) from infection, and after major preclinical safety issues have been resolved, it will be appropriate to begin testing in human beings. The first step will be to administer the vaccine to a small group of volunteers in order to obtain preliminary information about both short-term safety and immunogenicity. Whether members of AIDS risk groups or persons not at risk should be the first to receive the experimental vaccine is one of many issues that will require considerable discussion early in the process. In these initial trials, side effects of the vaccine will need to be monitored clinically and biologically with a variety of tests. Since the receptor site for this virus appears to be closely related to the T4 antigen on lymphocytes, special attention will have to be given to monitoring any antilymphocyte reactions in vaccine recipients. If the vaccine performs reasonably in these early studies, larger safety and immunogenicity trials could follow.

As immunogenicity data are being collected and the ideal dose and spacing of doses are being determined, efficacy trials could be planned. Groups of susceptible people at risk of infection would need to be identified and studied to determine the incidence of infection. For example, the Centers for Disease Control and the National Institutes of Health are conducting studies in several cities in which the incidence rates of HTLV-III/LAV infection in high-risk populations are being followed. From the incidence rates in these populations, sample-size estimates for double-blind, randomized, placebo-controlled trials could be made.

During efficacy trials, monitoring of participants may be complicated by the presence of persons who, because of recent infection or aberrant immune responses, may have negative serologic tests even though they are infected with HTLV-III/LAV and have viremia. If these persons received the AIDS vaccine, two outcomes could confuse vaccine evaluation. In the first case, seroconversion in such persons could be due to the preexisting infection rather than the vaccine. Secondly, and perhaps more important, if vaccine volunteers who were already infected with HTLV-III/LAV later acquired viremia or the signs and symptoms of AIDS, the safety of the vaccine would be questioned. However, viral isolation from selected participants and serologic testing for antibodies to viral antigens not contained in the vaccine should resolve any confusion on this score.

Application of an AIDS Vaccine

If a safe and effective AIDS vaccine is produced and made available, for whom should it be recommended? In the United States such decisions are usually made by the Immunization Practices Advisory Committee of the Public Health Service, the Immunization Committee of the American College of Physicians, and the Committee on Infectious Diseases of the American Academy of Pediatrics. These groups will probably have a key role in formulating a vaccination strategy for any AIDS vaccine, although it is also probable that a much broader public dialogue on the issues will occur in advance of formal recommendations by those committees. For example, there will almost surely be workshops sponsored by various government organizations, such as the Centers for Disease Control, the FDA, and the National Institutes of Health, and the Vaccine Advisory Committee of the FDA will undoubtedly discuss some of these issues during the investigational stages. To make recommendations, these committees will balance the infection risks of individual groups with the safety, efficacy, and cost of the vaccine. It will probably be easy to recommend the vaccine for uninfected persons from major AIDS risk groups, such as homosexual men, intravenous drug abusers, and sexual contacts of infected persons. But because of the potentially severe consequences of infection with this virus, the use of a vaccine may also be considered for those at lower risk of infection. For example, members of the health professions who care for infected patients appear to be rarely infected, yet even the rare transmission of HTLV-III/LAV to persons in this group might be prevented by a vaccine. Therefore, health care workers, along with other groups with a lower risk of infection, may be very interested in receiving the vaccine.

Ultimately, the goal of an AIDS vaccine program would be to halt the transmission of the causative virus. To accomplish this, all the people at risk of infection would have to be reached and successfully immunized before exposure. In the United States, we know now that personnel at the medical-access points for members of risk groups, such as sexually-transmitted-disease clinics for gay men and methadone clinics for intravenous drug abusers, see people far too late for prevention. By the time members of these groups visit such clinics, too many have already been infected. In the developing world, access to susceptible people will be even more difficult. For transmission to be interrupted successfully in all areas of the world, widespread immunization of large segments of the population of several countries may have to be considered.

In summary, a vaccine for AIDS is urgently needed because of the seriousness of the disease and the extent to which the causative virus has spread. The outlook for an AIDS vaccine is uncertain, but it has recently been brightened by the advent of an effective vaccine against another retrovirus, feline leukemia virus. However, there are a number of issues that need to be discussed and resolved before candidate AIDS vaccines will be ready for clinical testing. If a safe and effective AIDS vaccine is developed, wide use of the vaccine may be required to halt further transmission among members of high-risk groups and in the general population.

References

1. Barré-Sinoussi F, Chermann JC, Rey F, et al. Isolation of a T-lymphotropic retrovirus from a patient at risk for acquired immune deficiency syndrome (AIDS). Science 1983; 220:868-71.
2. Feorino PM, Kalyanaraman VS, Haverkos HW, et al. Lymphadenopathy associated virus infection of a blood donor–recipient pair with acquired immunodeficiency syndrome. Science 1984; 225:69-72.
3. Montagnier L, Chermann JC, Barré-Sinoussi F, et al. A new human T-lymphotropic retrovirus: characterization and possible role in lymphadenopathy and acquired immune deficiency syndromes. In: Gallo RC, Essex M, Gross L, eds. Human T-cell leukemia/lymphoma virus. Cold Spring Harbor, N.Y.: Cold Spring Harbor Laboratory Press, 1984: 363-70.
4. Gallo RC, Salahuddin SZ, Popovic M, et al. Frequent detection and isolation of cytopathic retroviruses (HTLV-III) from patients with AIDS and at risk for AIDS. Science 1984; 224:500-3.
5. Levy JA, Hoffman AD, Kramer SM, Landis JA, Shimabukuro JM, Oshiro LS. Isolation of lymphocytopathic retroviruses from San Francisco patients with AIDS. Science 1984; 225:840-2.
6. Ma P, Armstrong D, eds. The acquired immune deficiency syndrome and infections of homosexual men. New York: Yorke, 1984.
7. Jaffe HW, Bregman DG, Selik RM. Acquired immune deficiency syndrome in the United States: the first 1,000 cases. J Infect Dis 1983; 148:339-45.
8. Piot P, Quinn TC, Taelman H, et al. Acquired immunodeficiency syndrome in a heterosexual population in Zaire. Lancet 1984; 2:65-9.
9. Goedert JJ, Sarngadharan MG, Biggar RJ, et al. Determinants of retrovirus (HTLV-III) antibody and immunodeficiency conditions in homosexual men. Lancet 1984; 2:711-5.
10. Feorino PM, Jaffe HW, Palmer E, et al. Transfusion-associated acquired immunodeficiency syndrome: evidence for persistent infection in blood donors. N Engl J Med 1985; 312:1293-6.
11. Jaffe HW, Darrow WW, Echenberg DF, et al. Acquired immunodeficiency syndrome in a cohort of homosexual men: a 6-year follow-up study. Ann Intern Med 1985; 103:210-4.
12. Prevention of acquired immune deficiency syndrome (AIDS): report of inter-agency recommendations. MMWR 1983; 32:101-3.
13. Provisional Public Health Service inter-agency recommendations for screening donated blood and plasma for antibody to the virus causing acquired immunodeficiency syndrome. MMWR 1985; 34:1-5.
14. Where are we now with AIDS? Nature 1985; 313:254.
15. Wain-Hobson S, Sonigo P, Danos O, et al. Nucleotide sequence of the AIDS virus, LAV. Cell 1985; 40:9-17.
16. Ratner L, Hazeltine W, Patarca R, et al. Complete nucleotide sequence of the AIDS virus. HTLV-III. Nature 1985; 313:277-84.
17. Musing MA, Smith DH, Cabradilla CD, Benton CV, Lasky LA, Capon DJ. Nucleic acid structure and expression of the human AIDS/lymphadenopathy retrovirus. Nature 1985; 313:450-8.
18. Sanchez-Pescador R, Power MD, Barr PJ, et al. Nucleotide sequence and expression of an AIDS-associated retrovirus (ARV-2). Science 1985; 227:484-92.
19. Barin F, McLane MF, Allan JS, et al. Virus envelope protein of human T-cell leukemia virus type III (HTLV-III) represents major target antigen for antibodies in AIDS patients. Science 1985; 228:1094-6.
20. Kitchen LW, Barin F, Sullivan JL, et al. Aetiology of AIDS — antibodies to human T-cell leukaemia virus (type III) in haemophiliacs. Nature 1984; 312:367-9.
21. Schüpbach J, Haller O, Vogt M, et al. Antibodies to HTLV-III in Swiss patients with AIDS and pre-AIDS and in groups at risk for AIDS. N Engl J Med 1985; 312:265-70.
22. Ho DD, Rota TR, Hirsch MS. Antibody to lymphadenopathy-associated virus in AIDS. N Engl J Med 1985; 312:649-50.
23. McDougal JS, Cort SP, Kennedy MS, et al. Immunoassay for the detection and quantitation of infectious human retrovirus, lymphadenopathy-associated virus (LAV). J Immunol Methods 1985; 76:171-83.
24. Essex M. Feline leukemia: a naturally occurring cancer of infectious origin. Epidemiol Rev 1982; 4:189-203.
25. Olsen RG, Hoover EA, Schaller JP, et al. Abrogation of resistance to feline oncornavirus disease by immunization with killed feline leukemia virus. Cancer Res 1977; 37:2082-5.
26. Lewis MG, Mathes LE, Olsen RG. Protection against feline leukemia by vaccination with a subunit vaccine. Infect Immun 1981; 34:888-94.
27. Olsen RG, Lewis M, Mathes LE, et al. Feline leukemia vaccine: efficacy testing in a large multicat household. Feline Pract 1980; 10:13-6.
28. Miller JM, Van Der Maaten MJ, Schmerr MJF. Vaccination of cattle with binary ethylenimine-treated bovine leukemia virus. Am J Vet Res 1985; 44:64-7.
29. Patrascu IV, Coman S, Sandu I, et al. Specific protection against bovine leukemia virus infection conferred on cattle by the Romanian inactivated vaccine BL-VACC-RO. Rev Roum Med Viral 1980; 31:95-102.
30. Petricciani J. Old issues confront biotechnology and new products. Vaccine 1984; 2:235-6.
31. Mathes LE, Olsen RG, Hebebrand LC, et al. Immunosuppressive properties of a virion polypeptide, a 15,000-dalton protein, from feline leukemia virus. Cancer Res 1979; 39:950-5.
32. Alter HJ, Eichberg JW, Masur H, et al. Transmission of HTLV-III infection from human plasma to chimpanzees: an animal model for AIDS. Science 1984; 226:549-52.
33. Francis DP, Feorino PM, Broderson JR, et al. Infection of chimpanzees with lymphadenopathy-associated virus. Lancet 1984; 2:1276-7.
34. Gajdusek DC, Amyx HL, Gibbs CJ Jr, et al. Infection of chimpanzees by human T-lymphotropic retrovirus in brains and other tissues from AIDS patients. Lancet 1985; 1:55-6.

EDITORIAL

HTLV-III, AIDS, AND THE BRAIN

Paul H. Black, M.D.

TWO timely and important articles in this issue of the *Journal* deal with infection of the central nervous system by the human T-cell lymphotropic virus Type III (HTLV-III). The article by Ho et al.[1] indicates that acute infection of the central nervous system occurs with seroconversion to the HTLV-III agent. This study further indicates that certain patients with HTLV-III infection have had neurologic disease but no clinical manifestations of immunodeficiency, although this needs more precise documentation. The article by Resnick et al.[2] documents the presence within the blood–brain barrier of a specific immunoglobulin to HTLV-III in patients with neurologic complications of the acquired immunodeficiency syndrome (AIDS) or the AIDS-related complex. Careful quantitative and qualitative analysis of the antibody present in the cerebrospinal fluid — particularly the finding of unique oligoclonal IgG bands — indicates that the synthesis of IgG occurred intrathecally, providing further evidence that replication of HTLV-III can occur in the brain.

Both articles indicate that HTLV-III is probably directly responsible for some of the neurologic syndromes — such as chronic meningitis, dementia, and the so-called AIDS encephalopathy — that occur in certain patients with AIDS or the AIDS-related complex (the occurrence in patients with AIDS of central nervous system disease caused by a number of other organisms is well known).[3] The study by Resnick et al. also indicates that HTLV-III replication may occur in the brain without causing clinical neurologic disease.[2] These studies document the existence of another acute syndrome caused by HTLV-III (acute meningitis); an acute mononucleosis-like syndrome with seroconversion to HTLV-III had been described previously.[4] More important, the studies confirm that HTLV-III is neurotropic as well as lymphotropic.[5-7] Although the type or types of brain cells infected by HTLV-III are not now known, the finding that the virus infects and replicates in brain cells may not be surprising in view of the fact that HTLV-III is genetically and morphologically related to visna virus, a neurotropic retrovirus that causes a chronic degenerative disease in sheep and goats.[8] However, the neurotropism of HTLV-III raises many important questions about the nature, extent, and duration of infection of the central nervous system by this virus, and these must now be addressed.

It is curious that the brain, as well as other nervous tissue, is frequently involved in subacute, chronic, slow, or latent infections, particularly with viruses. Thus, after acute infection, the herpes simplex viruses and the varicella–zoster virus reside latently in nerve cells of the sensory ganglia; measles virus may persist in brain cells after acute measles infection and may cause subacute sclerosing panencephalitis many years later in a small number of persons; the human papovavirus (J.C. virus) presumably resides in the brain after initial infection and years later may cause progressive multifocal leukoencephalopathy in certain immunocompromised patients; and although little is known of their natural history, the spongiform encephalopathies — Creutzfeldt–Jakob disease, kuru, scrapie, and mink encephalopathy, diseases that are associated with the presence of proteinaceous particles called prions — tend to involve only the brain in a chronic progressive disease. Now, HTLV-III must be included with other viruses that can exist in the brain in the absence of clinical disease or that can directly cause chronic progressive neurologic disease.

The events that promote viral latency and persistence are not completely understood; they probably represent a combination of viral, cellular, and immune factors. The highly specialized structure and function of nerve cells make it almost certain that the pathogenesis of viral infections in the central nervous system is quite complex. A number of studies, both in vitro and in vivo, indicate that viruses may display tropism for distinct types of cells, such as neurons, myelin-forming cells, or astrocytes, or they may show varying degrees of virulence in the several cell types they infect.[9,10] Moreover, the stage of cellular differentiation may favor defective or incomplete viral assembly, which in turn may result in persistent infections of neurons.[9] In addition, the existence of a blood–brain barrier and the absence of a lymphatic circulation in the brain may render the brain an immunologically privileged site, favoring viral persistence.

Although it is unlikely that all the chronic infections of the central nervous system mentioned above involve the same mechanisms for maintaining persistence, one may speculate whether the viruses share any properties that are important with respect to persistence. One property shared by the measles virus, the visna virus, and HTLV-III is their combined lymphotropism and neurotropism. A recent study of patients with subacute sclerosing panencephalitis revealed the presence of measles virus RNA in lymphocytes of the central nervous system as well as in nerve cells, indicating both the lymphotropism and neurotropism of measles virus in subacute sclerosing panencephalitis and suggesting that lymphocytes were involved in the pathogenesis of the disease.[11] In experimental visna virus infection, viral replication first occurs in lymphocytes that reach the central nervous system during virus infection, viral replication first occurs in lymphocytes that reach the central nervous system during acute infection[12]; a similar series of events has been postulated in acute measles virus infection.[11] There is evidence that lymphocytes may pass through the blood–brain barrier and enter the central nervous system without there being an apparent lesion in the brain.[11] Presumably, lymphocytes may carry the infection to the brain in this way. In HTLV-III infection, virus replication occurs in T4 lymphocytes; when and how in the course of the infection the central nervous system becomes involved is unknown.

It is likely that in all these infections (although most of the experimental evidence relates to visna and measles) some degree of nonpermissiveness or host-cell restriction (i.e., partial expression of the viral genome resulting in incomplete synthesis of viral proteins) promotes persistence even in the absence of clinical manifestations, for years. Cells infected by the visna retrovirus and HTLV-III contain integrated proviral DNA for the life of the cell — a condition that would also promote persistence.[5] There is continued synthesis of virus or viral antigen in all these infections, since oligoclonal IgG specific for the virus may appear in the cerebrospinal fluid, indicating synthesis of immunoglobulin within the blood–brain barrier. Whether infected lymphocytes contribute to the persistence of these viruses in the central nervous system — and, if so, how — is not completely understood.[11,13]

Much evidence indicates that HTLV-III infection of the brain probably persists throughout the life of the patient. The persistence of viral infection would be further promoted by the immunosuppression caused by HTLV-III infection. The brain, therefore, may well provide a sanctuary for HTLV-III, as has been pointed out[1,2,5]; the question that remains is, To what extent is it also a reservoir for HTLV-III infection? The special features of persistent infection in the brain, coupled with the difficulty of bringing adequate concentrations of drugs to this locus across the blood–brain barrier, will make eradication of HTLV-III infection of the central nervous system very difficult, if not impossible.

Some insight into the timing and incidence of seeding of the central nervous system in asymptomatic seropositive persons could be gained by examining the cerebrospinal fluid for antibody to HTLV-III.[2] In addition, it will be important to know whether seroconversion to HTLV-III is accompanied by the appearance of intrathecal antibody to HTLV-III, particularly IgM. The presence of such antibody would be ominous, because it would indicate that the central nervous system was seeded with HTLV-III at the time of infection and that the virus was replicating there.

As the reports in this issue demonstrate, HTLV-III infection may alter the function of brain cells. One may speculate that a consequence of such alteration could be changes in the concentrations of certain neuromediators, neurotransmitters, or neurohormones released by these cells. Alteration may further modulate immune function both in the central nervous system and at other sites in the body, thereby contributing to the immunosuppression caused by HTLV-III.[14] It is clear that the two studies appearing in this issue of the *Journal* have raised many important and perplexing questions about infection of the central nervous system with HTLV-III.

References

1. Ho DD, Rota TR, Schooley RT, et al. Isolation of HTLV-III from cerebrospinal fluid and neural tissues of patients with neurological syndromes related to the acquired immunodeficiency syndrome. N Engl J Med 1985; 313:1493-7.
2. Resnick L, diMarzo-Veronese F, Schupbach J, et al. Intra-blood–brain-barrier synthesis of HTLV-III-specific IgG in patients with neurologic symptoms associated with AIDS or AIDS-related complex. N Engl J Med 1985; 313:1498-504.
3. Levy RM, Bredesen DE, Rosenblum ML. Neurological manifestations of the acquired immunodeficiency syndrome (AIDS): experience at UCSF and review of the literature. J Neurosurg 1985; 62:475-95.
4. Cooper DA, Gold J, Maclean P, et al. Acute AIDS retrovirus infection: definition of a clinical illness associated with seroconversion. Lancet 1985; 1:537-40.
5. Shaw GM, Harper ME, Hahn BH, et al. HTLV-III infection in brains of children and adults with AIDS encephalopathy. Science 1985; 227: 177-82.
6. Levy JA, Shimabukuro J, Hollander H, Mills J, Kaminsky L. Isolation of AIDS-associated retroviruses from cerebrospinal fluid and brain of patients with neurological symptoms. Lancet 1985; 2:586-8.
7. Harris AA, Segreti J, Levin S. Central nervous system infections in patients with the acquired immune deficiency syndrome (AIDS). Clin Neuropharm 1985; 8:201-10.
8. Gonda MA, Wong-Staal F, Gallo RC, Clements JE, Narayan O, Gilden RV. Sequence homology and morphological similarity of HTLV-III and visna virus, a pathogenic lentivirus. Science 1985; 227:173-7.
9. Dubois-Dalcq M, Rentier B, Hooghe-Peters E, Haspel MV, Knobler RL, Holmes K. Acute and persistent viral infections of differentiated nerve cells. Rev Infect Dis 1982; 4:999-1014.
10. Johnson RT. Selective vulnerability of neural cells to viral infections. Brain 1980; 103:447-72.
11. Fournier J-G, Tardieu M, Lebon P, et al. Detection of measles virus RNA in lymphocytes from peripheral-blood and brain perivascular infiltrates of patients with subacute sclerosing panencephalitis. N Engl J Med 1985; 313:910-5.
12. Nathanson N, Georgsson G, Pálsson PA, Najjar JA, Lutley R, Pétursson G. Experimental visna in Icelandic sheep: the prototype lentiviral infection. Rev Infect Dis 1985; 7:75-82.
13. Griffith JF. Subacute sclerosing panencephalitis and lymphocytes. N Engl J Med 1985; 313:952-4.
14. MacLean D, Reichlin S. Neuroendocrinology and the immune process. In: Ader R, ed. Psychoneuroimmunology. New York: Academic Press, 1981: 475-520.

CORRESPONDENCE

CUTANEOUS REACTION TO TRIMETHOPRIM–SULFAMETHOXAZOLE IN PATIENTS WITH AIDS AND KAPOSI'S SARCOMA

To the Editor: An epidemic of acquired immunodeficiency syndrome (AIDS) complicated by *Pneumocystis carinii* pneumonia, other opportunistic infections, and Kaposi's sarcoma is now occurring in the United States.[1-3] The combination of trimethoprim and sulfamethoxazole has been shown to be effective in both the treatment and prophylaxis of *P. carinii* pneumonia.[4-6]

We report a striking incidence of maculopapular cutaneous eruptions associated with the administration of trimethoprim–sulfamethoxazole in patients with AIDS with or without Kaposi's sarcoma. Of the patients with AIDS and Kaposi's sarcoma seen at University of California, Los Angeles, Medical Center and San Francisco General Hospital, 35 have received trimethoprim–sulfamethoxazole either therapeutically or prophylactically for *P. carinii* pneumonia. In 16 of 25 patients who received trimethoprim–sulfamethoxazole for documented *P. carinii* pneumonia, a diffuse skin rash developed soon after initiation of therapy. Similarly, 8 of 10 patients had cutaneous reactions after prophylactic therapy with trimethoprim–sulfamethoxazole.

Among the patients at University of California, Los Angeles, Medical Center, rash occurred a median of four days after initiation of therapy (range, one to nine days). No patient had previously reported allergies to sulfa or folate antagonists, and none had a notable history of atopy. All patients had prompt resolution of their skin rash when trimethoprim–sulfamethoxazole was discontinued. Two patients were also receiving ketoconazole at the time of development of their rash. This medication was continued without adverse effects after the cessation of trimethoprim–sulfamethoxazole. The median age, extent of Kaposi's sarcoma, total leukocyte count, and degree of depression in the helper/suppressor T-cell ratio were similar in patients who had reactions and in those who did not. All patients had elevated serum titers to cytomegalovirus, and of all but two cytomegalovirus was grown from the urine and semen samples.

P. carinii pneumonia occurs frequently in this population and is routinely treated with trimethoprim–sulfamethoxazole. We report a 69 percent incidence of cutaneous reactions to trimethoprim–sulfamethoxazole in these patients. This risk is considerably higher than the 2.2 percent estimated incidence of cutaneous reaction to trimethoprim–sulfamethoxazole in patients with other hematologic or neoplastic diseases (LaBraico J: personal communication), and warrants caution and close follow-up after administration in patients with AIDS and Kaposi's sarcoma.

Ronald Mitsuyasu, M.D.
Jerome Groopman, M.D.
University of California,
Los Angeles Medical Center
Los Angeles, CA 90024

Paul Volberding, M.D.
San Francisco General Hospital
San Francisco, CA 94110

References

1. Gottlieb MS, Schroff R, Schanker HM, et al. *Pneumocystis carinii* pneumonia and mucosal candidiasis in previously healthy homosexual men: evidence of a new acquired cellular immunodeficiency. N Engl J Med 1982; 305:1425-31.
2. Groopman JE, Gottlieb MS. Kaposi's sarcoma: an oncologic looking glass. Nature 1982; 299:103-4.
3. Follansbee SE, Busch DF, Wofsy CB, et al. An outbreak of *Pneumocystis carinii* pneumonia in homosexual men. Ann Intern Med 1982; 96:705-13.
4. Hughes WT. Treatment of *Pneumocystis carinii* pneumonitis. N Engl J Med 1976; 295:726-7.
5. Lau WK, Young LS. Trimethoprim–sulfamethoxazole treatment of *Pneumocystis carinii* pneumonia in adults. N Engl J Med 1976; 295:716-8.
6. Hughes WT, Kuhn S, Chaudhary S, et al. Successful chemoprophylaxis for *Pneumocystis carinii* pneumonitis. N Engl J Med 1977; 297:1419-26.

BONE-MARROW TRANSPLANTATION IN AIDS

To the Editor: The acquired immunodeficiency syndrome (AIDS) has a two-year mortality rate estimated to exceed 80 percent, with no reported cases of spontaneous recovery of normal immunologic function once opportunistic infections have appeared.[1] Our early experience[2] with the unrelenting course of AIDS in patients, despite our aggressive and prompt use of antimicrobial agents and our preliminary attempts at therapy using alpha interferon, thymosin fraction 5, and transfer factor, which failed to yield any measurable alteration of immune function, led us to further attempts to restore immunocompetence in our patients. Because a profound, apparently broad-based, progressive immunodeficiency is present,[2-5] we thought that an acute and irreversible insult to the lymphoid system at the level of some marrow stem cell

Table 1. Immunologic Indexes before and after Bone-Marrow Transplantation.*

	Case 1		Case 2		Normal Controls
	Before	After	Before	After	
Total white-cell count	1200	1400	4400	3700	7,800±3,00/μl
Total lymphocytes	50	25	800	600	1,000–4,800/μl
DTH skin tests	Absent	Absent	Absent	Absent	Present
Lymphocyte markers					
Leu 1 (%)	61	QNS	91	83	80±7
Leu 3/Leu 2	0.06	QNS	0.09	0.05	Greater than 1.00
Mitogen response					
Phytohemagglutinin	691	QNS	8045	1329	29,000±4,400 cpm
Concanavalin A	744	QNS	1489	623	21,000±6,200 cpm
Pokeweed mitogen	372	QNS	239	626	15,800±5,100 cpm
NK HSV-1 function	18	QNS	24	QNS	111 (52–239) lytic units/ml

*DTH denotes delayed-type hypersensitivity, Leu leucine, QNS quantity not sufficient, and NK HSV-1 natural-killer-cell activity against herpes simplex virus type 1.

might underlie AIDS. Both to test this hypothesis and to find a definitive therapeutic approach to the problem, we decided to attempt immunologic reconstitution through allogeneic bone-marrow transplantation. Successful transplantation would suggest that the initiating, presumably infectious, insult is transient and that a marrow-dependent cell system is a major target of the agent of AIDS.

Two homosexual men with Kaposi's sarcoma, recurrent opportunistic infections, and severe wasting were selected for study after human-subjects-committee approval and informed consent had been obtained. Each patient had an immunologically intact HLA-compatible family donor (father and sister) matched at HLA-DR and mutually unresponsive in mixed leukocyte culture. Both patients were profoundly immunodeficient; both had depression of natural-killer-cell activity against herpes simplex virus type 1, which is associated with a reduced risk of graft-versus-host disease in bone-marrow transplantation in severe, combined immunodeficiency[6] (Table 1). Consequently, no conditioning regimen was given to the recipients before or after bone-marrow transplantation. Each patient received more than 1×10^{10} marrow mononuclear cells. We found donor HLA-A (Case 1) or XX (Case 2) phenotypes in marrow two weeks after cell transfer, but these markers were undetectable at four weeks. Neither subject had regression of Kaposi's sarcoma, control of opportunistic infections, or a discernible improvement in immune function in the post-transplantation period (Table 1).

Our inability to reconstitute essential immunologic functions by allogeneic bone-marrow transplantation could be attributable to several factors, including the possible persistence of an immunosuppressive etiologic agent of AIDS or the presence of reactivated viruses potentially suppressive of donor cells. We found both patients to have circulating lymphocytotoxins that were reactive with donor cells, characterized as HLA-nonspecific, warm-reactive, complement-fixing antibodies, but plasmapheresis in Case 2 did not facilitate engraftment. These studies indicate that single large marrow infusions given late in the course of AIDS, without conditioning regimens, cannot be expected to reverse the disease process. It may still be justified to try bone-marrow transplantation, including multiple infusions of marrow or leukapheresis-derived donor cells, in earlier stages of the disease, when several of the problems we encountered may not yet be present.

Joseph M. Hassett, M.D.
Charles G. Zaroulis, M.D.
Michael L. Greenberg, M.D.
Frederick P. Siegal, M.D.
The Mount Sinai Medical Center
New York, NY 10029

References

1. Update on acquired immune deficiency syndrome (AIDS) — United States. MMWR 1982; 31:507-8, 513-4.
2. Siegal FP, Lopez C, Hammer GS, et al. Severe acquired immunodeficiency in male homosexuals, manifested by chronic perianal ulcerative herpes simplex lesions. N Engl J Med 1981; 305:1439-44.
3. Mildvan D, Mathur U, Enlow RW, et al. Opportunistic infections and immune deficiency in homosexual men. Ann Intern Med 1982; 96:700-4.
4. Friedman-Kien AE, Laubenstein LJ, Rubinstein P, et al. Disseminated Kaposi's sarcoma in homosexual men. Ann Intern Med 1982; 96:693-700.
5. Gottlieb MS, Schroff R, Schanker HM, et al. *Pneumocystis carinii* pneumonia and mucosal candidiasis in previously healthy homosexual men: evidence of a new acquired cellular immunodeficiency. N Engl J Med 1981; 305:1425-31.
6. Lopez C, Kirkpatrick D, Sorell M, et al. Association between pre-transplant natural kill and graft-versus-host disease after stem-cell transplantation. Lancet 1979; 2:1103-7.

INOCULATION OF CRYPTOCOCCOSIS WITHOUT TRANSMISSION OF THE ACQUIRED IMMUNODEFICIENCY SYNDROME

To the Editor: The risk of HTLV-III seroconversion in health-care workers sustaining a needle-stick injury while caring for patients with AIDS appears to be low.[1,2] There is only one report of seroconversion after a needle stick, which involved the inoculation of a small amount of blood.[3] The transmission of hepatitis B virus but not HTLV-III after percutaneous exposure has been described.[4] We report a similar case, which is of interest because (1) it again demonstrates the lack of HTLV-III seroconversion after percutaneous inoculation of enough HTLV-III antibody–positive blood to allow the transmission of another infectious agent, (2) it is a report of primary cutaneous cryptococcosis at the site of traumatic inoculation of *Cryptococcus neoformans,* and (3) it demonstrates that immunocompetent patients with primary cutaneous cryptococcosis can be successfully treated in a noninvasive fashion.

A 24-year-old medical student accidentally inoculated his right thumb with a needle contaminated with blood from a patient with cryptococcal fungemia and a positive HTLV-III serologic test. The puncture wound healed within several days. Ten days later, he noticed painful swelling and erythema of his thumb. Axillary lymphadenopathy was noted, and dicloxacillin was prescribed. Four days later, a felon of the right thumb was incised and drained. Culture of the aspirated material grew *C. neoformans*. At that time, the thumb was still swollen and erythematous. Tender right epitrochlear and axillary lymphadenopathy was present, and the incision site was granulating slowly. A chest roentgenogram, complete blood count, SMA-20 profile, urine cultures for fungus, and serum cryptococcal antigen were normal. A roentgenogram of the right thumb showed soft-tissue swelling. Therapy with flucytosine at a dose of 150 mg per kilogram of body weight per day was started and continued for six weeks, at which time there were no signs of inflammation. Antibodies to HTLV-III were negative both 1 and 26 months after inoculation. The patient remains in good health.

Primary inoculation cutaneous cryptococcosis has been documented in experimental models[5] but not in human beings. Although some investigators have recommended systemic evaluation of patients presenting with localized cutaneous cryptococcosis, including a lumbar puncture, and therapy with amphotericin B for patients who are also immunodeficient,[5,6] there is no overall consensus in the literature regarding the treatment of immunocompetent patients.[7,8] Our patient was cured with six weeks of flucytosine therapy (150 mg per kilogram of body weight per day). Central nervous system evaluation was not performed, since a known traumatic inoculation of *C. neoformans* had occurred at the site of his infection, and other instances of primary mycotic lymphocutaneous infection have resolved without therapy.[5,9] This case supports recent evidence that isolated percutaneous inoculation of blood from patients with AIDS poses a low risk of transmission of HTLV-III.

Jordan B. Glaser, M.D.
Adam Garden, M.D.
Staten Island Hospital
Staten Island, NY 10305

References

1. Hirsch MS, Wormser GP, Schooley RT, et al. Risk of nosocomial infection with human t-cell lymphotropic virus III (HTLV-III). N Engl J Med 1985; 312:1-4.
2. Centers for Disease Control. Prospective evaluation of health-care workers exposed via the parenteral or mucous-membrane route to blood or body fluids from patients with AIDS. MMWR 1985; 34:101-3.
3. Needlestick transmission of HTLV-III from a patient infected in Africa. Lancet 1984; 2:1376-7.
4. Gerberding JL, Hopewell PC, Kaminsky LS, Sande MA. Transmission of hepatitis B without transmission of AIDS by accidental needlestick. N Engl J Med 1985; 312:56-7.
5. Noble RC, Fajardo LF. Primary cutaneous cryptococcosis: review and morphologic study. Am J Clin Pathol 1972; 57:13-22.
6. Iacobellis FW, Jacobs MI, Cohen RP. Primary cutaneous cryptococcosis. Arch Dermatol 1979; 115:984-5.
7. Sarosi GA, Silberfarb PM, Tosh FE. Cutaneous cryptococcosis: a sentinel of disseminated disease. Arch Dermatol 1971; 104:1-3.
8. Brier RL, Mopper C, Stone J. Cutaneous cryptococcosis: presentation of a case and a review of previously reported cases. Arch Dermatol 1957; 75:262-3.
9. Moore M. Cryptococcosis with cutaneous manifestations. J Invest Dermatol 1957; 28:159-82.

FOLLOW-UP AT 4½ YEARS ON HOMOSEXUAL MEN WITH GENERALIZED LYMPHADENOPATHY

To the Editor: A longitudinal study of homosexual and bisexual men with persistent generalized lymphadenopathy was initiated in February 1981. After 30 months, 8 of 42 men (19 percent) had the acquired immunodeficiency syndrome (AIDS), as previously reported.[1] We now report our experience after 4½ years: 12 of 42 patients (29 percent) have had progression to AIDS — 7 with Kaposi's sarcoma, 2 with *Pneumocystis carinii* pneumonia, 1 with both these symptoms, and 1 with non-Hodgkin lymphoma. The mean duration of lymphadenopathy before diagnosis of AIDS was 25 months; before diagnosis of Kaposi's sarcoma, 19 months; before diagnosis of *P. carinii* pneumonia, 33 months. Kaposi's sarcoma and lymphoma were associated with lymph-node enlargement (four of eight patients), and *P. carinii* pneumonia with lymph-node regression (all of four patients).

Reports of longitudinal studies of homosexual men with lymphadenopathy have differed with respect to the frequency of progression to AIDS. Other studies conducted in New York City showed incidences of 8 percent in one year[2] and 18 percent in 18 months[3] — results very similar to ours. In contrast, a San Francisco study of lymphadenopathy found no cases of AIDS during 18 months of follow-up[4] and a 7 percent incidence after 36 months.[5] The variation between New York data and San Francisco data could be accounted for by differences in duration of infection with human T-cell lymphotropic virus Type III/lymphadenopathy-associated virus (HTLV-III/LAV) in the respective study populations, since the epidemic appeared in New York approximately one year before it began in San Francisco. Another, more exciting possibility — because it implies the potential for limiting the number of cases of AIDS that may occur — is that cofactors are responsible for the progression of lymphadenopathy to AIDS, and that these cofactors occur with differing frequency in the New York and San Francisco populations at high risk.

Additional observations on our cohort support the possible role of cofactors in disease manifestations of AIDS. Analysis at 30 months showed that a history of heavy or moderate use of nitrite inhalant before study entry was predictive of ultimate progression to AIDS.[1] After 4½ years, with the development of additional cases of *P. carinii* pneumonia, we find that the association between such nitrite use and the development of Kaposi's sarcoma remains significant ($P<0.05$), whereas no such association is observed for *P. carinii* pneumonia. Although based on small numbers, these findings are important since they were derived from longitudinal observations. An early case-control study of Kaposi's sarcoma detected a significant association with nitrite inhalants,[6] but a large case-control study of AIDS by the Centers for Disease Control did not confirm this finding.[7] Recently, however, Haverkos et al. reanalyzed the data from the Centers for Disease Control, according to disease manifestation, and found that heavy use of nitrite inhalant was the variable most strongly associated with Kaposi's sarcoma.[8]

Taken together, these findings point to the interpretation that nitrite inhalants may act alone or in combination with other, as yet unidentified cofactors after AIDS retrovirus-induced immunodeficiency, by promoting the specific disease manifestation of Kaposi's sarcoma.

Usha Mathur-Wagh, M.D.
Donna Mildvan, M.D.
and Ruby T. Senie, Ph.D.
Mt. Sinai School of Medicine
New York, NY 10003

References

1. Mathur-Wagh U, Enlow RW, Spigland I, et al. Longitudinal study of persistent generalised lymphadenopathy in homosexual men: relation to the acquired immunodeficiency syndrome. Lancet 1984; 1:1033-8.

2. Gold JWM, Sears CL, Henry S, et al. Lymphadenopathy in homosexual men and development of the acquired immunodeficiency syndrome. Clin Res 1983; 31:363A. abstract.
3. Fernandez R, Mouradian J, Metroka C, Davis J. The prognostic value of histopathology in persistent generalized lymphadenopathy in homosexual men. N Engl J Med 1983; 309:185-6.
4. Abrams DI, Lewis BJ, Beckstead JH, Casavant CH, Drew WL, Ammann AJ. Lymphadenopathy in homosexual men: endpoint or prodrome? Proc Am Soc Clin Oncol 1983; 2:47. abstract.
5. Abrams D, Mess T, Volberding P. Lymphadenopathy: endpoint or prodrome? Update of a 36 month prospective study. Presented at the International Conference on AIDS-Associated Syndromes, Irvine, Calif., December 8 and 9, 1984.
6. Marmor M, Friedman-Kien AE, Laubenstein L, et al. Risk factors for Kaposi's sarcoma in homosexual men. Lancet 1982; 1:1083-7.
7. Jaffe MW, Choi K, Thomas PC, et al. National case-control study of Kaposi's sarcoma and *Pneumocystis carinii* pneumonia in homosexual men. 1. Epidemiologic results. Ann Intern Med 1983; 99:145-51.
8. Haverkos HW, Pinsky PF, Drotman DP, Bregman DJ. Disease manifestations among homosexual men with acquired immunodeficiency syndrome (AIDS): a possible role of nitrites in Kaposi's sarcoma. Sex Transm Dis 1985; 12:203-8.

INACTIVATION OF HUMAN T-CELL LYMPHOTROPIC RETROVIRUS (HTLV-III) BY LD™

To the Editor: HTLV-III is a human retrovirus that has been implicated in the causation of AIDS.[1-3] With a high level of interest in the protection of health care personnel and in the decontamination of equipment used in the care of patients with AIDS and the AIDS-related complex, attempts are being made in various laboratories to find reagents that can completely inactivate HTLV-III/LAV. LD™ (Alcide, Norwalk, Conn.) is a unique two-component product used as a general laboratory disinfectant, which contains, at its standard-use dilution, 0.23 percent sodium chlorite and 1.26 percent lactic acid in a specialized formulation that confers stability. The mechanism of action is based on the controlled formation of chlorous acid and subsequent release of chlorine dioxide. To our knowledge, no known generic compound works by a similar mechanism.

We have studied the effect of LD™ on HTLV-III infectivity and find that it can completely inactivate HTLV-III at a 200-fold dilution of its standard-use dilution (Table 1). HTLV-III expression was detected by assaying for reverse transcriptase activity in the culture supernatant and by the detection of HTLV-III p15 and HTLV-III p24 in cells fixed with methanol:acetone (1:1) with use of monoclonal antibodies.[4] As shown in Table 1, LD™ was not toxic to the uninfected H9 cells, as evidenced by the growth of these cells after exposure to this compound at similar dilutions. On the basis of our results, we believe that LD™ is an effective disinfectant for use in hospitals and clinical laboratories involved in handling tissue specimens and in the care of patients with AIDS and the AIDS-related complex.

Table 1. Effect of LD™ on HTLV-III Replication in H9 Cells.*

LD™ Dilution	No. of Cells ($\times 10^{-6}$)	Reverse Transcriptase (cpm $\times 10^{-3}$ per reaction)	% Control	% IF p15	% Control	% IF p24	% Control
—	0.95	385	100	39	100	36	100
1:100	1.12	0.4	0	0	0	0	0
1:200	1.50	0.6	0	0	0	0	0
1:400	1.12	129	34	3	8	1.5	4

*The virus (HTLV-III and LD™ were added simultaneously to the H9 cells after exposure to Polybrene (2 μg per milliliter) as previously described.[4] Reverse transcriptase assays were carried out in the culture supernatant with (dT) $15(A)_n$ used as the template primer in the presence of magnesium as a divalent cation, and immunofluorescence assays were carried out with HTLV-III monoclonal antibodies to p15 and p24 as described.[4] The background counts for reverse transcriptase assays were 485 cpm per reaction. % IF denotes the percentage of cells showing immunofluorescence with monoclonal antibodies. Assays were carried out on Day 4 after infection, in duplicate. The results shown are the average of four experiments.

P.S. Sarin, Ph.D.
National Cancer Institute
Bethesda, MD 20205

D.I. Scheer
Yale University School of Medicine
New Haven, CT 06510

R.D. Kross
Alcide Corporation
Farmingdale, NY 11735

References

1. Gallo RC, Salahuddin SZ, Popovic M, et al. Frequent detection and isolation of cytopathic retroviruses (HTLV-III) from patients with AIDS and at risk for AIDS. Science 1984; 224:500-3.
2. Sarin PS, Gallo RC. Human T-lymphotropic retroviruses in adult T-cell leukemia-lymphoma and acquired immune deficiency syndrome. J Clin Immunol 1984; 4:415-23.
3. Wong-Staal F, Gallo RC. Human T-lymphotropic retroviruses. Nature 1985; 317:395-403.
4. Sarin PS, Taguchi Y, Sun D, Thornton A, Gallo RC, Oberg B. Inhibition of HTLV-III/LAV replication by foscarnet. Biochem Pharmacol 1985; 34: 4075-8.

EFFECT OF COHN FRACTIONATION CONDITIONS ON INFECTIVITY OF THE AIDS VIRUS

To the Editor: Intravenous gamma globulins prepared by means of Cohn fractionation have been reported to transmit non-A,non-B hepatitis viruses,[1-3] suggesting that the alcohol concentration, pH, and temperature used in this process do not completely inactivate these lipid-membrane-coated viruses. Since the virus causing AIDS (human T-cell lymphotropic virus Type III [HTLV-III], lymphadenopathy-associated virus, or AIDS-related virus), hereafter called the AIDS virus, may be present in plasma pools used for manufacturing blood derivatives,[4-6] it is important to determine whether the virus can survive the fractionation procedure.

We therefore performed the following experiment. Plasma from a small number of donors shown to be free of antibody to HTLV-III by enzyme-linked immunosorbent assay was pooled and fractionated according to the Cohn procedure for ethanol fractionation,[7,8] in routine use at the New York Blood Center. Supernatants from Cohn fraction I, containing 8 percent ethanol at pH 7.2, Cohn fraction II+III, containing 25 percent ethanol at pH 7.0, and Cohn fraction III, containing 17 percent ethanol at pH 5.4, were stored at −70°C. To aliquots of the above supernatants, which represent the potentially most inactivating conditions to which viruses are exposed during gamma globulin preparation, 0.1 volume of an AIDS virus stock was added. This stock consisted of RPMI-1640, 20 percent fetal-calf serum, and culture supernatant from H9/HTLV-III_β producer cells.[9] The virus was added after adjustment of the supernatants to the temperature at which they are normally held during Cohn fractionation: −2°C for fraction I supernatant, −5°C for fraction II+III supernatant, and −6°C for fraction III supernatant. After 2 and 24 hours at these temperatures, samples were transferred to a −8°C crushed-ice-sodium chloride bath. These mixtures and control mixtures of virus diluted in normal plasma were passed through a 20-ml Sephadex G-25 column precoated with human serum albumin and equilibrated with RPMI-1640 medium. Care was taken to pass the samples through these columns as rapidly as possible, in order to maintain low temperatures before the alcohol was removed. The void volumes were recovered, sterile-filtered, and assayed by inoculation of quadruplicate serial microtiter dilutions onto H9 cells.[10] After 14 days the culture supernatants were harvested and assayed for reverse transcriptase.[10] Little or no AIDS virus was inactivated under the conditions used.

Because of the long storage of liquid preparations of intramuscular immune serum globulin (ISG) between formulation and administration, intramuscular ISG may present little or no hazard of virus transmission, as has generally been concluded. However, the increasingly popular intravenous preparations of ISG are lyophilized immediately after formulation, are stored in the dry state, which preserves virus infectivity, and are given in large doses intravenously. This is probably the most sensitive route for infection with hepatitis or lymphotropic viruses. Thus, intravenous preparations of ISG are of particular concern, as shown for transmission of non-A,non-B hepatitis.[3]

Our findings suggest the desirability of applying virus-inactivation procedures to plasma subjected to Cohn ethanol fractionation, or to the resulting plasma derivatives, in order to sterilize them against non-A,non-B hepatitis viruses and also to inactivate the agent of AIDS.

Our results do not necessarily imply that intravenous gamma globulin preparations are unsafe, since some manufacturers have incorporated into their procedures steps that have the potential for inactivating these viruses.

Furthermore, it is possible that virus may fractionate predominantly into fractions other than the gamma globulin fraction, and that any virus in this fraction could be neutralized by antibody; also, it is possible that storage of intermediate fractions in the frozen state could inactivate virus.

Careful surveillance of recipients of intravenous gamma globulin preparations for development of antibodies to the AIDS virus is necessary. To date, no reports of such development have appeared.

These studies were partly supported under contracts (NO1-HB-3-7009 and NO1-HB-5-7007) with the National Heart, Lung, and Blood Institute.

Alfred M. Prince, M.D., Marcel P.J. Piet, M.D.,
and Bernard Horowitz, Ph.D.
Lindsley F. Kimball Research Institute
New York Blood Center
New York, NY 10021

References

1. Lane RS. Non-A,non-B hepatitis from intravenous immunoglobulin. Lancet 1983; 2:974-5.
2. Lever AML, Webster ADB, Brown D, Thomas HC. Non-A,non-B hepatitis after intravenous gammaglobulin. Lancet 1985; 1:587.
3. Ochs HD, Fischer SH, Virant FS, Lee ML, Kingdon HS, Wedgwood RJ. Non-A,non-B hepatitis and intravenous immunoglobulin. Lancet 1985; 1:404-5.
4. Pneumocystis carinii pneumonia among patients with hemophilia A. MMWR 1982; 31:365-7.
5. Vilmer E, Barre-Sinoussi F, Rouzioux C, et al. Isolation of new lymphotrophic retrovirus from two siblings with haemophilia B, one with AIDS. Lancet 1984; 1:753-7.
6. Evatt BL, Stein SF, Francis DP, et al. Antibodies to human T cell leukaemia virus-associated membrane antigens in haemophiliacs: evidence for infection before 1980. Lancet 1983; 2:698-701.
7. Cohn EJ, Strong LE, Hughes WL Jr, et al. Preparation and properties of serum and plasma proteins. I. A system of the separation into fractions of the protein and lipoprotein components of biological tissues and fluids. J Am Chem Soc 1946; 68:459-74.
8. Oncley JL, Melin M, Richert DA, Cameron JW, Gross PM Jr. The separation of the antibodies, isoagglutinins, prothrombin, plasminogen and β_1-lipoprotein into subfractions of human plasma. J Am Chem Soc 1949; 71:541-50.
9. Popovic M, Sarngadharan MG, Read E, Gallo RC. Detection, isolation, and continuous production of cytopathic retroviruses (HTLV-III) from patients with AIDS and pre-AIDS. Science 1984; 224:497-500.
10. Prince AM, Horowitz B, Dichtelmueller H, Stephan W, Gallo RC. Quantitative assays for evaluation of HTLV-III inactivation processes: Tri(*n*-butyl) phosphate: sodium cholate and β-propiolactone. Cancer Res 1985; 45: Suppl:4592S-4S.

Index

A

B

I